AF527266

DERMOSCOPY
Text and Atlas

DERMOSCOPY
Text and Atlas

Editor-in-Chief

Subrata Malakar
MD (Dermatology) DCH
Director
Rita Skin Foundation
Kolkata, West Bengal, India

Associate Editors

Priya Diwaker DDVL
Consultant Dermatologist
Rita Skin Foundation
Kolkata, West Bengal, India

Purva Mehta DNB
Consultant Dermatologist
Rita Skin Foundation
Kolkata, West Bengal, India

Samipa S Mukherjee
DDV DDVL FRGUHS (Ped Dermatology)
Consultant Pediatric Dermatologist and Dermatotrichologist
Cloud Nine Hospitals
Bengaluru, Karnataka, India
Rita Skin Foundation
Kolkata, West Bengal, India

Assistant Editors

Sushrut Save DNB
Consultant Dermatologist
Rita Skin Foundation
Kolkata, West Bengal, India

Anjali Pal MD
Consultant Dermatologist
Rita Skin Foundation
Kolkata, West Bengal, India

Surit Malakar MBBS PGT (Dermatology)
Rita Skin Foundation
Kolkata, West Bengal, India

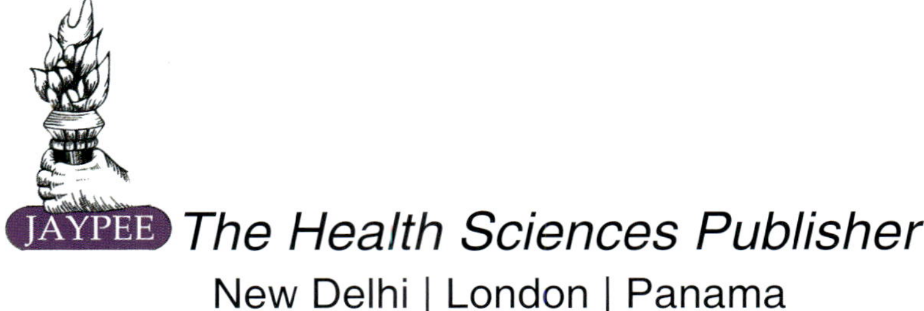

The Health Sciences Publisher
New Delhi | London | Panama

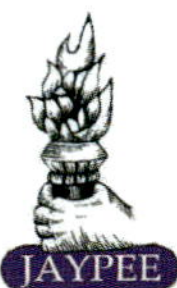

Jaypee Brothers Medical Publishers (P) Ltd

Headquarters
Jaypee Brothers Medical Publishers (P) Ltd.
4838/24, Ansari Road, Daryaganj
New Delhi 110 002, India
Phone: +91-11-43574357
Fax: +91-11-43574314
E-mail: jaypee@jaypeebrothers.com

Overseas Offices

JP Medical Ltd.
83, Victoria Street, London
SW1H 0HW (UK)
Phone: +44-20 3170 8910
Fax: +44(0)20 3008 6180
E-mail: info@jpmedpub.com

Jaypee-Highlights Medical Publishers Inc.
City of Knowledge, Bld. 235, 2nd Floor, Clayton
Panama City, Panama
Phone: +1 507-301-0496
Fax: +1 507-301-0499
E-mail: cservice@jphmedical.com

Jaypee Brothers Medical Publishers (P) Ltd.
17/1-B, Babar Road, Block-B, Shyamoli
Mohammadpur, Dhaka-1207
Bangladesh
Mobile: +08801912003485
E-mail: jaypeedhaka@gmail.com

Jaypee Brothers Medical Publishers (P) Ltd.
Bhotahity, Kathmandu, Nepal
Phone: +977-9741283608
E-mail: kathmandu@jaypeebrothers.com

Website: www.jaypeebrothers.com
Website: www.jaypeedigital.com

Inquiries for bulk sales may be solicited at: jaypee@jaypeebrothers.com

Dermoscopy: Text and Atlas

First Edition: **2019**

ISBN: 978-93-5270-394-4

Printed at: Ajanta Offset & Packagings Ltd., Faridabad, Haryana.

Dedicated to

My late wife Dr Rita Shah Malakar

Contributors

Balachandra S Ankad MD
Professor and Head
Department of Dermatology
SN Medical College
Bagalkot, Karnataka, India

Priya Diwaker DDVL
Consultant Dermatologist
Rita Skin Foundation
Kolkata, West Bengal, India

Niti Khunger MD
Professor and Consultant Dermatologist
Vardhman Mahavir Medical College
and Safdarjung Hospital
New Delhi, India

Shruti Kulkarni MD
Consultant Dermatologist
Rita Skin Foundation
Kolkata, West Bengal, India

Subrata Malakar MD
Director
Rita Skin Foundation
Kolkata, West Bengal, India

Surit Malakar MBBS PGT (Dermatology)
Rita Skin Foundation
Kolkata, West Bengal, India

Purva Mehta DNB
Consultant Dermatologist
Rita Skin Foundation
Kolkata, West Bengal, India

Samipa S Mukherjee
DDV DDVL FRGUHS (Ped Dermatology)
Consultant Pediatric Dermatologist
and Dermatotrichologist
Cloud Nine Hospitals
Bengaluru, Karnataka, India
Rita Skin Foundation
Kolkata, West Bengal, India

Balakrishna Nikam MD
Assistant Professor
Krishna Institute of Medical Sciences
Karad, Maharashtra, India

Anjali Pal MD
Consultant Dermatologist
Rita Skin Foundation
Kolkata, West Bengal, India

Jayasree Puravoor MD DNB
Consultant Dermatologist
Medical Trust Hospital
Cochin, Kerala, India

Sushrut Save DNB
Consultant Dermatologist
Rita Skin Foundation
Kolkata, West Bengal, India

Preface

Dermoscopy is fast gaining hold in clinical practice of dermatologists across India and the world. Since the inception of this science, a lot of work has been done in white skin especially cutaneous cancers. This text has been compiled by dermoscopy enthusiasts with a vision to guide the students and practitioners to learn and master the art and science of dermoscopy through a structured, detailed and a step-by-step approach. The idea for this exhaustive compilation was conceived when I noticed a dearth of literature in the skin of color, with regards to dermatological disorders apart from cutaneous malignancies. The authors of this book have made their maiden attempt to solve the diagnostic dilemmas and make treatment choices using this noninvasive method of dermoscopy.

The format of the book has been kept reader-friendly with uniform headings maintained throughout the text. The keynote message at the end of most of the topics summarizes the important dermoscopic features and the gist of the text elaborated. The plethora of images of a single condition from the author's personal collection gives a glimpse to the possible variations and presentations under dermoscopy in different clinical scenarios. Novel chapters like 'The Melanin Module' and 'Color Concept in Dermoscopy' serve as steady foundation for the reader. **In this part of the world (India), the incidence of melanoma is extremely rare, hence we have not included dermoscopy of melanoma in our book.**

Dermoscopy being a relatively new science, there are developments and newer observations being made everyday, and the authors have attempted to compile their newer findings in this book. It is certain that the readers, when they embark on their journey in dermoscopy, will make their own new observations as they go along and the authors solemnly support and appreciate their efforts and request them to share their work and knowledge which will help in enriching the subject.

We, the editorial team and the authors hope that this book will be a learning guide for all those who are practicing dermoscopy and serve as a boost and motivation for those who want to learn the art and science of dermoscopy, thereby delivering better healthcare to their patients through improvised diagnosis.

Subrata Malakar

Acknowledgments

We would like to acknowledge our patients who have inspired us to work on this project.

We acknowledge the support of Dr Uday Khopkar, Dr Uttam Banerjee, Dr Pratibha Pradhan, Dr SC Mondal, Dr Jayasree Puravoor and Dr Vivek Nigam who have been instrumental in the formation of the book.

We appreciate the efforts of Mr Suman Das for his technical assistance.

We would like to thank Shri Jitendar P Vij (Group Chairman), Mr Ankit Vij (Group President), Ms Chetna Malhotra Vohra (Associate Director–Content Strategy), Ms Ritika Chandna (Development Editor), Mr Sabyasachi Hazra (Commissioning Editor, Kolkata Branch) and the entire team of Jaypee Brothers Medical Publishers, New Delhi, India, for their tireless efforts in producing the book in its final form.

Contents

CHAPTER 1

Dermoscopy: A Window into Epidermis and Dermis

Purva Mehta, Subrata Malakar

INTRODUCTION

Dermoscopy or epiluminescence microscopy is a simple, noninvasive method to examine the subsurface features of the skin invisible to the naked eye. It serves as a telescope through which the intricate details of a lesion in the epidermis and superficial dermis can be appreciated at a greater magnitude. Normally, light is reflected and scattered by the stratum corneum thus making the structures in the epidermis and superficial dermis invisible to the eye. This pitfall is superseded by a dermoscope, which decreases scattering of light and increases transillumination either through polarized light or through linkage fluids; allowing visualization of subsurface structures.

The orange hue at dawn signals the advent of the rising sun. Similarly, colors on dermoscopy underline the depth and nature of the structure being observed.

The naked eye cannot appreciate the vascular morphology of lesions such as a hemangioma or pyogenic granuloma. It is through the dermoscope that we can identify various vascular structures such as lacunae or red homogeneous areas and understand what the color red stands for. In dermoscopic language, it indicates either vasculature or traumatic extravasation of blood. Dermoscope provides a telescopic view into the vascular world of subsurface. It enlightens us not only about the location of the blood vessels but also their course in the dermis. Vessels seen as dots or loops on dermoscopy are placed in the papillary dermis whereas linear vessels correspond to the subpapillary plexus. Also, linearity of the vessels on dermoscopy suggests that they run parallel to the epidermis whereas dotted vessels signify a perpendicular orientation to the epidermis.

A granulomatous lesion like lupus vulgaris or sarcoidosis or a xanthogranuloma presents clinically in varied forms. Dermoscopy in such cases noninvasively demonstrates orangish yellow structures, which indicate granulomas, and guides the clinician towards correct differentials.

A nevus to the naked eye looks like an innocent macule or nodule. Dermoscopy provides a window into its subsurface and designates the location of melanocytes and the need for biopsy. A pigmented or a globular network suggests junctional activity of the melanocytes whereas a cobblestone pattern indicates a dermal nest of melanocytes. A clinical view of a pigmented lesion in most cases is inadequate to classify it as benign or malignant. Magnification on dermoscopy provides vital clues; eccrine atypical network or irregular streaks or a bizarre dermoscopic image leaning toward malignancy. Dermoscopy also helps to allocate the location of chromophores in the skin. Melanin in the upper and lower epidermis is seen through a dermoscope as black and brown respectively, whereas melanin in the papillary and reticular dermis is seen as gray and bluish gray respectively.

The naked eye is incapable of visualizing the shaft or the root of the hair. Dermoscopy offers a visual window into the appendageal world. If the hair root is destroyed, it will be seen as a fibrotic white dot on trichoscopy indicating cicatrization. A circumscribed bald patch on the scalp clinically ignites the possibilities of alopecia areata, trichotillomania, etc. But it is the demonstration of exclamation mark hair or Pohl-Pinkus constriction through a dermoscope that indicates disease activity in alopecia areata thereby offering a trichoscopic confirmation of the disease as well.

Dermoscopy opens up a whole new world of the subsurface. It is an essential tool in day-to-day practice as it offers a telescopic view of pigment patterns, vascular patters and appendageal structures.

CHAPTER 2

Dermoscopy: A Missing Link between Clinical Dermatology and Histopathology

Samipa S Mukherjee, Subrata Malakar

INTRODUCTION

Dermoscopy saw its inception in the 1980s when it was predominantly used for pigmented lesions in the Caucasian skin primarily for the diagnosis of cutaneous carcinomas. The early 2000s saw a rapid advance in this noninvasive diagnostic modality not only in the field of cutaneous malignancies but in the diagnosis of dermatological and hair disorders. Being a noninvasive tool with almost nil downtime in the depiction of results, it quickly gained acceptance among dermatologists and is on its way to becoming indispensible in the evaluation of a dermatological disorder.

IMPORTANCE OF DERMATOSCOPY

Dermoscopy serves as a bridge between the clinical and histopathological tale in dermatological disorder. In instances where there is a clinical or histopathological dilemma, this instrument serves as an important jury in correlating the clinical and histopathological picture.

The need for dermoscopy as a bridge:

- Helps in providing corroborative evidence toward the diagnosis.
- Helps in arousing suspicion regarding the probability of a diagnosis.
- Helps in providing important clinical clues about the lesion under investigation when adequate history and findings may not be available.

It serves as the third eye for the dermatologist as it can see beyond the vision of the naked eye; thus, opening the window towards probable histopathologic changes, which are further correlated for a conclusive diagnosis. The histopathologic changes reflect the clinical manifestations of dermatological disorders whereas dermoscopy identifies various patterns like the melanocytic pattern, vascular pattern etc.

For example, the Auspitz sign seen clinically in psoriasis is correlated histopathologically as dilated tortuous vessels in the papillary dermis which can be seen through the dermoscope as red dots. Linear telangiectatic vessels seen in discoid lupus erythematosus results from thinning of the skin due to atrophy and visualization of the vessels located in the subpapillary plexus; this is depicted under the dermoscope as thin linear telangiectatic vessels.

Similarly, the melanin network or pattern seen under the dermoscope and clinically seen in melanocytic lesions can be correlated histopathologically with regards to the proliferation of melanocytes at various levels in the skin.

Another clinical scenario where the diagnosis may be elusive to the naked eye is the skin colored adnexal tumors. Although the lesion may appear as benign and naïve as a compound nevus dermoscopic examination of the lesion may reveal the vascular and melanocytic pattern of a more sinister condition like that of a basal cell carcinoma. Visualization of arborizing vessels all across the lesion with a kaleidoscopic color under the dermoscopic lens assists in arousing the suspicion of cutaneous malignancies.

Dermoscope, till date, although considered as an important adjuvant and aid in establishing the diagnosis is rapidly on its way to becoming a definitive diagnostic tool for certain dermatological disorder thus obviating the need for biopsy in those conditions. For example, the constellation of telangiectasia, white structureless area and follicular plugging establishes the diagnosis of discoid lupus erythematosus definitively without the further need of an invasive cutaneous investigation. Likewise, the demonstration of Wickham's striae under the dermoscopic lens in a scenario where lichen planus and other conditions are considered as differential diagnoses alleviates the need for biopsy and helps in establishing a definitive diagnosis.

Thus, it can be stated that the histopathologic reality is on its way to becoming a dermoscopic reality as well.

To conclude, clinico-dermoscopic-histopathologic correlation not only helps us in establishing a firm diagnosis in an otherwise dubious case but also helps in better understanding of the pathogenesis of the condition. In due course of time, establishment of more and more specific dermoscopic criterias will probably further obviate the need of biopsy which may be of immense importance in scenarios where invasive procedures may be difficult like in pediatric age groups, patients with bleeding disorders and noncooperative patients.

CHAPTER 3

The Dermoscope

Samipa S Mukherjee

INTRODUCTION

A dermoscope (dermatoscope) is a noninvasive, diagnostic tool which visualizes subtle clinical patterns of skin lesions and subsurface skin structures not normally visible to the naked eye. It has also been called a skin surface microscope, epiluminescence microscope or episcope. Basically, a dermoscope is functionally similar to a magnifying lens but with the added features of an inbuilt illuminating system, a higher magnification which can be adjusted, the ability to assess structures as deep as in the reticular dermis, and the ability to record images.[1] The most commonly used term "dermoscopy" was proposed by Friedman et al. in 1991.[2] In comparison to the hand lens that has been used over the decades, the dermoscope has the ability not just for magnification but also to look at the subsurface structures defining the patterns.

WORKING PRINCIPLE OF THE DERMOSCOPE

The basic principle of dermoscopy is transillumination of a lesion and studying it with a high magnification to visualize subtle features. Light incident on skin undergoes reflection, refraction, diffraction, and absorption. Most of the light incident on dry, scaly skin is reflected, but smooth, oily skin allows most of the light to pass through it, reaching the deeper dermis. Thus, the application of linkage fluids over the lesions to be studied improves the translucency of the skin. The scattering of light is overcome by polarized light in polarized dermoscopes and contact fluid in nonpolarized dermoscopes, allowing visualization of subsurface structures like those in the lower layers of epidermis, dermoepidermal junction, and upper dermis. Various linkage fluids used are oils (immersion oil, olive oil, and mineral oil), water, an antiseptic solution, and glycerin. Water or antiseptic solutions evaporate quickly and hence are less preferred than oils.

COMPONENTS OF A DERMOSCOPE

- *Achromatic lens*: Most handheld instruments provide 10X–20X magnification, but higher magnifications can be achieved with special lenses and advanced machines like Fotofinder, where a magnification of up to 180X can be reached.
- *Inbuilt illuminating system*: Light emitting diodes (LEDs) (Delta 20Ó, DermLiteÓ) provide high intensity white light and consume 70% less power than halogen lamps. Illumination can be altered by turning off a set of LEDs. They are also designed to emit lights of different colors for better visualization of the skin, as penetration of the skin by light is proportional to the wavelength of light (DermLite MSÓ). An orange light helps in enhancing the contrast between the natural skin color and the pigmented lesions which may be found in the newer equipment (DermLite DL3 and DL4).
- *Power supply*: Handheld instruments are usually powered by batteries, e.g. lithium ion battery (DermLite DL100Ó, DermLite platinumÓ), rechargeable lithium battery (DermLite MSÓ, DermLite Pro DP-RÓ), AA battery (mini 2000

dermatoscopeÓ), and rechargeable handles (DELTA 20Ó). Video dermoscopes are powered directly via the USB cable attached.

Additional facilities in some dermoscopes are an inbuilt photography system, trichoanalysis, body mapping and imaging, softwares for calculating area of involvement and severity scoring.

TYPES OF DEVICES

Nonpolarized Devices

These devices require a contact fluid with a refractive index equal to that of the skin, which optically links the skin surface with the face plate of the dermoscopes.

Polarized Devices

Polarized devices have two filters in a process called cross polarization, one filter is placed between the light source and skin and the second one is placed between the skin and light detector. This cross polarization enables excellent visibility by absorbing all the scattered light allowing light only in a single plane to pass through. They can be used without the contact fluid.

Hybrid Devices

These devices incorporate both polarized and nonpolarized light. The need for both the modes in a single device arises from the fact that nonpolarized mode helps in clearly demonstrating structures on the surface whereas polarized mode demonstrates pigmentary and vascular changes better. The latest in the series include DermLite DL3, DL4, and Fotofinder.

DERMATOSCOPY IMAGE CHARACTERISTICS AND DIFFERENCES AMONG COMMONLY USED STANDARD DERMATOSCOPES

We have compared the four commonly used standard dermatoscopes, viz. Heine Delta 20 (Heine optotechnik, Herrsching, Germany), Heine Delta 20 plus (Heine optotechnik, Herrsching, Germany), DermLite DL3 (3Gen Inc, USA) and Fotofinder (Fotofinder® Dermoscope studio). Heine Delta 20 plus, DermLite DL3, and Fotofinder have both polarized and nonpolarized modes. Heine Delta 20 has only nonpolarized mode, which requires a contact fluid. Nonpolarized dermatoscope helps in the detection of superficial structures in the skin, whereas a polarized dermatoscope allows deeper visualization. Though polarized dermatoscopes do not require contact fluid, images captured by them are sharper in the presence of interface fluid.[3]

Images taken with nonpolarized mode offer better visualization of dermatoscopic findings in lesions with surface abnormalities. Also, most of the studies in the earlier period of dermatoscopy were done on dermoscopes with nonpolarizing mode.

Vascular lesions are better characterized under the polarized mode as the light in this mode penetrates deeper. Visualization of regular red dots in psoriasis is superior with earlier devices, viz. Heine Delta 20, where images are less bright and have a relatively white tone. However, these devices are less efficient in picking up the background erythema as compared to Heine Delta 20 plus and DermLite DL3.[4]

The warmer tone in images of Heine Delta 20 plus dermatoscope and Fotofinder is attributed to higher color rendering index values of the device.

The magnification of images using the Fotofinder is up to 180X whereas with the other instruments is up to 20X which can be further accentuated by the zoom in facility of the digital and smart phone cameras. Fotofinder is an excellent research tool that can be used to document the details of the lesion/hair as the case may be. It can be used for calculating psoriasis area severity index (PASI) in psoriasis, melasma area severity index (MASI) in melasma and so on.

DIGITAL IMAGING AND DERMOSCOPY

Dermoscopy is the art and science of viewing surface and subsurface structures of the skin thereby aiding in diagnosis. The device was evolved primarily to detect melanomas and prior to biopsy of suspicious lesions. Recently it has found application in diagnosis of papulosquamous disorders, pigmentary disorders other than melanoma, and other benign conditions.

The upper layers of the skin have a reflective property whereas the lower layers have a refractive and absorptive property. Dermoscopes make use of the two most important color giving molecules in the skin, hemoglobin, and melanin. When we look at a skin lesion with a magnifying loupe with lighting, most of the light is scattered due to the reflective property of the stratum corneum. There are two ways to overcome this problem so as to allow more light to pass through the stratum corneum, enabling us to look deeper into the skin to visualize the pigment and vascular patterns among other things. One is by using a fluid medium as an interface and a transparent glass contact plate and the other is by using a cross polarized light.[5]

CHOICE OF THE INSTRUMENT

A number of factors need to be taken into account, namely, quality, budget, need for documentation, and even the major types of cases that one encounters. The most commonly used dermoscopes are the independent handheld units (Figs. 1 to 3) (these do not need to be connected to a monitor to visualize skin lesions), which usually have a magnification of around 10X–20X. Photographs in these devices can be recorded via smart phone cameras, point and shoot as well as digital SLRs, (Figs. 4A and B) using adapters. The image thus captured can be further cropped and magnified to view the minor details.

The other category of dermoscopes is one that needs to be connected to a viewing monitor (Fig. 5), usually with a USB connection. A larger view is obtained which can also be shared with the patients, if needed, for counseling purposes and images can be stored easily along with printed reports that can be given to the patients to carry home. Advanced versions of the video dermoscopes also incorporates whole body imaging and mapping systems, inbuilt trichoanalysis software and serial dermoscopic image recording facilities, however their use is restricted by cost factors.

POINTS TO BE BORNE IN MIND WHILE PRACTICING DERMOSCOPY IN VIVO[6]

- *The choice between wet and dry dermoscopy*: It is always a good idea to start with dry dermoscopy first to visualize the scales followed by wet dermoscopy to visualize the subsurface structures. Wet dermoscopy is more useful for the demonstration of vasculature and pathology in the upper dermis. The choice of linkage fluid in wet dermoscopy could range from immersion oil to water to ultrasound gel based on availability, cost, and feasibility. Dry dermoscopy is especially useful in scaly conditions, for viewing nail anomalies and to see the surface structures like in seborrheic keratosis.
- It must be borne in mind that the investigator must familiarize himself with the normal skin of the affected individual and proceed toward the diseased skin or scalp. This helps in picking up the abnormalities specific to the affected individual.
- The area to be examined must be stabilized to avoid out of focus images and findings.
- In practice, contact dermoscopy can be avoided for infected/infective lesions. The use of disposable contact caps, food wraps, adhesive tapes, and using 70% ethanol as the interface fluid help to avoid cross infection in contact dermoscopy.[7]
- While practicing contact dermoscopy, it is important to avoid excess pressure over the lesion, so as to avoid blanching effect.
- The use of polarized and nonpolarized mode will depend on whether the investigator wishes to demonstrate the surface (nonpolarized mode) or subsurface structures (polarized mode).
- The use of additional facilities like pigment boost could be explored while dealing with hyper/hypopigmentary disorders.

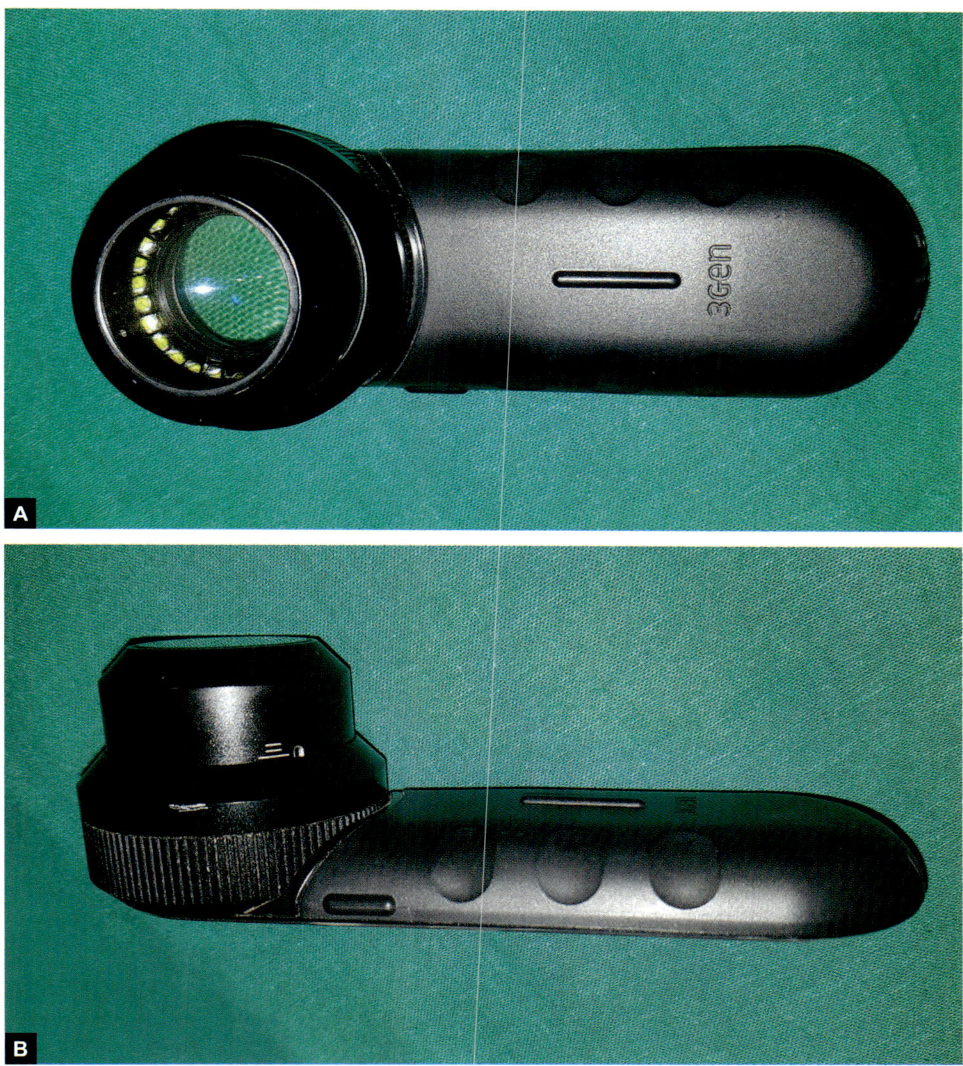

Figs. 1A and B: DermLite DL3.

- Few devices also have UV light as an additional feature, which facilitates in monitoring conditions like vitiligo.
- Special imaging techniques are required while doing dermoscopy on mucosal surface in order to avoid soiling of instrument and transmission of disease and maintain hygiene. Using of cellophane tape or glass slide as the interface medium in mucosal dermoscopy are widely used methods. However, usage of glass slide has clear advantages over cellophane. Glass slide helps in dispersing the collected smegma/fluid/discharge on the mucosal area thus providing a clear field of vision. Also the number of artifacts due to reflectance is lesser with glass slide as compared to the cellophane sheets.

TAKING A GOOD QUALITY IMAGE

While documenting dermoscopic image, do not forget to take a good quality clinical image. Clinical image is of vital importance for a clinic dermoscopic correlation and future reference like in monitoring of treatment or before and after therapy. Also, using the inbuilt measuring scale available in most units give an idea of the size of the lesion. For clinical image capture, one must select the right lesion, decide on whether or not to use the facility of flash in the camera,

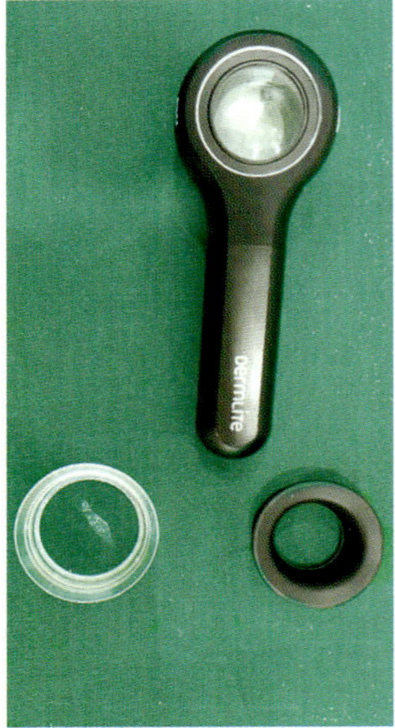

Fig. 2: DermLite DL4.

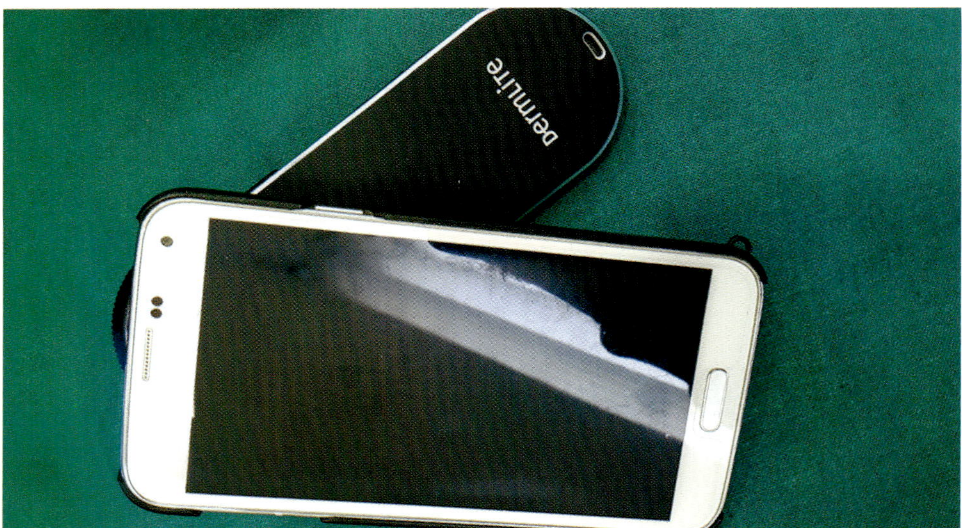

Fig. 3: DermLite with smart phone attachment.

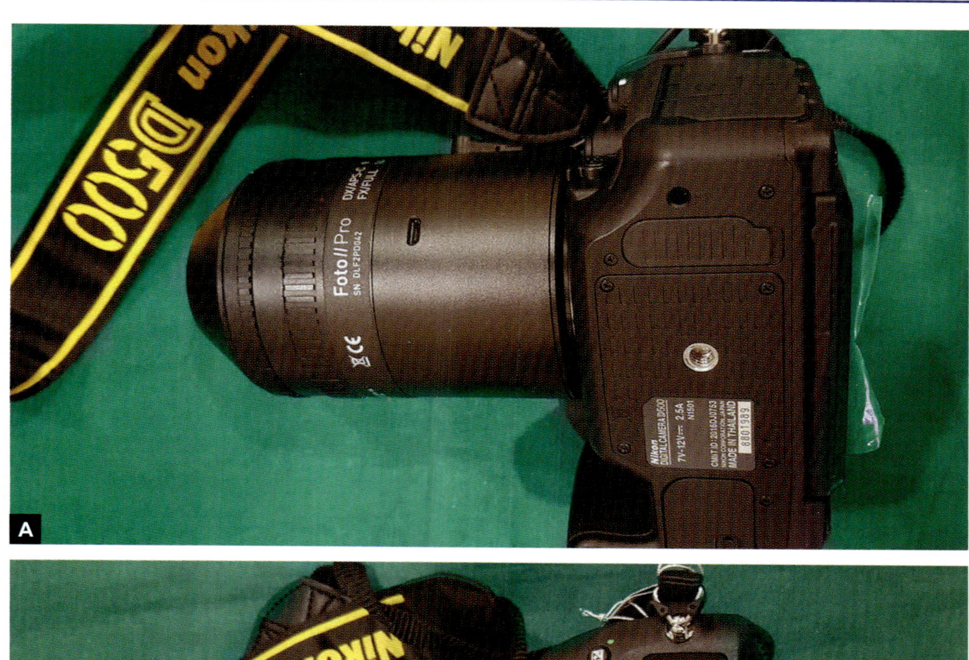

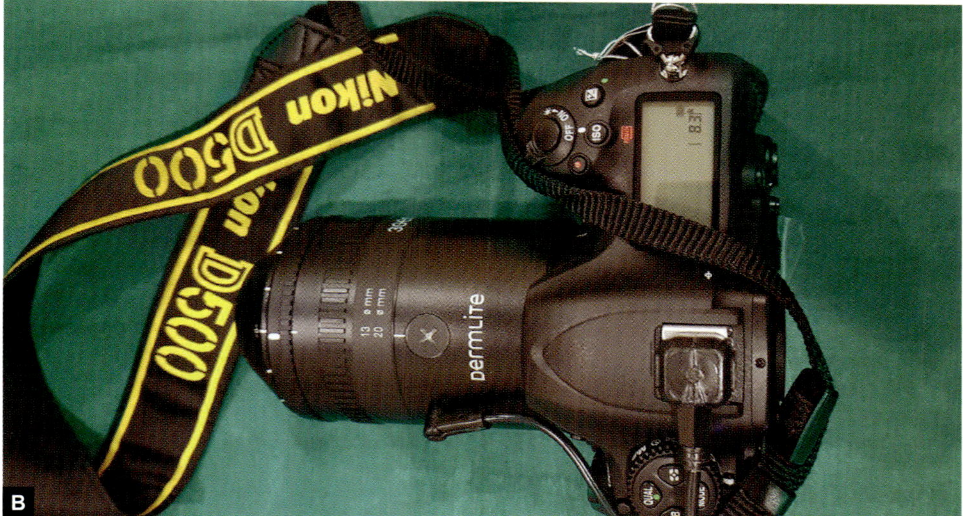

Figs. 4A and B: DermLite Photo II Pro.

eliminate background chaos to focus on the lesion in question and thereby frame the lesion while capturing image. Stability of hand taking the photograph is of immense importance to avoid shaky or blurred images.

Capturing good quality dermoscopic images may be a matter of practice and expertise with time. It may be a good idea to have an assistant at hand who can help to stabilize the lesion, add linkage fluid, stretch the skin, and assist in capturing the image. While practicing contact dermoscopy and capturing the image special importance should be given to avoid excess pressure since that leads to blanching of the lesion. In the author's view, it is a good idea to use both hands while capturing images through a handheld dermoscope in the smart phone cameras. The non-dominant hand is used for stabilizing the camera while the dominant hand may be used to manipulate and maneuver the dermoscope for focusing on the lesion of interest.

STORAGE OF DIGITAL IMAGES

Digital images can be store in the smart phones, computers, tablets or on cloud after appropriate labeling with patient details, clinical image, and related dermoscopic findings. It may be a good idea to clearly label the relevant dermoscopic findings using arrows or circles with a color that has sufficient contrast compared to the background.

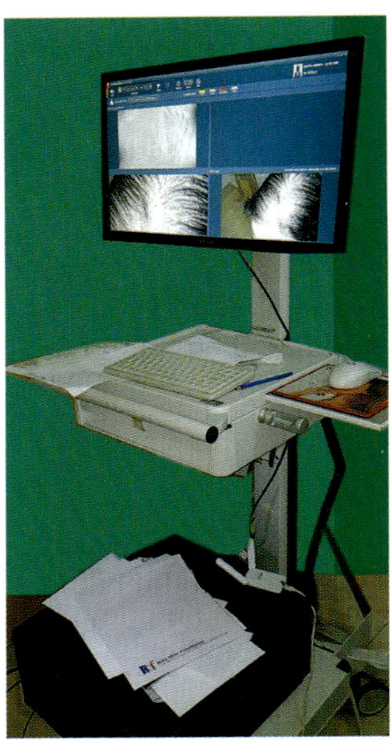

Fig. 5: Fotofinder.

REFERENCES

1. Nischal KC, Khopkar U. Dermoscope. Indian J Dermatol Venereol Leprol. 2005;71:300-3.
2. Friedman RJ, Rigel DS, Silverman MK, et al. Malignant melanoma in the 1990s: the continued importance of early detection and the role of physician examination and self-examination of the skin. CA Cancer J Clin. 1991;41:201-26.
3. Pan Y, Gareau DS, Scope A, et al. Polarized and nonpolarized dermoscopy: the explanation for the observed differences. Arch Dermatol. 2008;144:828-9.
4. Nirmal B. Dermatoscopy image characteristics and differences among commonly used standard dermatoscopes. Indian Dermatol Online J. 2017;8:233-4.
5. Kaliyadan F. The scope of the dermoscope. Indian Dermatol Online J. 2016;7:359-63.
6. Mukherjee SS, Malakar S. Taking the dermoscope from bench to practice. Int J Dermoscop. 2017;1(2):4-6.
7. Kaliyadan F, Kuruvilla J. Using transparent adhesive tape to prevent cross infection during contact dermoscopy. Indian J Dermatol Venereol Leprol. 2016;82:744.

CHAPTER 4

Recognition of Patterns

Sushrut Save, Purva Mehta, Subrata Malakar

4A. MELANOCYTIC PATTERNS

Sushrut Save, Subrata Malakar

INTRODUCTION

The first step in the algorithm in dermoscopy is to primarily identify whether a lesion is melanocytic or nonmelanocytic. Recognition and interpretation of various dermoscopic structures and colors enable us in diagnosing benign melanocytic lesions and differentiating them from malignant lesions.

Colors play a very important role in dermoscopy. Melanin is the most crucial chromophore present in skin and in the various melanocytic neoplasms, and depending upon the anatomic location and concentration of melanin in the skin, various colors can be appreciated on dermoscopy, such as light brown, dark brown, black, blue, blue-gray, etc.[1]

If the melanin is located in the stratum corneum and the upper epidermis, then black color can be perceived on dermoscopy of the lesion. Melanin, when present in multiple layers in the skin, may also appear black. Light to dark brown indicates that the melanin is located in the epidermis or at the dermoepidermal junction. Gray to gray-blue, depending on the density, corresponds to melanin in the papillary dermis. Blue color is appreciated when the pigmentation is confined to the reticular dermis, as the portions of visible light with shorter wavelengths (blue-violet end of spectrum) are more dispersed.[1,2]

DERMOSCOPIC STRUCTURES

The identification of specific dermoscopic structures in different regions of the same lesion contributes to the diagnosis of melanocytic lesions and is called local patterns. They include pigment network, parallel pattern, homogeneous pigmentation, pigmented globules and dots, cobblestone pattern, streaks, their appearance is presented below. The predominant presence of some of these local patterns can determine some global patterns.[3]

Pigment Network

The typical pattern of pigment network is a regular mesh or a grid of intersecting pigmented "lines" along with intervening angulated hypopigmented "holes" forming a honeycomb pattern (Figs. 1 and 2). These intersecting lines basically represent the melanin in the keratinocytes and melanocytes present in the epidermal rete ridges following the contours of the dermoepidermal junction, while holes are a reflection of the tips of dermal papillae and the overlying suprapapillary epidermis.[1,4] The other variations of pigment network pattern are:

- *Atypical network*: There is a variation in the thickness of the intersecting lines of the pigment network along with irregular holes and is a reflection of dysplastic changes resulting in fusion of the rete ridges (Fig. 3).[4]

- *Pseudonetwork*: The melanocytic network on the face is replaced by a pseudonetwork wherein there is diffuse pigmentation along with intervening nonpigmented follicular or adnexal openings. This pattern is appreciated in both melanocytic and nonmelanocytic lesions.
- *Negative pigment network (inverse network)*: The network shows comparatively lighter areas apparently made up of serpiginous intersecting lines and comparatively darker areas, resembling globular structures, filling the apparent holes. Histologically it corresponds to the thin elongated rete ridges along with large melanocytic nests within a widened papillary dermis. The presence of negative network signifies that the lesion is of melanocytic origin. It is most often associated with Spitz nevi and melanoma, and rarely congenital nevi.[1,5]

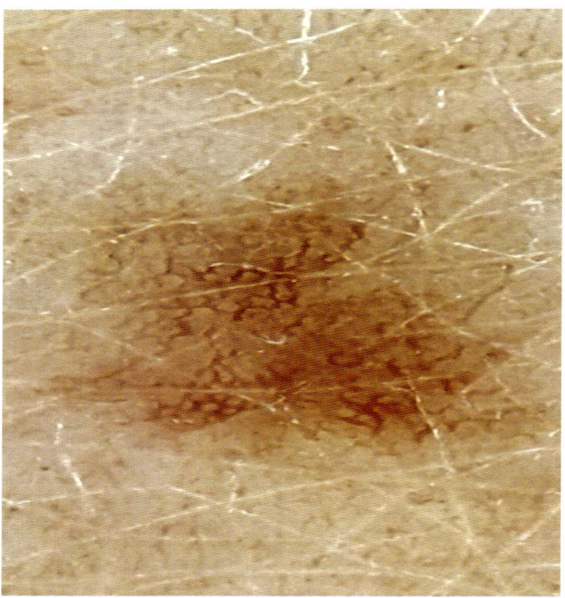

Fig. 1: Normal melanocytic network.

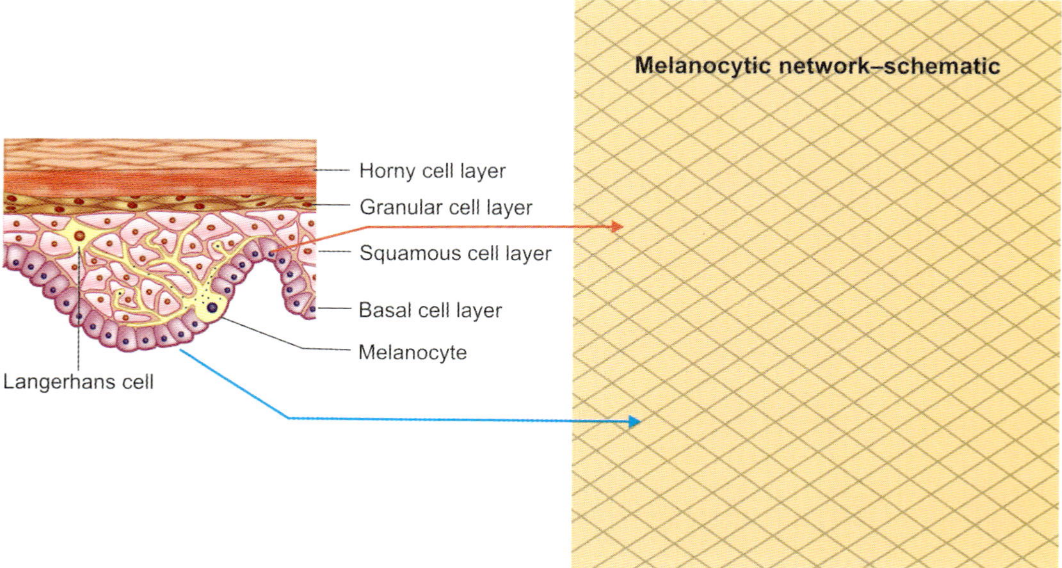

Fig. 2: Normal melanocytic network consisting of intersecting lines. These lines correspond to rete ridge melanocytes whereas the holes correspond to the dermal papillae where concentration of melanocytes is comparatively less.

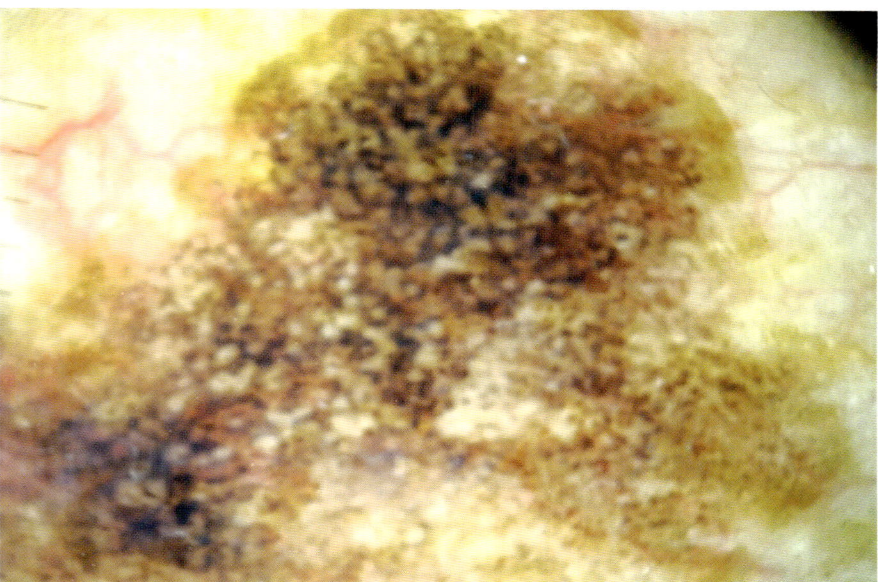

Fig. 3: Atypical pigment network.

Parallel Pigment Pattern

The palmar-plantar skin has a thick and compact stratum corneum, that has dermatoglyphics, formed by furrows and ridges and the pigmentation is seen on the parallel furrows or fissures of the skin markings (other variations of this pattern include the globular subtype and the double-lined subtype) (Fig. 4).[6]

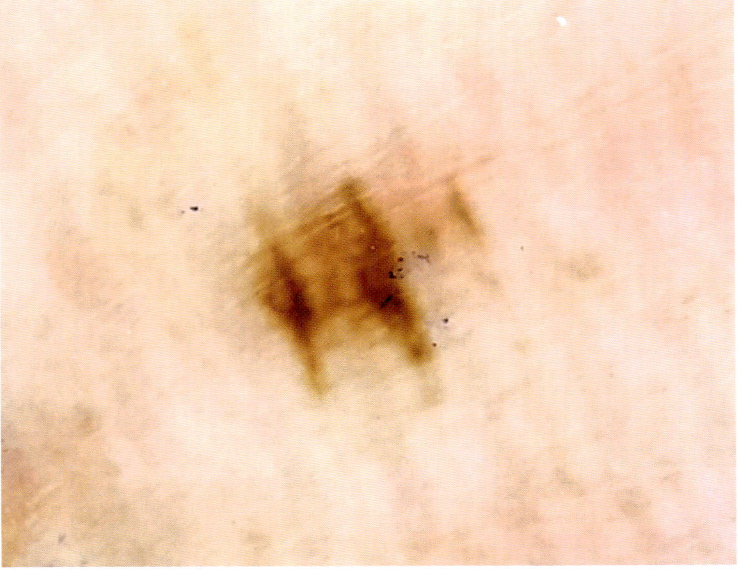

Fig. 4: Parallel pigment pattern is found over palms and soles.

Dots and Pigmented Globules[1]

Dots are round or oval structures, less than 0.1 mm in diameter and may be black, brown, gray or bluish in color. They represent free melanin or melanin containing melanocytes or keratinocytes. Globules are round or oval structures of more than 0.1 mm in diameter, and like dots, their color also ranges from black to brown to blue-gray. Histologically they represent nests of melanocytes in the lower epidermis, dermoepidermal junction or papillary dermis.

- Because both the dots and globules are frequently observed together (Fig. 5) and they represent melanocyte nests, a combined name "dots and globules" is coined for them.
- Dermoscopically, nevi and melanoma both may have dots and globules.
- Depending on the depth and concentration of the melanin in the skin, following types of dots and globules may be seen:
  - Black dots/globules represent melanin/nests of melanocytes in the stratum corneum or in the upper parts of the epidermis.
  - Brown dots/globules represent focal accumulations of melanin/nests of melanocytes in the stratum spinosum or dermoepidermal junction.
  - Gray-blue dots or peppering are seen when melanin is present in the superficial dermis. Melanin may be present either within the melanophages or as extracellular dust.

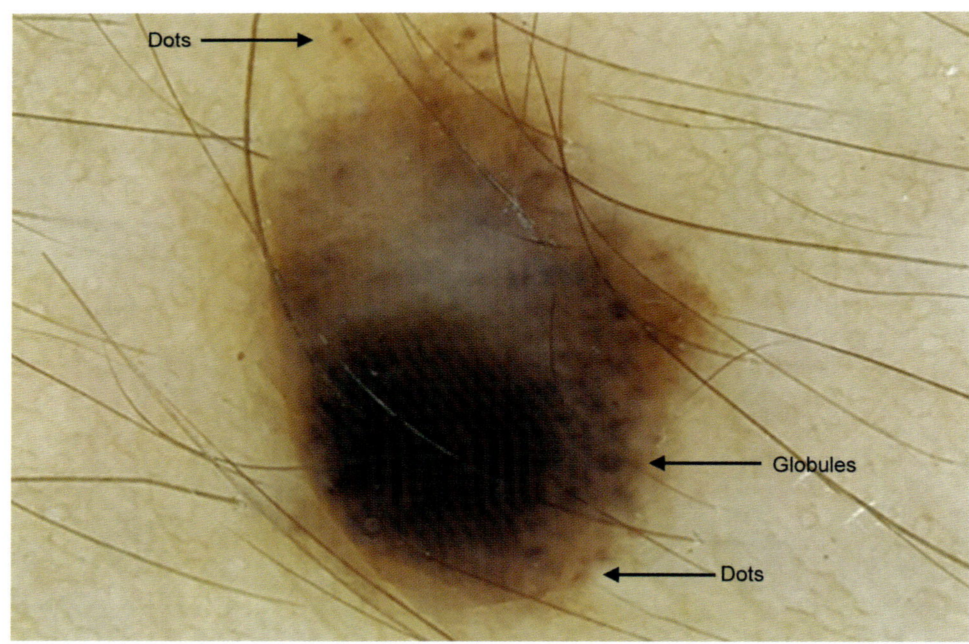

Fig. 5: Dots and globules in a melanocytic lesion.

Cobblestone Pattern[4]

It appears as closely aggregated angulated brown globules resembling cobblestones. It is a reflection of large dermal nests on histopathology and is observed in dermal melanocytic nevi.

Homogeneous Pigmentation

It refers to various shades of diffuse but patchy hyperpigmentation that obscure the ability to appreciate other dermoscopic features, such as melanocytic network, dots, etc. Histopathologically, characterized by prominent melanin aggregation throughout the epidermis and dermis.

Homogeneous blue pigmentation is seen in blue nevi and is characterized by structureless blue areas throughout the lesion, representing heavily pigmented nests of dermal melanocytes (Fig. 6).[1,7]

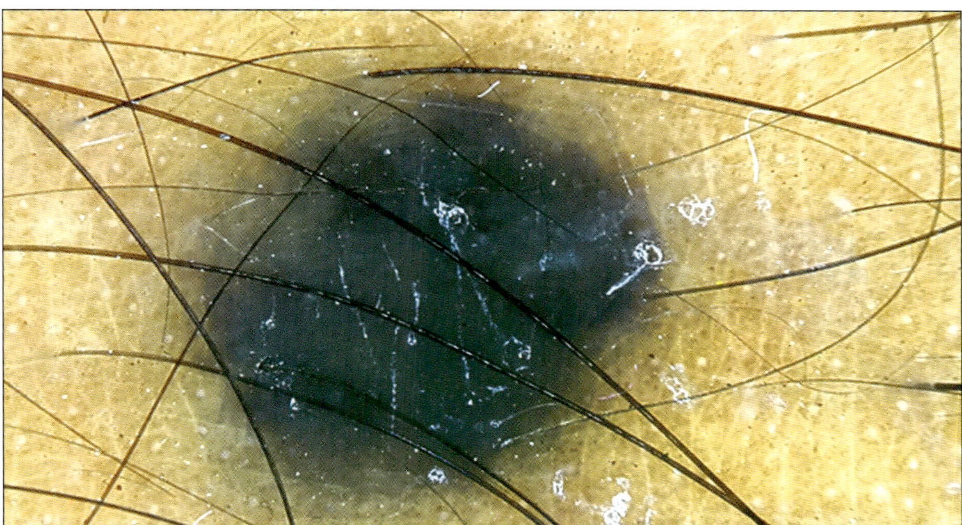

Fig. 6: Homogeneous blue pigmentation in blue nevus.

Streaks[1]

They are pigmented linear projections arranged radially at the periphery of the lesion (Fig. 7). Both pseudopods and radial streaming are the variations of streaks.

Histopathologically, streaks show confluent nests of melanocytes at the dermoepidermal junction.

In Spitz nevi, streaks are distributed symmetrically around the entire lesion; whereas melanoma has streaks only focally at the periphery of the lesion.

Pseudopods: Finger-like structures of brown to black pigment situated at the periphery of the lesion. The finger-like structures have small nobs at their tips. The pseudopods are attached centrally to a blotch or pigmented network. Pseudopods are one of the specific criteria to diagnose superficial spreading melanoma.

Histopathologically pseudopods represent confluent nests of melanocytes at the dermoepidermal junction.

Radial streaming: When parallel linear lines are arranged radially at the perimeter, it is called radial streaming.

Histopathologically it corresponds to confluent nests of melanocytes at the dermoepidermal junction.

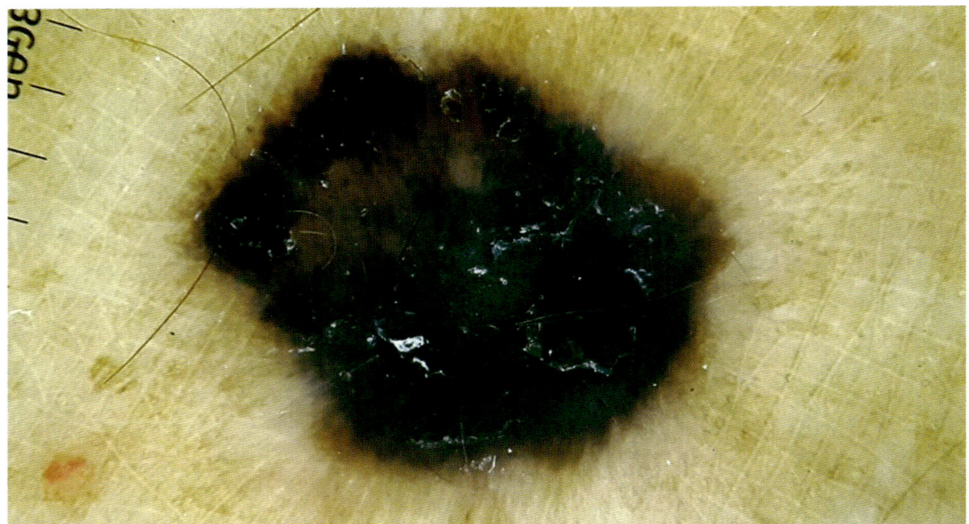

Fig. 7: Streaks.

Multicomponent Pattern[8]

It is represented by three or more patterns, namely (1) reticular, (2) globular, and (3) homogeneous. The homogeneous areas are either "blotches" or "structureless areas". These nevi may also exhibit other structures such as network, streaks, negative pigmented network, chrysalis, etc. In dysplastic nevus, these structures are distributed symmetrically and in an organized manner, while if their distribution is asymmetric and in a disorganized fashion, melanoma is the diagnosis.

Blue-White Veil

- Dermoscopic description—it is a confluent blue-white pigmentation with an overlying translucent ground-glass appearance (Fig. 8).[1]
- Histopathologically it represents compact orthokeratosis and acanthosis overlying a densely pigmented area, such as an agglomeration of melanin laden melanocytes or melanophages in the upper dermis.[9]
- In the case of melanoma, the blue-white veil is heterogeneous, conspicuous and asymmetric, while in the case of nevi, it is usually homogeneous with a light hue and located centrally (Fig. 8).[10]
- Melanoma is a life-threatening disease. Therefore, it is imperative that all lesions, which are clinically and/or dermoscopically suspicious for melanoma, should be diagnosed early using dermoscopy and removed, while minimizing the excision of benign lesions.
- Based on the Consensus Net Meeting on Dermoscopy (CNMD) the following 3-point checklist was proposed for early diagnosis of melanoma using a dermoscope.[11]
- 3-point checklist (presence of two or more is suggestive of suspicious lesion).[11]
  - *Asymmetry*: Asymmetry of color and structure in one or two perpendicular axes
  - Atypical network
  - *Blue-white structures*: Any type of blue and/or white color, i.e. combination of blue-white veil and regression structures.

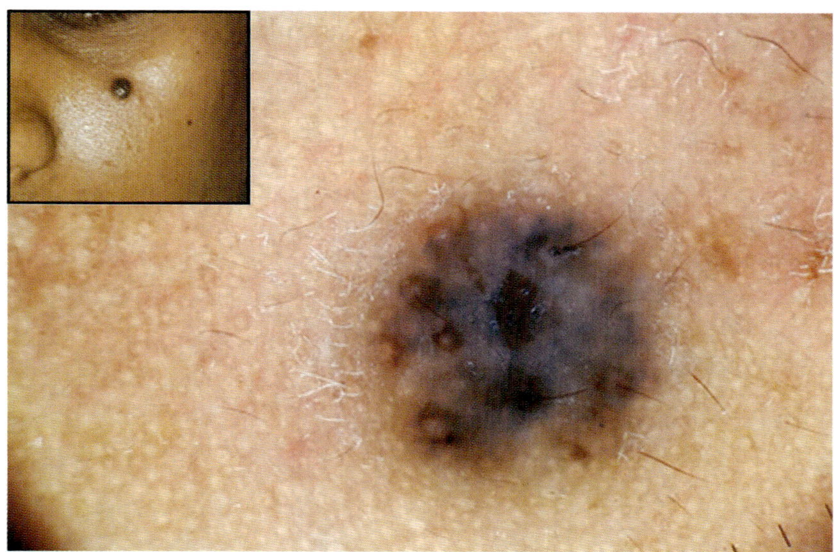

Fig. 8: Blue-white veil is defined as confluent blue pigmentation with an overlying white ground glass haze. In nevi, it is homogeneous with a light hue and is located toward the center of the lesion.

REFERENCES

1. Braun RP, Scope A, Marghoob AA, et al. Histopathologic tissue correlations of dermoscopic structures. In: Marghoob AA, Malvehy J, Braun RP (Eds). An Atlas of Dermoscopy, 2nd edition. London: Informa Healthcare; 2012. pp. 58-69.
2. Ferrara G, Soyer HP, Malvehy J, et al. The many faces of blue nevus: a clinicopathologic study. J Cutan Pathol. 2007;34:543-51.
3. Argenziano G, Soyer HP, De Giorgio V, et al. Interactive Atlas of Dermoscopy. Milan, Italy: EDRA Medical Publishing and New Media; 2000.
4. Bowling J. Regression in melanoma. In: Diagnostic Dermoscopy: The Illustrated Guide, 2nd edition. United States: Wiley-Blackwell; 2012. p. 54.
5. Pizzichetta MA, Talamini R, Marghoob AA, et al. Negative pigment network: an additional dermoscopic feature for the diagnosis of melanoma. J Am Acad Dermatol. 2013;68:552-9.
6. Saida T, Miyazaki A, Oguchi S, et al. Significance of dermoscopic patterns in detecting malignant melanoma on acral volar skin: results of a multicenter study in Japan. Arch Dermatol. 2004;140:1233-8.
7. de Giorgi V, Massi D, Salvini C, et al. Dermoscopic features of combined melanocytic nevi. J Cutan Pathol. 2004;31:600-4.
8. Ashfaq A, Marghoob AA, Kopf AW. Benign melanocytic lesions. In: Marghoob AA, Malvehy J, Braun RP (Eds). An Atlas of Dermoscopy, 2nd edition. London: Informa Healthcare; 2012. pp. 159-70.
9. Menzies SW, Crotty KA, Ingvar C, et al. An Atlas of Surface Microscopy of Pigmented Skin Lesions: Dermoscopy, 2nd edition. Sydney: McGraw-Hill Book Company; 2003.
10. Yadav S, Vossaert KA, Kopf AW, et al. Histopathologic correlates of structures seen on dermoscopy (epiluminescence microscopy). Am J Dermatopathol. 1993;15:297-305.
11. Argenziano G, Soyer HP, Chimenti S, et al. Dermoscopy of pigmented skin lesions: results of a consensus meeting via the Internet. J Am Acad Dermatol. 2003;48:679-93.

4B. VASCULAR PATTERNS

Purva Mehta, Subrata Malakar

INTRODUCTION

The identification of vascular patterns on dermoscopy is of vital significance as they provide important clues in the diagnosis of clinical lesions. A two pronged approach is used to decipher vascular patterns on dermoscopy, namely the shape of the vessel and its structural arrangement. A dermoscope gives an insight not only regarding the course of the vessels but also determines the location of the vessels in the dermis.

PRELIMINARY GROUNDWORK

At the outset, some basics regarding vascular patterns in dermoscopy need to be understood. The shape of the vessel indicates its course along the dermis. The linearity of a vessel indicates that it runs a course parallel to the skin surface since a dermatoscope is held horizontal to the skin surface (Fig. 1).

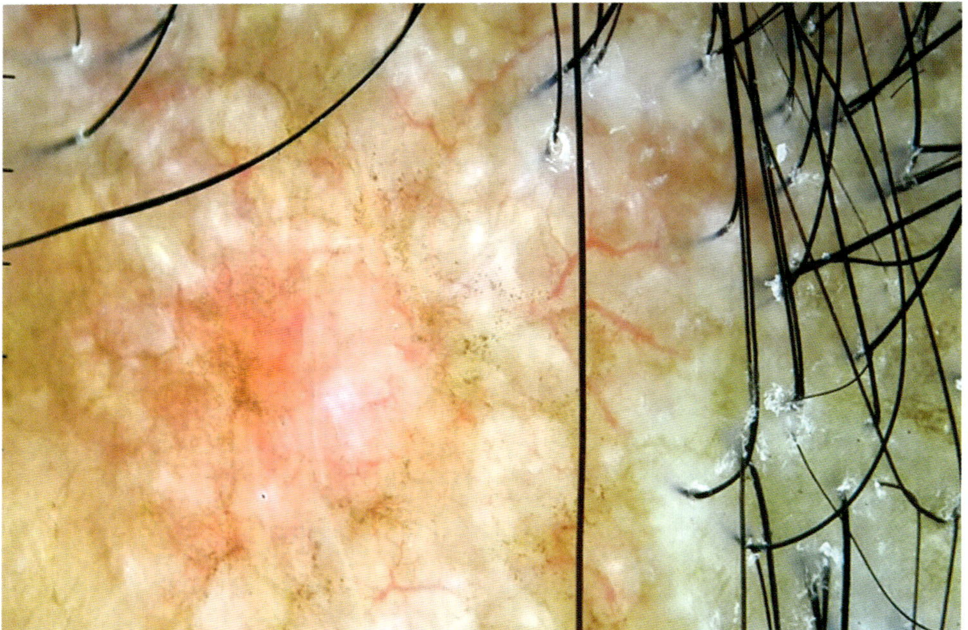

Fig. 1: Vessels parallel to skin surface are linearly oriented.

Similarly, if the vessel is dotted or looped, it shows that the vessel is oriented perpendicular to the surface of the skin (Fig. 2).[1]

The color and prominence of vascular patterns on dermoscopy delineate the location of the vessels in the dermis. The vessels which are just below the epidermis appear bright red, prominent and in focus owing to their proximity to the skin surface (Fig. 3).

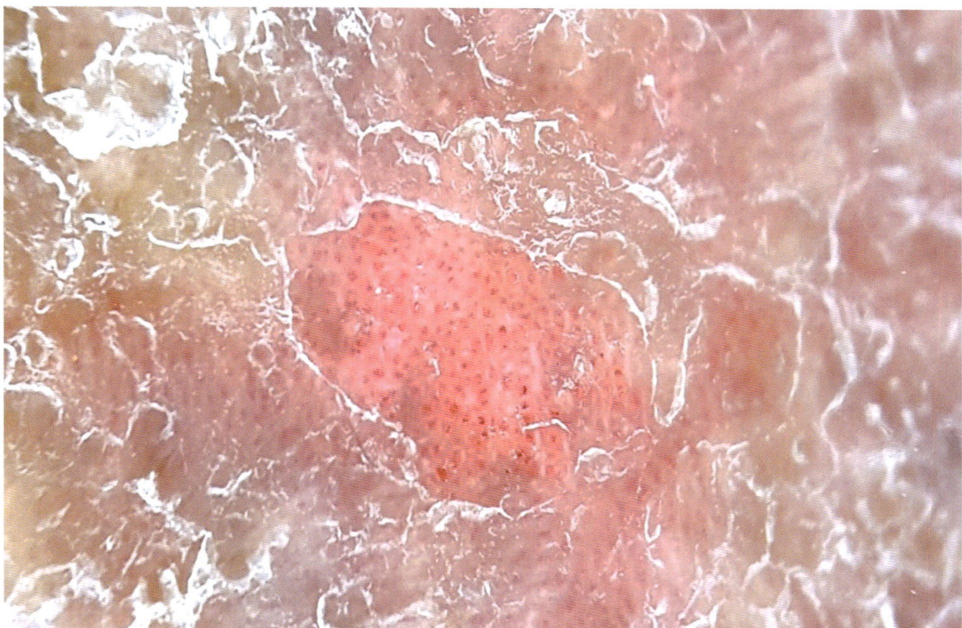

Fig. 2: Vessels perpendicular to skin surface appear as dots or loops.

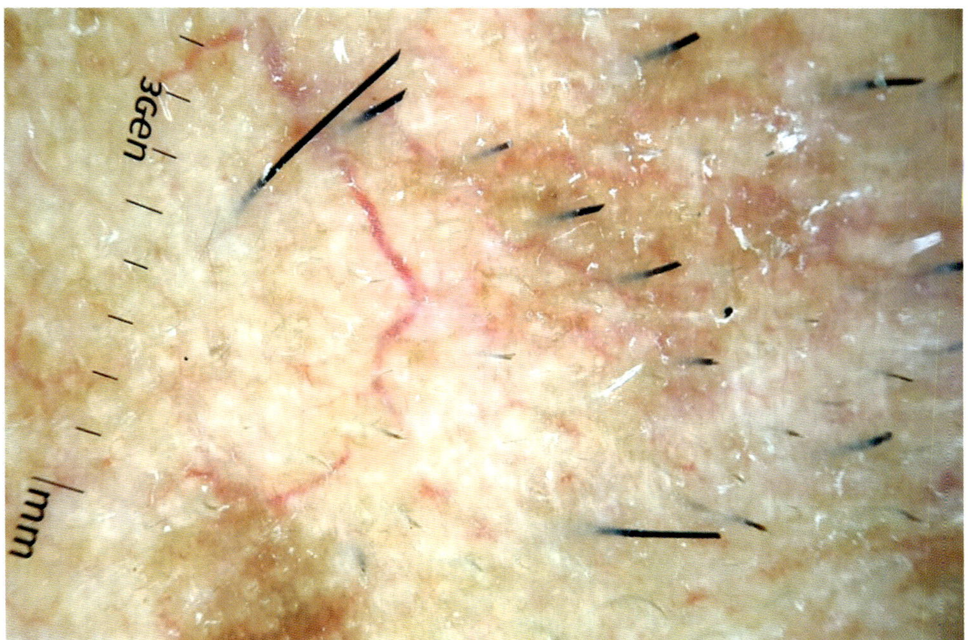

Fig. 3: Superficial vessels appear bright red and in focus on dermoscopy.

Comparatively, the connective tissue present in the deeper dermis causes dispersion of light due to which the deeper dermal vessels appear pink in color, less prominent and out of focus (Fig. 4).[2]

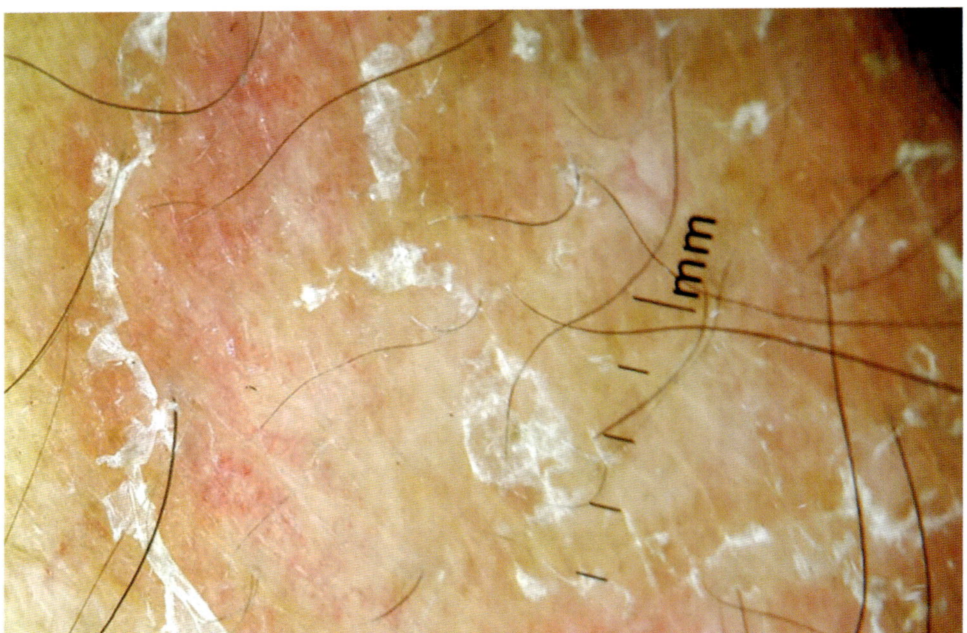

Fig. 4: Deep vessels appear pink and out of focus.

Two pronged approach to vascular dermoscopic patterns is given in Table 1.[2-4]

Table 1: Pattern, description, and arrangement of the vessels.

Pattern of the vessel	*Description*	*Arrangement of the vessels*		
Dotted vessels	Rounded, small diameter vessels resembling a pinhead	Regular arrangement, e.g. psoriasis	Patchy arrangement, e.g. eczema	Dotted vessels arranged linearly resembling a "string of pearls", e.g. clear cell acanthoma
Comma vessels	Curved vessels with one end being thicker than the other	Isolated arrangement, e.g. dermal nevi or compound nevi		
Hairpin vessels	Loop vessels with a U shaped bend	Peripheral, irregular arrangement, e.g. keratoacanthoma squamous cell carcinoma	Coursing throughout the lesion: seborrheic keratosis	
Crown vessels	Vessels along the periphery, rarely branch and never cross the midline	Radial arrangement, e.g. sebaceous hyperplasia, molluscum contagiosum		
Arborizing vessels	Prominent large bore vessels dividing into finer vessels	Branching throughout the lesion, e.g. basal cell carcinoma, adnexal tumors		
Glomerular vessels	Vessels curling up on each other in a tortuous manner	Clustered arrangement, e.g. Bowen's disease, stasis dermatitis		
Corkscrew vessels	Linear vessels arranged spirally/helically	Irregular arrangement, e.g. melanoma, melanoma metastasis		
Linear irregular vessels	Straight vessels	Irregular arrangement, e.g. melanoma, squamous cell carcinoma		
Coral vessels	Vessels in a flowery arrangement resembling the tentacles of a coral	Superficial arrangement, e.g. secondary milia		
Lacunae	Well demarcated, round to oval, reddish blue structures	Solitary/clustered arrangement, e.g. angiokeratoma, hemangioma		
Polymorphous vessels	Various patterns coexisting in the same lesion	Irregular arrangement, e.g. melanoma, carcinomas		

Dotted Vessels

- Dotted vessels in a regular distribution are the dermoscopic hallmark for psoriasis (Fig. 5). They correspond histopathologically to the capillaries in the dermal papillae. They serve as a therapeutic marker as their density decreases on clinical improvement.[5]
- Dotted vessels albeit in a patchy distribution are seen in eczematous conditions.

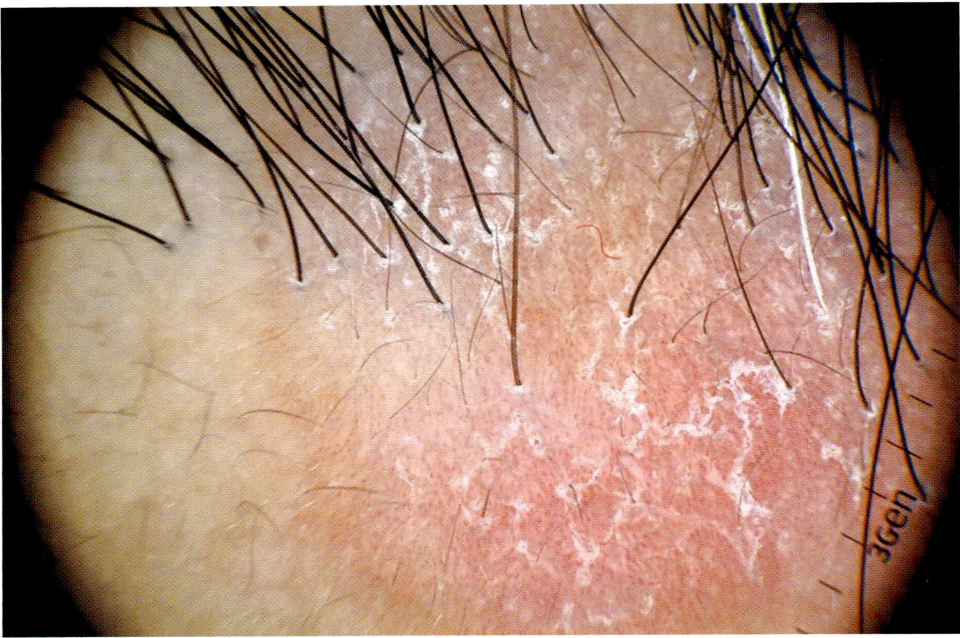

Fig. 5: Regularly distributed red dots in a case of scalp psoriasis.

- Dotted vessels arranged in a linear, "string of pearls" distribution is highly characteristic of clear cell acanthoma (Fig. 6).[6]
- Dotted vessels are commonly seen in nevi. In benign nevi, such as dermal melanocytic nevi or Spitz nevi, their arrangement is regular whereas the arrangement becomes regular to irregular in dysplastic nevi. In malignant melanoma (thin lesions), the distribution is completely irregular.[3,7,8]

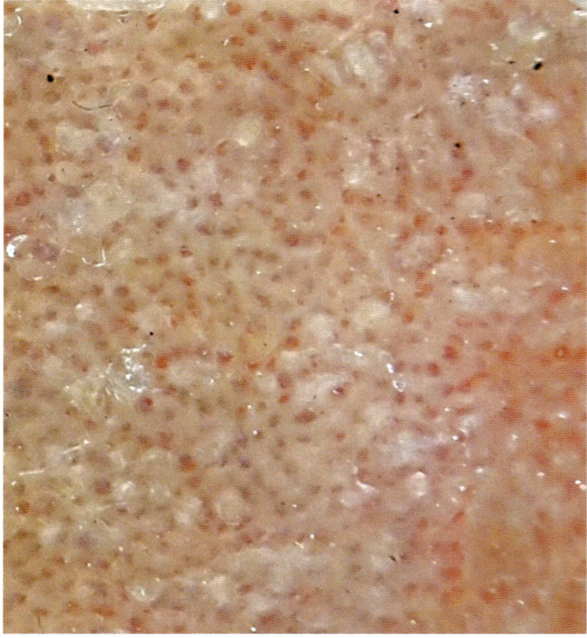

Fig. 6: Dotted vessels arranged in a linear, "string of pearls" distribution in a case of clear cell acanthoma.

Comma Vessels

- The key dermoscopic feature for the diagnosis of mature melanocytic nevi is the presence of comma vessels (Fig. 7).
- However, comma vessels are a negative predictive factor in cases of melanoma, almost ruling out its possibility.[3,8]
- Comma vessels are also found in other conditions, such as dysplastic nevi, dermatofibroma, etc.

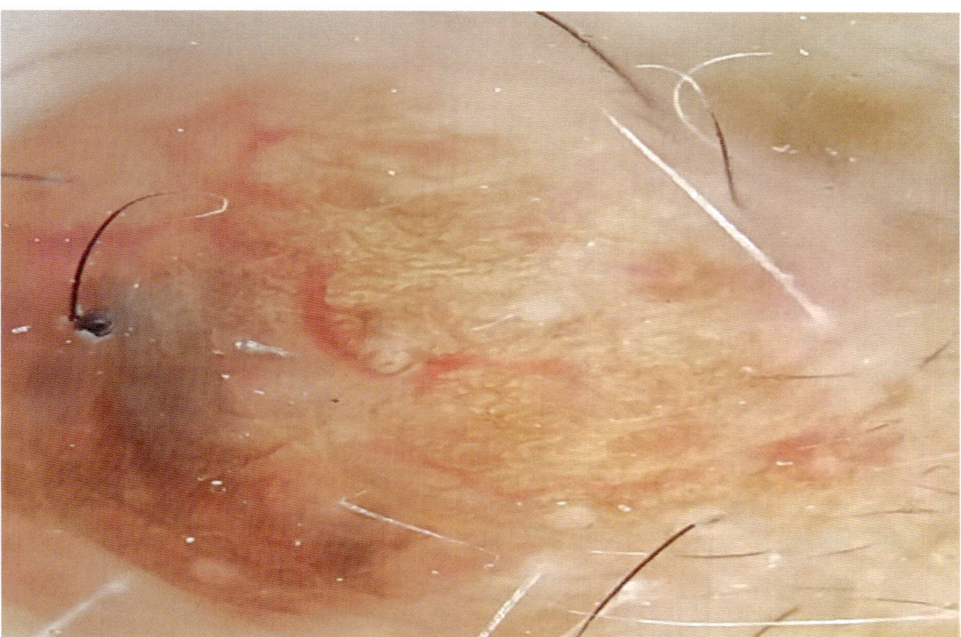

Fig. 7: Dermoscopic image of comma vessels in a case of compound nevus.

Hairpin Vessels (Fig. 8)

Hairpin vessels on dermoscopy are characteristic of keratinizing tumors such as seborrheic keratosis, keratoacanthoma, squamous cell carcinoma, etc. In such cases, there is a whitish halo surrounding the hairpin vessels, which is a dermoscopic marker for keratinization. The presence of this halo helps to differentiate hairpin vessels in keratinizing tumors from hairpin vessels in melanoma which lack this halo.[1,3]

The hairpin vessels have a characteristic peripheral arrangement in keratoacanthoma and this helps to distinguish hairpin vessels in seborrheic keratosis where they are dispersed throughout the lesion.[2]

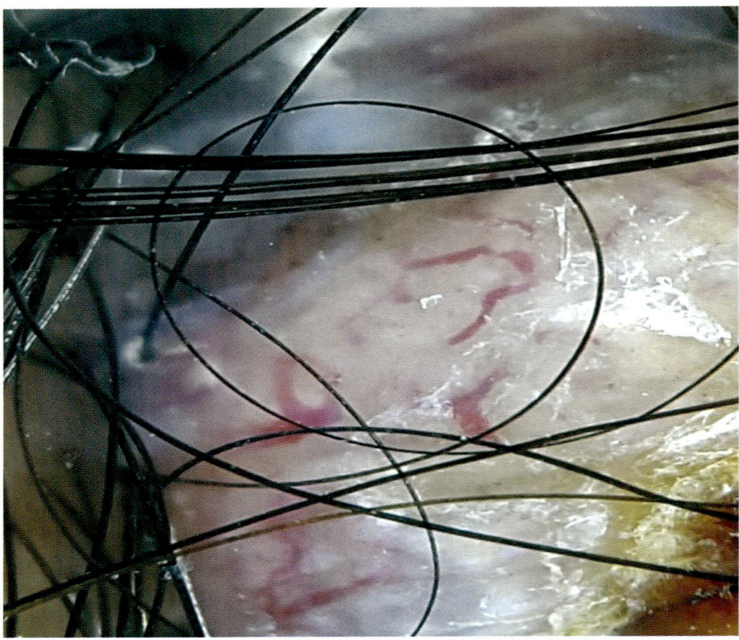

Fig. 8: Hairpin vessels.

Crown Vessels (Fig. 9)

Crown vessels on dermoscopy are seen in sebaceous hyperplasia and molluscum contagiosum. In both these conditions, they are distributed radially at the periphery of the lesion and do not cross the midline.[9,10] In both, crown vessels surround a central whitish-yellow lobulated area or crateriform area which corresponds to sebaceous lobules in sebaceous

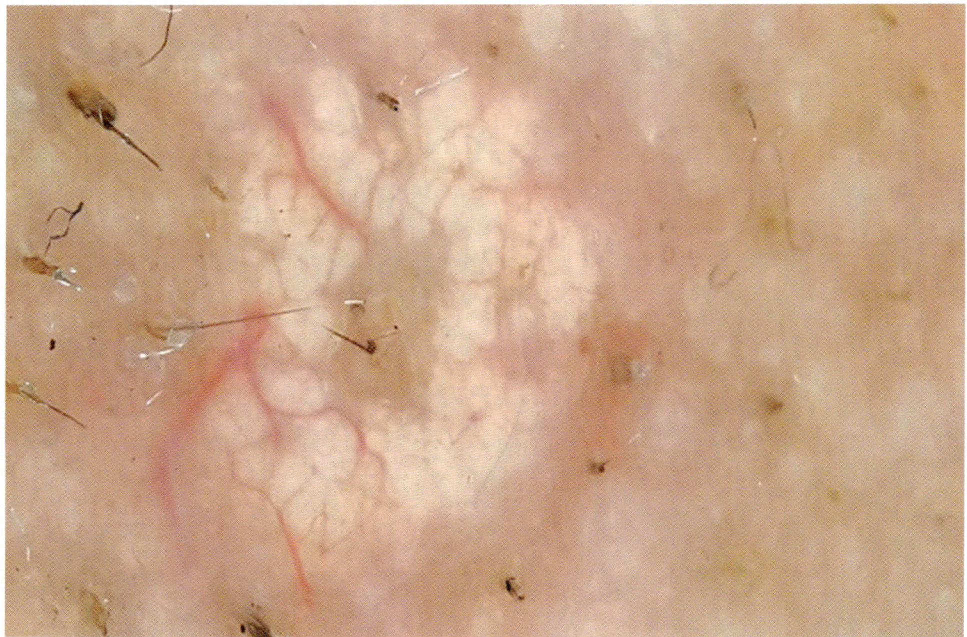

Fig. 9: Crown vessels in a radial distribution classically seen in sebaceous hyperplasia and molluscum contagiosum.

hyperplasia and to lobules of squamous epithelium filled with molluscum bodies in molluscum contagiosum. As the sebaceous lobules or the molluscum bodies expand, the dermis is displaced and hence the dermal vessels are pushed to the periphery resulting in crown vessels.[1]

Arborizing Vessels

These large bore vessels branch at abrupt irregular intervals into finer vessels. Arborizing vessels are a vascular dermoscopic hallmark for basal cell carcinoma, especially nodular basal cell carcinoma and adnexal tumors.[1,3,11] The arborizing vessels in these cases are usually bright red in color, prominent and "in focus" indicating their location to be just below the epidermis (Fig. 10). These are the feeding vessels of the tumor essential for its growth and correlate to dilated vessels in the superficial dermis histopathologically.[1]

Arborizing vessels are also seen in other malignancies such as squamous cell carcinoma and melanoma.

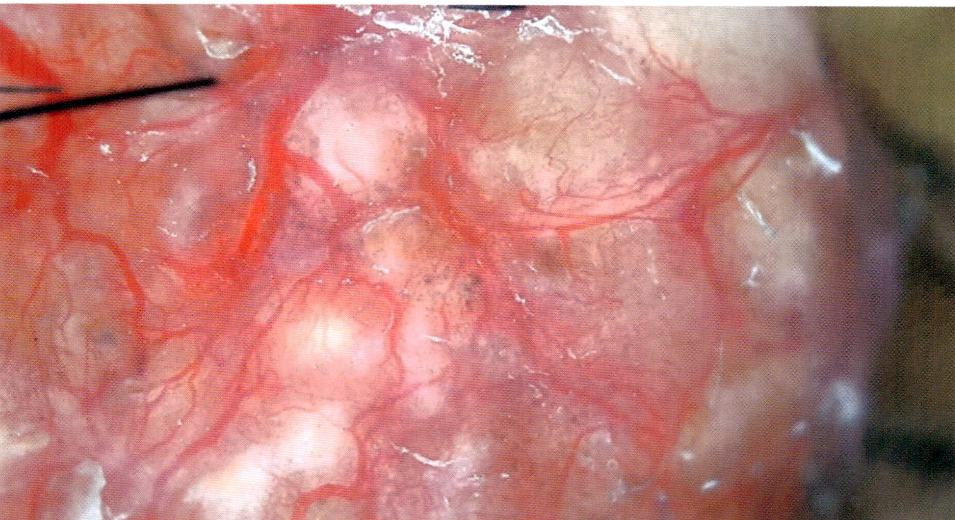

Fig. 10: Arborizing vessels, bright red, sharp and in focus. They are feeding vessels to nodular basal cell carcinoma in this case.

Glomerular Vessels

They are tortuous vessels, curling upon each other and are named after the glomerular apparatus of the kidney owing to their resemblance to it. Glomerular vessels are seen most commonly in Bowen's disease where they are packed together and thus have a clustered distribution (Fig. 11). They are commonly associated with surface scaling in Bowen's. Stasis eczema over the legs is another differential to be considered for the presence of dermoscopic glomerular vessels.[12,13]

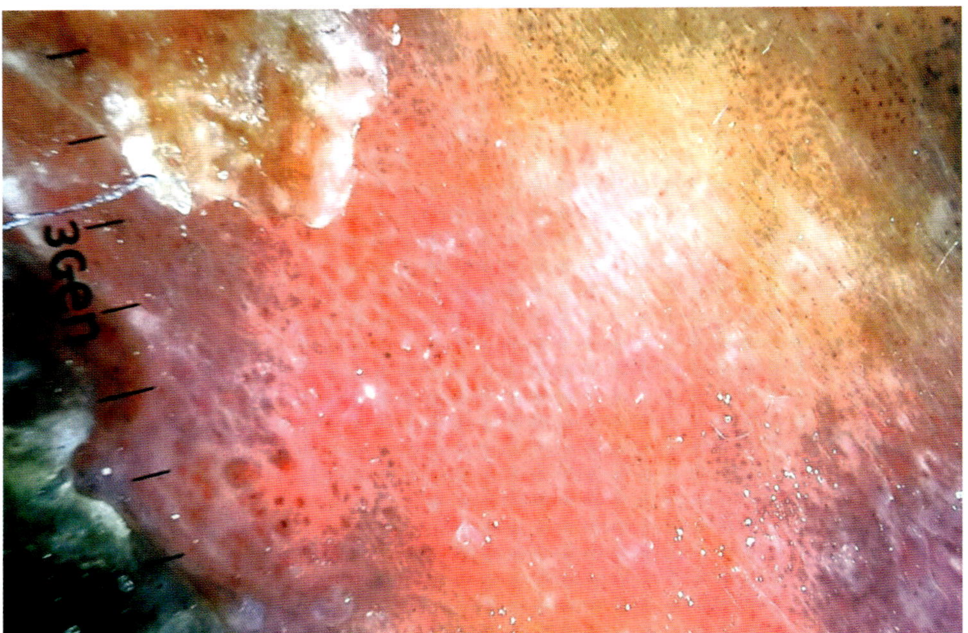

Fig. 11: Glomerular vessels in a clustered distribution.

Corkscrew Vessels

Corkscrew vessels are a dermoscopic indicator of melanoma and more commonly melanoma metastasis. They are helically designed and distributed irregularly throughout the lesion.[14]

Linear Irregular Vessels

Irregularly arranged linear vessels are seen on dermoscopy in premalignant conditions such as actinic keratosis, Bowen's disease and in frankly malignant conditions such as squamous cell carcinoma, melanoma, etc.[2]

Coral Vessels

These vessels loop in a peculiar manner resembling the tentacles of oceanic corals and have been identified in secondary milia (Fig. 12). Stretching of the skin over the surface of secondary milia as a part of the postinflammatory process causes the vessels to branch and loop extensively resulting in a coral pattern (Author's observation).

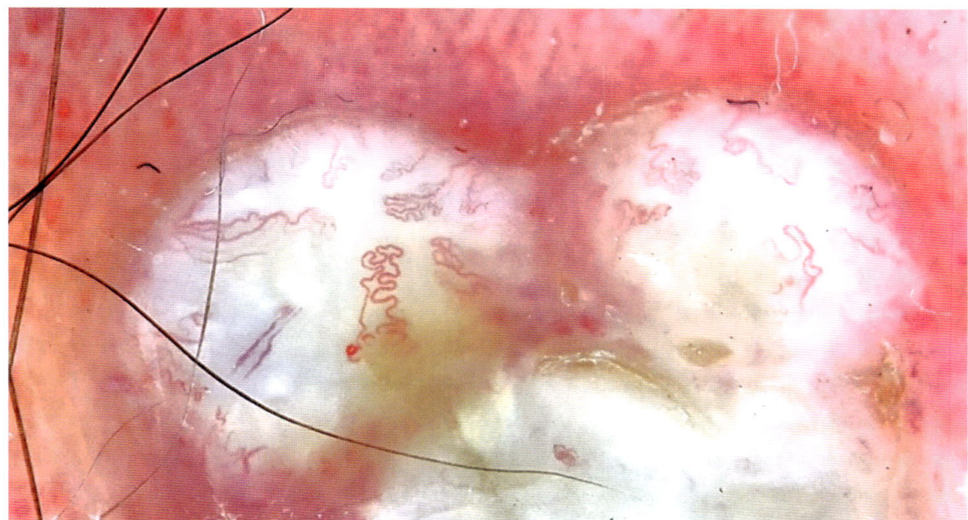

Fig. 12: Coral vessels seen on the surface of secondary milia.

Lacunae

Lacunae are round to oval, well defined, reddish or reddish-blue structures (Fig. 13). They are characteristically seen on dermoscopy in solitary angiokeratomas, hemangiomas, angioma serpiginosum, and lymphangioma circumscripta.[4,15,16] Lacunae correspond to dilated vascular spaces in the superficial dermis on histopathology. They are either singularly placed or arranged in clusters and vary in color depending on the underlying condition.[15] Thrombosed hemangiomas

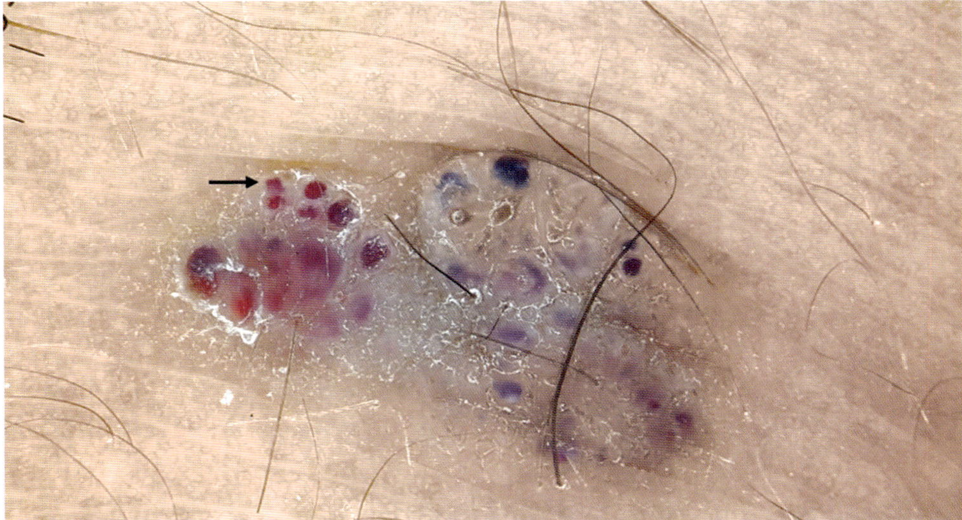

Fig. 13: Well demarcated, round to oval, red to blue lacunae (arrow) in solitary angiokeratoma.

tend to have dark lacunae whereas regressing hemangiomas have a whitish scar like appearance.[4] The lacunae in angioma serpiginosum are bright red in color whereas those in lymphangioma circumscripta are yellow to brown surrounded by a pale septa.[1,16]

Polymorphous Vessels

Polymorphous vessels on dermoscopy indicate that more than one vascular pattern coexists in the same lesion. Vascular polymorphism is not restricted to malignancies but has been documented in adnexal tumors, dermatofibroma, irritated seborrheic keratosis, etc.[1]

Recognition of these vascular patterns on dermoscopy is of utmost importance as they highlight features invisible to the naked eye and thus aid in clinical diagnosis.

REFERENCES

1. Martin JM, Bella-Navarro R, Jordá E. Vascular patters in dermoscopy. Actas Dermosifiliogr. 2012;103:357-75.
2. Zalaudek I, Kreusch J, Giacomel J, et al. How to diagnose nonpigmented skin tumors: a review of vascular structures seen with dermoscopy. Part I. Melanocytic skin tumors. J Am Acad Dermatol. 2010;63:361-74.
3. Argenziano G, Zalaudek I, Corona R, et al. Vascular structures in skin tumors: a dermoscopy study. Arch Dermatol. 2004;140:1485-9.
4. Wolf IH. Dermoscopic diagnosis of vascular lesions. Clin Dermatol. 2002;20:273-5.
5. Micali G, Lacarrubba F, Musumeci ML, et al. Cutaneous vascular patterns in psoriasis. Int J Derm. 2010;49:249-56.
6. Bugatti L, Filosa G, Broganelli P, et al. Psoriasis-like dermoscopic pattern of clear cell acanthoma. J Eur Acad Dermatol Venereol. 2003;17:452-5.
7. Ferrara G, Argenziano G, Soyer HP, et al. The spectrum of Spitz nevi: a clinicopathologic study of 83 cases. Arch Dermatol. 2005;141:1381-7.
8. Menzies SW, Kreusch J, Byth K, et al. Dermoscopic evaluation of amelanotic and hypomelanotic melanoma. Arch Dermatol. 2008;144:1120-7.
9. Zaballos P, Ara M, Puig S, et al. Dermoscopy of sebaceous hyperplasia. Arch Dermatol. 2005;141:808.
10. Zalaudek I, Kreusch J, Giacomel J, et al. How to diagnose nonpigmented skin tumors: a review of vascular structures seen with dermoscopy: Part II. Nonmelanocytic skin tumors. J Am Acad Dermatol. 2010;63:377-86.
11. Menzies SW, Westerhoff K, Rabinovitz H, et al. Surface microscopy of pigmented basal cell carcinoma. Arch Dermatol. 2000;136:1012-6.
12. Zalaudek I, Argenziano G, Leinweber B, et al. Dermoscopy of Bowen's disease. Br J Dermatol. 2004;150:1112-6.
13. Zaballos P, Salsench E, Puig S, et al. Dermoscopy of venous stasis dermatitis. Arch Dermatol. 2006;142:1526.
14. Minagawa A, Koga H, Sakaizawa K, et al. Dermoscopic and histopathological findings of polymorphous vessels in amelanotic cutaneous metastasis of pigmented cutaneous melanoma. Br J Dermatol. 2009;160:1134-6.
15. Zaballos P, Daufi C, Puig S, et al. Dermoscopy of solitary angiokeratoma: a morphological study. Arch Dermatol. 2007;143:318-25.
16. Kalisiak MS, Haber RM. Angioma serpiginosum with linear distribution: case report and review of the literature. J Cutan Med Surg. 2008;12:180-3.

4C. OTHER NOTABLE PATTERNS

Subrata Malakar

WHITE STARBURST PATTERN[1,2]

It has been defined as a dermoscopic finding of radially arranged whitish lines (Fig. 1) on a reddish-brown background in cases of prurigo nodularis (PN). This pattern is a useful clue to distinguish PN from its closed differentials such as hypertrophic lichen planus, nodular scabies, multiple keratoacanthoma, and reactive perforating collagenosis. Moreover, the incidental detection of starburst pattern in regressing lesions is very useful in diagnosing PN retrospectively.

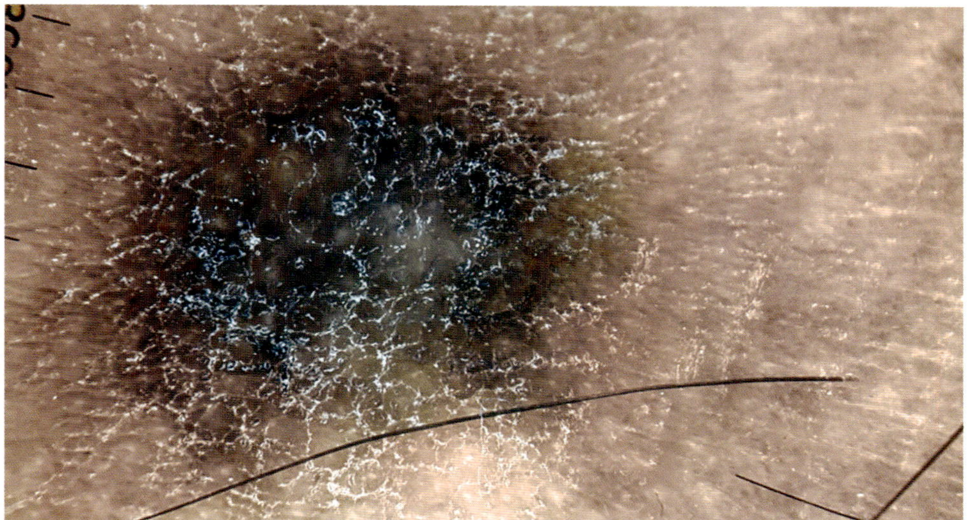

Fig. 1: White starburst pattern in prurigo nodularis on dermoscopy. Note the radially arranged whitish lines.

Dermoscopy: Histopathology Correlation

Radially arranged whitish lines correspond to papillary dermal fibrosis. The thickened collagen fibers are arranged perpendicular to the skin surface in the papillary dermis. When viewed dermoscopically, they appear as whitish lines or projections especially at the periphery.

PALISADE PIGMENTATION PATTERN

Dermoscopically a distinct structure is observed in discoid lupus erythematosus (DLE) characterized by a band of pigmentation surrounding the entire lesion, which resembles a fence of wooden sticks fixed to the ground, forming an enclosure (Figs. 2 and 3). This pigmentation is observed mainly in the late stage of DLE.

Palisade pigmentation represents pigmentary incontinence histopathologically. The incontinence may not involve the entire dermis but is present focally or segmentally due to focal interface vacuolar degeneration of basal layer (Fig. 4). As the pigmentation is present only at the border of the lesion, it is viewed as palisade pigmentation on dermoscopy.

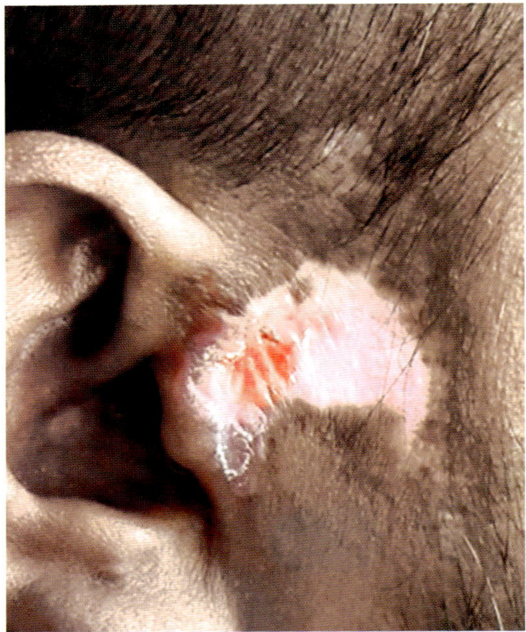

Fig. 2: A case of discoid lupus erythematosus (DLE).

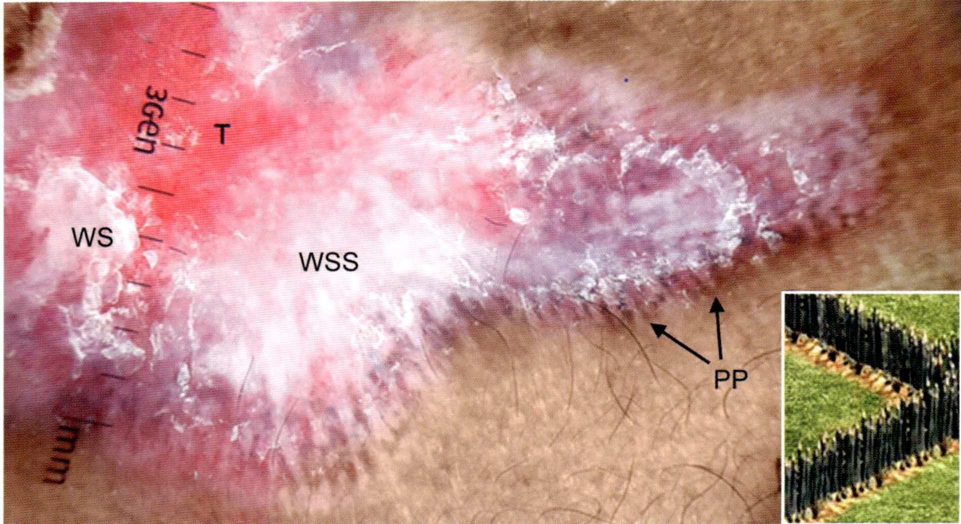

Fig. 3: Palisade pigmentation (PP) in a case of discoid lupus erythematosus (DLE). Note other features of the disease such as white shiny structures (WSS), telangiectasis (T) and scales. Inset shows a picture of palisade arrangement.

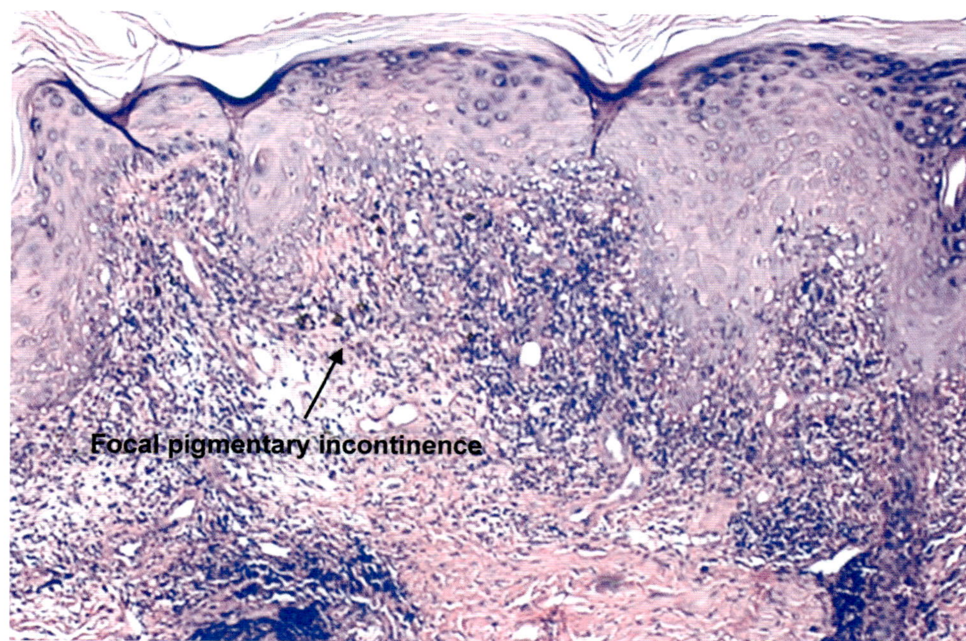

Fig. 4: Focal pigmentary incontinence on histology corresponds to palisade pigmentation on dermoscopy.

BOUQUET OF WHITE ROSES PATTERN

Dermoscopy demonstrates a very characteristic finding in hypertrophic lichen planus showing a conglomeration of white structures resembling a bunch of white roses. The white structures are in a curvilinear arrangement and spiral towards the apex in each of them. Magnification of these structures digitally mimics a bouquet of white roses. This phenomenon corresponds histologically to the hyperkeratosis atop wedge-shaped hypergranulosis enclosed within the hyperplastic appendages.[3]

"Corn pearls" have been described in hypertrophic lichen planus along with rippled surface, comedo-like structures with keratin plugs.[4] The corn pearls increase in number as the lesions become more hypertrophic. As more number of corn pearls hypertrophy, they conglomerate to form "bouquet of white roses" (Figs. 5A to F).

Hence, a new dermoscopic metaphor, "bouquet of white roses" is being proposed for hypertrophic lichen planus. This sign will not be seen in other forms of lichen planus as the degree of hyperkeratosis essential to produce a conglomeration of such structures is absent. The hyperkeratosis in hypertrophic lichen planus lies atop follicular or acrosyringeal openings and this is not the scenario in PN and lichen simplex chronicus.[5] Hence, the hyperkeratosis with underlying wedge-shaped hypergranulosis centered atop hyperplastic appendages in hypertrophic lichen planus produces the "bouquet of white roses" on dermoscopy and this sign is absent in other hypertrophic conditions.

ROAD TO BOUQUET OF WHITE ROSES

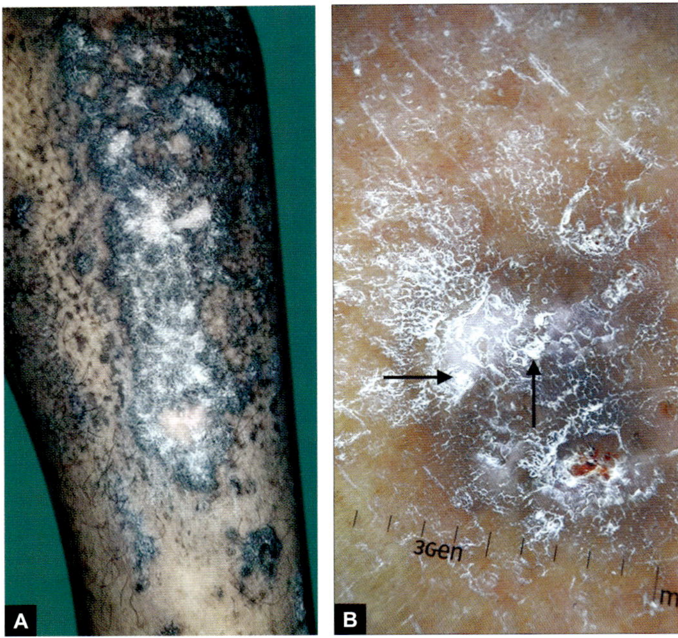

Figs. 5A and B: (A) Clinical picture of hypertrophic lichen planus; (B) A few corn pearls (arrows).

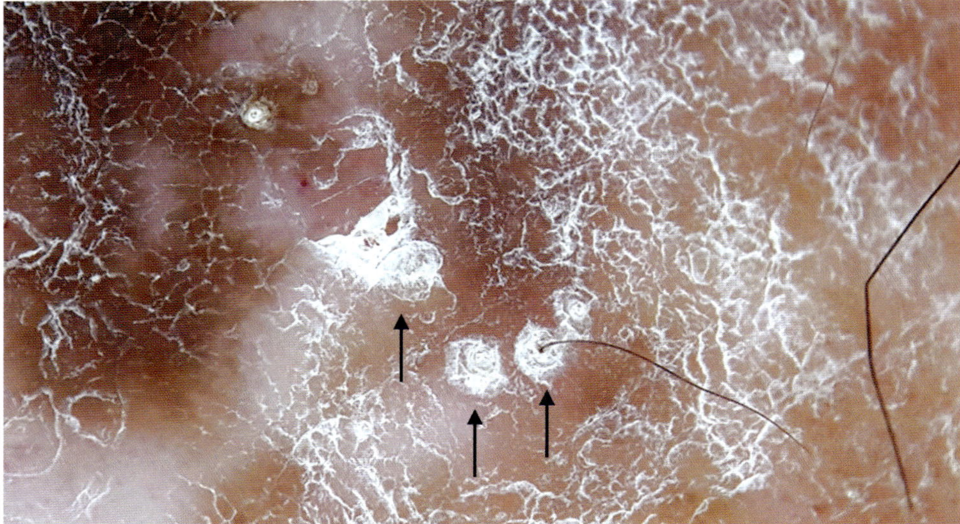

Fig. 5C: Corn pearls increasing in number (arrows).

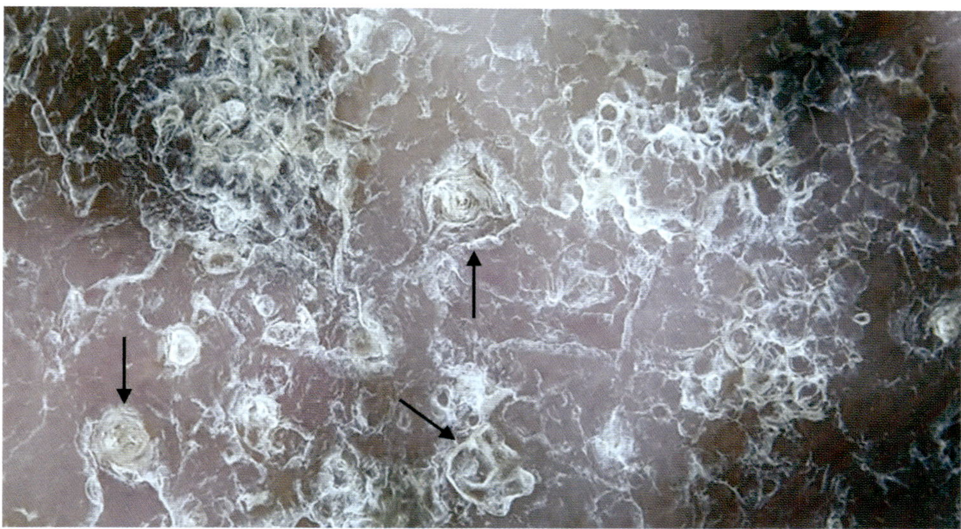

Fig. 5D: Corn pearls increasing in number and beginning to hypertrophy (arrows).

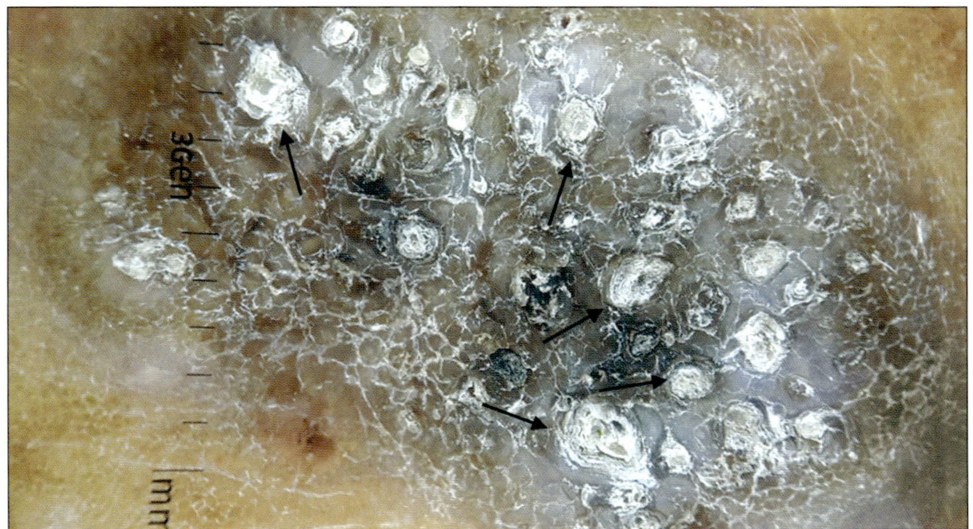

Fig. 5E: Hypertrophied corn pearls beginning to aggregate (arrows).

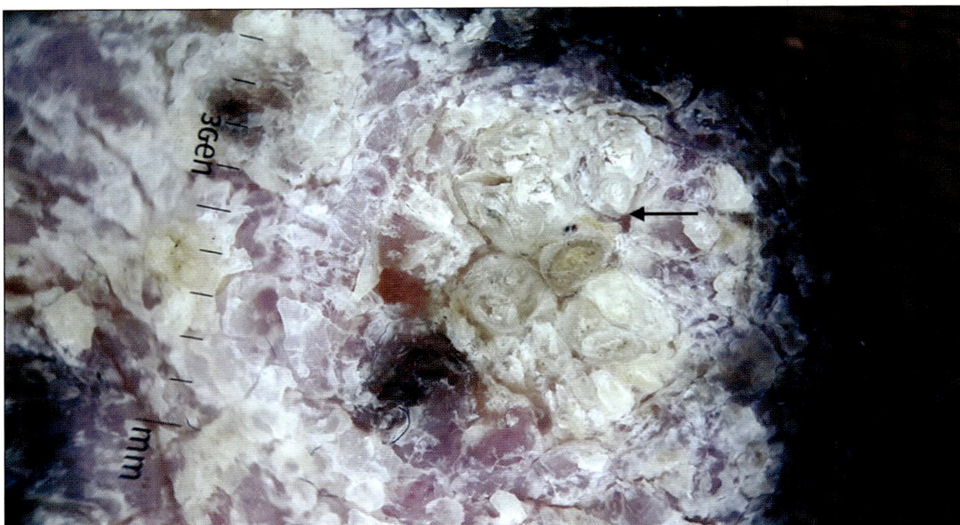

Fig. 5F: Conglomeration of corn pearls to form a "bouquet of white roses" (arrow).

RED STARBURST PATTERN

In some long-standing cases of DLE, dermoscopy reveals radially arranged red lines on an erythematous background that appear as red starburst and "red starburst pattern" has been coined for this pattern. Few pigment dots and globules may also be interwoven with the radial red lines (Fig. 6).

Long-standing cases of DLE histopathologically show telangiectasia, pigmentation changes and diffuse dermal fibrosis.[6] All these features combine to represent red starburst pattern.

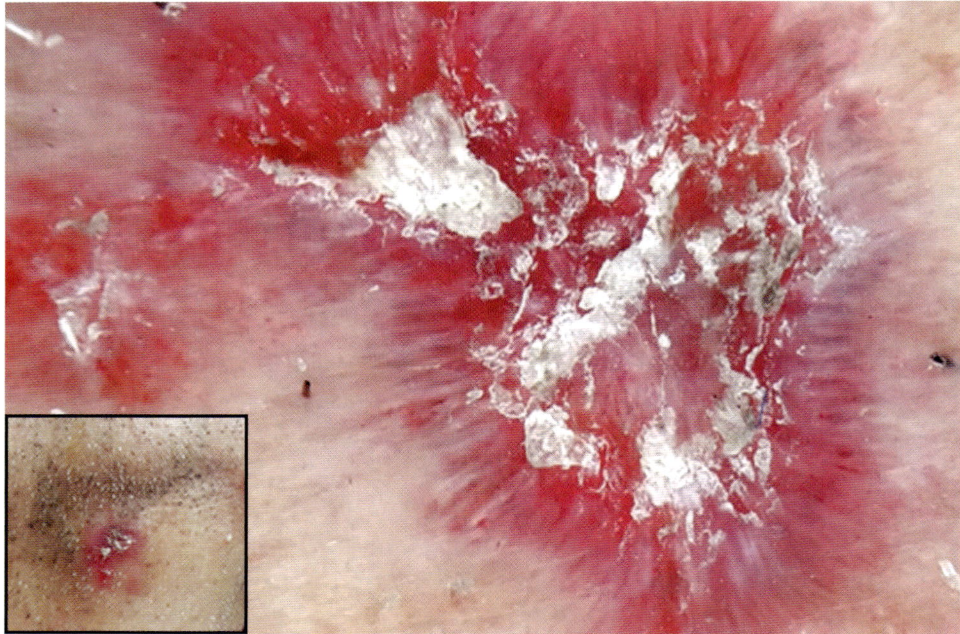

Fig. 6: Dermoscopy reveals a new pattern, the "red starburst pattern". Telangiectasia is usually a late feature of discoid lupus erythematosus (DLE). The combination of telangiectasias, epidermal hyperplasia and diffuse dermal fibrosis may be the cause of this red starburst pattern. Thick white scales and follicular plugging are also evident in this dermoscopic field.

CLOUDY SKY PATTERN[7]

This pattern is classically described in syringomas. Dermoscopy of them reveal homogeneous or and ivory white areas, which is akin to cloudy sky, that is the reason for this metaphoric term "cloudy sky" pattern (Figs. 7 and 8). The homogeneous white areas can be histologically correlated with the fibrous and sclerotic stroma around the eccrine ducts, the origin of the syringomas (Fig. 9).

Similarly in juvenile xanthogranuloma yellow orange clouds are noted more commonly in comparison to the classically described setting sun appearance in the skin of color.

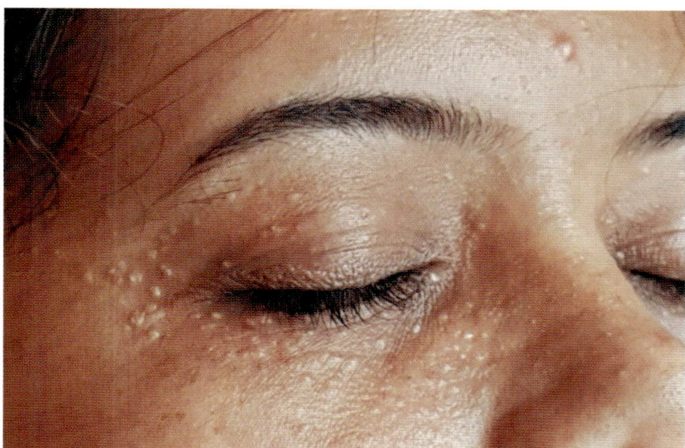
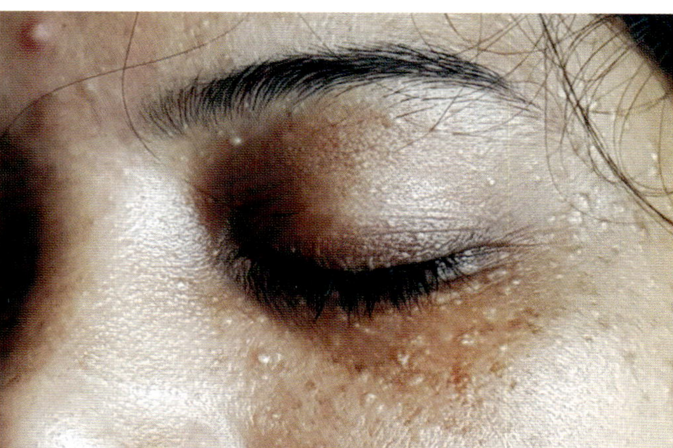

Fig. 7: Syringomas

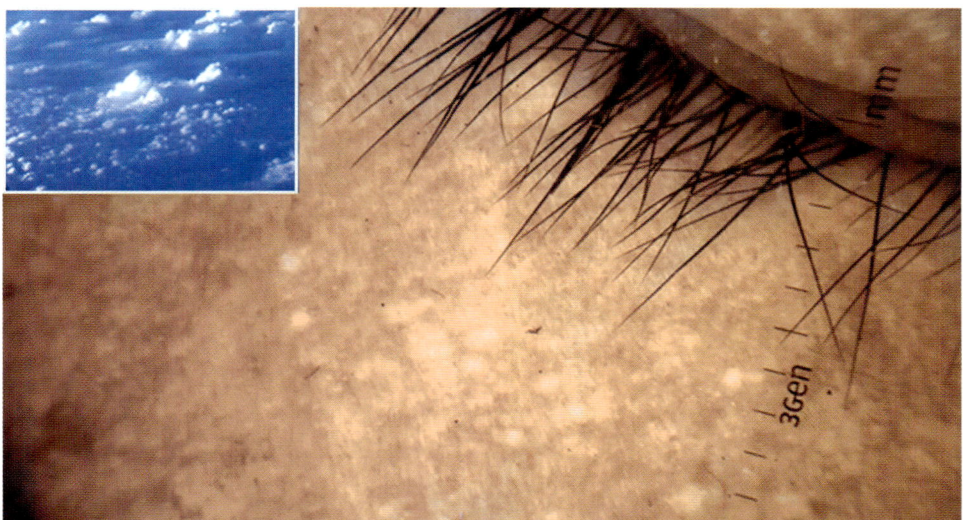

Fig. 8: Dermoscopy of syringoma showing cloudy sky pattern

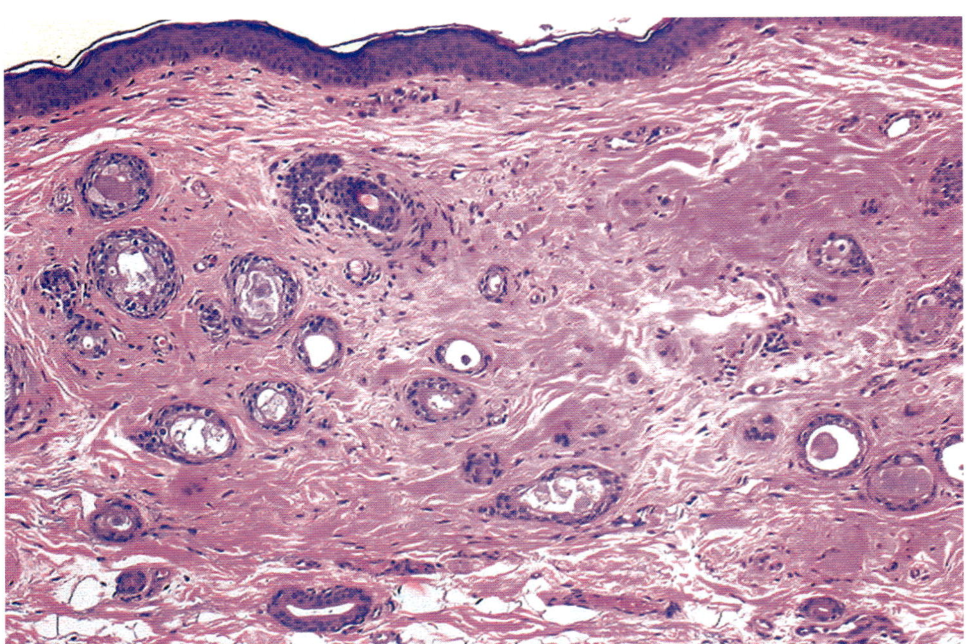

Fig. 9: Histopathology demonstrates numerous small ducts in a sclerotic stroma. Note the tadpole shaped ducts. Usually the walls of these ducts are lined by two rows of cuboidal epithelial cells.

REFERENCES

1. Errichetti E, Piccirillo A, Stinco G. Dermoscopy of prurigo nodularis. J Dermatol. 2015;42:1-3.
2. Ankad BS, Beergouder SL. Hypertrophic lichen planus versus prurigo nodularis: a dermoscopic perspective. Dermatol Pract Concept. 2016;6:9-15.
3. Vázquez-López F, Manjón-Haces JA, Maldonado-Seral C, et al. Dermoscopic features of plaque psoriasis and lichen planus: new observations. Dermatology. 2003;207:151-6.
4. Lallas A, Giacomel J, Argenziano G, et al. Dermoscopy in general dermatology: practical tips for the clinician. Br J Dermatol. 2014;170:514-26.
5. Weedon D. The lichenoid reaction pattern (interface dermatitis). In: Weedon D (Ed). Weedon's Skin Pathology, 2nd edition. London: Churchill Livingstone; 2002. pp. 31-74.
6. McKee P, Calonje E, Granter S. Idiopathic connective tissue disorders. In: McKee P (Ed). Pathology of the Skin with Clinical Correlations, 3rd edition. Amsterdam: Elsevier Mosby; 2005. pp. 775-803.
7. Rodríguez SS, Ciancio RM, Cabo H. Dermoscopic study of periorbital syringoma. Med Cutan Iber Lat Am. 2015;43(2):132-5.

CHAPTER 5

Dermoscopic Dialogues

Subrata Malakar, Shruti Kulkarni

ARBORIZING VESSELS: SCHEMATIC

Dermoscopic description: They are large caliber vessels (diameter 0.2 mm or more) and branch into finer secondary vessels that are similar in appearance to the branches of a tree.[1] These vessels are sharply in focus due to their superficial location in the upper dermis. Histologically they represent dilated arterial circulation (Figs. 1 to 4).[2,3]

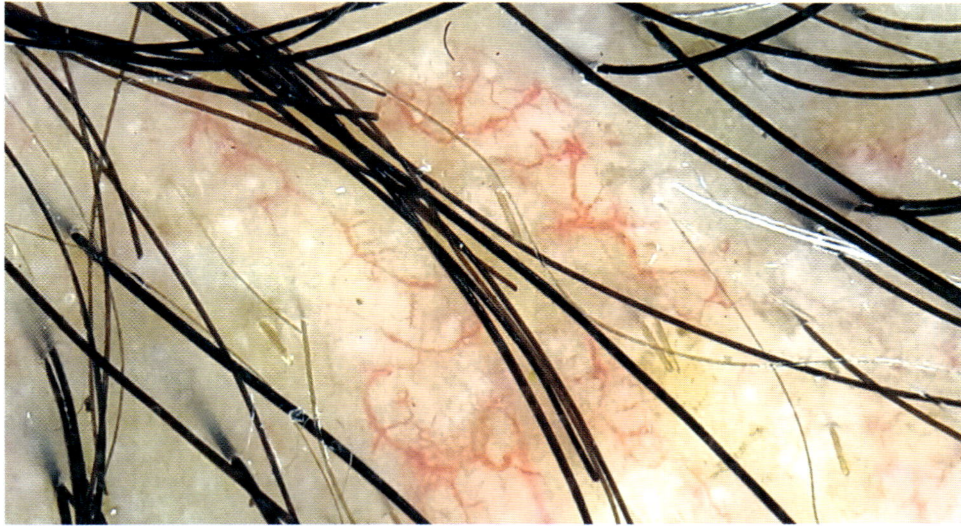

Fig. 1: A few arborizing vessels (ARV) may be found in healthy individual on scalp.

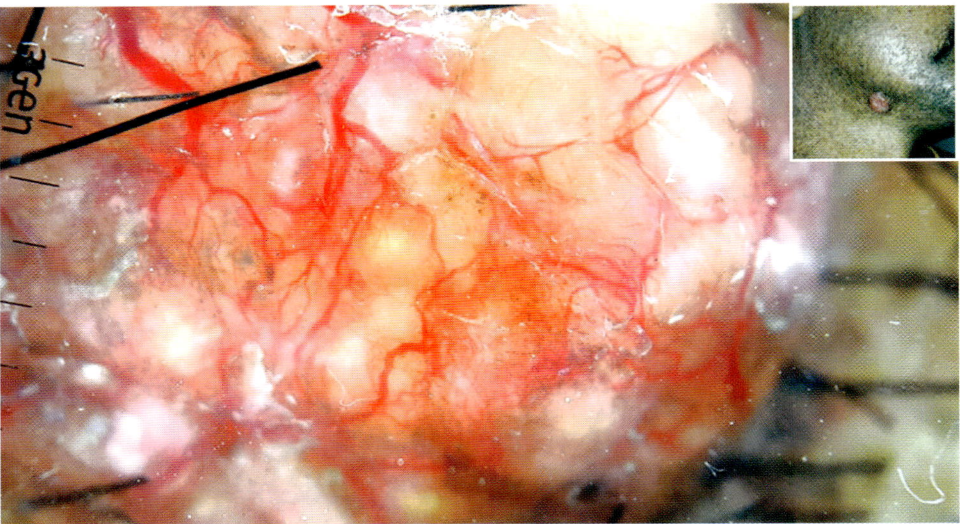

Fig. 2: Arborizing vessels (ARV) are present in more than 80% basal cell carcinomas where its positive predictive value is 94%.

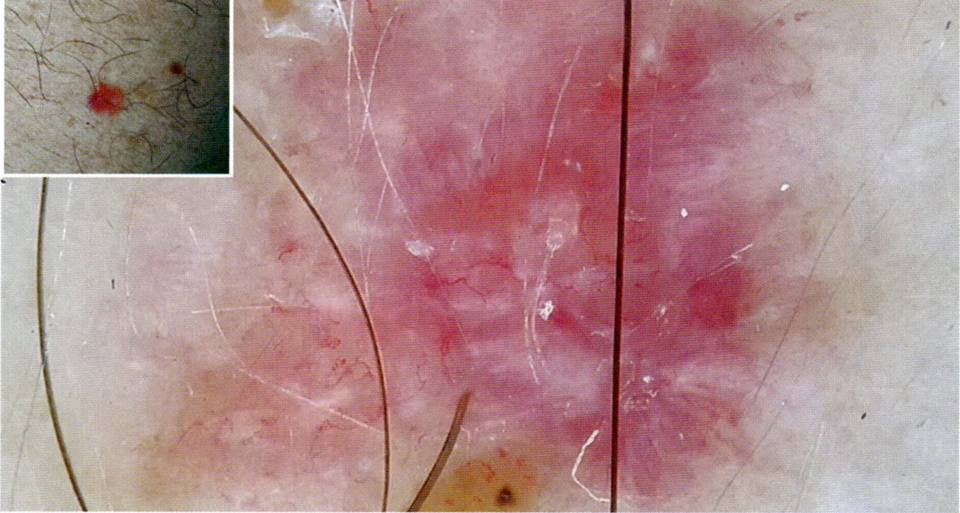

Fig. 3: In non-pigmented basal cell carcinoma arborizing vessels (ARV) are the hallmark for diagnosing the condition.

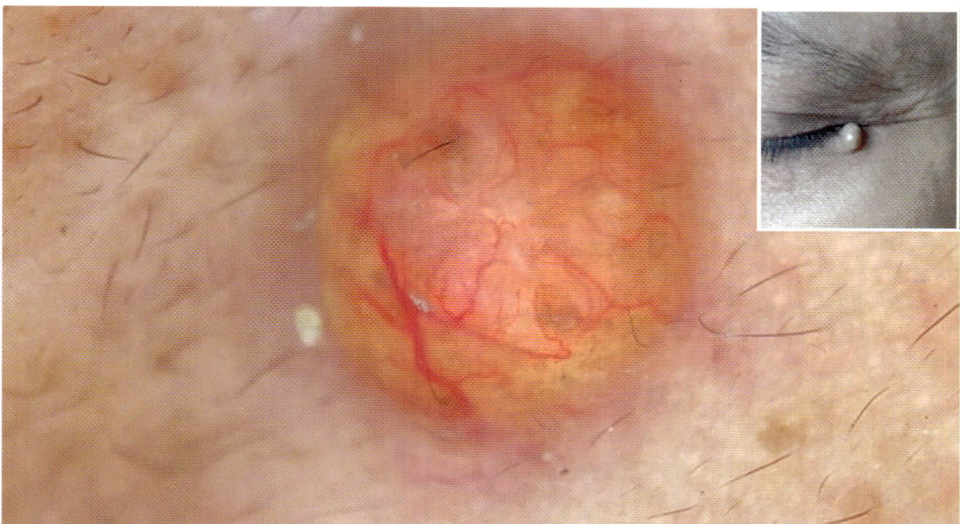

Fig. 4: Arborizing vessels (ARV) can sometimes be seen in milia.[3]

REFERENCES

1. Argenziano G, Zalaudek I, Corona R, et al. Vascular structures in skin tumors: a dermoscopy study. Arch Dermatol. 2004;140:1485-9.
2. Soyer HP, Argenziano G, Hoffmann-Wellenhoff R, et al. Pattern analysis. In: Dermoscopy: The Essentials, 2nd edition. United Kingdom: Elsevier/Saunders; 2012. p. 107.
3. Malakar S, Mukherjee SS. Vascular pattern of milia on dermatoscopy. Our Dermatol Online. 2017;8:497-8.

BLOTCHES

Blotches refer to various shades of diffuse hyperpigmentation that obscure the ability to appreciate other dermoscopic features, such as melanocytic network, dots, etc.[1] Histopathologically, blotches are characterized by conspicuous melanin pigmentation throughout the epidermis and dermis.

The blotches, which are homogeneously brown or dark, located in the center of the lesion and have regular borders are designated as regular blotches (Fig. 5). They are suggestive of benign lesions. Whereas those blotches, which are located off-center, have heterogeneous dark hues with irregular borders are termed irregular blotches.[2] These blotches favor the diagnosis of malignant lesions.

Pseudoblotch[3] refers to a blotch-like structure that is observed in an activated nevi and is due to pronounced concentration of melanin in the stratum corneum. The black blotch correlates histopathologically to pigmented parakeratosis of an otherwise conventional junctional nevus. This pigment can easily be stripped off using tape-stripping procedure, which allows the recognition of the underlying regular network.

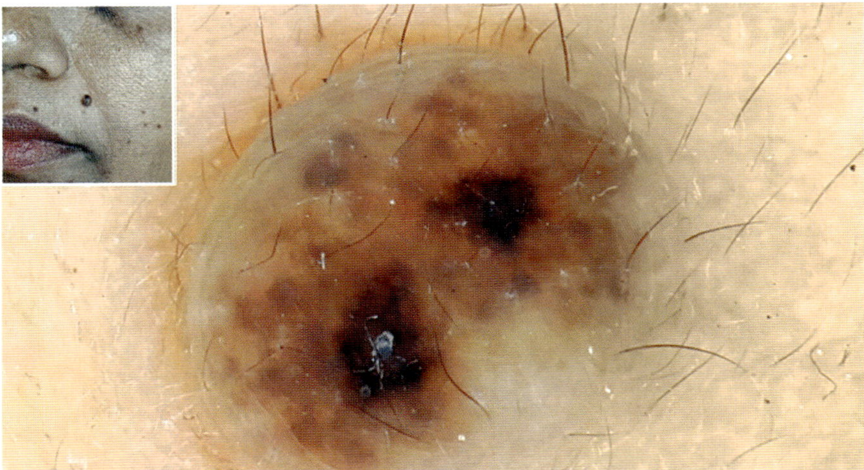

Fig. 5: Blotches that are homogeneously brown or dark, located in the center of the lesion and have regular borders are designated as regular blotches. They are suggestive of benign lesions.

REFERENCES

1. Soyer HP, Argenziano G, Hoffmann-Wellenhoff R, et al. Pattern analysis. In: Dermoscopy: The Essentials, 2nd edition. United Kingdom: Elsevier/Saunders; 2012. p. 107.
2. Argenziano G, Fabbrocini G, Carli P, et al. Epiluminescence microscopy for the diagnosis of doubtful melanocytic skin lesions. Comparision of the ABCD rule of dermatoscopy and a new 7-point checklist based on pattern analysis. Arch Dermatol. 1998;134:1563-70.
3. Guillod JF, Skaria AM, Salomon D, et al. Epiluminescence videodermoscopy: black dots and brown globules revisited by stripping the stratum corneum. J Am Acad Dermatol. 1997;36:371-7.

BLUE-GRAY BLOTCHES (BLUE-GRAY OVOID NESTS)

- *Dermoscopic description*: They are pigmented round to oval areas and are larger than globules.
- Histopathologically, they represent heavily pigmented aggregates of basaloid cells in the papillary dermis.[1]
- These blotches are highly suggestive of pigmented basal cell carcinoma especially in the absence of melanocytic network (Fig. 6).[1]

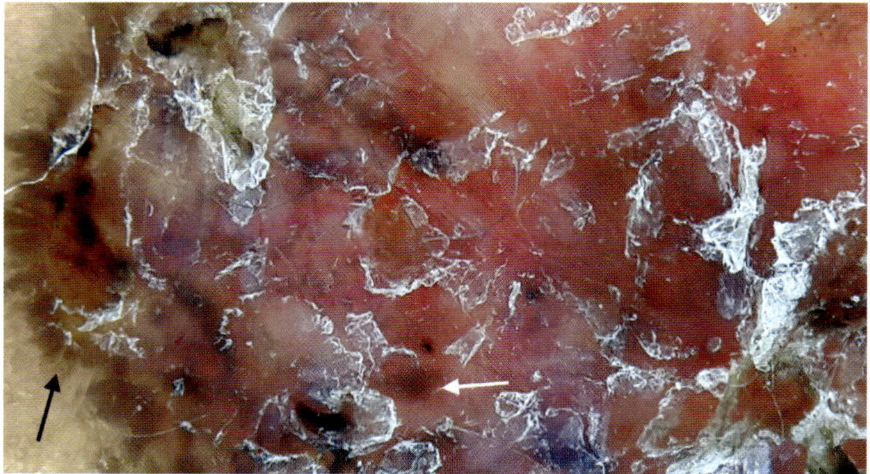

Fig. 6: Blue-gray blotches (white arrow) signify it to be a case of basal cell carcinoma. Note the leaf-like pattern (black arrow).

REFERENCE

1. Menzies SW. Dermoscopy of pigmented basal cell carcinoma. Clin Dermatol. 2002;20:268-9.

BLUE-WHITE VEIL

- *Dermoscopic description*: It is confluent blue-white pigmentation with an overlying translucent ground-glass appearance.[1]
- Histopathologically, it represents compact orthokeratosis and acanthosis overlying a densely pigmented area such as an agglomeration of melanin-laden melanocytes or melanophages in the upper dermis.[2]
- Blue-white areas should be differentiated from regression structures because both the conditions show blue-white color by dermoscopy. Clinically, the surface will be palpable in blue-white veil whereas the surface is flat in regression structures.[3]
- In melanoma, the blue-white veil is present focally in an ill-defined area. Conversely, it occupies the entire surface and has a uniform color in blue nevus (Figs. 7 and 8).

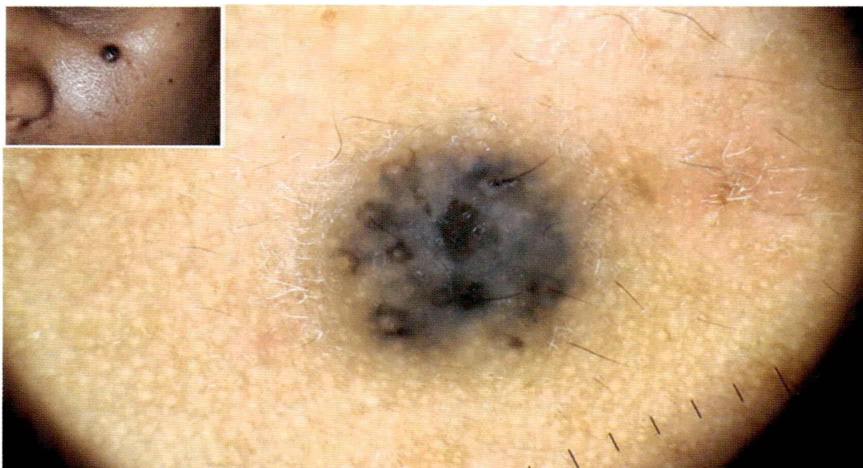

Fig. 7: Blue-white veil is defined as confluent blue pigmentation with an overlying white ground glass haze. In nevi, it is homogeneous with a light hue and is located toward the center of the lesion.

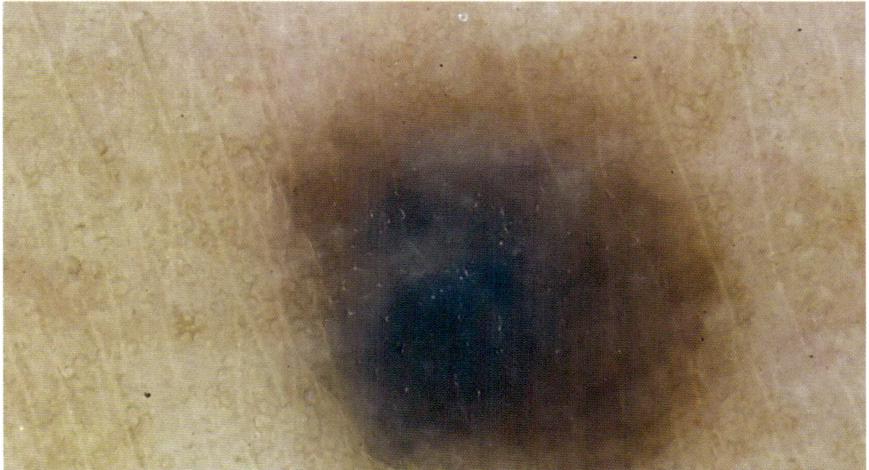

Fig. 8: A central blue-white veil is usually found in benign nevus.

REFERENCES

1. Menzies SW, Crotty KA, Ingvar C, et al. An Atlas of Surface Microscopy of Pigmented Skin Lesions. Sydney: McGraw-Hill Book Company; 2003.
2. Yadav S, Vossaert KA, Kopf AW, et al. Histopathologic correlates of structures seen on dermoscopy (epiluminescence microscopy). Am J Dermatopathol. 1993;15:297-305.
3. Braun RP, Scope A, Marghoob AA, et al. Histopathologic tissue correlations of dermoscopic structures. In: Marghoob AA, Malvehy J, Braun RP (Eds). Atlas of Dermoscopy, 2nd edition. London: Informa Healthcare; 2012. pp. 10-32.

CEREBRIFORM PATTERN (BRAIN-LIKE APPEARANCE)[1,2]

- *Dermoscopic description*: This pattern appears as multiple fissures and ridges, which resemble the sulci and gyri of the brain. Sulci and gyri are thick digitate, linear, and curvilinear branched structures. During evolution, they are seen as oval or round structures.
  - Cerebriform pattern is most commonly observed in seborrheic keratosis and may even be the only finding. Rarely, it may be seen in dermal nevi.
  - Histopathologically, the fissures correlate to wedge-shaped invaginations of the epidermis filled with keratin (Figs. 9 and 10).

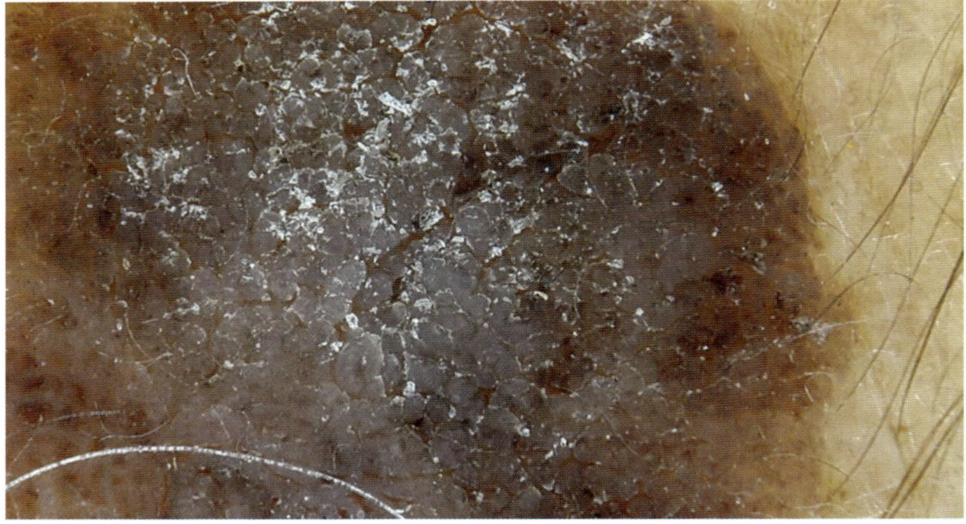

Fig. 9: Multiple fissures (sulci) and ridges (gyri) produce a cereberiform pattern where the structures mimic sulci and gyri of the brain.

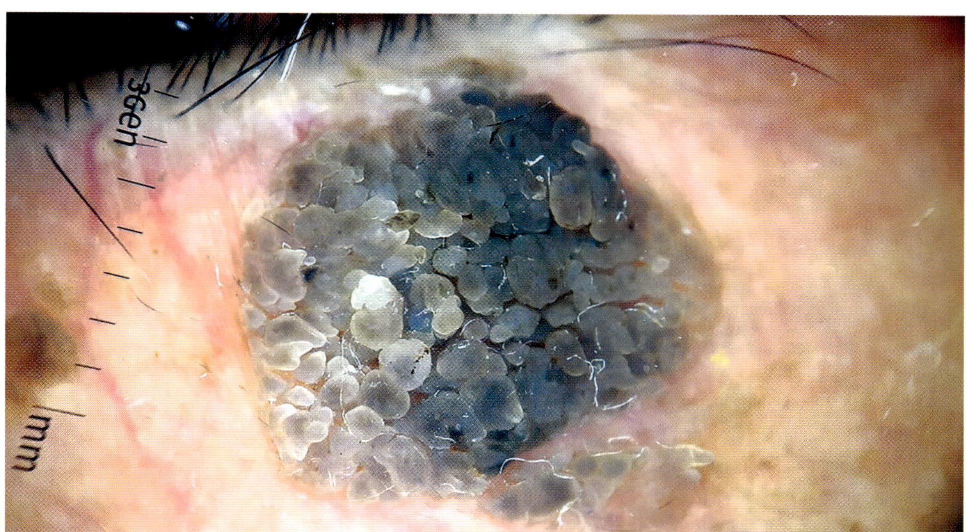

Fig. 10: The cerebriform pattern is created by the ridges and sulci.

REFERENCES

1. Wang SQ, Marghoob AA, Rabinovitz HS, et al. Solar lentigines, seborrheic keratosis and lichen planus-like keratosis. In: Marghoob AA, Malvehy J, Braun RP (Eds). Atlas of Dermoscopy, 2nd edition. London: Informa Healthcare; 2012. pp. 58-69.
2. Braun RP, Rabinovitz H, Krischer J, et al. Dermoscopy of pigmented seborrheic keratosis. Arch Dermatol. 2002;138:1556-60.

CHRYSALIS STRUCTURES (CRYSTALLINE STRUCTURES)

- *Dermoscopic description*: They are shiny white streaks seen under polarizing devices. Nonpolarized dermoscopes fail to demonstrate this phenomenon.[1] They are observed in tumors with a dermal component such as dermatofibroma, basal cell carcinoma, Spitz nevus, and melanoma. Chrysalis structures can also be found in scars (Fig. 11).
- Histopathologically, they represent altered collagen in the dermis. Collagen appears shiny white due to its rapid randomization of polarized light.

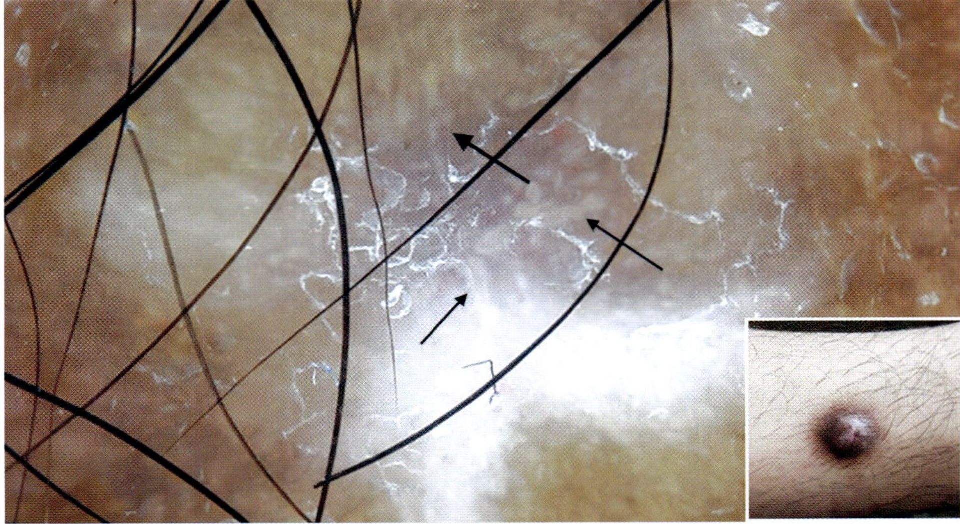

Fig. 11: White chrysalis structure in dermatofibroma (arrows). They are oriented parallel or sometimes orthogonal.

REFERENCE

1. Marghoob AA, Cowell L, Kopf AW, et al. Observation of chrysalis structures with polarized dermoscopy. Arch Dermatol. 2009;145:168.

COBBLESTONE PATTERN[1]

- *Dermoscopic description*: It appears as closely aggregated angulated brown globules resembling cobblestones. It is considered to be a variation of globular pattern. Both globules and cobblestones may be seen within the same lesion dermoscopically. Cobblestone pattern is observed in dermal melanocytic nevi (Fig. 12).
- Histopathologically, cobblestone morphology represents large dermal nests of melanocytes.

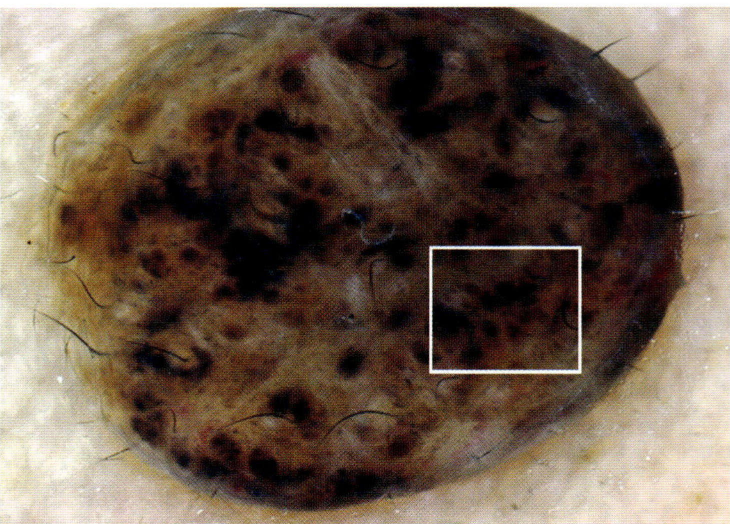

Fig. 12: Dermoscopy of this melanocytic nevus showing cobblestone morphology (appears as angulated circles). On histology, cobblestoning reflects large dermal nests of melanocytes.

REFERENCE

1. Bowling J. Regression in melanoma. In: Diagnostic Dermoscopy: The Illustrated Guide, 2nd edition. United States: Wiley-Blackwell; 2012. p. 19.

COMEDO-LIKE OPENINGS[1,2]

- *Dermoscopic description*: Dermoscopically they appear as round to ovoid dark brown structures resembling comedo-like openings. These structures are usually seen in seborrheic keratosis (SK). Rarely, they are observed in melanocytic nevus with a congenital pattern (Fig. 13).[2]
- Histopathologically, they correspond to keratin plugs within dilated follicular openings.

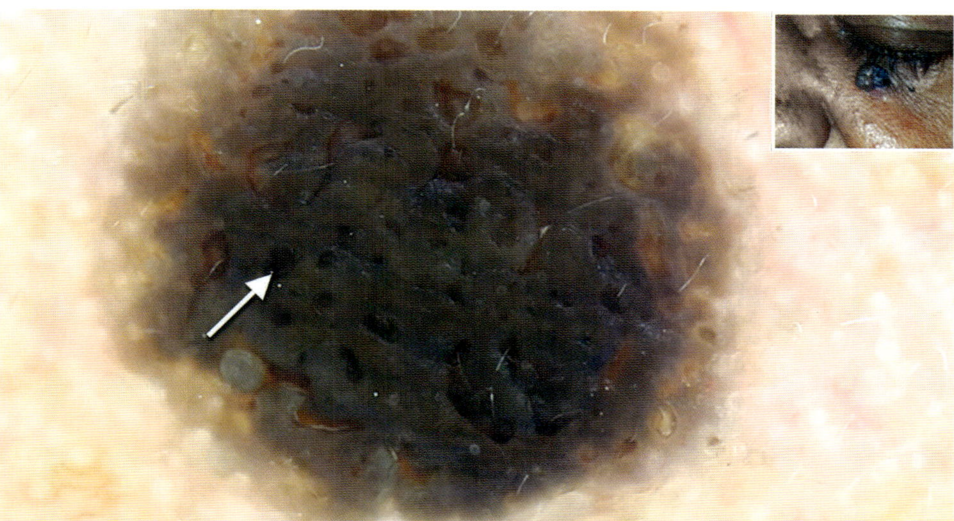

Fig. 13: Comedo-like openings (CLOs) (arrow) in a case of seborrheic keratosis. CLOs are round to ovoid craters that have black or brown comedo-like plugs.

REFERENCES

1. Braun RP, Rabinovitz H, Krischer J et al. Dermoscopy of pigmented seborrheic keratosis. Arch Dermatol 2002;138:1556-60.
2. Wang SQ, Marghoob AA, Rabinovitz HS, et al. Solar lentigines, seborrheic keratosis and lichen planus-like keratosis. In: Marghoob AA, Malvehy J, Braun RP (Eds). Atlas of Dermoscopy, 2nd edition. London: Informa Healthcare; 2012. pp. 58-69.

COMMA VESSELS[1-3]

- *Dermoscopic description*: They are thick, curved red lines with little branching; not uncommonly one end is thicker than the other appearing to take the shape of a "comma". The vessels may have a deeper location in the dermis and consequently appear slightly off-focus.
- They are found most commonly in dermal nevi and compound nevi (Fig. 14).

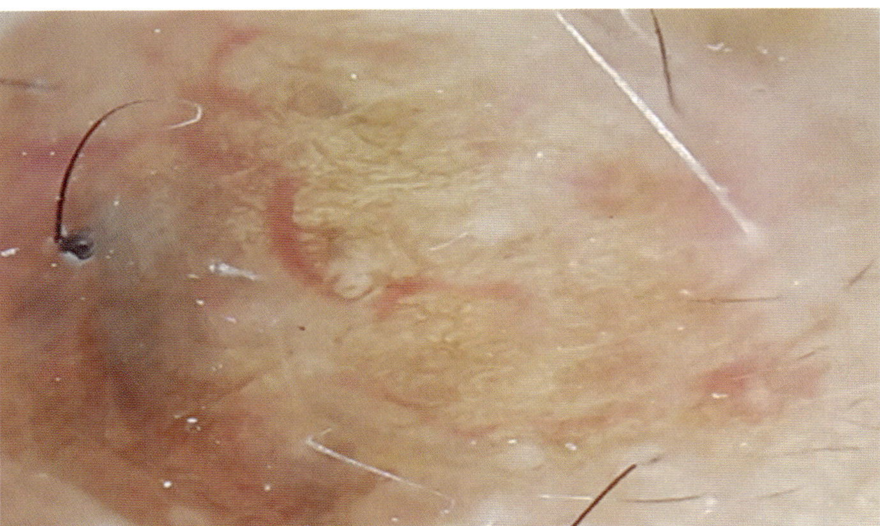

Fig. 14: Comma vessels in a case of compound melanocytic nevus. Comma vessles are highly suggestive of benign nevi; dermal nevi, most commonly followed by compound nevi.

REFERENCES

1. Marghoob AA, Liebman TN. Vascular structures. In: Marghoob AA, Malvehy J, Braun RP (Eds). Atlas of Dermoscopy, 2nd edition. London: Informs Healthcare; 2012. pp. 337-50.
2. Braun RP, Oliviero M, Kolm I, et al. Dermoscopy: what's new? Clin Dermatol. 2009;27:26-34.
3. Martin JM, Bella-Navarro R, Jordá E. Vascular patterns in dermoscopy. Actas Dermosifiliogr. 2012;103:357-75.

CROWN VESSELS[1]

- They are minimally branching peripheral vessels extending toward the center of the lesion without crossing it. This arrangement of the vessels gives the appearance of a "crown", justifying the name crown vessels.
- They are found in sebaceous hyperplasia and molluscum contagiosum (Figs. 15 to 17).

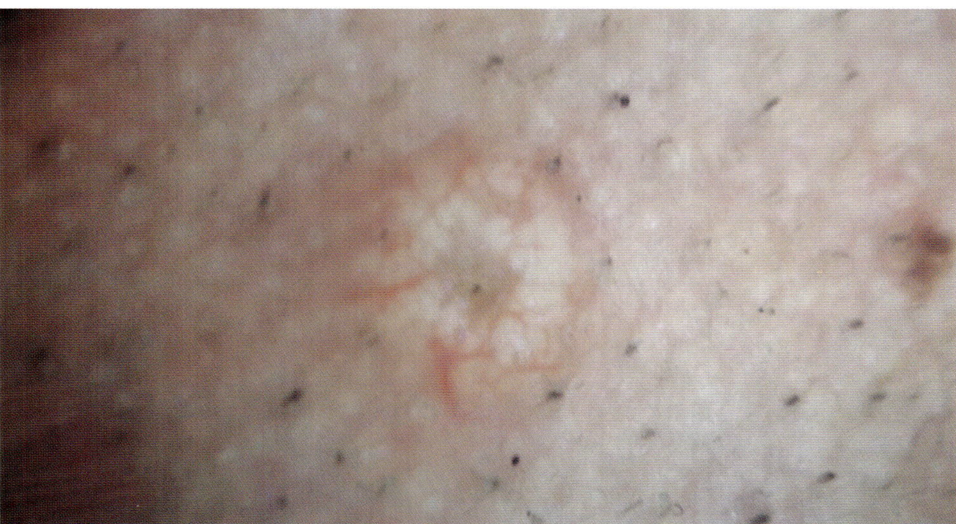

Fig. 15: Typical crown vessels at the periphery of the sebaceous gland that do not crosses the central crater of the gland.

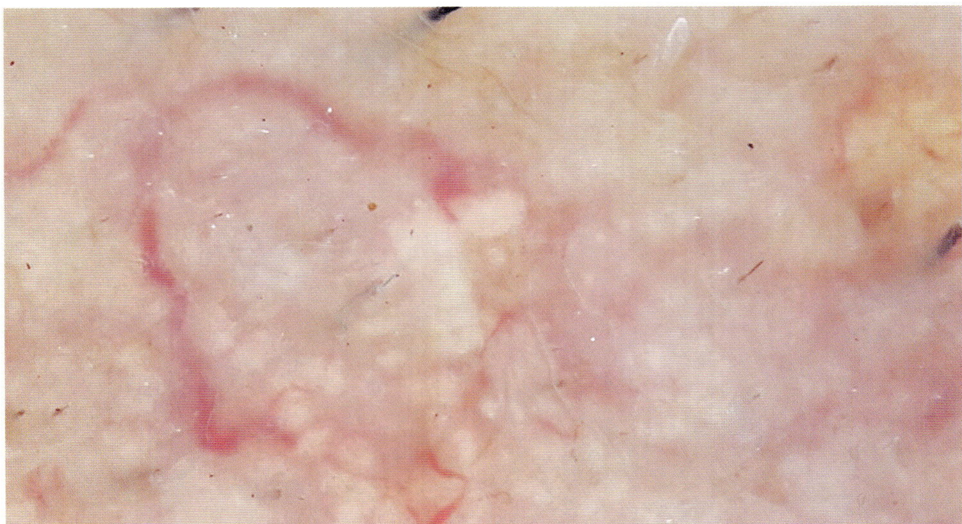

Fig. 16: Crown vessels are very prominent which rarely branch and do not cross the center of the sebaceous gland.

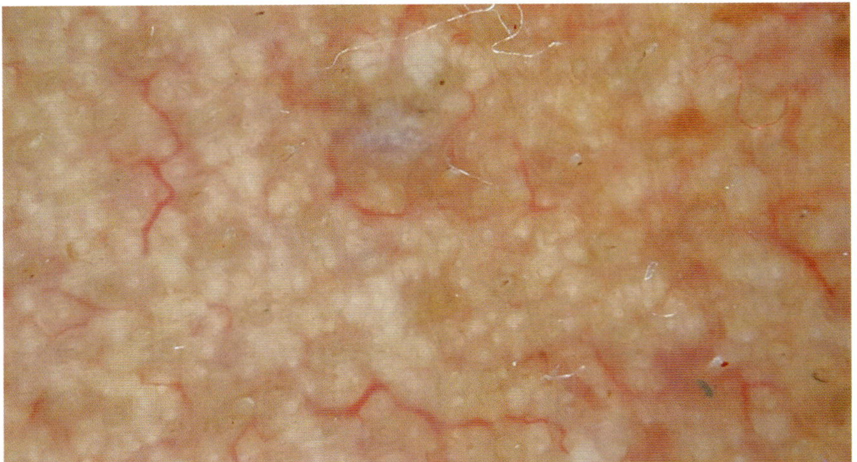

Fig. 17: Multiple sebaceous glands are seen in this field with crown vessels at the periphery of all the sebaceous glands.

REFERENCE

1. Martin JM, Bella-Navarro R, Jordá E. Vascularizacion en dermatoscopia. Actas Dermosifiliogr. 2012;103:357-75.

DOTS

- Dots are tiny round structures of less than 0.1 mm in diameter, their color ranging from black to brown to blue-gray according to the depth and concentration of melanin in the skin.[1]
- Black dots represent melanin in the stratum corneum or in the upper parts of the epidermis.
- Brown dots represent focal accumulations of melanin in the stratum spinosum or dermoepidermal junction. Histopathologically they correspond to junctional nests of melanocytes.
- Histologically when nests of nevus are located at the tips of the rete ridges, the dots are found over the network lines.[2] Whereas if the dots are situated within the holes of the network, the nevus nests are found to be in the papillary dermis.
- Gray-blue dots or peppering are seen when melanin is present in the superficial dermis. Melanin may be present either within the melanophages or as extracellular dust. Peppering or gray-blue dots are found to be associated with regression structures (Fig. 18).[3]

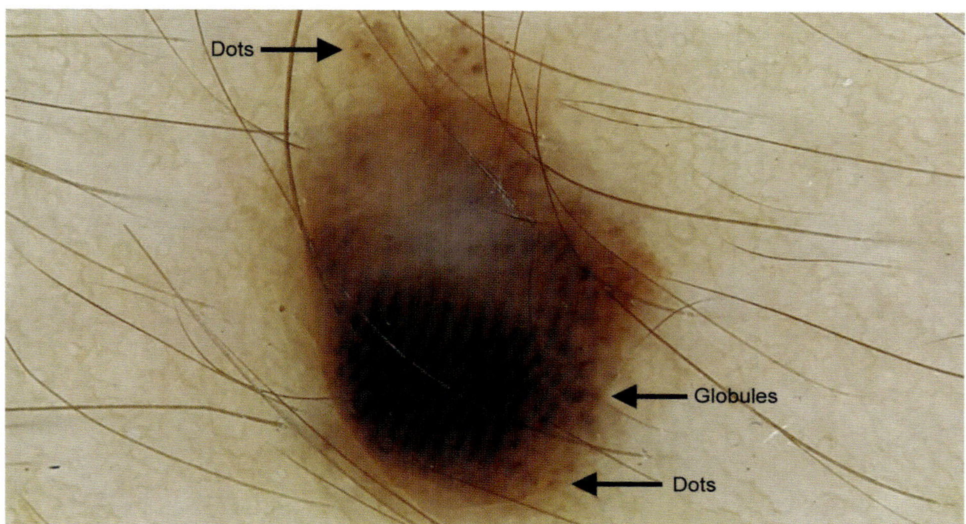

Fig. 18: As dots and globules are frequently seen together in a lesion, it is better to call them together as "dots and globules".

REFERENCES

1. Menzies SW, Crotty KA, Ingvar C, et al. Dermoscopy an Atlas. Sydney: McGraw-Hill; 2009.
2. Puppin D Jr, Salomon D, Saurat JH. Amplified surface microscopy. Preliminary evaluation of a 400-fold magnification in the surface microscopy of cutaneous melanocytic lesions. J Am Acad Dermatol. 1993;28:923-7.
3. Braun RP, Gaide O, Oliviero M, et al. The significance of multiple blue-grey dots (granularity) for the dermoscopic diagnosis of melanoma. Br J Dermatol. 2007;157:907-13.

DOTTED VESSELS[1]

- They are seen as tiny red dots of diameter 0.01–0.02 mm, which correspond histologically to the tips of perpendicular vessels in the papillary dermis.
- Dotted vessels are found both in the melanocytic and non-melanocytic lesions (Fig. 19).
- Among the melanocytic conditions, dotted vessels are observed in melanoma, dermal/congenital nevi, Clark's nevi, and Spitz nevi. In benign nevi, dotted vessels represent vessels at the tips of papillary dermis, thus on dermoscopy they are seen within the holes of the melanocytic network. In melanoma, dotted vessels are found along with the other vessel types, and they usually occupy the center of the lesion.
- Among the non-melanocytic lesions, dotted vessels are usually found in psoriasis, squamous cell carcinoma and clear cell acanthoma. Dotted vessels in psoriasis are uniform in size and are distributed regularly. In clear cell acanthoma, dotted vessels are arranged in a characteristic “string of pearls” fashion. In squamous cell carcinoma, dotted vessels are present focally along with adherent scales (Fig. 20).

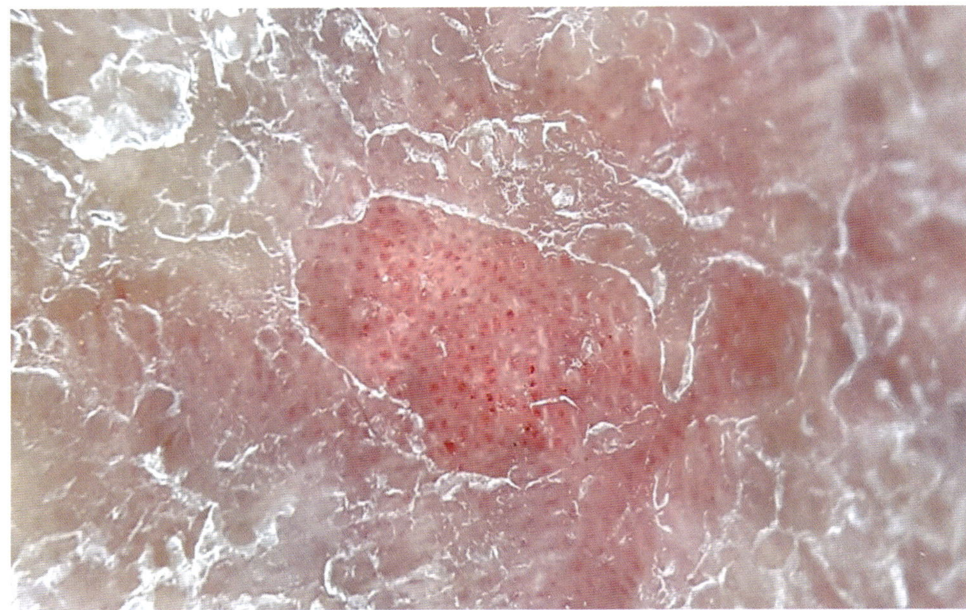

Fig. 19: Classically dotted vessels in regular distribution are found in psoriasis. Note the white scales which are also a feature of the disease.

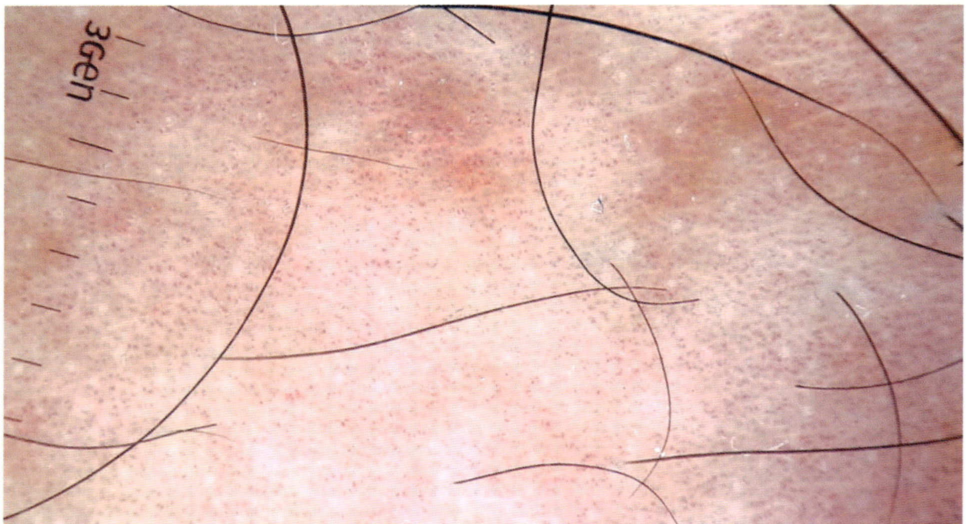

Fig. 20: Regular red dots is a dermoscopic hallmark of psoriasis. The absence of white scales indicate the psoriasis is undergoing treatment and is improving.

REFERENCE

1. Martin JM, Bella-Navarro R, Jordá E. Vascularizacion en dermatoscopia. Actas Dermosifiliogr. 2012;103:357-75.

FAT FINGERS

- They are thick, digitate, linear or curvilinear, branched dermoscopic structures usually observed in seborrheic keratosis (SK) where they correspond to the gyri of the cerebriform surfaces.[1]
- The recognition of fat fingers is very useful in the dermoscopic diagnosis of SK, particularly if the classic criteria of SK such as milia-like cysts, comedo-like openings, moth-eaten appearance, hairpin vessels, etc. are absent.
- Fat fingers are wider in comparison to other linear dermoscopic structures, e.g. melanocytic network, streaks, etc. The length of fat fingers varies from very short and miniature finger-like projections to half of the diameter of the lesion. They may have color variations from brown to blue-gray to hypopigmented. They may present with various shapes achievable using one's own finger such as linear like a straight finger; curvilinear resembling bent finger; branched like the letters "V" and "W" by extending two or three fingers and so on.[1]
- Histologically, cross-section done perpendicular to the gyrus shows protrusions of epidermis and papillary dermis (gyrus) surrounded by furrows (sulci) on each side packed with keratinous material (Fig. 21).

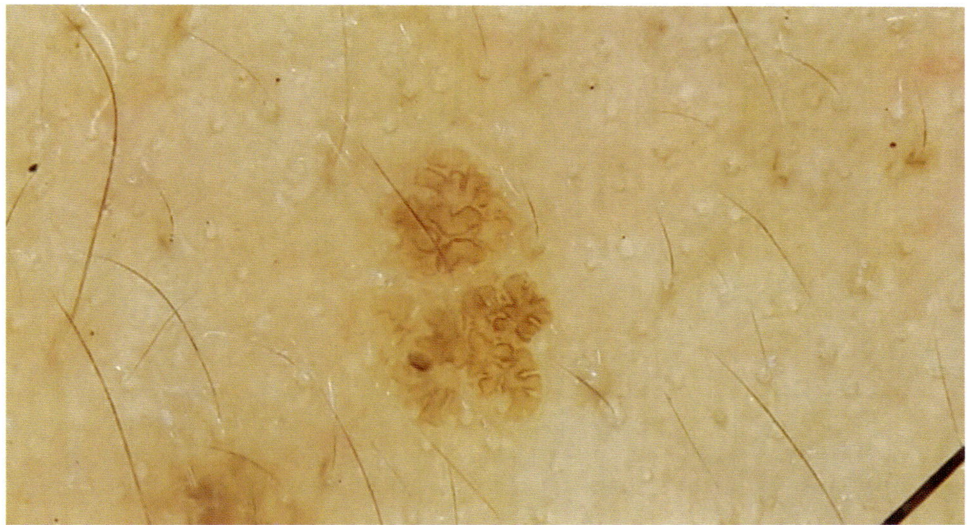

Fig. 21: Fat fingers may have variable shapes such as the letters "V", "W", etc. Their recognition is of utmost importance because in the absence of other features of seborrheic keratosis fat fingers are useful to diagnose the condition.

REFERENCE

1. Kopf AW, Rabinovitz H, Marghoob AA, et al. "Fat fingers:" a clue in the dermoscopic diagnosis of seborrheic keratoses. J Am Acad Dermatol. 2006;55(6):1089-91.

FINGERPRINT-LIKE STRUCTURES[1,2]

- They are light brown tiny ridges running parallel to each other resembling fingerprints. They are seen in solar lentigines and some flat seborrheic keratosis.
- These structures most likely correspond histologically to thin elongated epidermal ridges (Fig. 22).

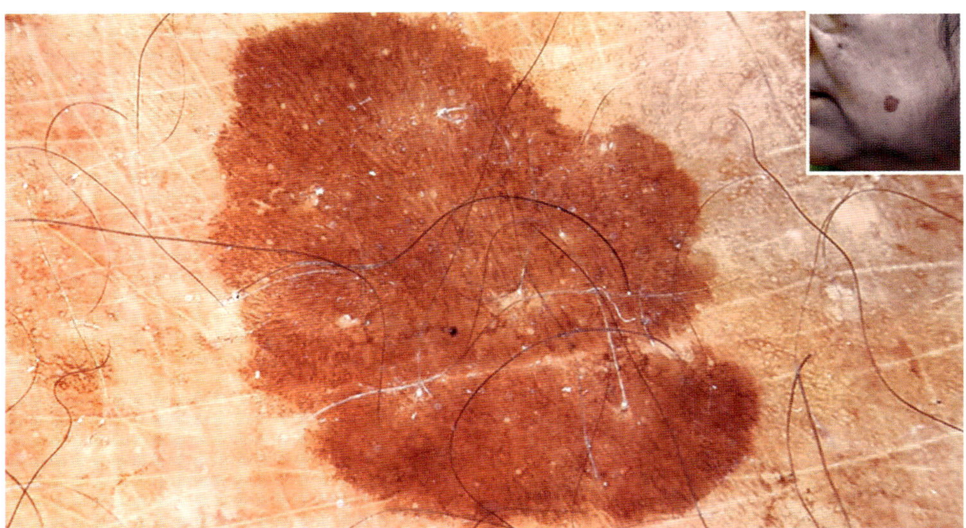

Fig. 22: Fingerprint-like structures in a case of solar lentigines.

REFERENCES

1. Braun RP, Scope A, Marghoob AA, et al. Histopathologic tissue correlations of dermoscopic structures. In: Marghoob AA, Malvehy J, Braun RP (Eds). Atlas of Dermoscopy, 2nd edition. London: Informa Healthcare; 2012. pp. 10-32.
2. Braun RP, Rabinovitz H, Krischner J, et al. Dermoscopy of pigmented seborrheic keratosis. Arch Dermatol. 2002;138:1556-60.

GLOBULES[1]

- Globules are round or oval structures of more than 0.1 mm in diameter, and like dots. Their color also ranges from black to brown to blue-gray according to the depth and concentration of the melanin in the skin.
- Histologically, they represent nests of melanocytes in the lower epidermis, dermoepidermal junction or papillary dermis.
- Because both the dots and globules are frequently observed together and they represent melanocyte nests, a combined name "dots and globules" is coined for them.
- Dermoscopically nevi and melanoma both may have dots and globules.
- Dots and globules are brown in color and uniform in shape and size in case of nevi; they are also evenly distributed throughout the lesion. Whereas in melanoma, dots and globules are usually situated focally at the periphery of the lesion and their color, shape and size are not uniform; they are distributed irregularly in the lesion (*see* Fig. 18).

REFERENCE

1. Braun RP, Scope A, Marghoob AA, et al. Histopathologic tissue correlations of dermoscopic structures. In: Marghoob AA, Malvehy J, Braun RP (Eds). Atlas of Dermoscopy, 2nd edition. London: Informa Healthcare; 2012. pp. 10-32.

GLOMERULAR VESSELS

- They appear as large-caliber reddish dots and are formed by tortuous capillaries curled up into a ball.[1] They are named glomerular vessels because the vascular pattern resembles the glomerular apparatus of kidney.
- Histologically, the vessels represent the dilated capillaries in the papillary dermis.[2]
- Most commonly, glomerular vessels are found in Bowen's disease and superficial squamous cell carcinoma. They are also seen in many other conditions such as stasis dermatitis, invasive squamous cell carcinoma, clear cell acanthoma, psoriasis, seborrheic dermatitis, eccrine poroma, and keratoacanthoma (Fig. 23).[1]

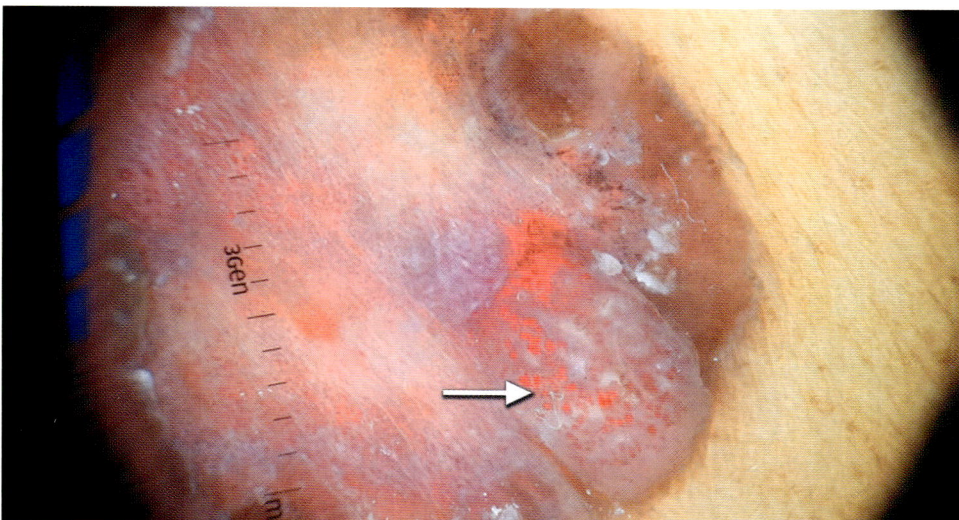

Fig. 23: Glomerular vessels (arrow) in a patchy distribution are observed in Bowen's disease.

REFERENCES

1. Martin JM, Bella-Navarro R, Jordá E. Vascularizacion en dermatoscopia. Actas Dermosifiliogr. 2012;103:357-75.
2. Felder S, Rabinovitz H, Oliviero M, et al. Dermoscopic differentiation of a superficial basal cell carcinoma and squamous cell carcinoma in situ. Dermatol Surg. 2006;32:423-5.

HAIRPIN VESSELS

- The hairpin vessels have a sharp bend at one end and appear as "U"-shaped blood vessels on dermoscope. The diameter of the vessels remains fixed throughout the lesion as 0.01–0.03 mm.[1] Usually they are accompanied by a whitish halo around the lesion in case of non-melanocytic tumors;[2] however, this phenomenon cannot be observed in melanocytic lesions.[3]
- Hairpin vessels are seen in non-melanocytic lesions such as seborrheic keratosis, keratoacanthoma, and squamous cell carcinoma. Hairpin vessels are also present in melanomas where they are surrounded by a pink halo.[4,5] The vessels can also be observed in warts, basal cell carcinomas, dermal nevi, and Spitz nevi.[1,3] Occasionally they are found in pilomatrixoma where the vessels coexist with glomerular and atypical linear vessels (Fig. 24).[6]

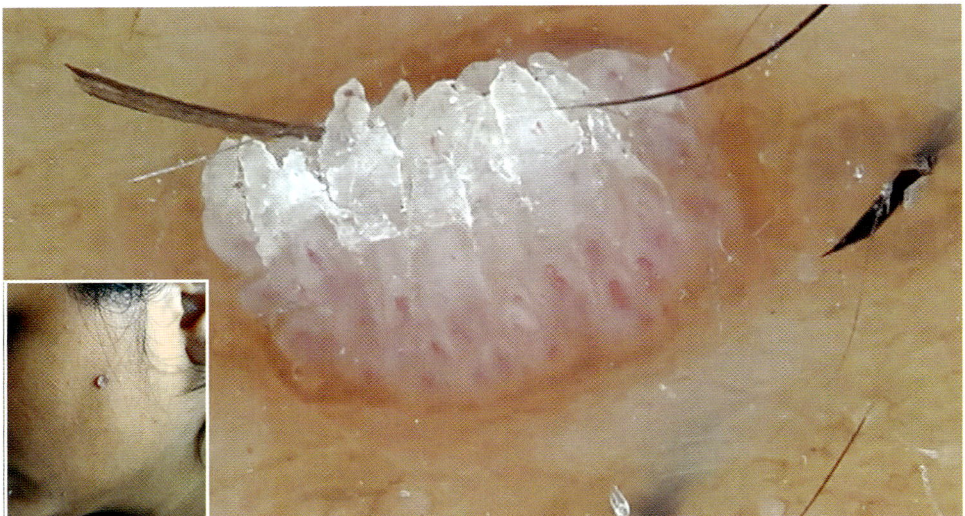

Fig. 24: A case of filiform warts showing hairpin vessels.

REFERENCES

1. Kreusch JF. Vascular patterns in skin tumors. Clin Dermatol. 2002;20:248-54.
2. Zalaudek I, Argenziano G, Oliviero M, et al. Dermoscopy of nonpigmented skin tumors. In: Thiers BH, Lang PG Jr (Eds). Year Book of Dermatology and Dermatologic Surgery 2007. Philadelphia: Elsevier Mosby; 2007. pp. 23-38.
3. Argenziano G, Zalaudek I, Corona R, et al. Vascular structures in skin tumours. A dermoscopy study. Arch Dermatol. 2004; 140:1485-9.
4. Malvehy J, Puig S, Argenziano G, et al. Dermoscopy report: proposal for standardization. Results of a consensus meeting of the International Dermoscopy Society. J Am Acad Dermatol. 2007;57:84-95.
5. Stoecker WV, Stolz W. Dermoscopy and the diagnostic challenge of amelanotic and hypomelanotic melanoma. Arch Dermatol. 2008;144:1207-10.
6. Zaballos P, Llambrich A, Puig S, et al. Dermoscopic findings of pilomatricomas. Dermatology. 2008;217:225-30.

LACUNAE[1,2]

They are clustered, well-demarcated red to dark blobs of round or oval shape. Histologically, they represent dilated vascular spaces in the dermis. The darker the lacunae, higher the degree of thrombosis within the vascular spaces. They are seen in angiomas and angiokeratomas (Figs. 25 and 26).

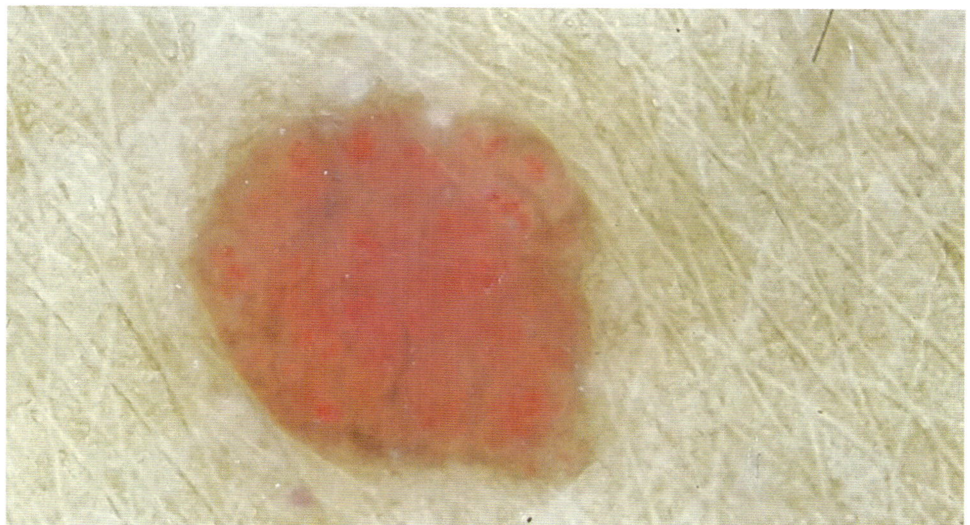

Fig. 25: They are multiple clustered, well-demarcated red/maroon/blue blobs with round or oval shape. The lacunae correspond to cavernous dilated blood vessels. In angiokerotoma the lacunae are blue black in color.

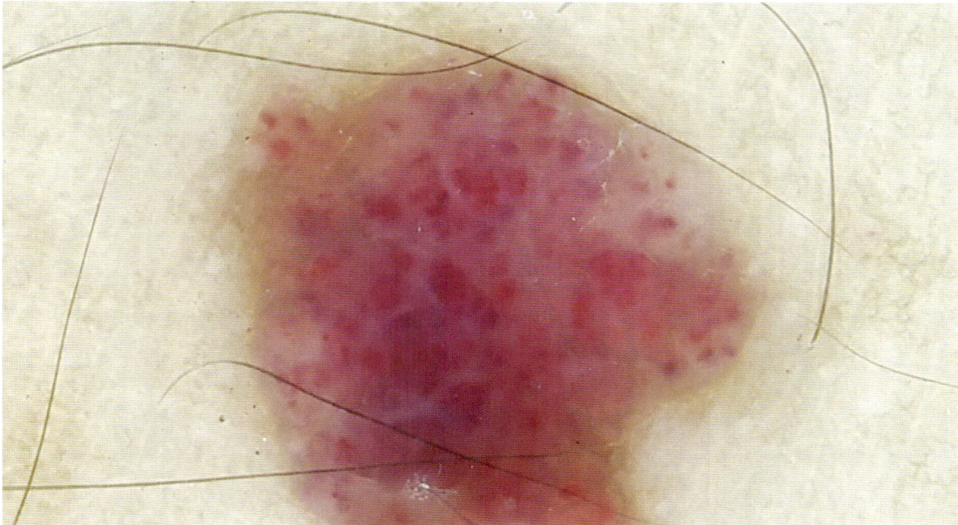

Fig. 26: Blood-filled lacunae.

REFERENCES

1. Zaballos P, Daufi C, Puig S, et al. Dermoscopy of solitary angiokeratomas: a morphological study. Arch Dermatol. 2007;143: 318-25.
2. Braun RP, Scope A, Marghoob AA, et al. Histopathologic tissue correlations of dermoscopic structures. In: Marghoob AA, Malvehy J, Braun RP (Eds). Atlas of Dermoscopy, 2nd edition. London: Informa Healthcare; 2012. pp. 10-32.

LEAF-LIKE AREAS[1]

- *Dermoscopic description*: They are brown to gray-blue discrete bulbous structures that often take the shape of a leaf. Sometimes there may be streaky extensions located at the periphery which tend to be broad and fuzzy. These extensions converge toward base and thus create a leaf-like structure. Leaf-like areas are highly specific for basal cell carcinoma.
- Histopathologically, they represent nests of pigmented epithelial nodules of basal cell carcinoma. These nodules are usually associated closely with the undersurface of the epidermis (Fig. 27).

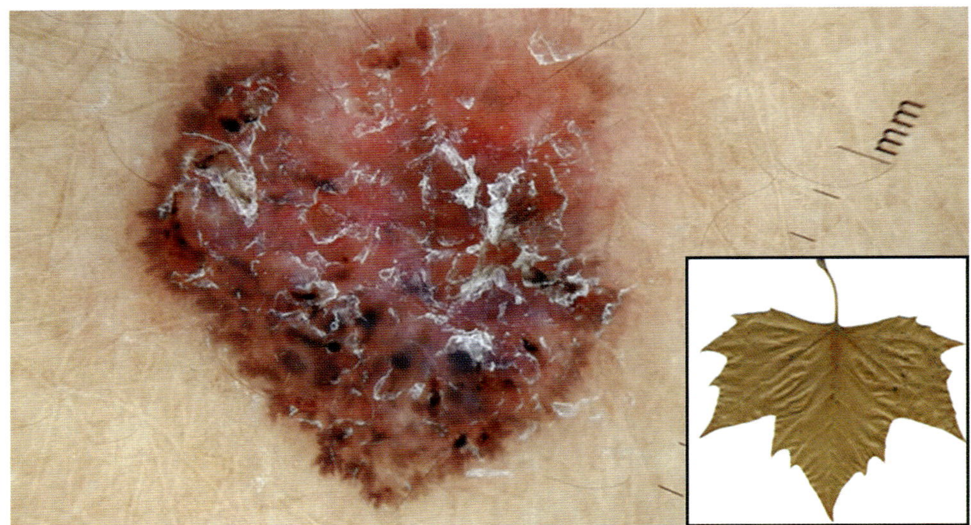

Fig. 27: Brown/gray-blue bulbous structures that often create the shape of a leaf; this leaf-like area is highly specific for basal cell carcinoma.

REFERENCE

1. Menzies SW. Dermoscopy of pigmented basal cell carcinoma. Clin Dermatal. 2002;20:268-9.

MELANOCYTIC NETWORK

- *Dermoscopic description*: The melanocytic network or pigment network appears as pigmented intersecting lines with holes resembling honeycomb. The network signifies that the lesion is usually of melanocytic origin.
- Histologically, the lines of the network correspond to rete ridge melanocytes and the holes represent the tips of the dermal papillae which are comparatively less pigmented.
- In the typical melanocytic network, the pigment lines are regular and have uniform color which gradually tend to fade towards the periphery. It is present in nevi.
- Whereas atypical pigment network shows irregular intersecting lines with holes of variable diameters and shapes. It has foci of darker and wider pigment lines which end abruptly at the periphery. It is associated with dysplastic nevi and melanoma.
- The melanocytic networks over palms and soles show a parallel pattern.[1] The network on the face is replaced by a pseudonetwork pattern (Figs. 28 and 29).[2]

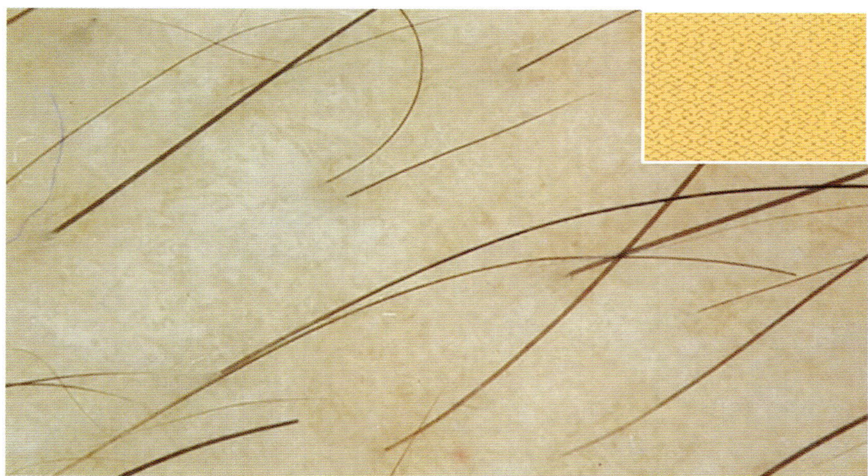

Fig. 28: Normal melanocytic network. It consists of intersecting pigmented lines and hypopigmented holes.

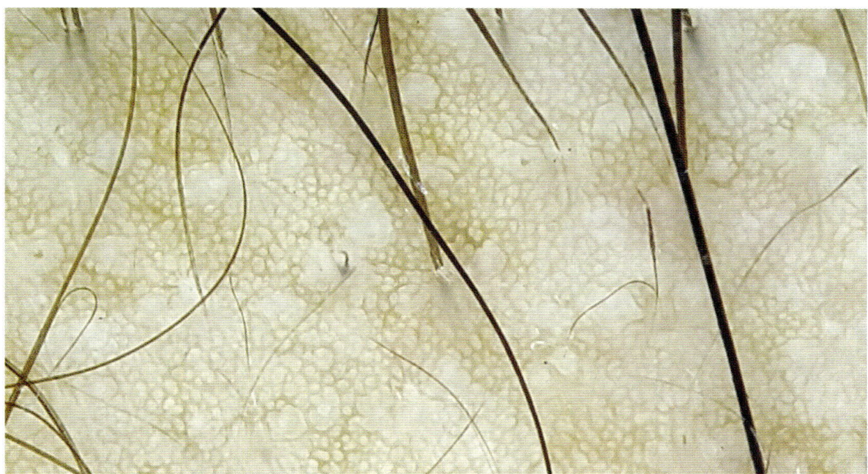

Fig. 29: Honeycomb pattern. This is also normal melanocytic network that appears on scalp. The holes represent the tips of the dermal papillae and are less pigmented whereas the grid of intersecting pigmented lines corresponds to rete ridge melanocytes.

REFERENCES

1. Saida T, Miyazaki A, Oguchi S, et al. Significance of dermoscopic patterns in detecting malignant melanoma on acral volar skin: results of a multicenter study in Japan. Arch Dermatol. 2004;140:1233-8.
2. Schiffner R, Schiffner-Rohe J, Vogt T, et al. Improvement of early recognition of lentigo maligna using dermatoscopy. J Am Acad Dermatol. 2000;42:25-32.

MILIA-LIKE CYSTS

- They appear as white to yellow, round or oval structures under both polarized and non-polarized dermoscopy.[1] But they tend to shine under non-polarized mode and resemble stars in the sky when present in groups (multiple milia-like cysts).
- Histologically, they are intraepidermal cysts of keratin.
- They are very commonly found in seborrheic keratosis. Milia-like cysts can also be seen in melanocytic lesions such as congenital nevi and melanoma (Figs. 30 and 31).

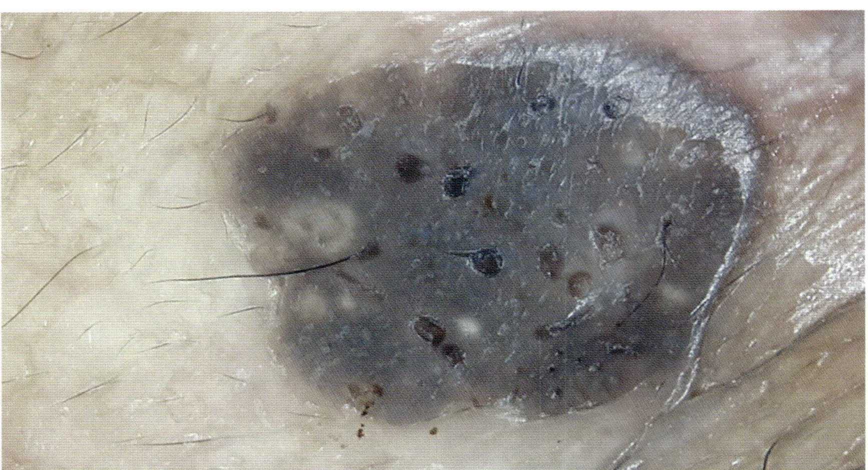

Fig. 30: Multiple large and small milia are seen in a case of seborrheic keratosis.

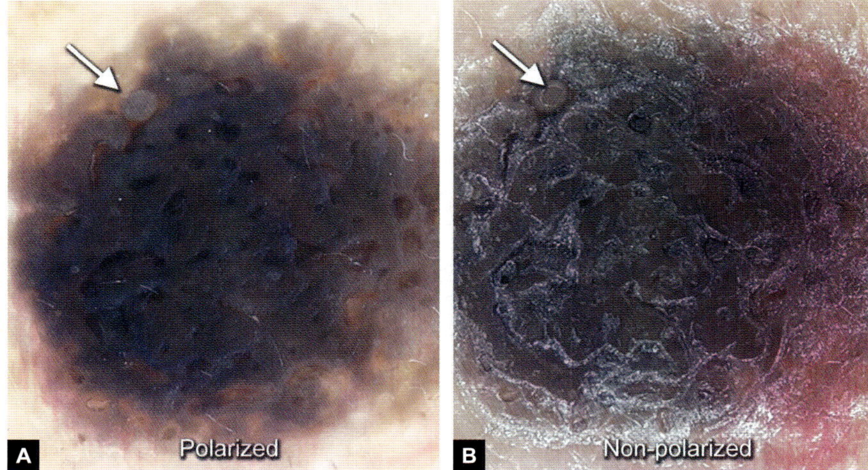

Figs. 31A and B: Appreciate the difference in dermoscopic appearance of the seborrheic keratosis (SK) lesion with the use of different modes of dermoscope. A milium (arrow) becomes more prominent in the non-polarized mode. The comedo-like openings show the keratin plugs in the non-polarized mode, whereas in the polarized mode the keratin plugs cannot be appreciated.

REFERENCE

1. Braun RP, Rabinovitz H, Krischner J, et al. Dermoscopy of pigmented seborrheic keratosis. Arch Dermatol. 2002;138:1556-60.

MOTH-EATEN BORDER[1]

- It is the concave invagination of the lesional border producing a pattern that resembles a moth-eaten garment.
- It can be observed in solar lentigo and seborrheic keratosis (Fig. 32).

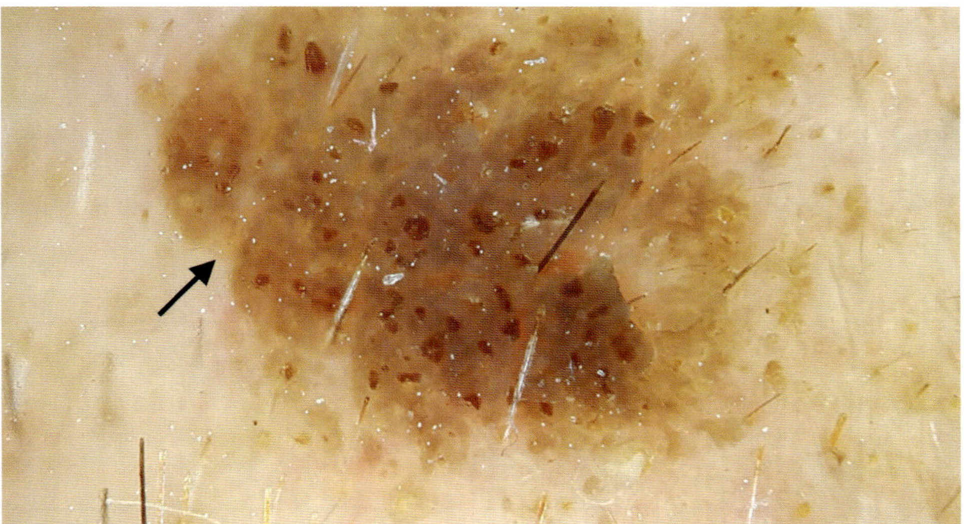

Fig. 32: Moth-eaten borders (arrow) are concave invaginations of the lesional border in a case of seborrheic keratosis.

REFERENCE

1. Menzies SW, Crotty KA, Ingvar C, et al. An Atlas of Surface Microscopy of Pigmented Skin Lesions. Sydney; McGraw-Hill Book Company; 2003.

MULTICOMPONENT PATTERN[1]

- *Dermoscopic description*: It has three or more components which include (1) reticular network, (2) globular, and (3) homogeneous areas. The homogeneous areas are either "blotches" or "structureless areas".
- It has also been defined as a lesion having three or more of the following components: (i) melanocytic network, (ii) dots and globules, (iii) blue-white veil, (iv) blotches, (v) streaks, (vi) structureless areas, (vii) negative network, and (viii) chrysalis structures. In dysplastic nevus, these structures are distributed symmetrically and in an organized manner. If their distribution is asymmetric and in a disorganized fashion, melanoma is the diagnosis.

REFERENCE

1. Ashfaq A, Marghoob AA, Kopf AW. Benign melanocytic lesions. In: Marghoob AA, Malvehy J, Braun RP (Eds). Atlas of Dermoscopy, 2nd edition. London: Informa Healthcare; 2012, pp. 159-70.

NEGATIVE PIGMENT NETWORK[1,2]

- *Dermoscopic description*: The network shows comparatively lighter areas apparently made of the intersecting lines and comparatively darker areas filling the apparent holes. It is a type of atypical network which shows a white reticular pattern seen as a negative of the pigmented network.
- Histopathologically, it represents thin elongated rete ridges along with large melanocytic nests within a widened papillary dermis.
- The presence of negative network signifies that the lesion is of melanocytic origin.
- The negative network may be seen in growing melanocytic nevi where the network is diffuse and symmetrical. Sometimes it may be found in Spitz nevi and dysplastic nevi. Most commonly it is associated with melanoma where the negative network is focal and asymmetric.
- Thus, dermoscopy is a highly precious tool in differentiating benign from alarming skin lesions.

REFERENCES

1. Connolly D, Silverstein DI. Dermoscopy and the negative pigment network. J Am Acad Dermatol. 2014;70:29-30.
2. Pizzichetta MA, Talamini R, Marghoob AA, et al. Negative pigment network: an additional dermoscopic feature for diagnosis for melanoma. J Am Acad Dermatol. 2013;68:552-9.

PEPPERING[1]

- *Dermoscopic description*: It is the accumulation of speckled blue-gray dots of sizes less than 0.1 mm. Usually it is present over a small area of the lesion, but the picture is confusing if the confluent granularity is seen over a large area.
- Histopathologically, peppering corresponds to melanin in the superficial dermis.
- In melanocytic nevi, peppering is seen in less than 10% of the lesion. Whereas in the case of melanoma, it is spread over 50% of the lesion (Fig. 33).

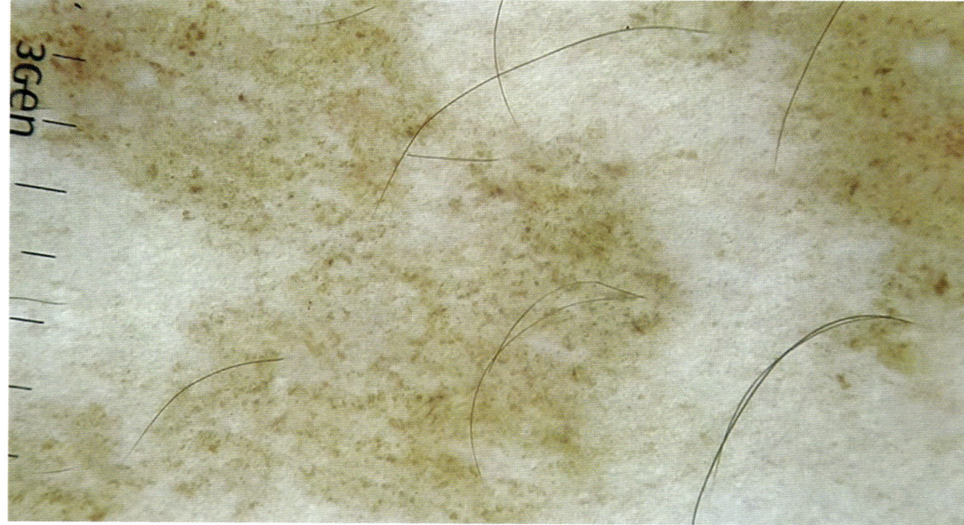

Fig. 33: Peppering are tiny blue-gray granules which histologically correspond to melanin particles in the dermis.

REFERENCE

1. Braun RP, Scope A, Marghoob AA, et al. Histopathologic tissue correlations of dermoscopic structures. In: Marghoob AA, Malvehy J, Braun RP (Eds). Atlas of Dermoscopy, 2nd edition. London: Informa Healthcare; 2012. pp. 10-32.

PSEUDONETWORK[1]

- The melanocytic network on the face is replaced by a pseudonetwork which is characterized by diffuse pigmentation interspersed with nonpigmented adnexal openings. As a result, the melanocytic lesions of face usually do not reveal a typical network pattern on dermoscopic examination.
- Histologically, the pigment of this network in the epidermis or dermis is interrupted by follicular and adnexal openings on the face.
- This pattern is observed in both melanocytic and non-melanocytic pigmented lesions of the face.
- Facial skin shows two distinct patterns—(1) annular and (2) reticular. The annular pattern has small circles correlating with follicular and other adnexal openings. These circles are surrounded by varying densities of pigment and are seen in solar lentigines and melanocytic neoplasms with junctional component.
- The reticular pattern is usually seen in solar lentigines and shows finer lines but does not form a clear network (Fig. 34).

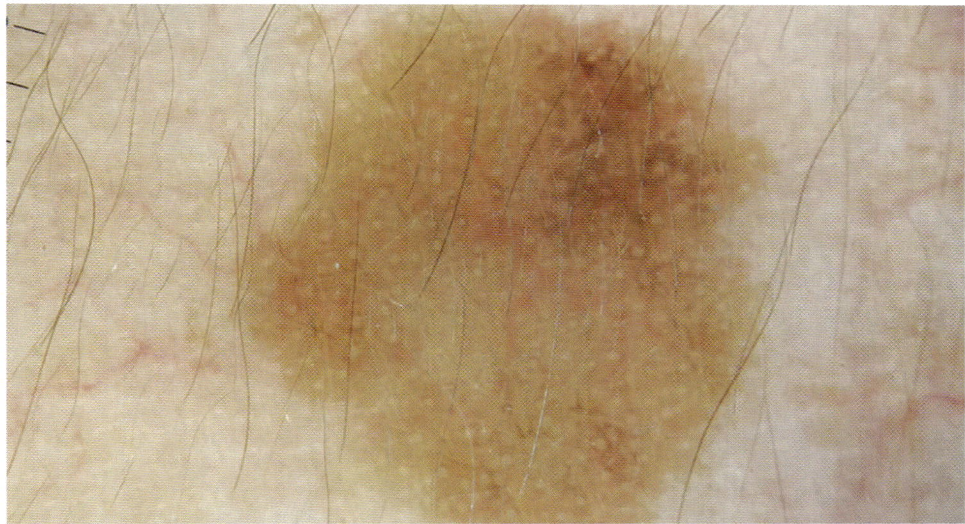

Fig. 34: Pseudonetwork is found in facial lesions. The diffuse pigmentation is interrupted by nonpigmented adnexal openings giving rise to the appearance of a pseudonetwork.

REFERENCE

1. Braun RP, Scope A, Marghoob AA, et al. Histopathologic tissue correlations of dermoscopic structures. In: Marghoob AA, Malvehy J, Braun RP (Eds). Atlas of Dermoscopy, 2nd edition. London: Informa Healthcare; 2012. pp. 10-32.

POLYMORPHOUS VESSELS

- *Dermoscopic description*: Two or more vascular patterns are seen dermoscopically, most frequent being dotted and linear-irregular; this combination is highly specific for amelanotic/hypomelanotic melanoma.[1] In eccrine poroma, combination of dotted and linear vessels may be found.[2]
- Combination of arborizing, linear-irregular, and hairpin-like vessels is highly suggestive of thick amelanotic and melanoma metastasis.[3,4]
- In squamous cell carcinoma and pilomatrixoma, combination of hairpin-like vessels and linear-irregular vessels are seen.[5]

REFERENCES

1. Eubanks LE, McBurney EI. Videomicroscopy of port-wine stains: correlation of location and depth of lesion. J Am Acad Dermatol. 2001;44:948-51.
2. Zalaudek I, Hoffmann-Wellenhoff R, Argenziano G. Dermoscopy of clear-cell acanthoma differs from dermoscopy of psoriasis. Dermatology. 2003;207:428.
3. Sgambato A, Zalaudek I, Ferrara G, et al. Nodules with a prominent vascular component. Arch Dermatol. 2008;144:702.
4. Menzies SW, Ingvar C, Crotty KA, et al. Frequency and morphologic characteristics of invasive melanomas lacking specific surface microscopic features. Arch Dermatol. 1996;132:1178-82.
5. Minagawa A, Koga H, Sakaizawa K, et al. Dermoscopic and histopathological findings of polymorphous vessels in amelanotic cutaneous metastasis of pigmented cutaneous melanoma. Br J Dermatol. 2009;160:1134-6.

REGRESSION STRUCTURES[1,2]

- *Dermoscopic description*: They appear as white scar like depigmentation and/or peppering. It is a dynamic process and there is a gradual involution of the melanocytic network; the network will be replaced by two components: (1) white structures and (2) multiple small blue-gray dots (peppering). The white structures correspond to fibrosis in papillary dermis and the gray structures represent melanophages.
- Histopathology shows fibrosis, variable amount of melanophages and sparse lymphocytic infiltration. The dermoepidermal junction becomes flattened.
- The presence of regression structure is a warning that the lesion may be melanoma.

REFERENCES

1. Braun RP, Scope A, Marghoob AA, et al. Histopathologic tissue correlations of dermoscopic structures. In: Marghoob AA, Malvehy J, Braun RP (Eds). Atlas of Dermoscopy, 2nd edition. London: Informa Healthcare; 2012. pp. 10-32.
2. Bowling J. Regression in melanoma. In: Diagnostic Dermoscopy: The Illustrated Guide, 2nd edition. United States: Wiley-Blackwell; 2012. p. 54.

RETICULOGLOBULAR PATTERN

- *Dermoscopic description*: This is one of the melanocytic patterns that exhibits peripheral melanocytic network along with central globules.[1]
- This pattern is usually seen in congenital melanocytic nevus (Fig. 35).

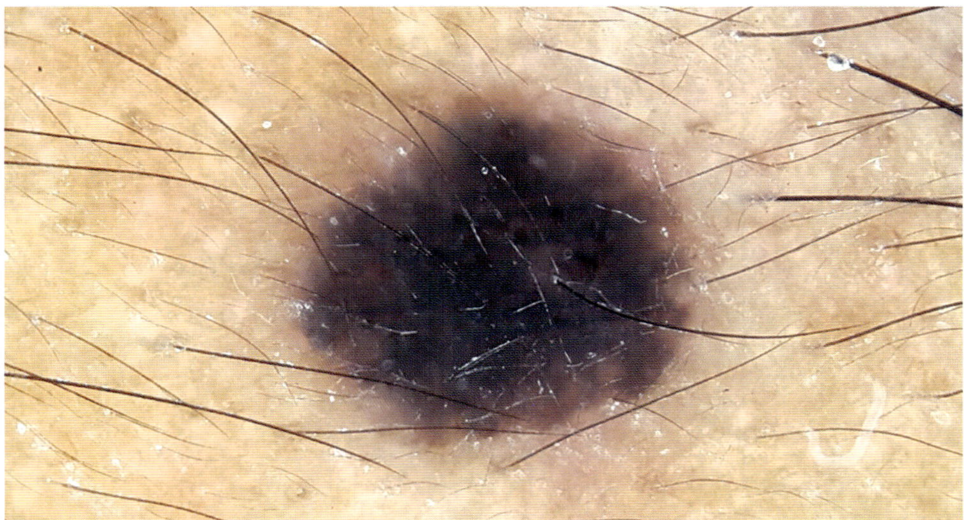

Fig. 35: Reticuloglobular pattern.

REFERENCE

1. Marghoob AA. Benign melanocytic lesions. In: Marghoob AA, Malvehy J, Braun RP (Eds). Atlas of Dermoscopy, 2nd edition. London: Informa Healthcare; 2012. pp. 147-58.

SPOKE-WHEEL STRUCTURES

- *Dermoscopic description*: Well-circumscribed projections of brown-gray-blue color that radiate out from a dark brown central hub. In the absence of pigment network, spoke-wheel pattern is highly specific of basal cell carcinoma.[1]
- Histopathologically spoke-wheel pattern represents pigmented aggregates of basal cell carcinoma that radiate from the undersurface of the dermoepidermal junction; they have multiple projections in the dermis (Fig. 36).

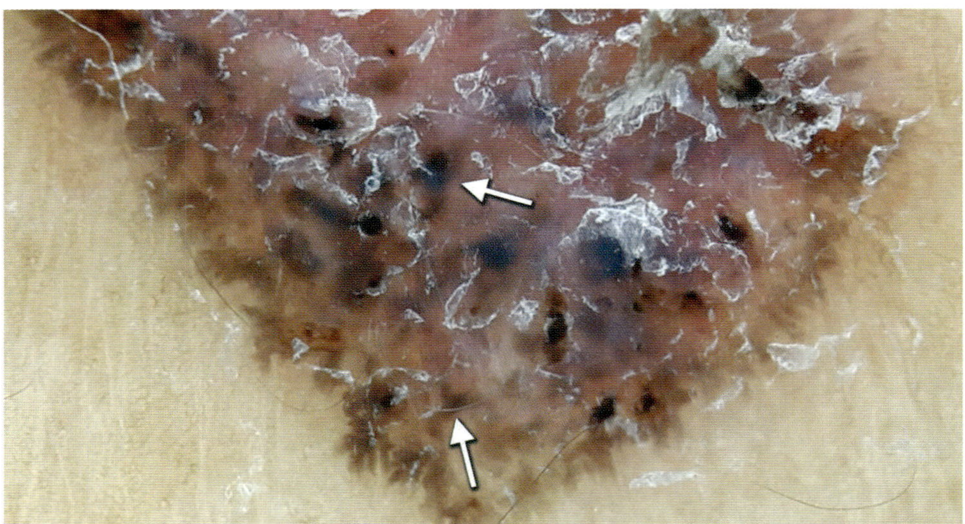

Fig. 36: A gray-blue radial projection meeting at a darker brown central hub (arrows) resembling the spoke-wheel; this structure highly signifies basal cell carcinoma.

REFERENCE

1. Menzies SW. Dermoscopy of pigmented basal cell carcinoma. Clin Dermatol. 2002;20:268-9.

STARBURST PATTERN

Dermoscopic Description

Dysplastic nevi and other nevi:[1] Multicomponent pattern usually observed in dysplastic nevi. This pattern presents in one of the two ways:

1. The peripheral globules tiered over one another with the center of the lesion having normal melanocytic network.
2. In an alternate presentation, streaks instead of globules are seen in the entire periphery of the lesion (Fig. 37).

Both the above presentations are observed in Spitz nevi; type 2 may also be seen in dysplastic nevi with spitzoid features.

Prurigo nodularis: Whitish starburst pattern seen (personal observation).

Discoid lupus erythematosus (DLE): Red starburst pattern (personal observation).

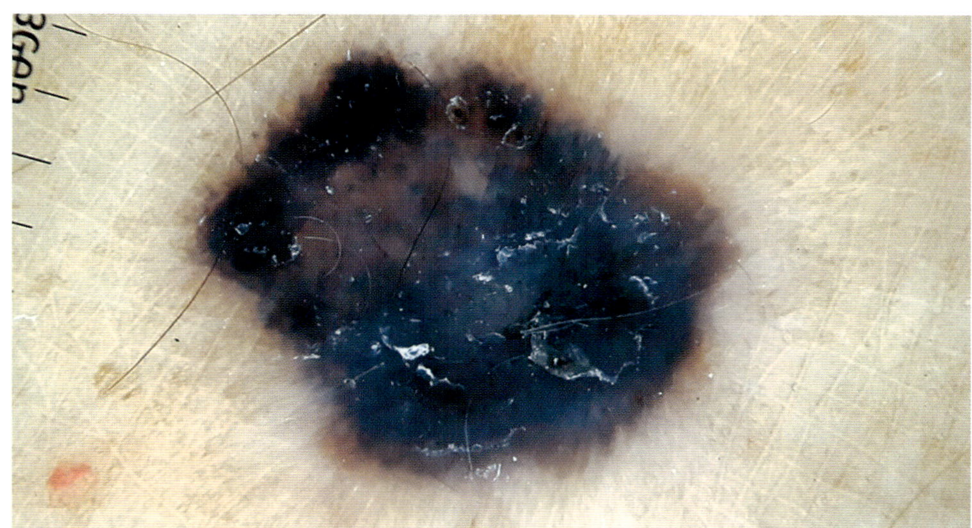

Fig. 37: Radial streaming present around the lesion resembling an exploding star. It may be found in dysplastic nevi, Spitz nevi, etc.

REFERENCE

1. Ashfaq A, Marghoob A, Kopf AW. Benign melanocytic lesions. In: Marghoob AA, Malvehy J, Braun RP (Eds). Atlas of Dermoscopy, 2nd edition. London: Informa Healthcare; 2012. pp. 159-70.

STREAKS[1]

- They are pigmented linear projections arranged radially at the periphery of the lesion. Both pseudopods and radial streaming are the variations of streaks.
- Histopathologically, streaks show confluent nests of melanocytes at the dermoepidermal junction.
- The presence of streaks means that the lesion has originated from melanocytes. In Spitz nevi, streaks are distributed symmetrically around the entire lesion; whereas melanoma has streaks only focally at the periphery of the lesion.

Pseudopods

- They are defined as finger-like structures of brown to black pigment situated at the periphery of the lesion. The finger-like structures have small nobs at their tips. The pseudopods are attached centrally to a blotch or pigmented network. Pseudopods are one of the specific criteria to diagnose superficial spreading melanoma.
- Histopathologically, pseudopods represent confluent nests of melanocytes at the dermoepidermal junction.

Radial Streaming

- When parallel linear lines are arranged radially at the perimeter, it is called radial streaming.
- Histopathologically, it corresponds to confluent nests of melanocytes at the dermoepidermal junction.

REFERENCE

1. Braun RP, Scope A, Marghoob AA, et al. Histopathologic tissue correlations of dermoscopic structures. In: Marghoob AA, Malvehy J, Braun RP (Eds). Atlas of Dermoscopy, 2nd edition. London: Informa Healthcare; 2012. pp. 10-32.

STRING OF PEARL VESSELS[1]

- *Dermoscopic description*: This is a vascular pattern in which glomerular vessels or dotted vessels are arranged linearly in a pattern that resembles a string of pearls.
- They are highly diagnostic of clear cell acanthoma (Fig. 38).

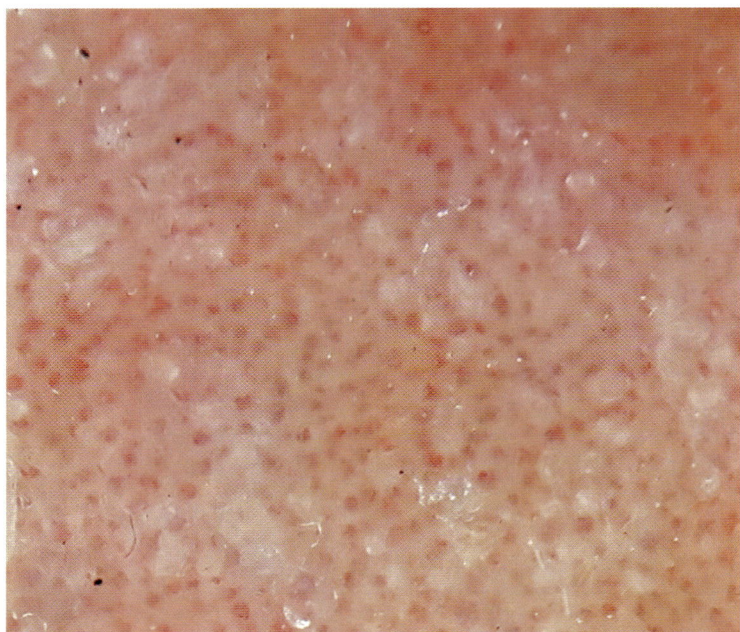

Fig. 38: Dotted vessels arranged linearly in a pattern which resembles a string of pearls. It is found in clear cell acanthoma.

REFERENCE

1. Wang SQ, Duzsa SW, Scope A, et al. Differences in dermoscopic images from non-polarized dermoscope and polarized dermoscope influence the diagnostic accuracy and confidence level: a pilot study. Dermatol Surg. 2008;34:1389-95.

STRUCTURELESS AREAS

- *Dermoscopic description*: This pattern is in contrast to 'blotches' which show uniform dark area.
- Structureless areas are hypopigmented in comparison to the rest of the lesion but not in comparison to the normal skin. By definition the size of the areas should be at least 10% of the lesional surface areas.[1,2]
- If it is observed within a lesion, it is a nevus whereas in melanoma the structureless area is found at the periphery of the lesion.[3]
- Histopathologically, these areas correspond to the flattening of the rete ridges with scattered atypical melanocytes (pagetoid cells) in the suprabasal epidermis.

REFERENCES

1. Stolz W, Braun-Falco O, Bilek P, et al. Color Atlas of Dermatoscopy. Berlin: Blackwell Wissenschafts-Verlag; 2002.
2. Stolz W, Schiffner R, Burgdorf WH. Dermatoscopy for facial pigmented skin lesions. Clin Dermatol. 2002;20:276-8.
3. Annessi G, Bono R, Sampogna F, et al. Sensitivity, specificity, and diagnostic accuracy of three dermoscopic algorithmic methods in the diagnosis of doubtful melanocytic lesions: the importance of light brown structureless areas in differentiating atypical melanocytic nevi from thin melanomas. J Am Acad Dermatol. 2007;56:759-67.

TWISTED RED LOOPS[1]

- *Dermoscopic description*: They appear as multiple coils or loops in a homogeneous distribution; the loops are more or less evenly spaced.
- This pattern is usually found in scalp psoriasis but can also be seen in seborrheic dermatitis and around the affected follicles in folliculitis decalvans (Fig. 39).

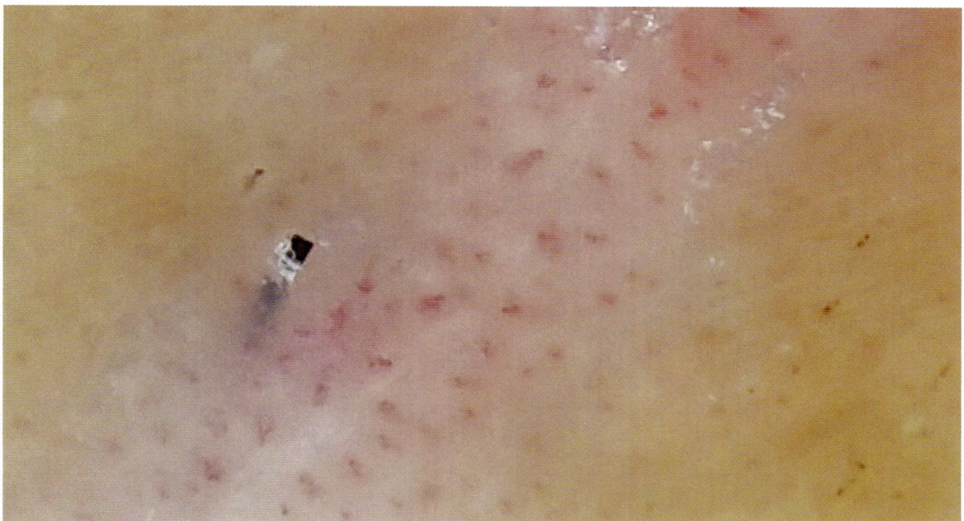

Fig. 39: Twisted red loops are found dermoscopically in a case of seborrheic dermatitis.

REFERENCE

1. Vazquez-Lopez F, Kreusch J, Marghoob AA. Dermoscopic semiology: further insights into vascular features by screening a large spectrum of nontumoral skin lesions. Br J Dermatol. 2004;150:226-31.

WICKHAM STRIAE

- *Dermoscopic description*: They appear as pearly-whitish structures of round, linear or reticular pattern on a purple to reddish background. Wickham striae (WS) may extend into thin arboriform projections surrounded by dotted or linear vessels.[1]
- They are highly sensitive and specific criteria for diagnosing lichen planus.
- Histopathologically, WS represent compact orthokeratosis, wedge-shaped hypergranulosis and acanthosis (Fig. 40).[2]

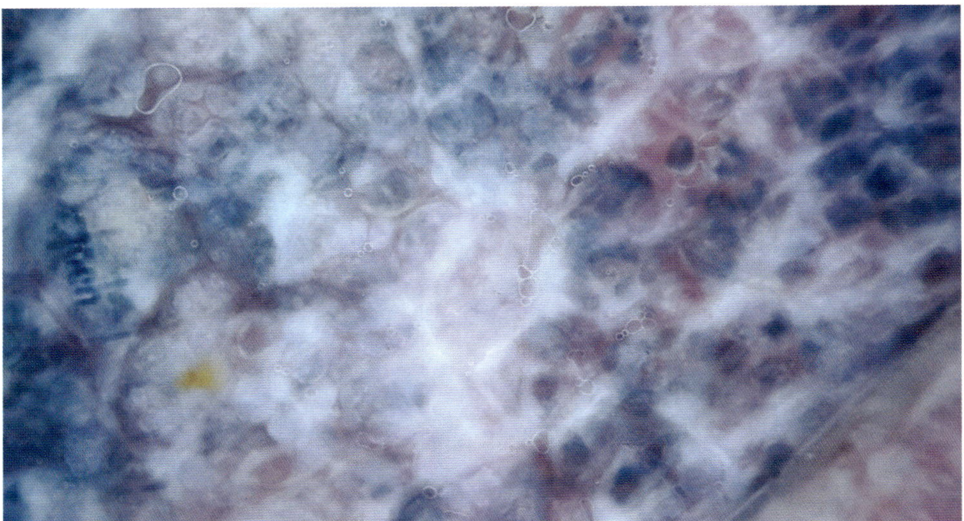

Fig. 40: Dermoscopy reveals reticular Wickham striae in a case of lichen planus.

REFERENCES

1. Zalaudek I. Dermoscopy in general dermatology. In: Marghoob AA, Malvehy J, Braun RP (Eds). Atlas of Dermoscopy, 2nd edition. London: Informa Healthcare; 2012. pp. 323-36.
2. Jung J, Cho E, Park E, et al. Atypical dermoscopic findings in patients diagnosed with lichen planus by histological examination. Dermatologica Sinica. 2017;35:20-4.

WOBBLE SIGN[1]

During the dermoscopic examination of a nodular pigmented skin lesion, when the contact plate of the dermoscope is firmly pressed down in vertical direction against the lesion and at the same time is slightly moved horizontally, parallel to the surface, the following may be observed:

- The lesion may appear stuck to the contact plate and the entire lesion moves with the dynamic dermoscope. This is seen in case of seborrheic keratosis.
- In case of papillomatous dermal nevi, the lesion does not move en block, on the contrary, it rolls back and forth. So, it can be said that the dermal nevi wobble.
- Because the melanomas are firm and fixed to the skin surface, they are not easily moveable (Figs. 41A to C).

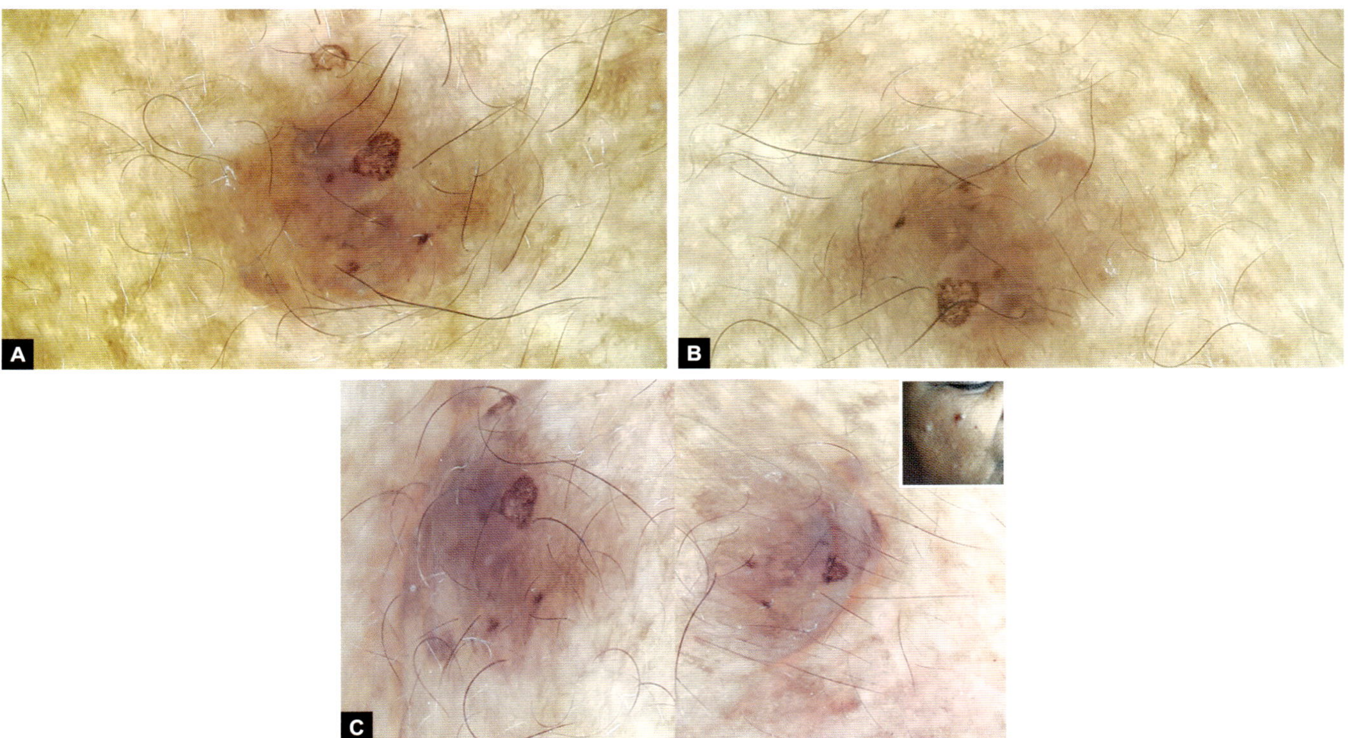

Figs. 41A to C: Dermoscopic demonstration of wobble sign. In case of dermal melanocytic nevi, they move back and forth during the dermoscopic examination of the nevi so it can be inferred that dermal nevi wobble.

REFERENCE

1. Wang SQ, Rabinovitz HS, Oliviero MS, et al. Solar lentigines, seborrheic keratosis and lichen planus-like keratosis. In: Marghoob AA, Malvehy J, Braun RP (Eds). Atlas of Dermoscopy, 2nd edition. London: Informa Healthcare; 2012. pp. 58-69.

CHAPTER 6

Color Concept through Dermoscopy

Subrata Malakar, Samipa S Mukherjee, Surit Malakar

INTRODUCTION

- Color seen through the dermoscope may be a diagnostic clue and points toward the diagnosis.
- Color through the dermoscope should not surprise the clinician and mislead them to a wrong diagnosis rather than a determined diagnosis.
- Different colors seen through the dermoscope depend upon the different chromophores and various structures present in the skin.
- Color merely may be an artifact and results from the reflection of light due to different positions of the dermoscope.
- Dermoscope can recognize colors and structures.
- Colors perceived through dermoscope may provide clue to morphologic information (Table 1).
- Benign lesions show one or two colors.
- Melanoma may reveal three or more colors.

Color concept through dermoscopy has been divided into six sections:

1. Color due to melanin
2. Color due to hemoglobin
3. White shiny structures
4. Yellow and orange color
5. Rainbow pattern
6. Color as an artifact.

SECTION 1: COLOR DUE TO MELANIN

THE MELANIN MODULE

The use of dermatoscopy in dermatological consultation extends the total time of the examination by only about 72 seconds,[1] thereby making it worth as an assessment tool for any lesion on the body of the patient during a routine dermatology checkup. Dermatoscopy is characterized by 83% sensitivity and 69% specificity for the detection of melanomas.[2]

Although melanin was one of the first chromophore to be explored so vividly in the field of dermoscopy, the diagnosis of melanocytic lesions still remains complicated with regards to the patterns and structures present in the lesion. One of the authors (Malakar) therefore felt the need for coding the location of melanin on histopathology, which can be correlated with dermoscopy and easily represented to denote the location of the pigment in the layers of the skin thereby leading to the inception of "melanin module".

Dermoscopic color detection of melanin depends upon its location and concentration in the different layers of the skin; the colors range from black to brown in the epidermis, and gray to blue in the dermis. If melanin is present in the stratum corneum or just below the color of the lesion, appear as black on dermoscopy. When melanin is present at dermoepidermal junction or lower epidermis, the color of the melanin appear as light brown to dark brown.

When located at the papillary dermis, the color of melanin is gray on dermoscopy. When located in the deeper dermis melanin appears blue in color.[3,4]

The concept of melanin module originated from this varied location of the pigment giving rise to different colors. Thereby English alphabets from A-D were allotted to dermoscopic level of melanin thereby giving rise to the melanin module. Thus, the module can be explained as follows (Fig. 1).

Henceforth, pigmented/melanocytic lesions can be described using the code for the color seen under the dermoscope. We explain this with the help of different cases:

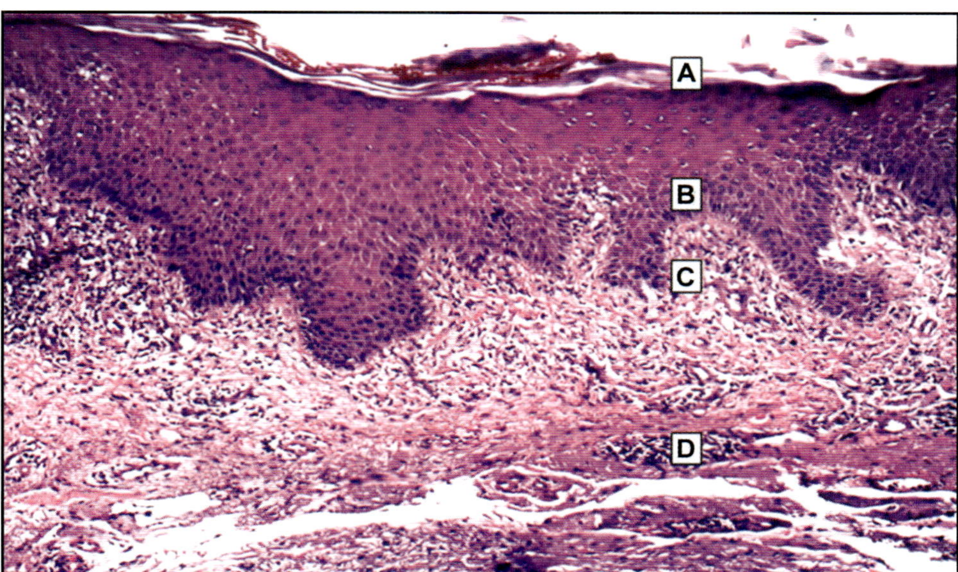

Fig. 1: Melanin module. A: Black—melanin in stratum corneum/just below; B: Light to dark brown—melanin in lower epidermis/dermoepidermal junction; C: Gray—melanin in the papillary dermis; D: Blue—melanin in deeper dermis

CONCLUSION

The melanin module will help in easy coding of the level of pigment in the skin based on the color as seen on dermoscopy thereby providing clue to the diagnosis. Also referring to the depth of the pigment in vivo on dermoscopy (Figs. 2 to 7) and its correlation ex vivo on histopathology will be simplified by this method. Further, this module can be utilized to group the lesions based on the level of pigment (Fig. 1).

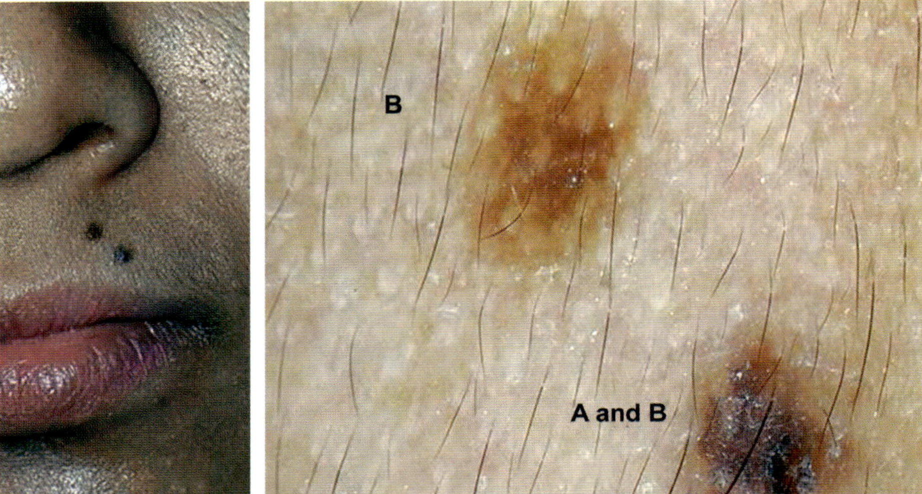

Fig. 2: A 20-year-old lady presented with twin pigmented lesions over the left upper lip since childhood, which showed very slow increase in the size and were asymptomatic. Dermoscopic examination using the melanin module revealed melanin deposition at level B in the upper lesion and A and B in the lower lesion thereby denoting that melanin was present in the superficial layers of epidermis excluding the stratum corneum for the upper lesion and in the lower lesion melanin level is at epidermis and dermoepidermal junction thereby confirming the diagnosis of epidermal nevus and junctional nevus, respectively.

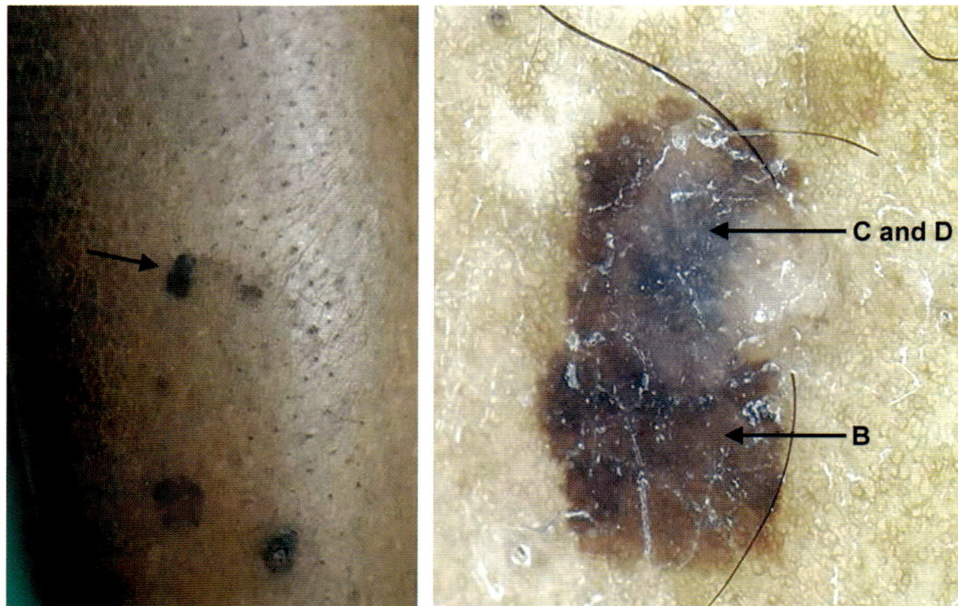

Fig. 3: A 32-year-old male presented with pigmented lesion over the left shin (arrow) of 5 years duration slowly increasing in size which was otherwise asymptomatic. Clinical examination revealed well-defined hyperpigmented macule over the anterior shin of the left shin. For the sake of convenience, the lesion was divided into upper and lower half. Dermoscopic examination using the melanin module revealed melanin deposition at level C and D in the upper half whereas lower half revealed melanin at level B. This denotes that melanin was at the level of papillary dermis and deeper dermis in the upper half of the lesion and at the level of lower epidermis/dermoepidermal junction in the lower half of the lesion.

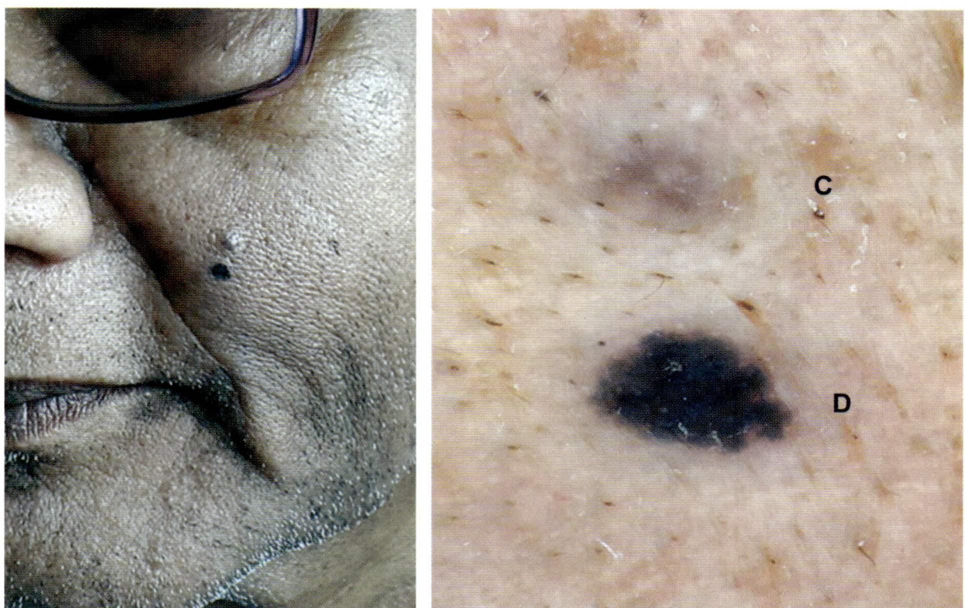

Fig. 4: Dermoscopic level of these two very close nevi demonstrate melanin at level C and D.

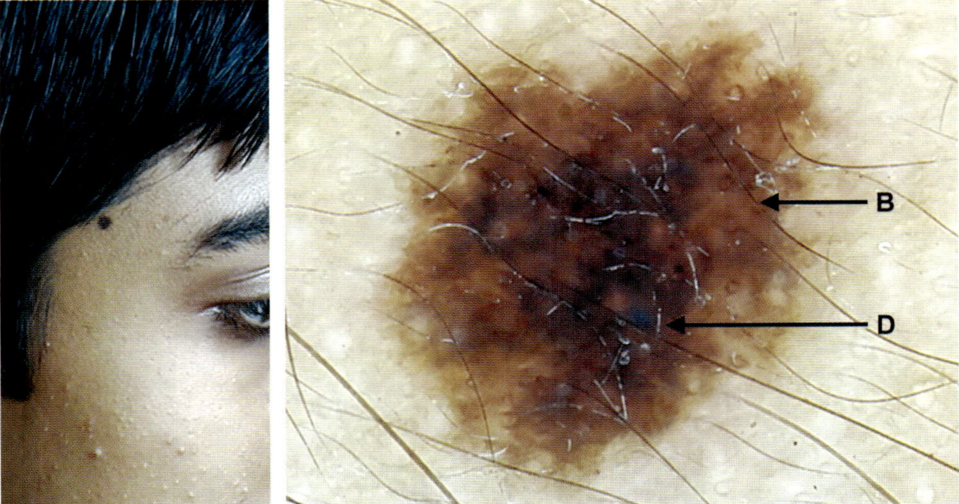

Fig. 5: In a single melanocytic nevus, melanin level can vary which can be demonstrated in the melanocytic nevus of this child. B and D are the levels of melanin according to the melanin module.

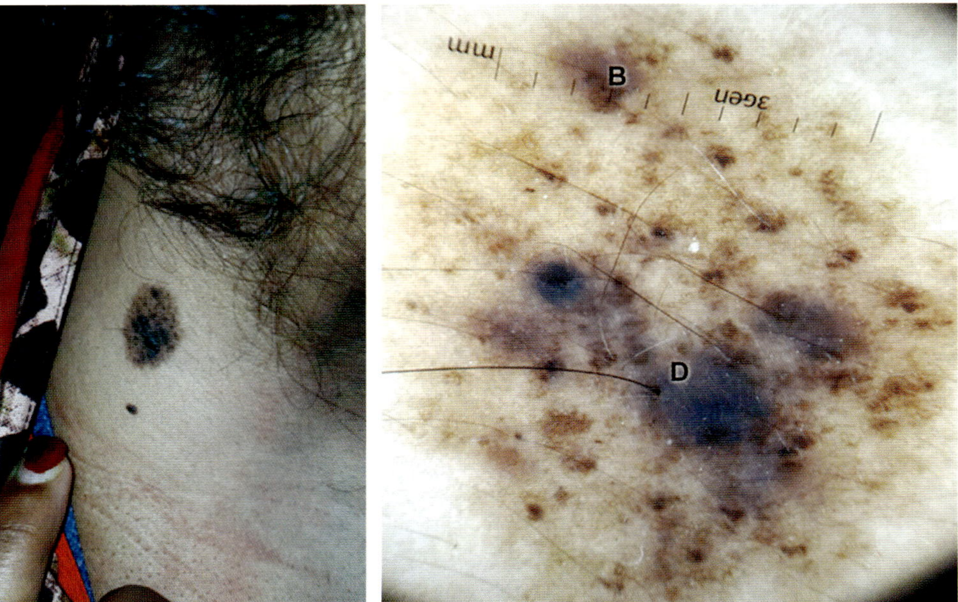

Fig. 6: The melanocytic nevus has melanin in the B and D level according to the melanin module.

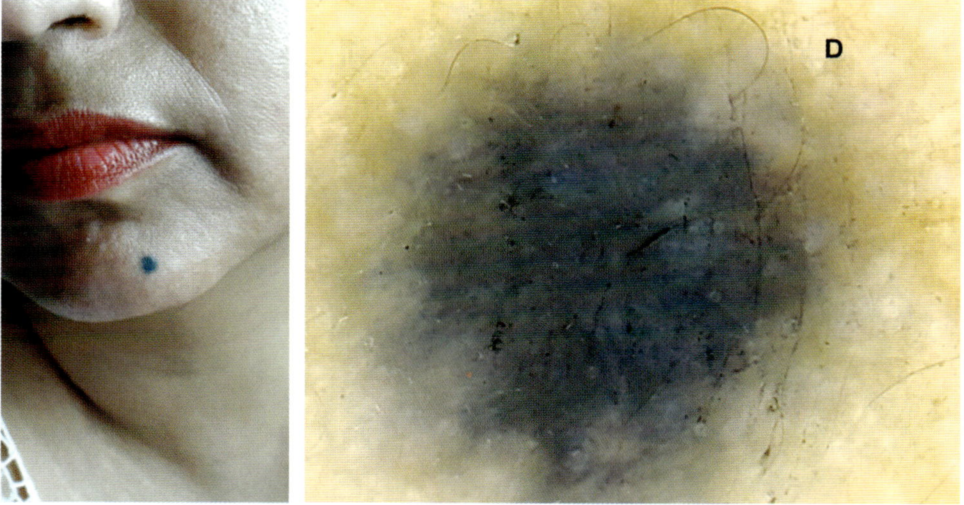

Fig. 7: Blue nevus in a case of middle-aged lady. According to the melanin module the level of pigment is D.

REFERENCES

1. Zalaudek I, Kittler H, Marghoob AA, et al. Time required for a complete skin examination with and without dermoscopy: a prospective, randomized multicenter study. Arch Dermatol. 2008;144:509-13.
2. Blum A, Hofmann-Wellenhof R, Luedtke H, et al. Value of the clinical history for different users of dermoscopy compared with results of digital image analysis. J Eur Acad Dermatol Venereol. 2004;18:665-9.
3. Binder M, Braun RP. Principles of dermoscopy. In: Marghoob AA, Braun RP, Kopf AW (Eds). Atlas of Dermoscopy. London: Taylor & Francis; 2005. pp. 7-10.
4. Carli P, De Giorgi V, Soyer HP, et al. Dermatoscopy in the diagnosis of pigmented skin lesions: a new semiology for the dermatologist. J Eur Acad Dermatol Venereol. 2000;14:353-69.

SECTION 2: COLOR DUE TO HEMOGLOBIN

INTRODUCTION

- Red color seen through the dermoscope is due to the chromophore hemoglobin that can reveal red, bluish, or even purple hues (Fig. 8).
- The different hues or tones depend upon the depth and degree of oxidation of hemoglobin, and also on the presence or absence of thrombosis.
- The red color shows up better in hypopigmented or nonpigmented lesions; also can be visualized better in the lighter areas of pigmented tumor.
- Dermoscope shows a horizontal view of the skin, as a result, the vessels that run perpendicular to the skin surface are viewed as dots or loops; whereas the vessels that run parallel to the surface are seen as lines (Fig. 9).
- Vessels closer to the skin surface are bright red in color and in focus; (Fig. 10) whereas, the vessels located in the dermis are usually pink and out of focus due to the dispersion of light through the connective tissue of the dermis (Fig. 11).
- Dermoscopic perception of red color depends also upon the skin type of the patient. Vessels can easily be seen in fair-skinned individuals in comparison to the darker skin.
- In certain areas of the body, especially breasts and buttocks the vasculature is very clear and the dermatologist must be cautious to avoid wrong diagnosis.
- In elderly patients, due to marked elastoses, normal vessels look prominent (Fig. 12) that may create confusion with the vessels of any skin tumors.

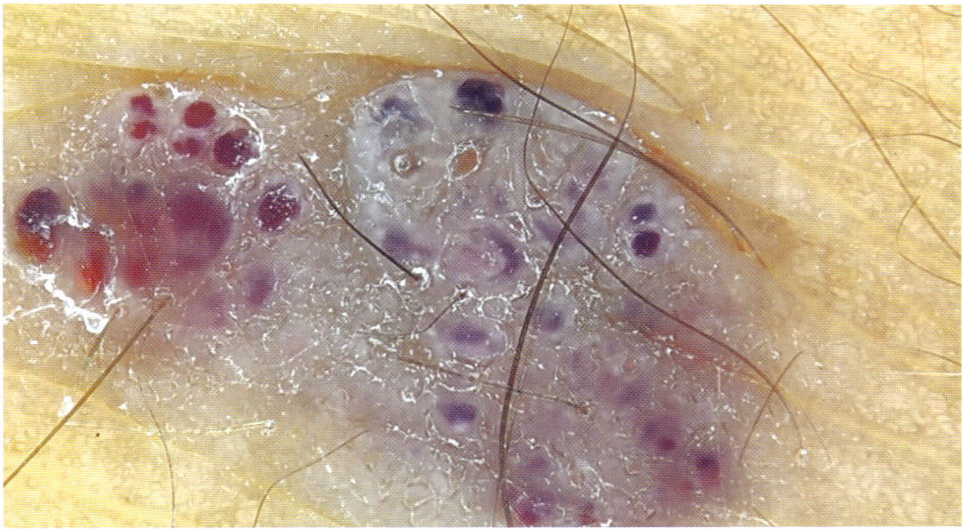

Fig. 8: Red and purple dots and clods. The purple clods represent thrombosed vessels.

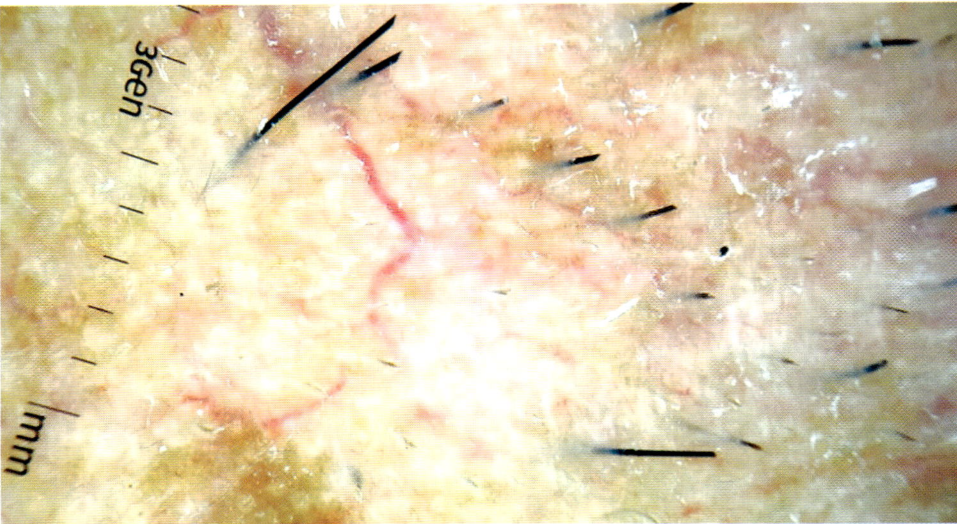

Fig. 9: Linear vessel that is in-focus suggesting the superficial nature of the vessel.

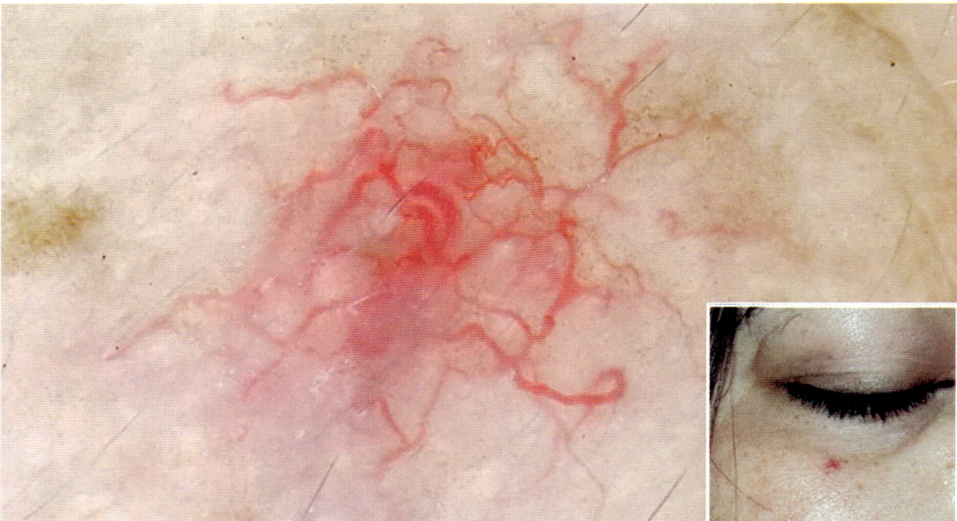

Fig. 10: A case of spider angioma showing radiating bright red in-focus vessels on dermoscopy.

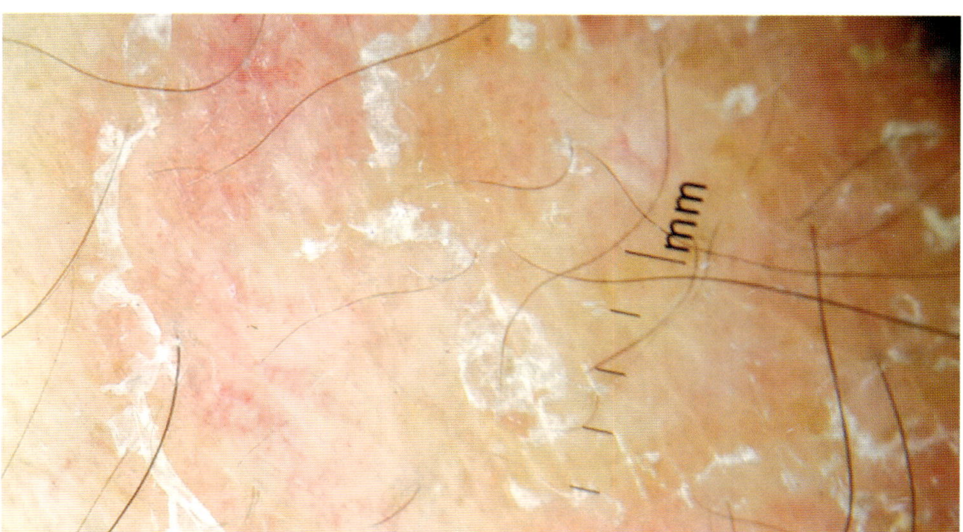

Fig. 11A: An erythematous hue without any well-defined vessels suggesting that the vessels are out of focus due to deeper location.

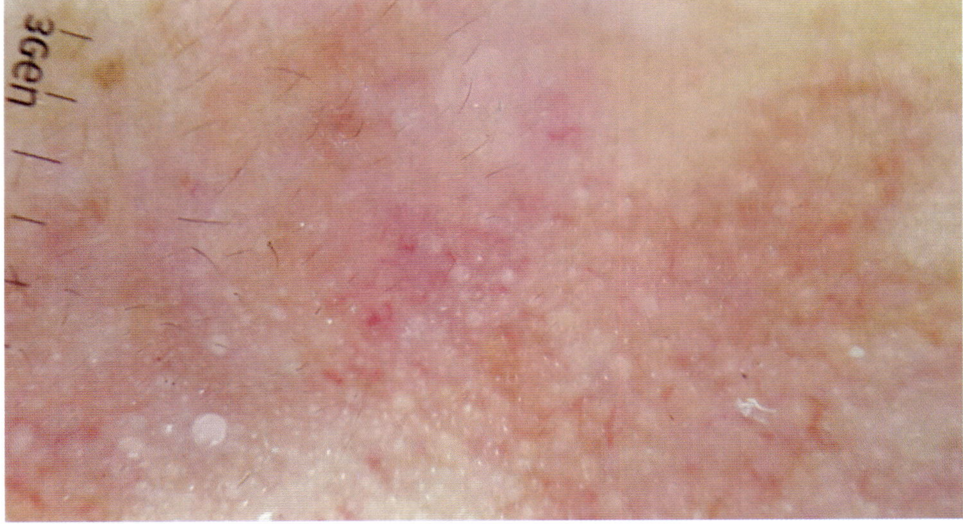

Fig. 11B: Pinkish hue along with out of focus blood vessels suggesting vascular structures are in the deeper dermis.

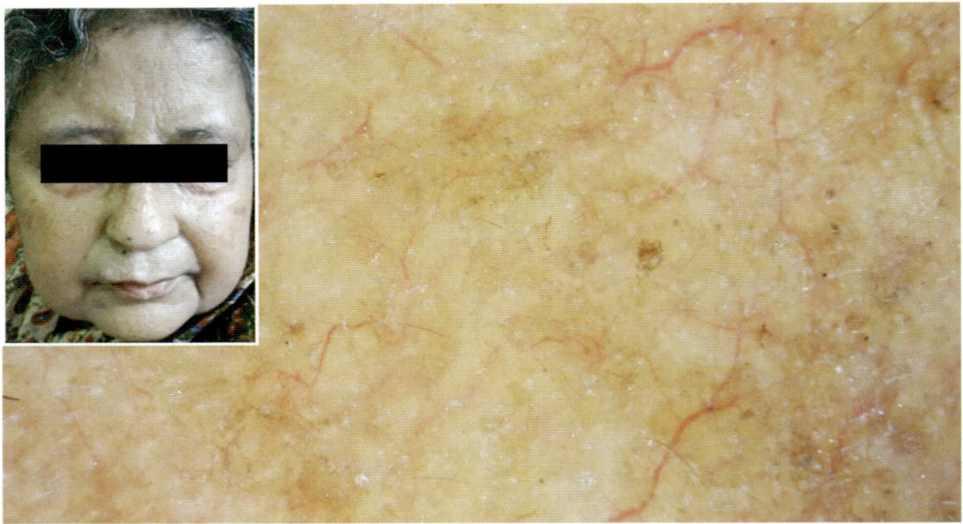

Fig. 12: Marked elastoses in an elderly patient. Note the yellow-orange hue and telangiectasis.

SECTION 3: WHITE SHINY STRUCTURES

INTRODUCTION

- White shiny structures can only be seen under polarized dermoscopy (Figs. 13 to 21).
- They appear as bright, white, shiny structures (Figs. 14, 15, 19, 20 and 21) and can take on a wide range of morphologies depending upon the lesional type. Three types of morphologies have been defined which include (1) white shiny lines, (2) white shiny areas, (3) and rosettes.
- The frequently used term chrysalis is a misnomer for describing the shiny structures and henceforth these structures are referred to as "crystalline structures".[5-7]
- White shiny areas represent white shiny clods/larger structureless areas having a bright shiny appearance.
- Rosettes are characterized by four bright white points grouped together that mimic four-leaf clover (Figs. 13, 16, 17, 18)[8]

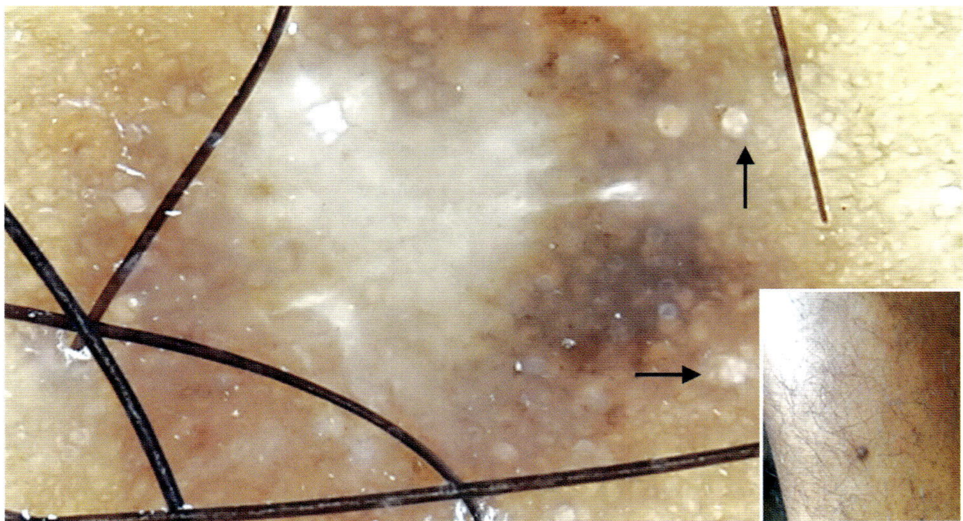

Fig. 13: Central white scar-like areas and rosettes (arrows) in dermatofibroma (DF).

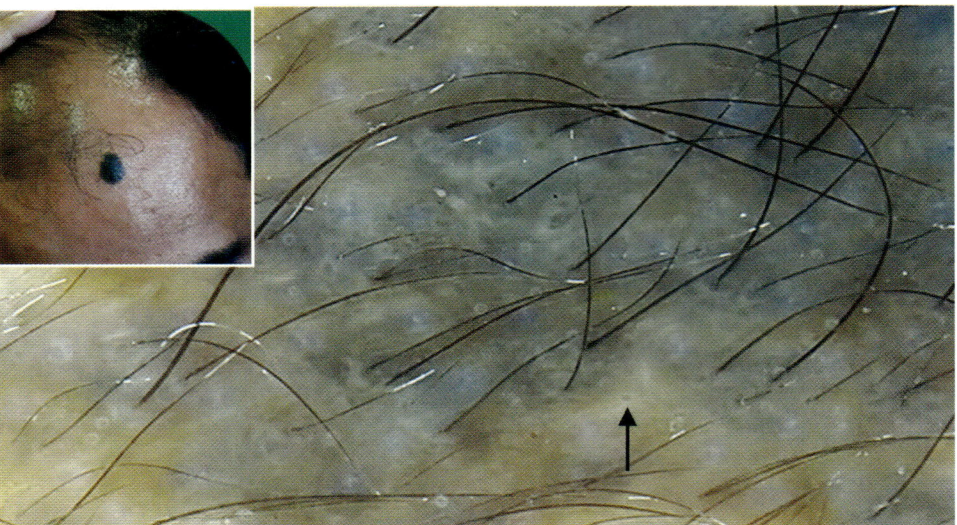

Fig. 14: Congenital melanocytic nevi (CMN) with white shiny lines and areas (arrow).

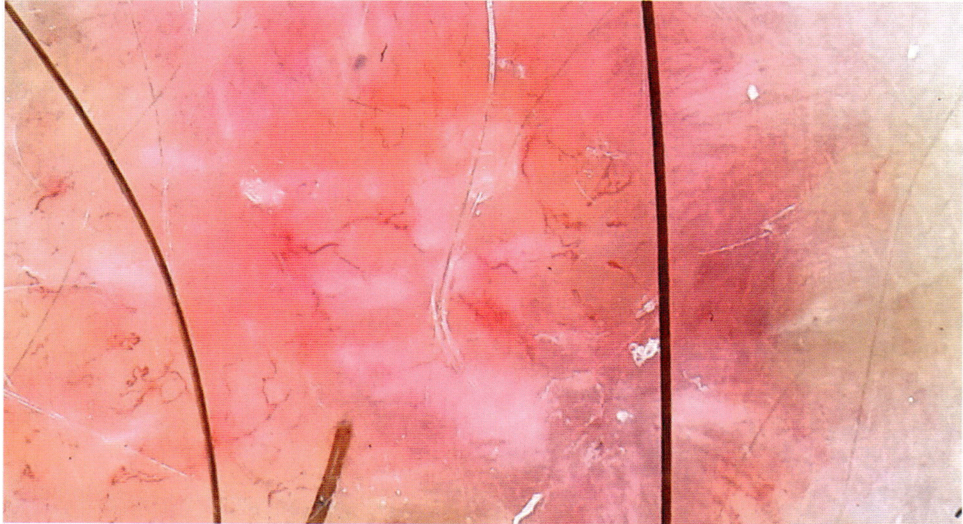

Fig. 15: White shiny structures are also seen in basal cell carcinoma. Note the arborizing blood vessels.

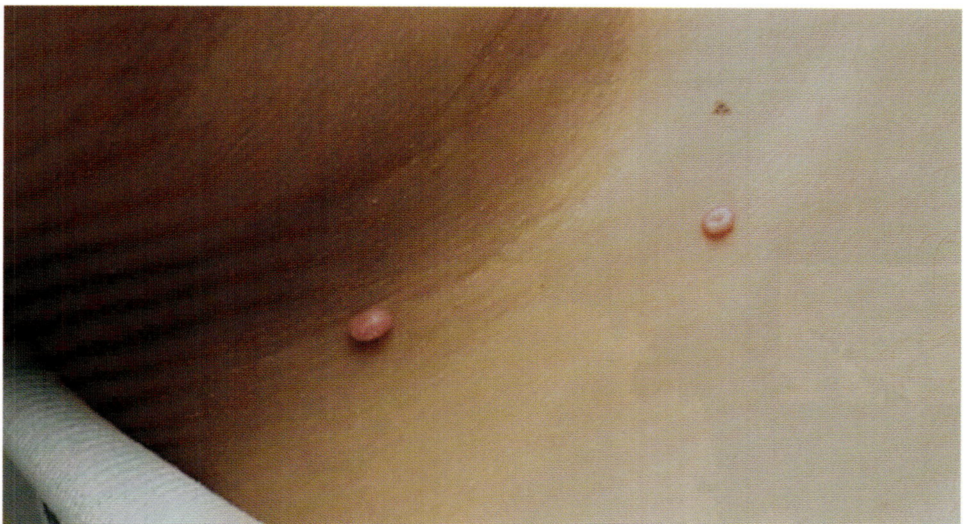

Fig. 16: A child with molluscum contagiosum lesions on the neck and upper chest area.

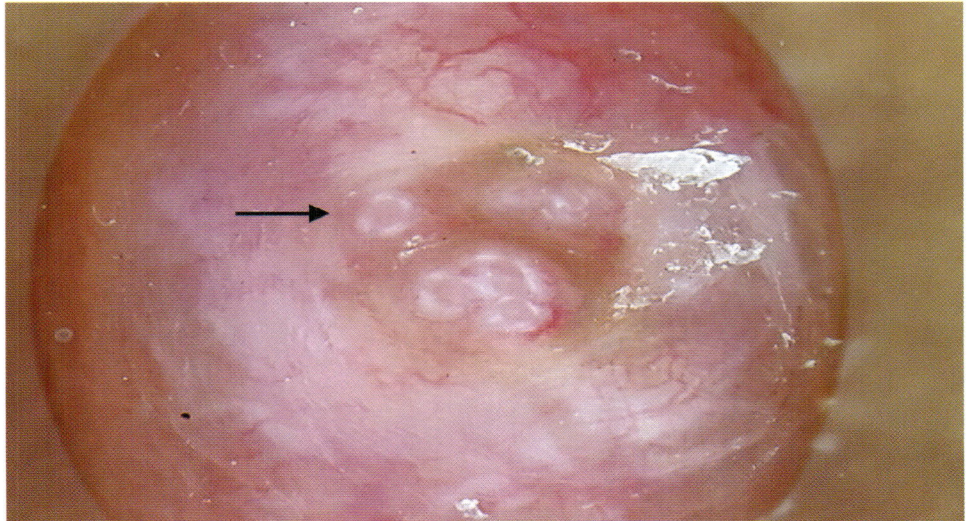

Fig. 17: Note the rosettes (arrow) in addition to crown vessels and central yellow white area (Previous patient).

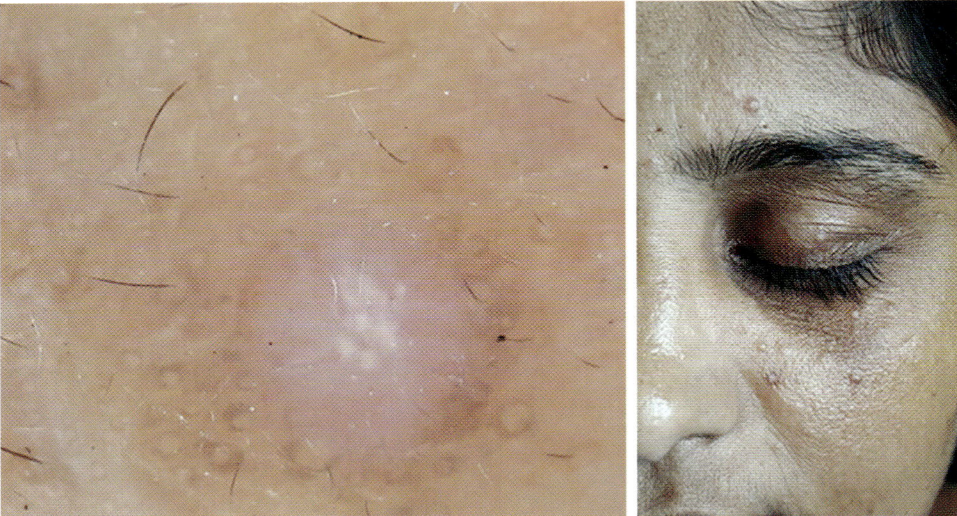

Fig. 18: A case of papular sarcoid showing skin colored smooth surfaced flat-topped papules on the face. Note the prominent rosette against a faint pink background.

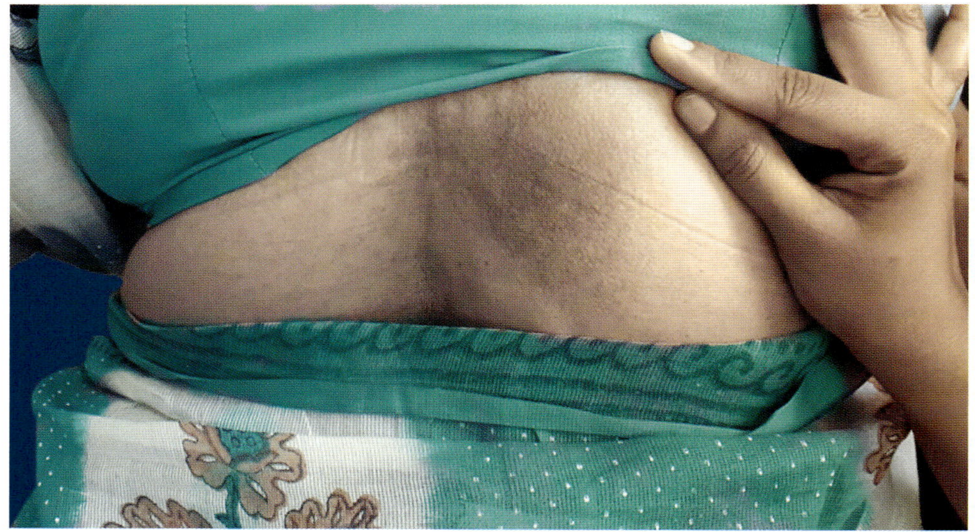

Fig. 19: A case of notalgia paresthetica (NP) in an elderly lady. NP usually presents unilaterally which clinically mimics macular amyloidosis (MA). The main difference with MA is its unilateral presentation and some associated symptoms like itching, burning, and unusual sensations. The most accepted hypothesis is compression of the nerves at the vertebral spinous openings.

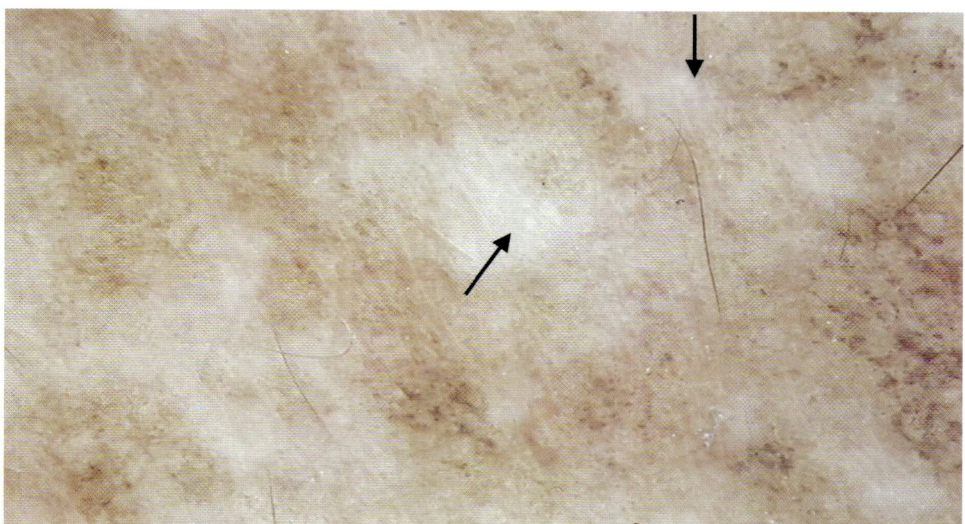

Fig. 20: (Dermoscopy of previous patient) White shiny streaks shown by arrows represent amyloid fibrils which due to its birefringent property under polarized light present as shiny white structures.

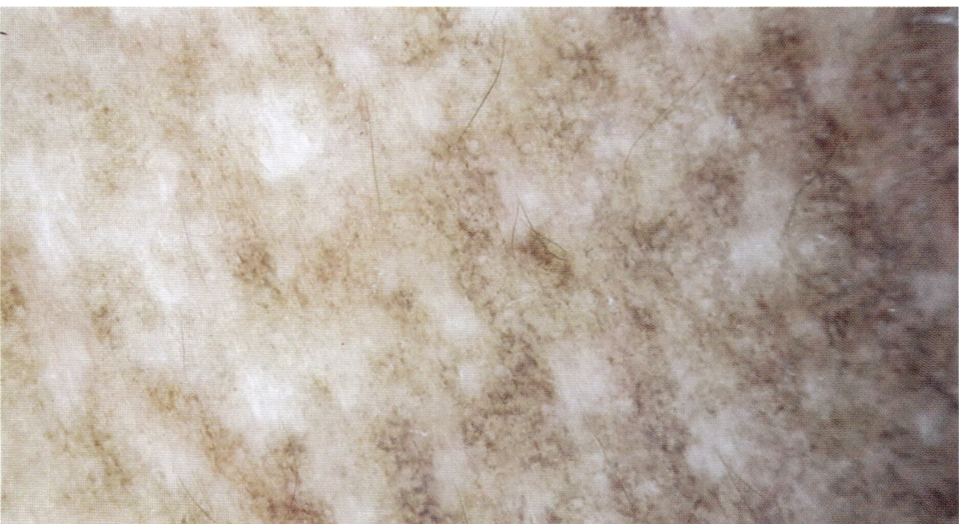

Fig. 21: Another field showing shiny white streaks. Pigmentation of various patterns revealed by dermoscopy corresponds to the basal pigmentation and scattered melanophages or pigmentary incontinence.

REFERENCES

5. Marghoob AA, Cowell L, Kopf AW, et al. Observation of chrysalis structures with polarized dermoscopy. Arch Dermatol. 2009;145:618.
6. Di Stefani A, Campbell TM, Malvehy J, et al. Shiny white streaks: an additional dermoscopic finding in melanomas viewed using contact polarised dermoscopy. Australas J Dermatol. 2010;51:295-8.
7. Liebman TN, Rabinovitz HS, Dusza SW, et al. White shiny structures: dermoscopic features revealed under polarized light. J Eur Acad Dermatol Venereol. 2012;26:1493-7.
8. Cuellar F, Vilalta A, Puig S, et al. New dermoscopic pattern in actinic keratosis and related conditions. Arch Dermatol. 2009;145:732.

SECTION 4: YELLOW AND ORANGE COLOR

INTRODUCTION

In clinical dermatology, color plays an important role to aid the diagnosis of a particular condition. For example, blue color has been associated with cyanosis, red color with inflammation, lilac color in morphea, and violaceous hue in lichen planus. Similarly in dermoscopy, color can provide a clue towards the dermatological diagnosis or can be an adjunct in the diagnosis. Thus, yellow and orange may serve as very important clues to the diagnosis. Way back dermoscopic diagnosis started with the recognition of different colors for melanoma.

We have classified the yellow-orange structures into three categories summarizing the features of the commonly encountered conditions.

Common yellow conditions seen in dermoscopy:

1. *Sebaceous hyperplasia*: Crown vessels and yellow lobular structures.[9]
2. *Nevus sebaceous of Jadassohn*: Peripheral telangiectasia and yellow lobular-like structure.
3. *Callus and clavus (corn)*: Callus—homogeneous yellow color and clavus—translucent core and yellow rim.[10]
4. *Pityriasis rosea*: Patchy dotted vessels with peripheral white scales and an orange yellow background.[11]
5. *Seborrheic dermatitis*: Yellowish scales and multicomponent vessels.[12]
6. *Nummular eczema*: Yellow clods and patchy dotted vessels.[13]
7. *Solar elastosis*: Waxy tone, homogeneous yellow background.[10]
8. *Juvenile xanthogranuloma*: Clouds of pale yellow globules/setting sun appearance but please note that in brown skin, a setting sun appearance is rarely seen and mostly we get clouds of pale yellow globules.[14]
9. *Yellow tattoo*: Homogeneous yellow area usually mixed with other colors like orange and black.
10. *Milia*: Homogeneous yellow white areas with linear arborizing vessels crossing the surface of the lesion.[15]
11. *Cutaneous lymphangioma circumscriptum*: Whitish-yellow lacunae with paler septa and hypopyon-like structure.[16]

Common orange conditions seen in dermoscopy:

1. Juvenile xanthogranuloma.
2. *Pigmented purpuric dermatoses*: Purpuric dots and globules and orange brown/orange yellow background.[17]
3. *Extragenital bullous lichen sclerosus*: Orange-yellow areas, white shiny structures, follicular plugging, and white shiny areas.
4. Granulomatous lesions like lupus vulgaris, granulomatous rosacea, necrobiosis lipoidica, sarcoidosis, granuloma annulare, cutaneous leishmaniasis; the hallmark of granulomatous skin disease is the orange yellow patches under dermoscopy, linear or branching vessels may be associated.[17]

Conditions where both yellow and orange are seen simultaneously under dermoscope:

- Granulomatous diseases such as cutaneous sarcoidosis, lupus vulgaris, cutaneous leishmaniasis, and granulomatous rosacea. Linear/branching vessels are typical additional feature of the above diseases under dermoscopy. However, a biopsy is the gold standard to differentiate between these entities.

  Although granuloma annulare represents nonspecific features on dermoscopy, the fact that usually it does not exhibit yellow-orange patches might help to rule out above granulomatous conditions[17] (Figs. 22 to 30).
- Juvenile xanthogranuloma
- Tattoo
- Pityriasis rosea
- Solar elastosis
- Cutaneous mastocytosis.

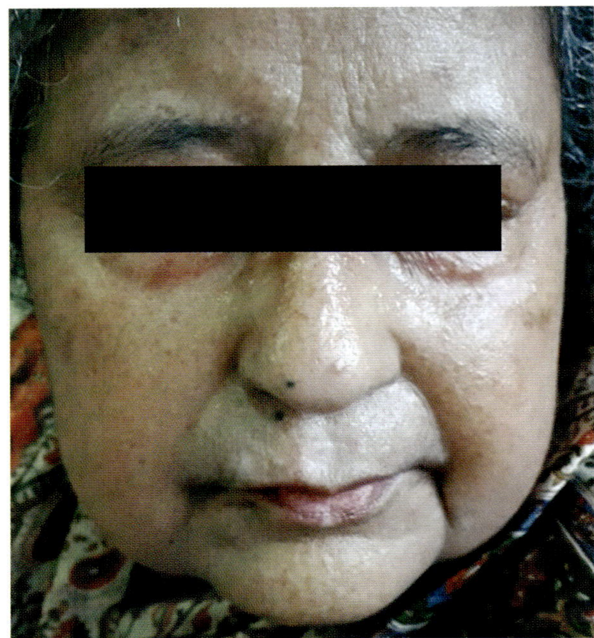

Fig. 22: Solar elastosis occurs as a result of the cumulative effects of prolonged and excessive sun exposure a process known as photoaging. On histopathology, dermis shows an accumulation of abnormal elastin. This 68-year-old lady shows yellow and thickened appearance of her skin with a waxy tone as a result of sun damage.

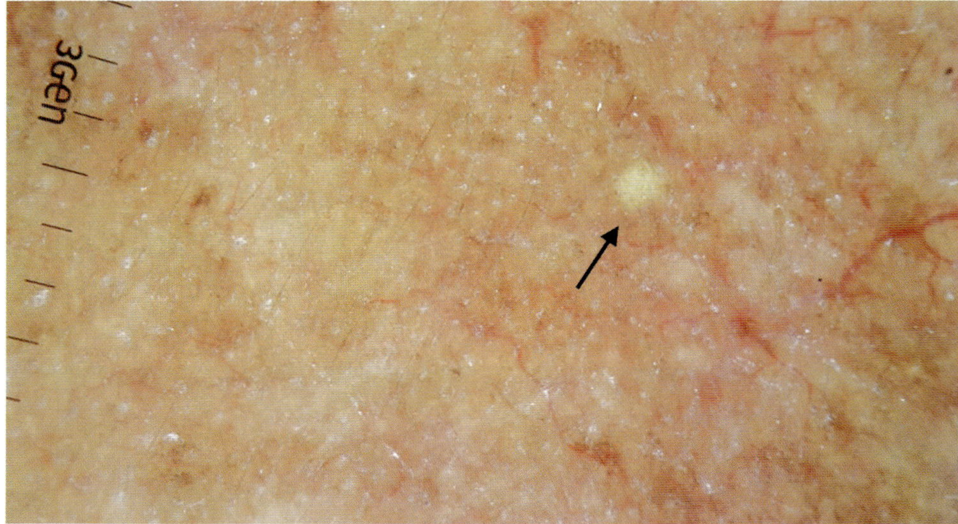

Fig. 23: Dermoscopy of the previous patient shows yellowish orange background with prominent telangiectasias seen in solar elastosis. A milium with a uniform yellow color is also visible in the field (arrow).

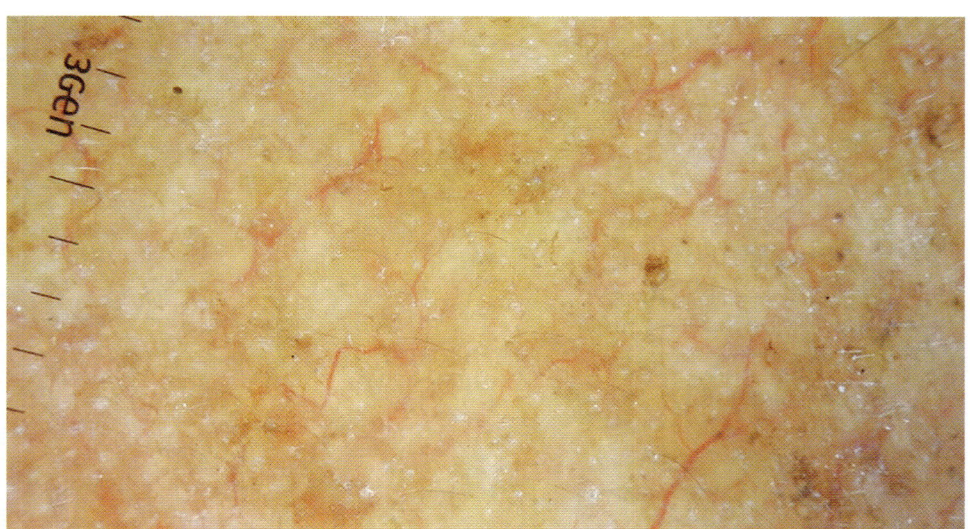

Fig. 24: Another field showing that the linear telangiectatic vessels are in focus suggesting they are superficial against a yellow orange background.

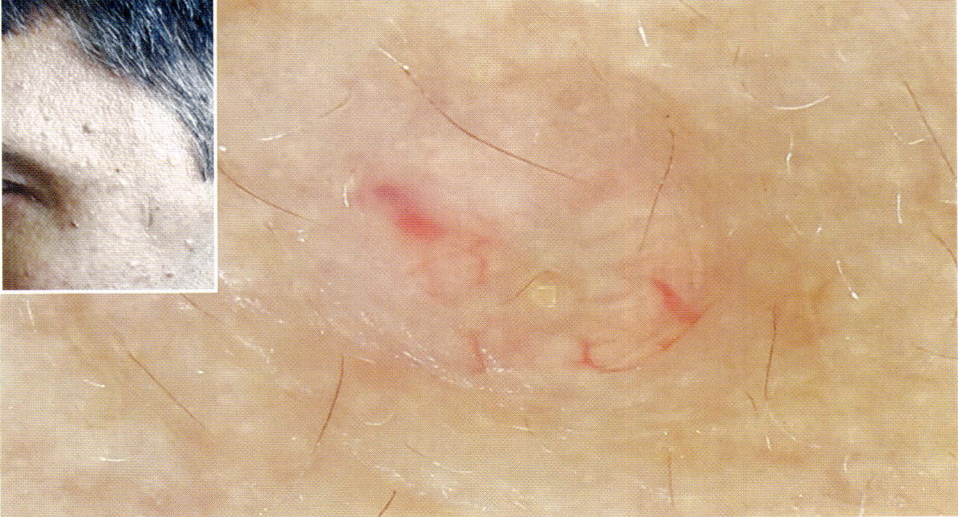

Fig. 25: This 49-year-old man shows multiple skin-colored waxy papules over the left temporal area. On dermoscopy, crown vessels are seen with well-demarcated yellow lobules suggestive of sebaceous hyperplasia.

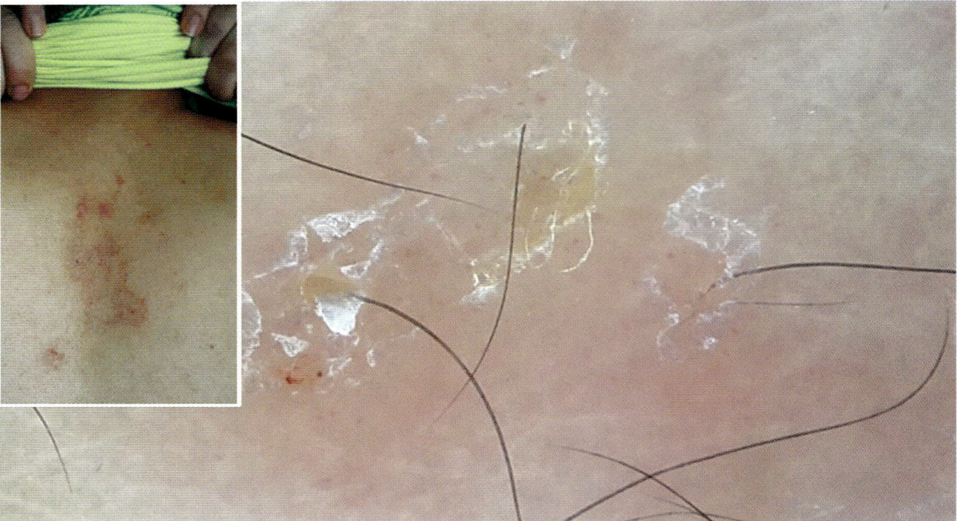

Fig. 26: On dermoscopy seborrheic dermatitis of the interscapular area reveals yellowish scales and some vascular patterns.

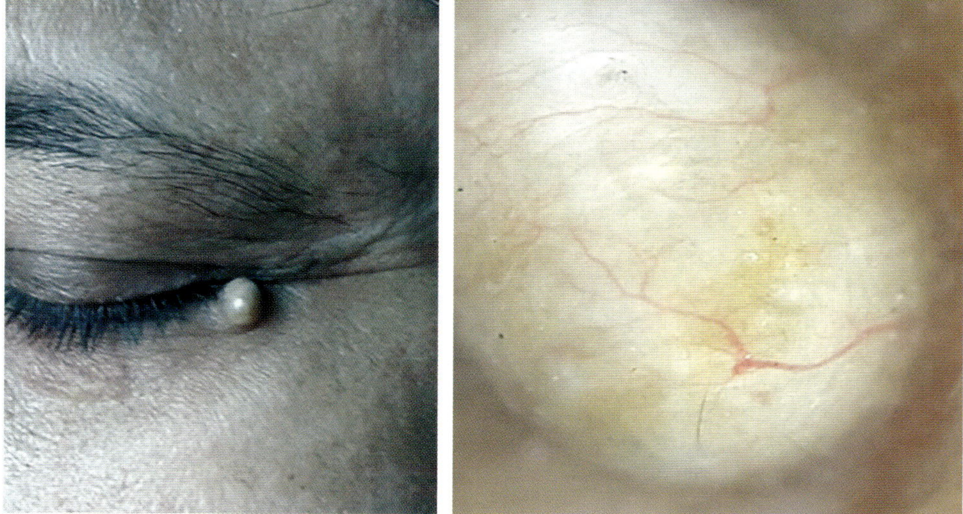

Fig. 27: A milium demonstrating yellow white structureless areas with linear arborizing vessels crossing the surface of the lesion.

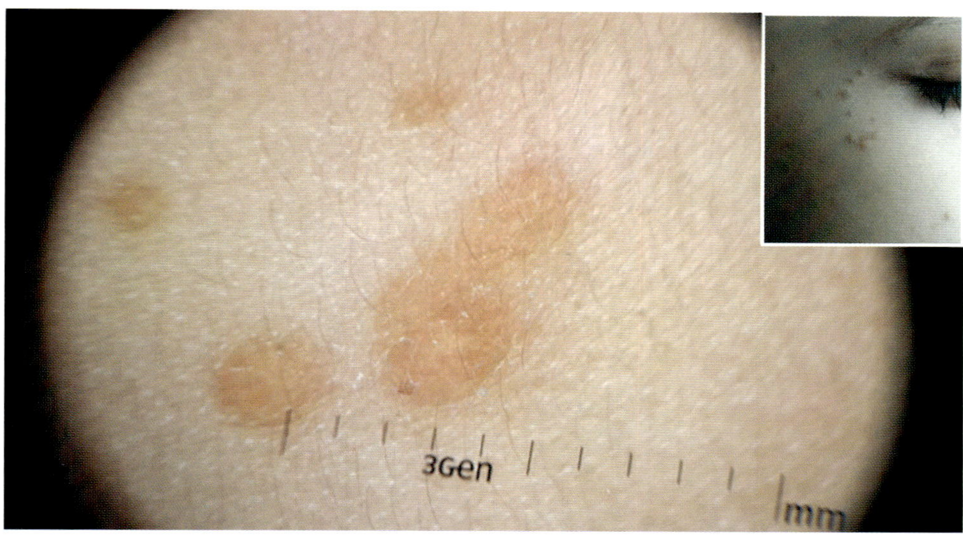

Fig. 28: Juvenile xanthogranuloma on dermoscopy shows yellow cloud-like appearance. Please note that classical description of setting sun appearance may not be appreciable in the skin of color.

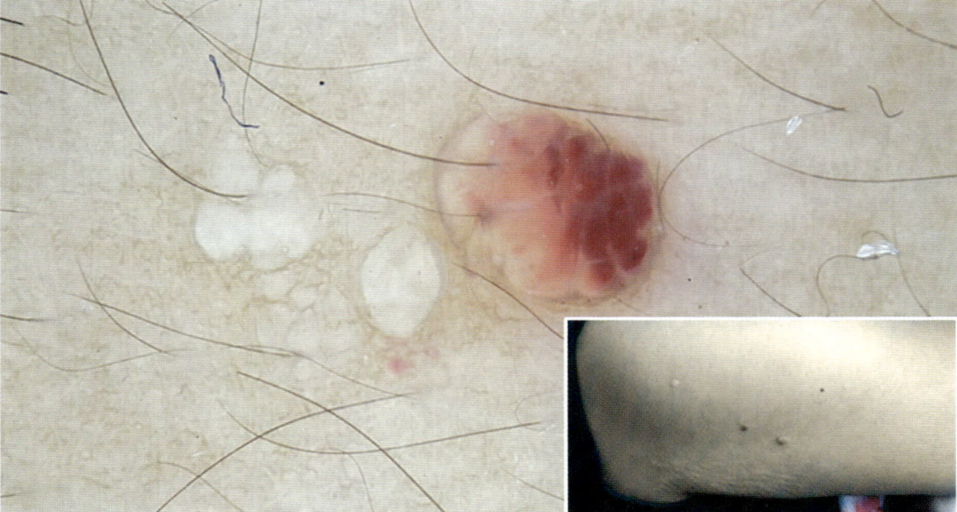

Fig. 29: Dermoscopy of lymphangioma circumscriptum reveals yellow lacunae with septa. Note one red hypopyon-like structure at the center of the dermoscopic field.

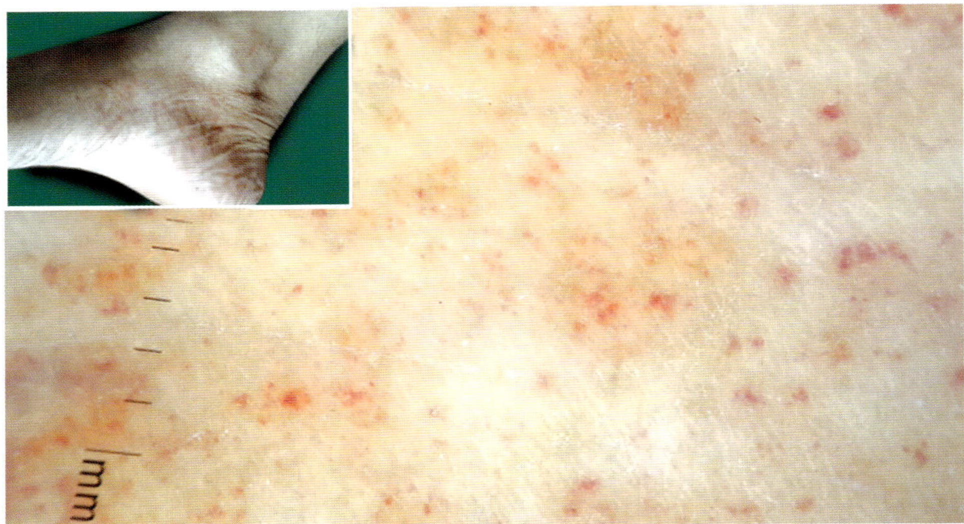

Fig. 30: Pigmented purpuric dermatoses showing yellow-brown/yellow-orange areas with red clods suggestive of purpura.

DISCUSSION

These colors seen under dermoscopy provide a clue to the diagnosis. The origin of these colors has not been fully explored till date. Lipid laden macrophages may explain the yellow color of xanthomas whereas at other times quinacrine and bilirubin may be responsible for the yellowish discoloration of the skin.

Color in skin lesions through dermoscopy can provide important clue for morphological information (Table 1).

Table 1: Color in skin lesions through dermoscopy.

Location on the skin	*Color on dermoscopy*
Stratum corneum	Yellow
Areas of sebaceous differentiation	Yellow/yellow hue
Blood vessels and vascular volume	Red/pink hue
Fibrosis, alteration in collagen matrix, keratinous cysts	White
Coagulated blood	Jet black color
Serum in erosions or superficial ulcers	Orange hue
The detailed account of brown, black, blue and gray colors has been discussed in the "Melanin module"	

There is difficulty in distinguishing yellow and orange color more often than not and especially this fact is more complicated in the skin of color where since the melanocytes predominate, the orange color is easily masked, as in juvenile xanthogranuloma; sunset appearance which consists of orange hue is rarely seen.

KEYNOTES

The take home points with clinical relevance of color in dermoscopy are the following:
Dermoscopic yellow color has been linked to keratin and lipids. Consequently this color is seen most frequently in tumors with sebaceous differentiation, juvenile xanthogranuloma, and keratinizing tumors, whereas orange color has been attributed to granulomatous skin diseases.

REFERENCES

9. Oztas P, Polat M, Oztas M, et al. Bonbon toffee sign: a new dermatoscopic feature for sebaceous hyperplasia. J Eur Acad Dermatol Venereol. 2008;22:1200-2.
10. Bae JM, Kang H, Kim HO, et al. Differential diagnosis of plantar wart from corn, callus and healed wart with the aid of dermoscopy. Br J Dermatol. 2009;160:220-2.
11. Errichetti E, Stinco G. Dermoscopy in general dermatology: a practical overview. Dermatol Ther (Heidelb). 2016;6:471-507.
12. Malakar S. Scalp psoriasis, seborrheic dermatitis and sebopsoriaisis. In: Malakar S (Ed). Trichoscopy: A Text and Atlas. 2017. pp. 275-86.
13. Lallas A, Kyrgidis A, Tzellos TG, et al. Accuracy of dermoscopic criteria for the diagnosis of psoriasis, dermatitis, lichen planus and pityriasis rosea. Br J Dermatol. 2012;166:1198-205.
14. Song M, Kim SH, Jung DS, et al. Structural correlations between dermoscopic and histopathological features of juvenile xanthogranuloma. J Eur Acad Dermatol Venereol. 2011;25:259-63.
15. Malakar S, Mukherjee SS. Vascular pattern of milia on dermatoscopy. Our Dermatol Online. 2017;8(4):497-8.
16. Amini S, Kim NH, Zell DS, et al. Dermoscopic-histopathologic correlation of cutaneous lymphangioma circumscriptum. Arch Dermatol. 2008;144:1671-2.
17. Lallas A, Giacomel J, Argenziano G, et al. Dermoscopy in general dermatology: practical tips for the clinician. Br J Dermatol. 2014;170:514-26.

SECTION 5: RAINBOW PATTERN

INTRODUCTION

Recently this pattern has been described as a dermoscopic feature of Kaposi's sarcoma. In this pattern, red to violet colors are juxtaposed next to each other. This pattern is mostly visible under 10× magnification.
Key dermoscopic features of Kaposi's sarcoma:

- Bluish red coloration
- Rainbow pattern
- Scaly surface
- Small brown globules.

DISCUSSION

Hu et al. described rainbow pattern in Kaposi's sarcoma as a specific pattern. Although histology remains the gold standard for diagnosis, they proposed dermoscopic examination as an adjunct to clinical examination may highlight the accuracy in the preoperative diagnosis of Kaposi's sarcoma. But shortly after this report, Cheng et al. encountered the rainbow pattern in some other conditions like stasis dermatitis, lichen planus, hemosiderotic dermatofibroma, and melanoma.

It is postulated that the optical phenomenon of diffraction gives rise to the rainbow pattern. Diffraction refers to the phenomenon of bending of waves around small obstacles or openings. Diffraction causes white light to split when light passes through a series of openings or slits that are closely spaced parallel to each other. Average thickness of endothelial cells is about 200 nm and visible light corresponds to a wavelength of 400–700 nm. Histology of Kaposi's sarcoma shows the vascular lumina lying in back-to-back arrangement. Therefore, the closely set honeycomb like pattern of vascular spaces in Kaposi's sarcoma mimics a diffraction device.

Another hypothesis states that it is a luminescence phenomenon related to light in different states of polarization, and its interaction with superficial and or deep structures within the lesion.

SECTION 6: COLOR AS AN ARTIFACT

INTRODUCTION

Color seen on polarized dermoscopy is due to reflection of light by the structures and components of the skin. For example, altered collagen gives rise to white shiny structures, lipid laden macrophages gives a yellowish hue or deposition of amyloid can give rise to shiny white structures.

Similarly exogenous deposition of chemicals on the skin in the form of makeup, topical applications, home remedies, etc. can give rise to different colors under dermoscope which may mislead the treating physician.

While practicing non-polarized dermoscopy, the addition of linkage fluid also can give rise to similar artifacts. Likewise while investigating an infective condition the use of cellophane paper or glass slide as an interface between the lesion and the face plate of the dermoscope may give rise to variegated colors (Figs. 31 to 34).

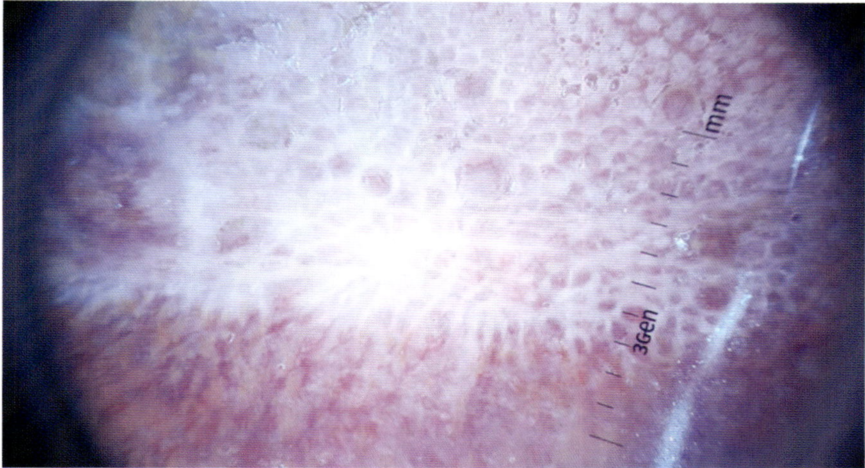

Fig. 31: Dermoscopy of tongue usually is done by putting a glass slide or cellophane paper in-between the dermoscopic lens and the object. The linear blue color light at the right side of the field is a color-artifact.

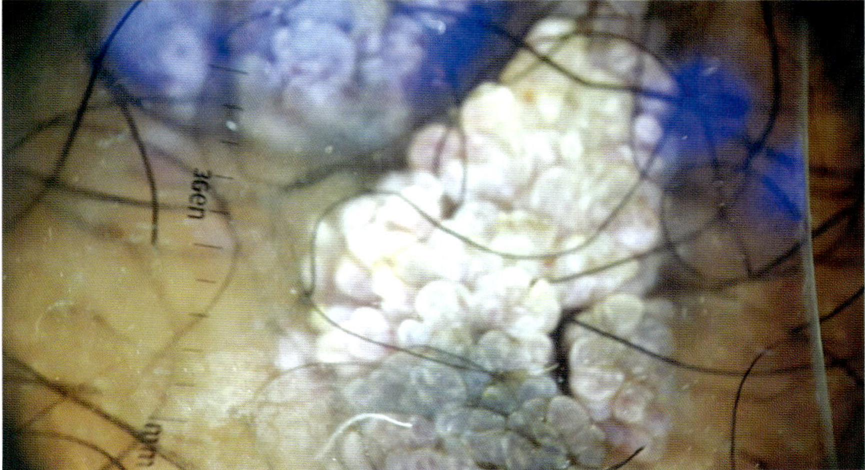

Fig. 32: Anogenital warts should always be examined by putting glass slide between dermoscopic lens and the lesion to avoid transmission of infection. Due to the interaction of polarized light from dermoscope and glass slide the blue light is created which is a color artifact.

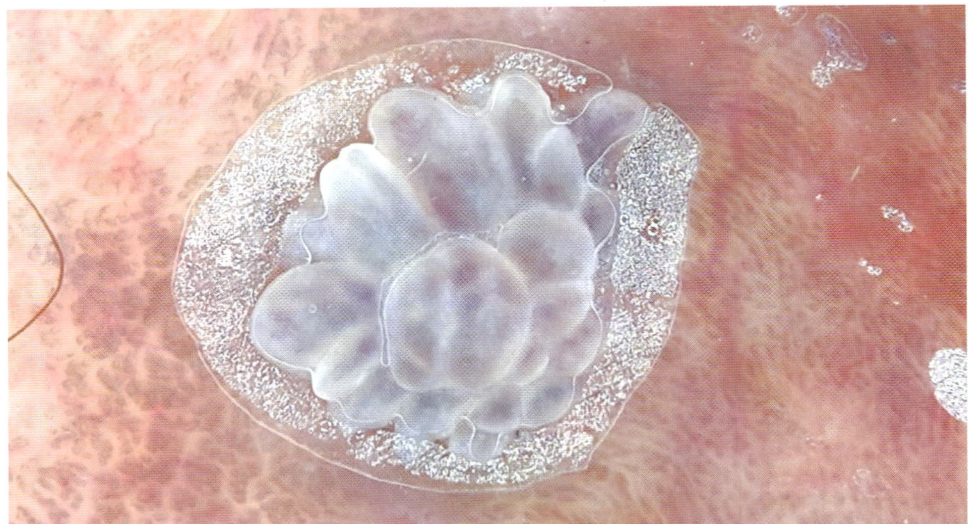

Fig. 33: Appearance of coral is truly an artifact due to the interaction of polarized light from dermoscope and the intervening cellophane paper. Clinically this is a case of condylomata acuminata which is a highly infectious viral infection.

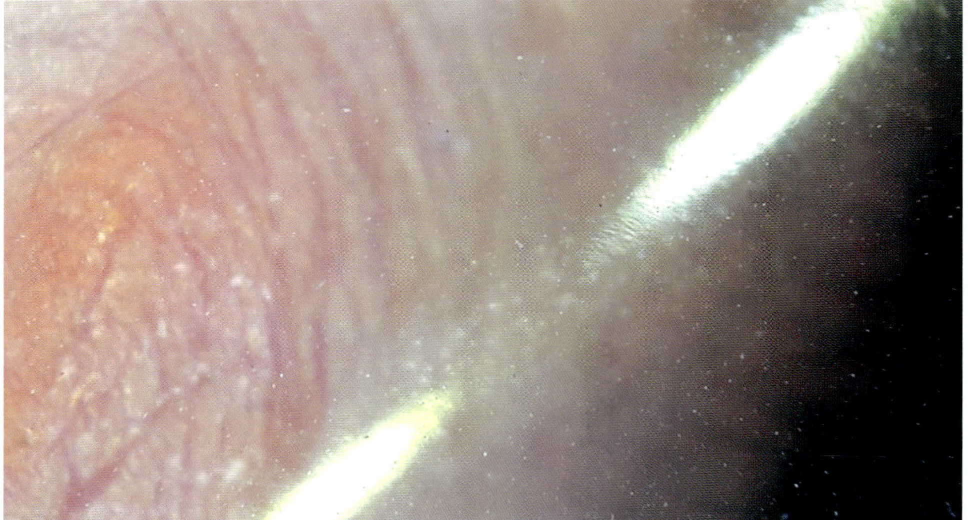

Fig. 34: This diagonal bright color artifact can immediately be recognized.

CHAPTER 7

Papulosquamous Disorders

Subrata Malakar

DERMATITIS

INTRODUCTION

Dermatitis includes a wide spectrum of conditions such as atopic dermatitis, allergic contact dermatitis and nummular eczema.

KEY DERMOSCOPIC FEATURES

- Dotted vessels in a patchy distribution
- Yellow clods (serocrusts).

DISCUSSION

The most noticeable dermoscopic features of dermatitis are dotted vessels in a patchy distribution and yellow serocrust ("yellow clod" sign).[1-3] Depending on disease duration, eczematous dermatitis display a spectrum of scaling and vascular changes with acute exudative lesion predominantly exhibiting yellow serocrusts whereas chronic and lichenified lesions typically show dotted vessel in a patchy distribution with scaling[1,3,4] (Figs. 1 and 2).

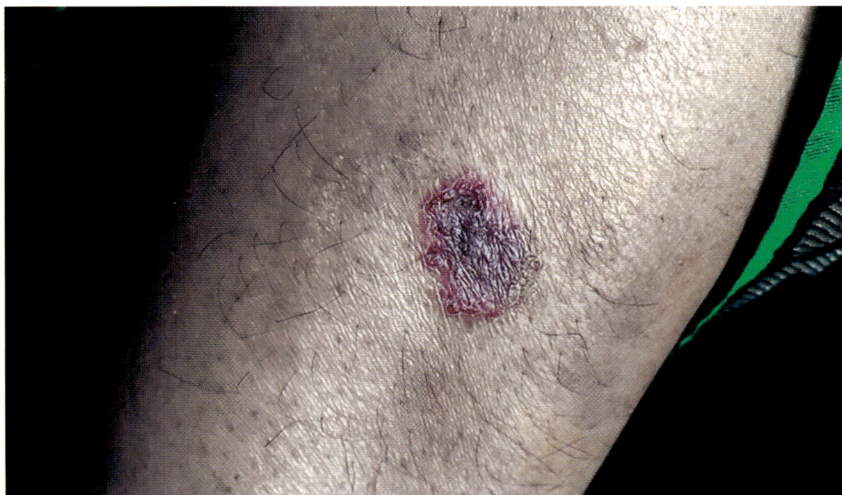

Fig. 1: Nummular dermatitis is an inflammatory condition characterized by the round or oval erythematous desquamative patches or plaques.

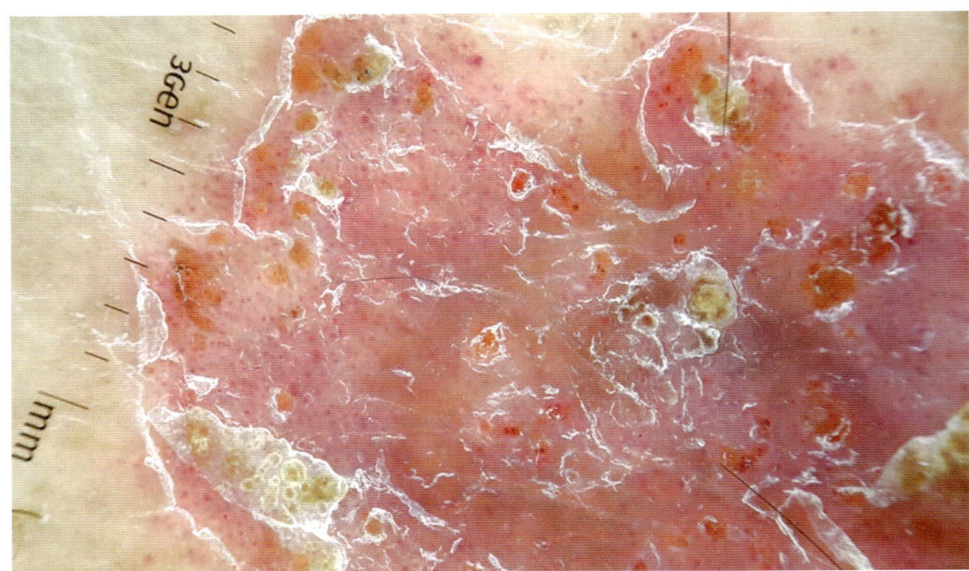

Fig. 2: Dermoscopy shows dotted vessels in a patchy distribution and yellow serocrusts (yellow clods). In chronic and lichenified lesions the yellow clods are not observed.

KEYNOTE

The most useful clues for differentiating dermatitis with other mimickers are the yellow clods and the patchy distribution of dotted vessels.

REFERENCES

1. Lallas A, Kyrgidis A, Tzellos TG, et al. Accuracy of dermoscopic criteria for the diagnosis of psoriasis, dermatitis, lichen planus and pityriasis rosea. Br J Dermatol. 2012;166:1198-205.
2. Lallas A, Argenziano G, Apalla Z, et al. Dermoscopic patterns of common facial inflammatory skin diseases. J Eur Acad Dermatol Venereol. 2013;(in press).
3. Lallas A, Apalla Z, Lefaki I, et al. Dermoscopic patterns of early stage mycosis fungoides. J Eur Acad Dermatol Venereol. 2013;27:617-21.
4. Navarini AA, Feldmeyer L, Tondury B, et al. The yellow clod sign. Arch Dermatol. 2011;147:1350.

LICHEN PLANUS

INTRODUCTION

Dermoscopic findings are confirmatory in the diagnosis of lichen planus (LP) in most of the cases and thus dermoscopy can replace histopathology.

KEY DERMOSCOPIC FEATURES[1,2]

- Wickham's striae (WS)
- Dotted/linear vessels at the periphery of the lesion
- Structureless homogeneous brown-gray areas or gray dots in regressing lesions of LP
- Comedo-like structures in hypertrophic LP
- "Bouquet of white roses."

DISCUSSION

We will follow the five dermoscopic parameters (Table 1) as a guide to describe each lesion of LP.

Table 1: Five dermoscopic parameters.
• Wickham's striae
• Pigment patterns
• Vascular patterns
• Background color
• Special features

The hallmark dermoscopic features of LP are WS which have been regarded as a highly specific and sensitive criterion for its diagnosis. WS appear as pearly whitish structures and may develop thin or broad arboriform projections, surrounded by dotted or linear vessels.[3,4] The morphological pattern of WS is usually reticular (Box 1); the other patterns being linear, round, annular, or displaying a "radial streaming" pattern, "starry sky" pattern or "leaf venation".[3,5,6]

Box 1: The morphological patterns of Wickham's striae (WS). Color of the WS may be white, yellow, and blue-white.
Patterns of Wickham's striae
• Reticular
• Linear
• Radial streaming
• Circular
• Globular
• Perpendicular
• Veil like
• Combined
• Invisible

Wickham's striae correspond histopathologically to compact orthokeratosis overlying the zones of wedge-shaped hypergranulosis.[7]

The main vascular patterns seen on dermoscopy of LP are dotted and linear vessels (Boxes 2 and 3). They are usually localized to the periphery of the lesion.[3,4] The background is commonly violet, pink or reddish.

The regressing lesions of LP show either structureless homogeneous brown-gray areas or gray dots (Box 4).[8] The gray dots correspond histopathologically to melanophages in the dermis. These two dermoscopic patterns of regressing LP help in monitoring and follow-up of the disease. The gray dots reflect persisting lesions whereas the homogeneous pattern tends to be self-limiting and transient.

Some special patterns such as "bouquet of white roses", pallisade pigmentation and red starburst pattern are also observed (Box 5).

Box 2: Vascular patterns of lichen planus.

- Red dots and globules
- Radial linear
- Peripheral homogeneous

Box 3: Background color.

- Violet
- Red
- Pink
- Brown
- Black
- Yellow

Box 4: Pigment patterns of lichen planus.

- Dots and globules
- Peppering
- Perifollicular
- Circular
- Homogeneous cloud like
- Circular
- Cobblestone

Box 5: Special patterns.

- Bouquet of white roses
- Starburst pattern
- Comedo-like structures

CASE 1 (FIGS. 3A AND B)

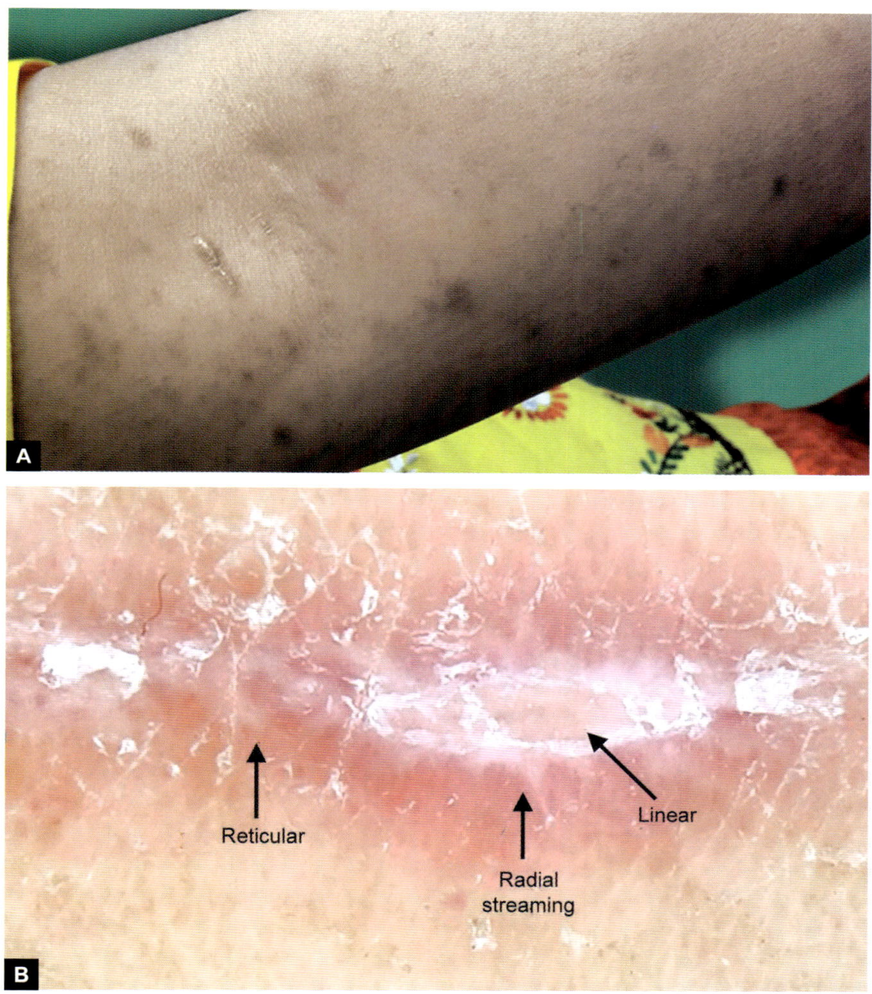

Figs. 3A and B: Lichen planus (LP) commonly starts developing on the flexural surfaces of the limbs. After a few weeks it starts spreading and a generalized eruption develops within a month or two. In more than 50% of patients, the lesions resolve within 6 months. Koebnerization is seen in this patient in the antecubital fossa (A); The surface of LP may exhibit white lines in a variable configuration known as Wickhams striae (WS) that correspond to orthokeratosis with underlying wedge-shaped hypergranulosis.[7-10] Dermoscopy in this patient shows combination of linear, radial streaming and reticular WS (B).

CASE 2 (FIGS. 4A TO C)[7,9]

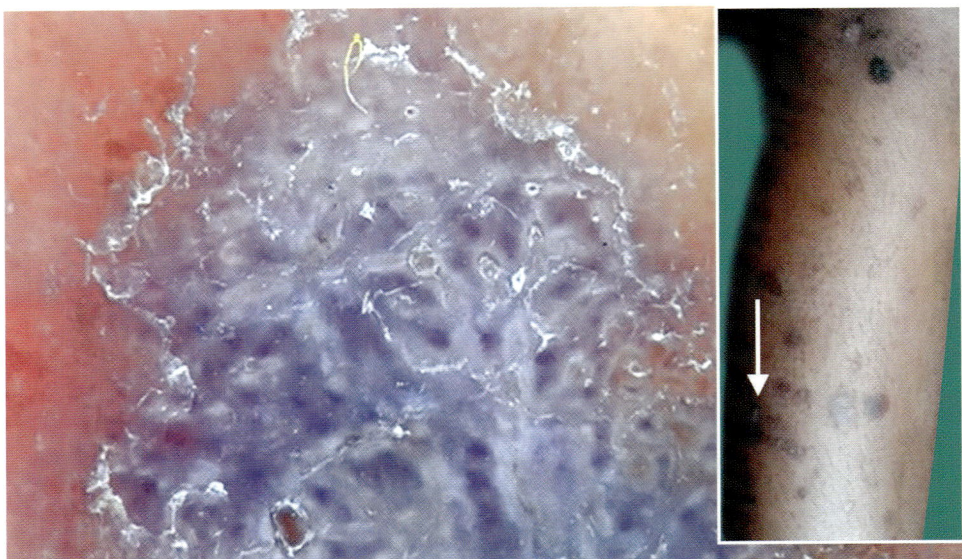

Fig. 4A: Patient of LP frequently shows active and healed lesions together. The papular lesion (arrow) on dermoscopy reveals WS in reticular pattern. This pattern is often seen in classical LP. WS is typically observed as white crossing lines and defined as "reticular pattern WS".

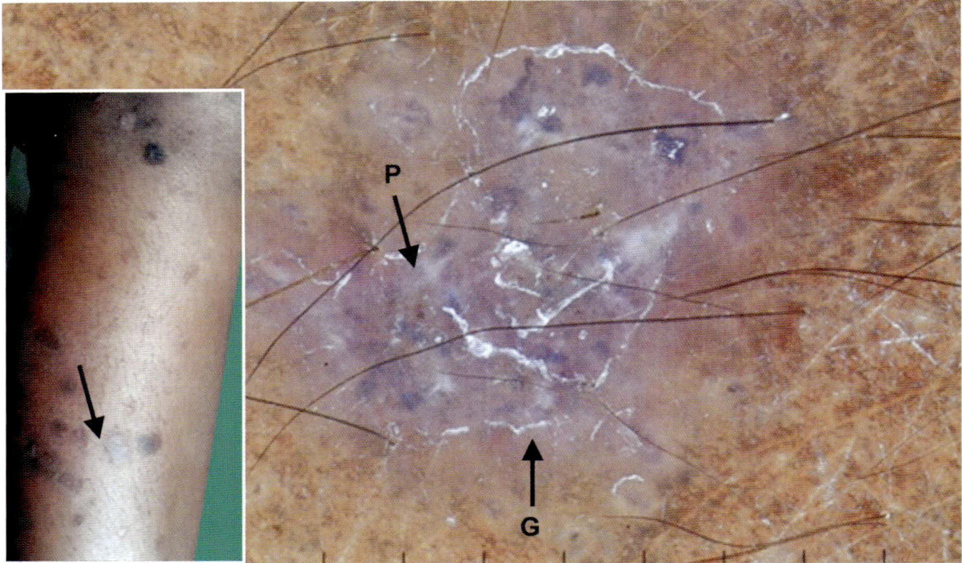

Fig. 4B: This healed lesion of LP (arrow) on dermoscopy shows white veil-like WS, perpendicular (P) and globular (G) WS. Pigment patterns observed are dots and globules, and pigment clods.

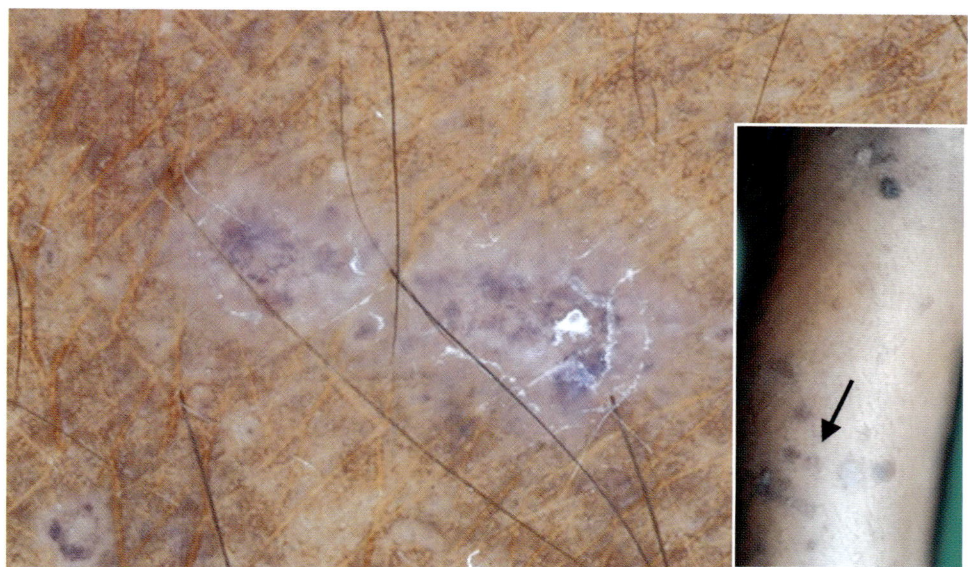

Fig. 4C: Dual lesions which have healed (arrow); on dermoscopy shows similar findings as the previous image. White veil-like is the predominant WS pattern; other WS patterns have almost resolved proving the fact that WS can be used as an activity marker.

CASE 3 (FIG. 5)

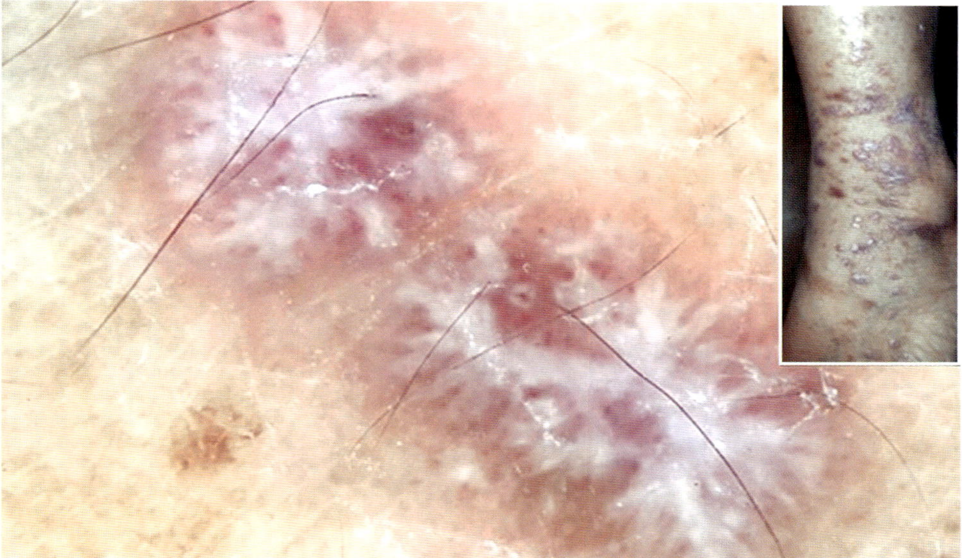

Fig. 5: A patient of classical lichen planus (LP) on dermoscopy shows radial streaming Wickham's striae (WS), erythematous background and peripheral red dots.

CASE 4 (FIG. 6)

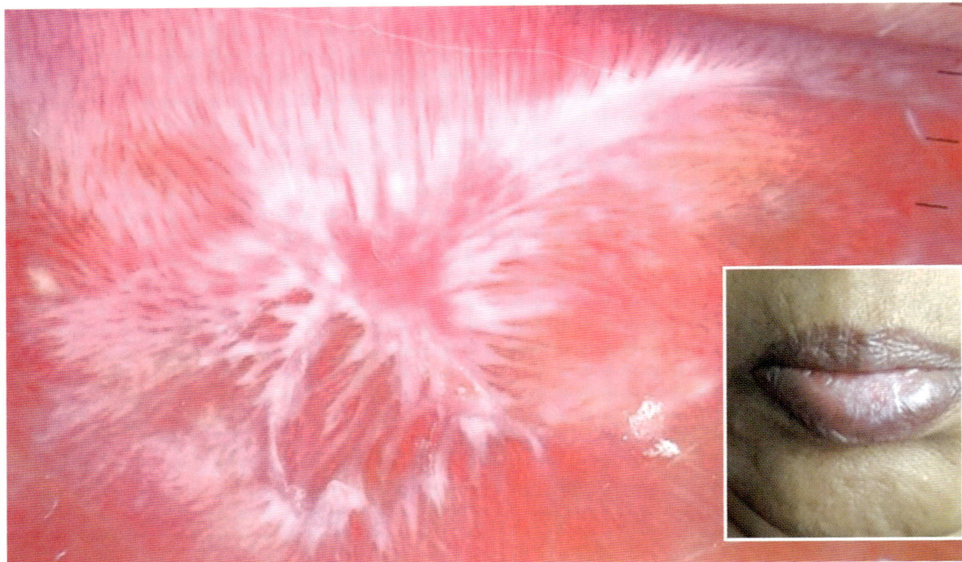

Fig. 6: Mucosal lichen planus (LP) has a variety of clinical presentations such as white striations, papules or plaques on labial mucosa, tongue or buccal mucosa. Erythema, erosion, and ulceration may also be present. A plaque of LP on lower labial mucosa of this lady on dermoscopy shows radial streaming Wickham's striae (WS) with peripheral linear vessels perpendicular to WS. Hairpin vessels are also obvious surrounding the radial streaming.

CASE 5 (FIG. 7)

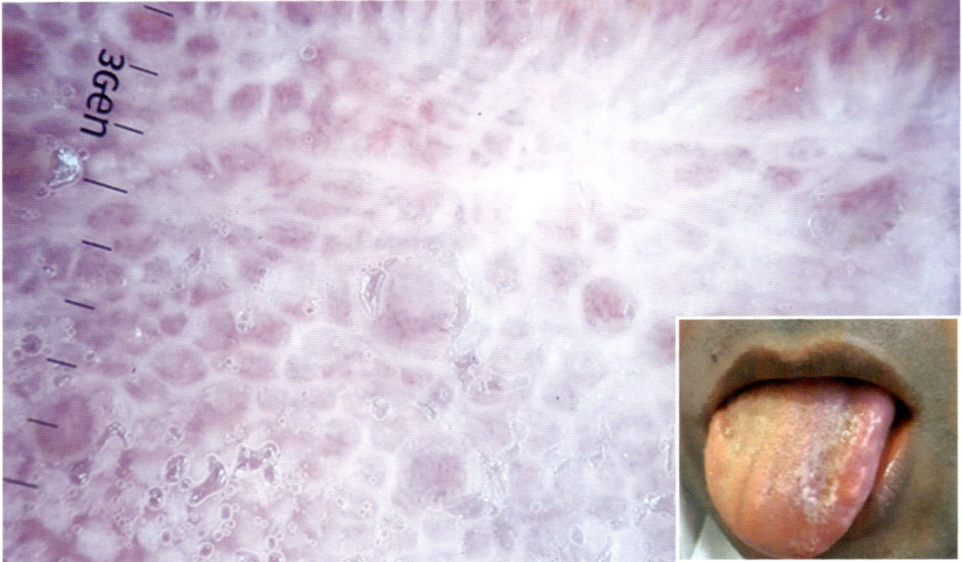

Fig. 7: A plaque of lichen planus (LP) on the left side of anterior tongue. A glass slide is used in-between the lens of the dermoscope and the tongue to avoid direct contact. Reticular pattern Wickham's striae (WS) is observed in the entire field.

CASE 6 (FIG. 8)

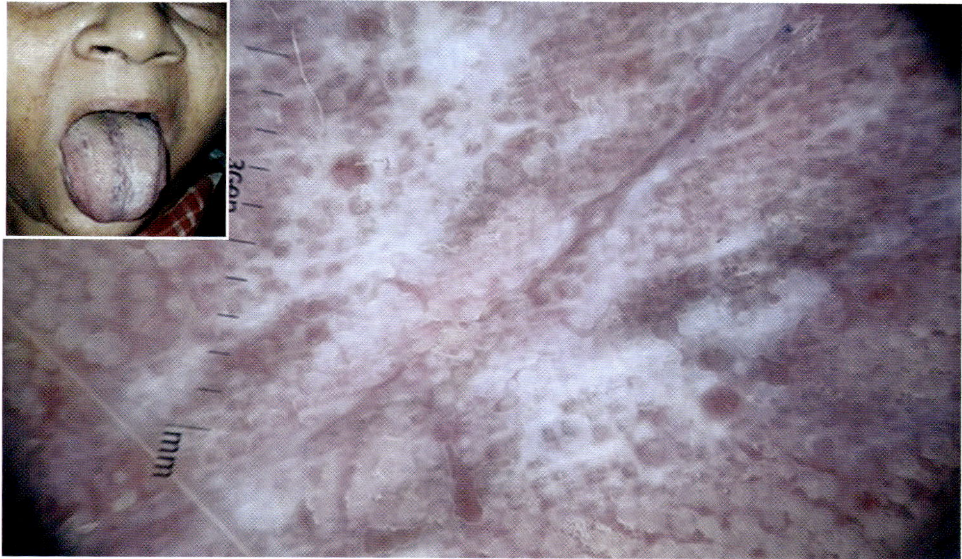

Fig. 8: The lady presented with a white plaque over the tongue for the last 7 months. On dermoscopy, patchy reticular pattern of Wickham's striae (WS) was observed confirming the diagnosis of oral lichen planus.

CASE 7 (FIG. 9)

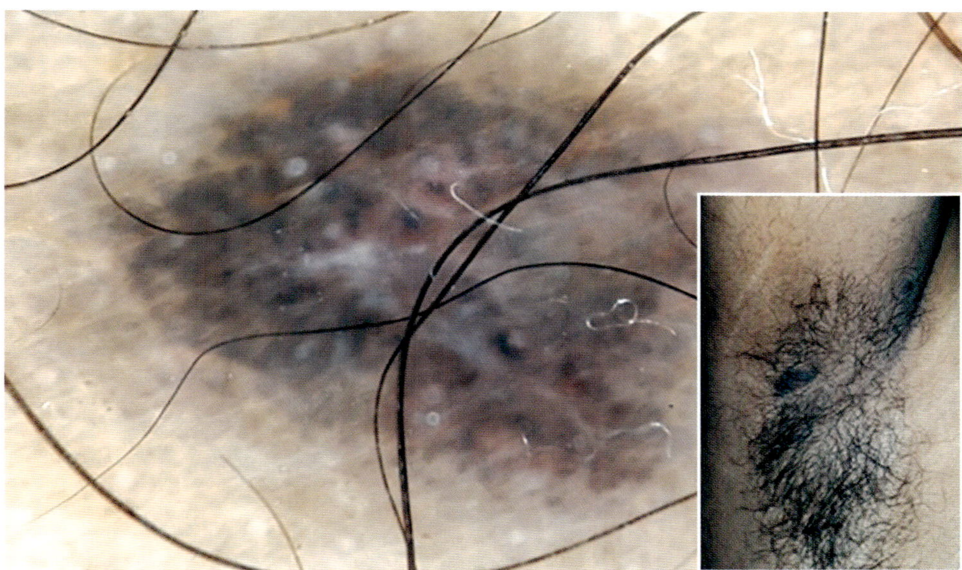

Fig. 9: A 42-year-old male presented with a small hyperpigmented plaque on the right axilla. A combination of linear, perpendicular, and veil-like Wickham's striae (WS) was found on dermoscopic examination. Background color is black. After careful examination, few classical lesions of lichen planus (LP) were found in the lower extremity, which also showed WS dermoscopically.

CASE 8 (FIG. 10)

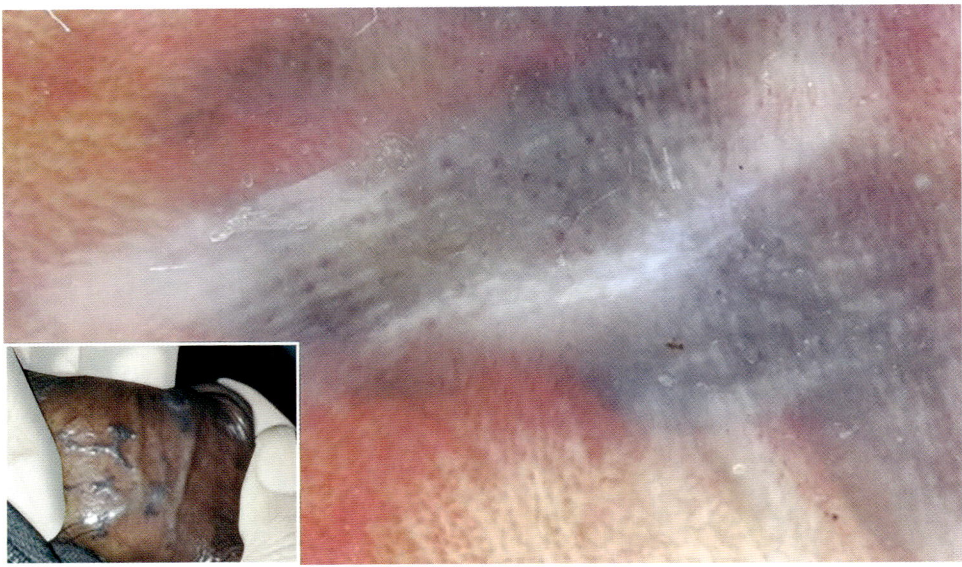

Fig. 10: Lichen planus (LP) on the prepuce and glans penis for the past 6 months. Dermoscopy reveals linear and veil-like Wickham's striae (WS) and dotted vessels at the periphery; the background has a violet and black hue.

CASE 9 (FIGS. 11A AND B)

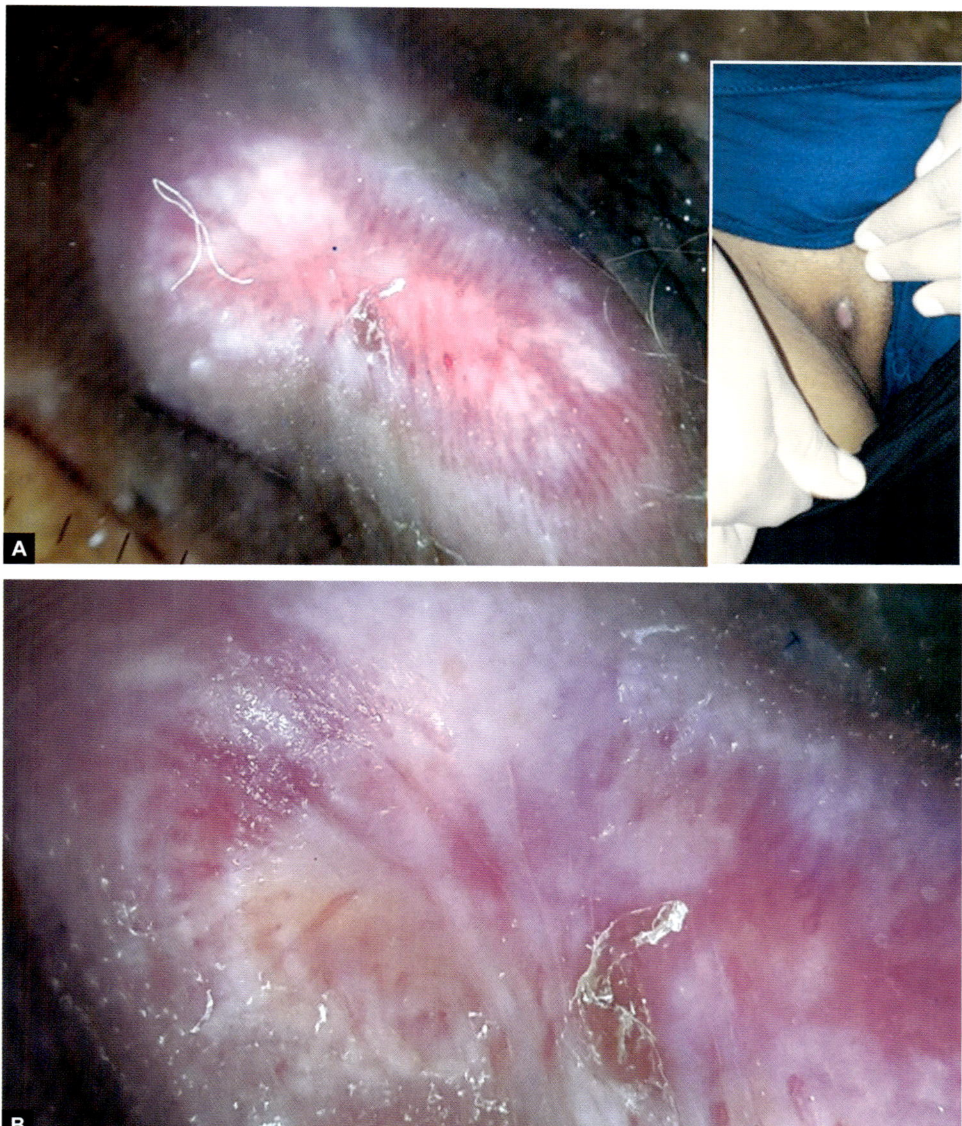

Figs. 11A and B: (A) Small itchy plaque on the vulva for 5 months. Dermoscopy demonstrates radial streaming Wickham's striae (WS) with peripheral linear vessels against a violaceous background. Histopathology confirmed the diagnosis of lichen planus; (B) Magnified view showing peripheral linear vessels, which appear as hairpin vascular pattern. Radial WS and violaceous background are more prominent in this image.

CASE 10 (FIGS. 12A TO F)[2]

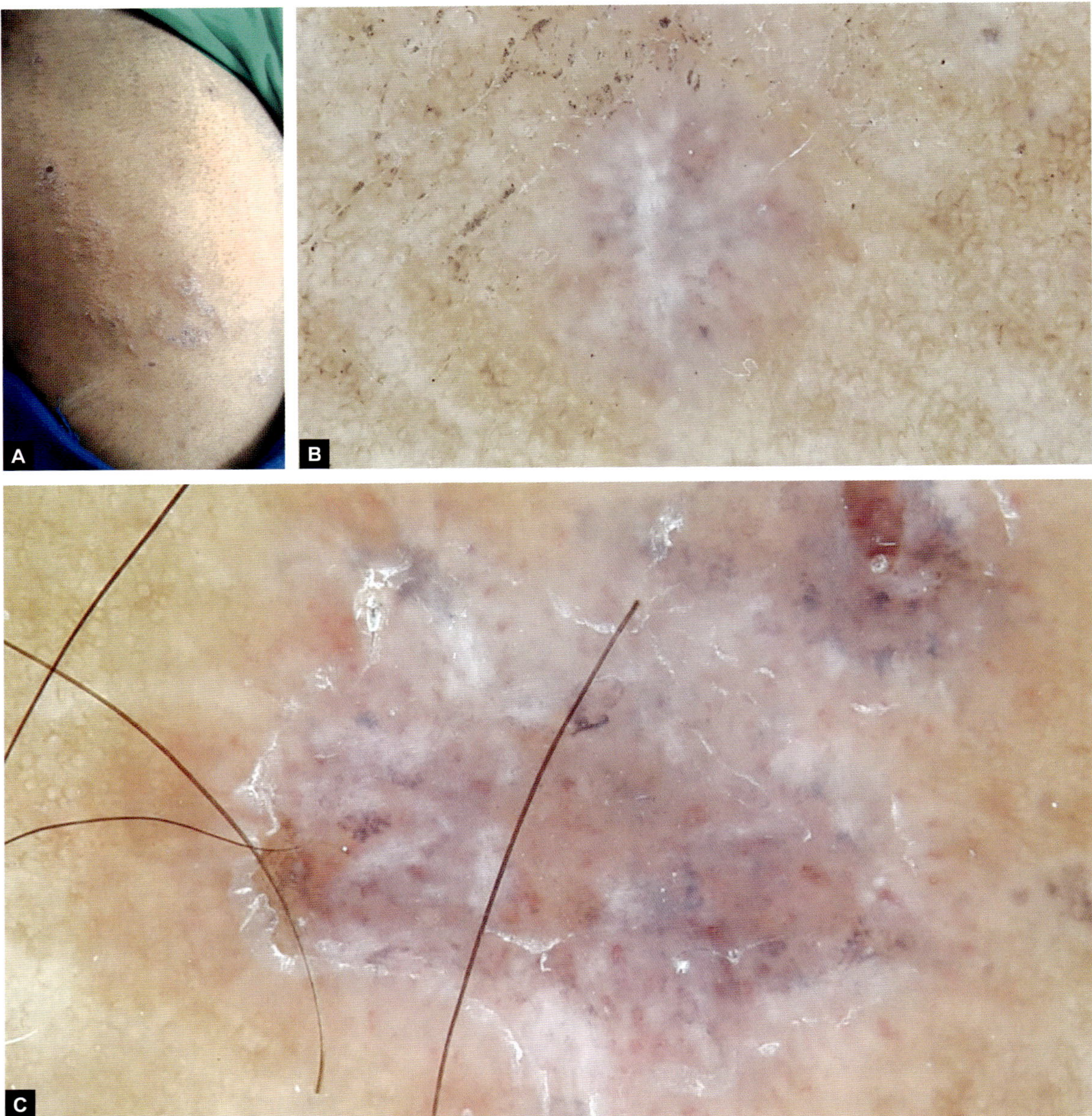

Figs. 12A to C: (A) Lichen planus (LP) following blaschkoid distribution; (B) Dermoscopy of a plaque over the upper part of the thigh shows linear Wickham's striae (WS). Pigment pattern consists of peripheral dots and globules, linear pigmentation is also observed; (C) Veil-like and radial streaming WS seen. Pigment pattern composes of diffuse dots and globules, with some irregular configurations.

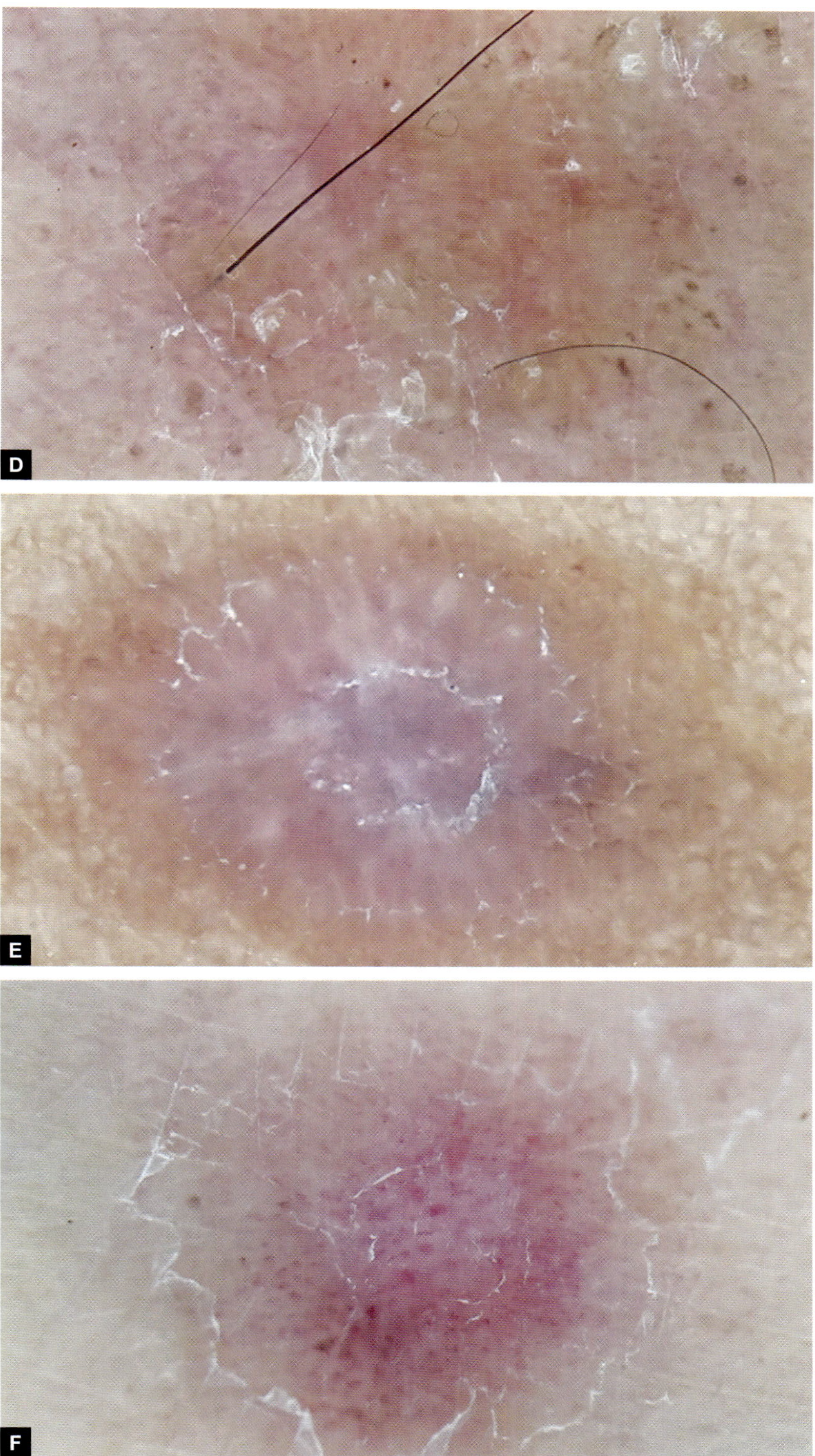

Figs. 12D to F: (D) WS disappeared after 3 weeks of topical steroid. WS has been suggested as an activation marker in LP lesions.[2] Some background erythema and peripheral peppering along with scales is observed; (E) Mostly radial streaming and few globular WS, violaceous background, and starburst pattern seen; (F) Central WS with no defined pattern and an erythematous background seen. Vascular pattern consists of peripheral dotted and central linear vessels.

CASE 11 (FIGS. 13A AND B)

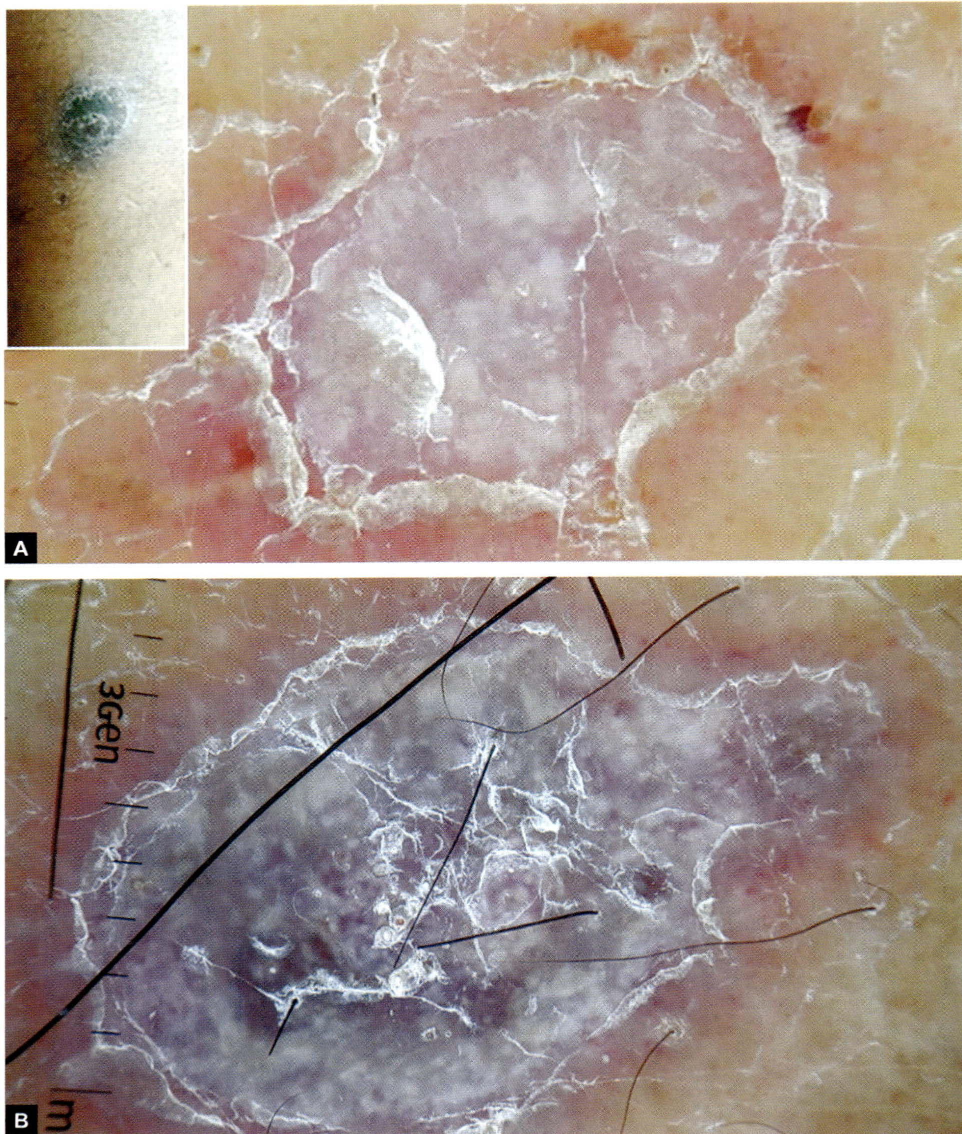

Figs. 13A and B: (A) Globular Wickham's striae (WS), peripheral dotted vessels against a violaceous background and a starburst pattern observed; (B) Globular as well as perpendicular WS, violaceous background, peripheral dotted vessels, and starburst pattern seen.

CASE 12 (FIG. 14)

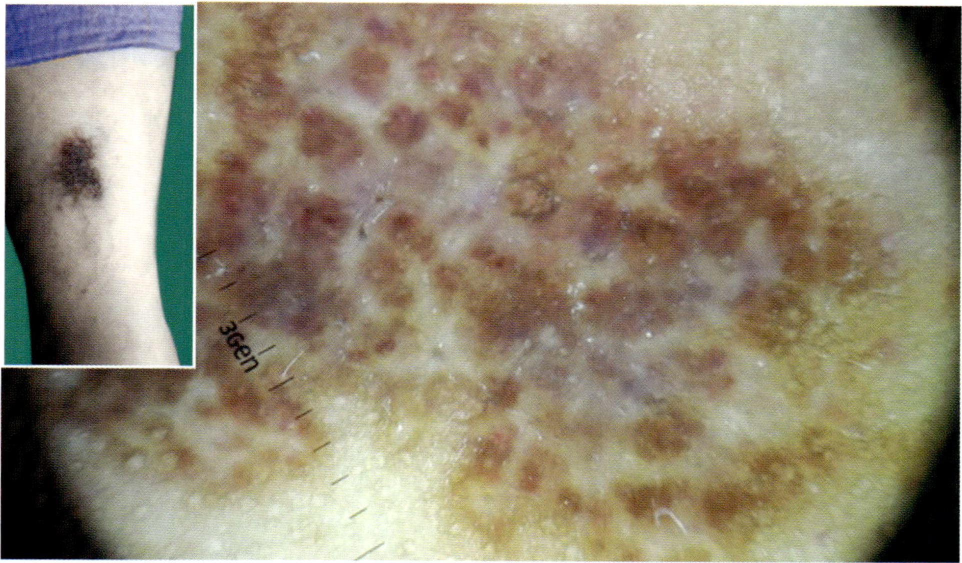

Fig. 14: Veil-like Wickham's striae (WS) on a yellowish-brown background.

CASE 13 (FIGS. 15A TO C)

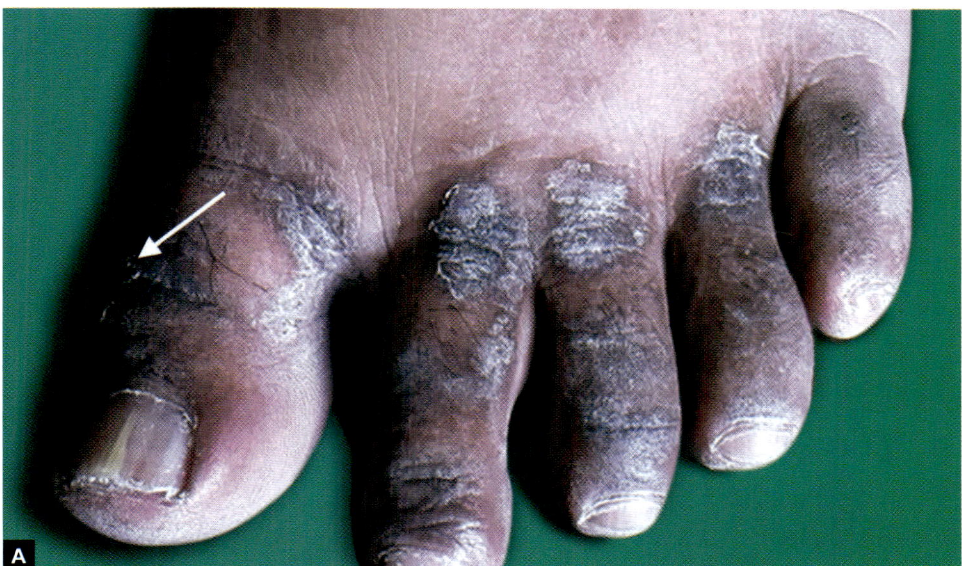

Fig. 15A: Hyperkeratotic, moderately itchy lesions (arrow) over the left foot. The patient had similar lesions over the right foot. Differential diagnoses were lichen simplex and lichen planus. Dermoscopy is difficult in such cases owing to the hyperkeratotic nature of the lesions.

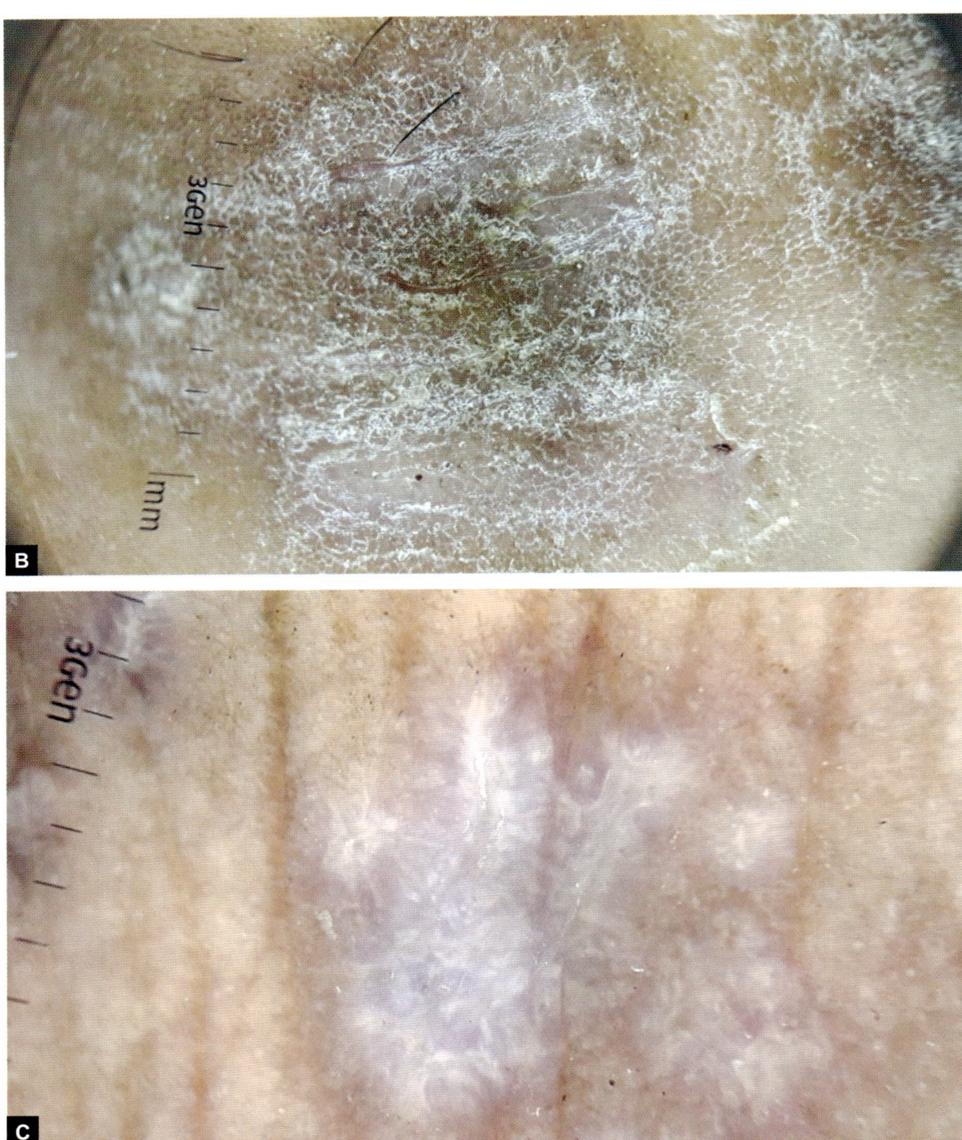

Figs. 15B and C: (B) Not much is visible in this dermoscopic field except for rippled scales due to the hyperkeratotic nature of the lesions; (C) In another field of dermoscopy where hyperkeratosis is comparatively much less, Wickham's striae (WS) is observed that shows radial streaming pattern.

CASE 14 (FIGS. 16A TO C)

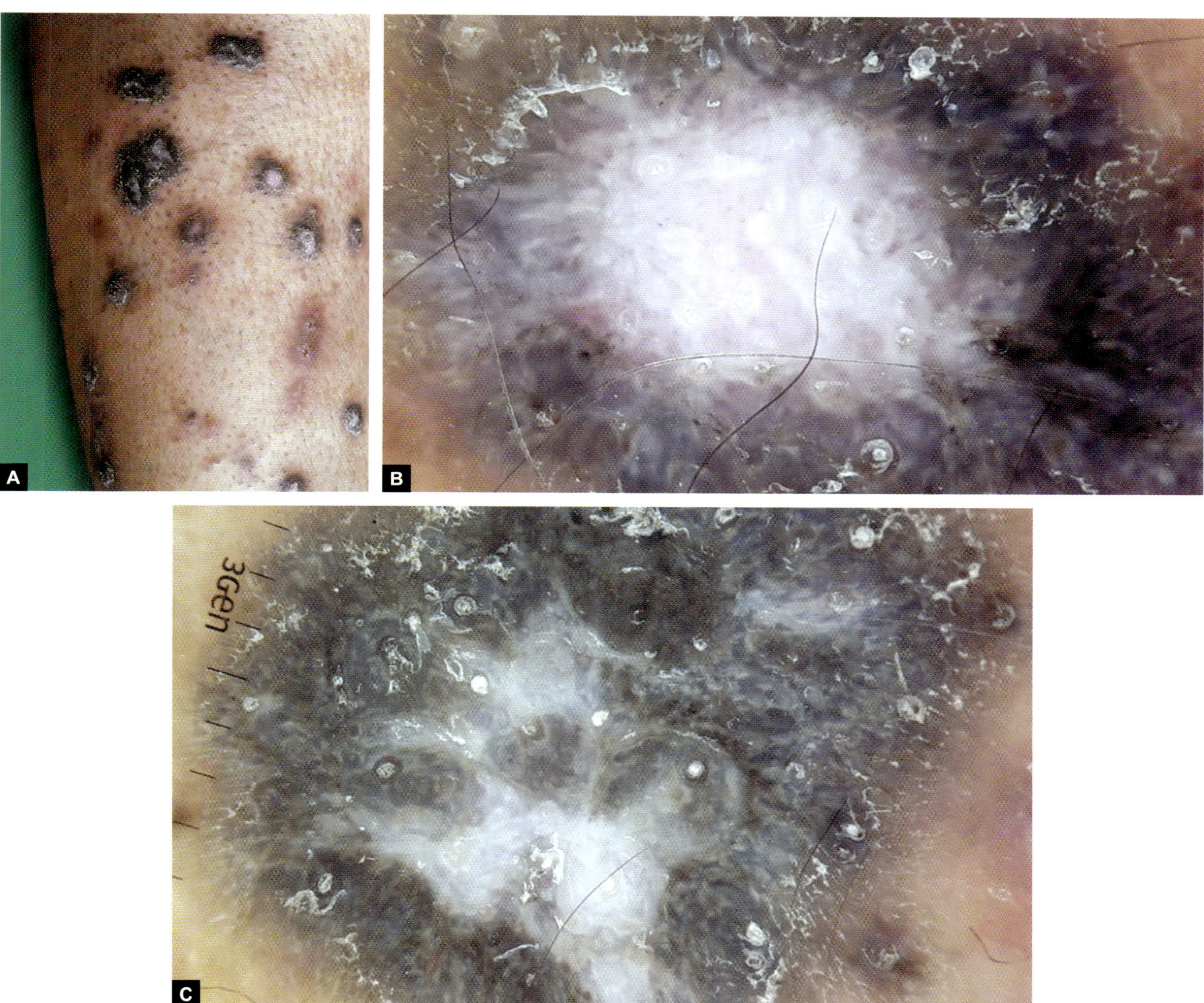

Figs. 16A to C: (A) Hyperkeratotic lichen planus (LP). The patient presented with extremely pruritic, hyperkeratotic lesions on the extensor surface of the lower extremities. These lesions typically were chronic healing with residual pigmentation and scarring; (B) Dermoscopy shows combination pattern Wickham's striae (WS) such as radial streaming, globular and few linear WS. Vascular patterns show dotted and linear vessels; the red color of the vessels is less prominent due to associated thick WS. Several comedo-like structures filled with keratinous plugs are also visible; (C) In another field, dermoscopic WS and comedo-like structures are seen.

CASE 15 (FIGS. 17A TO C)[10]

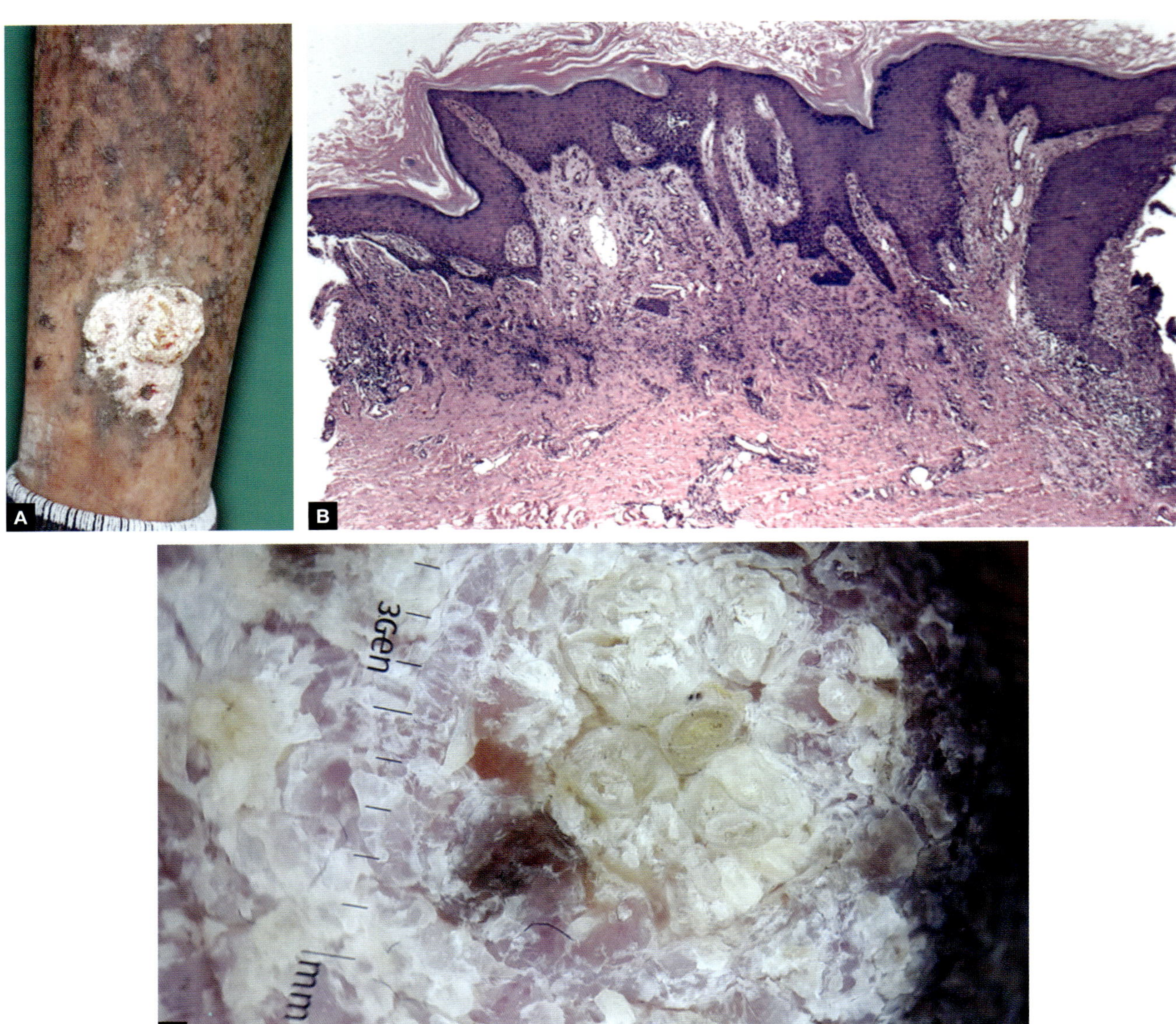

Figs. 17A to C: (A) Hypertrophic lichen planus (LP). This patient presented with itchy, hyperkeratotic lesions on the lower extremities for the past 2 years. The solitary nodule developed in the last 7 months. Biopsy was advised to exclude squamous cell carcinoma. Knackstedt reported cutaneous hypertropic LP resulting in squamous cell carcinoma in a series of 38 patients;[11] (B) Biopsy shows moderately dense superficial perivascular lymphocytic infiltrate along with irregular epidermal hyperplasia. The infiltrate tends to be denser around the hyperplastic appendages and encroaches upon them obscuring the dermoepidermal junction. The dermoepidermal junction at those spots shows occasional colloid bodies. Wedge-shaped hypergranulosis is seen within hyperplastic appendages. The report ruled out malignancy and is consistent with hypertrophic LP; (C) Dermoscopy reveals conglomeration of white lamellar structures resembling petals of white roses, which collectively form a pattern that metaphorically can be termed "Bouquet of white roses" (personal observation). Hyperkeratosis atop wedge-shaped hypergranulosis enclosed within hyperplastic appendages on histopathology correspond to the "bouquet of white roses" dermoscopically.

CASE 16 (FIGS. 18A TO C)

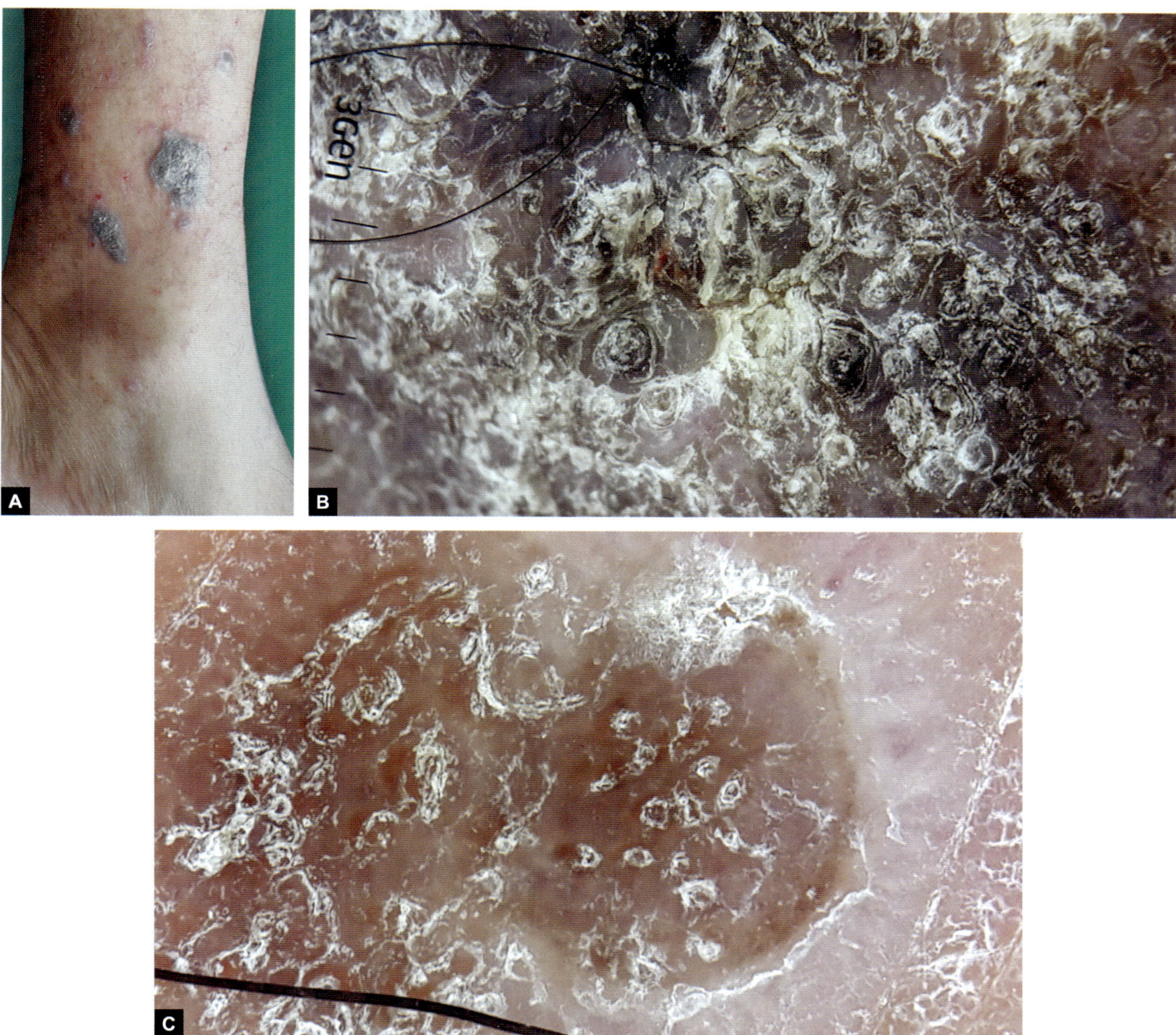

Figs. 18A to C: (A) Lichen planus (LP) presenting with papular and hypertrophic lesions; (B) Dermoscopy of the hypertrophic lesions shows a special pattern "bouquet of white roses"; the background color is violet and black; (C) A lesion of LP evolving into a hypertrophic lesion shows an incomplete "bouquet of white roses" pattern associated with radial streaming Wickham's striae (WS).

CASE 17 (FIGS. 19A AND B)

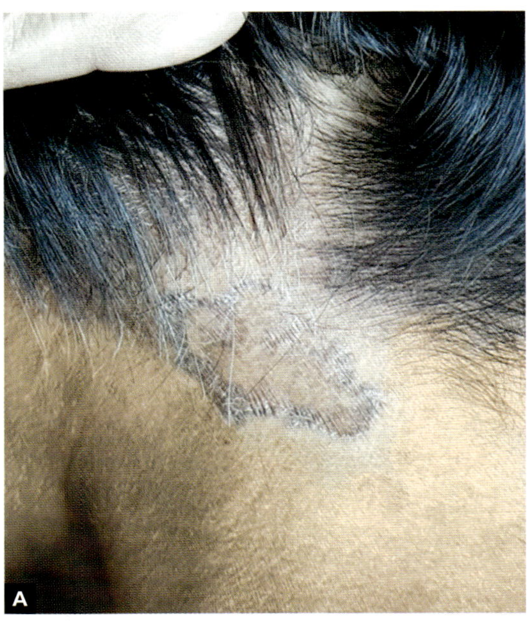

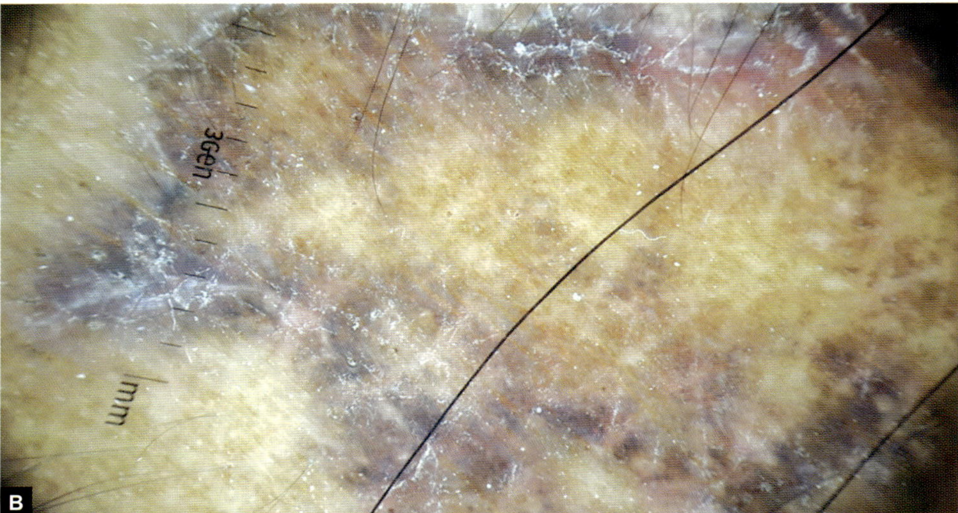

Figs. 19A and B: (A) The lady presented with this singular asymptomatic annular lesion on the neck since the last 5 months. Keeping in mind porokeratosis, annular sarcoid along with other clinical differentials of annular dermatoses, dermoscopy was performed; (B) Dermoscopy reveals circular white Wickham's striae (WS) and peripheral homogeneous cloud-like pigmentation confirming the diagnosis of annular lichen planus (LP); note this is an uncommon location for annular LP. Biopsy was also consistent with LP. Dermoscopy of the close clinical mimic porokeratosis presents with "white track" structure, i.e. annular peripheral whitish hyperkeratotic structure that corresponds on histology to cornoid lamella.

CASE 18 (FIGS. 20A TO G)

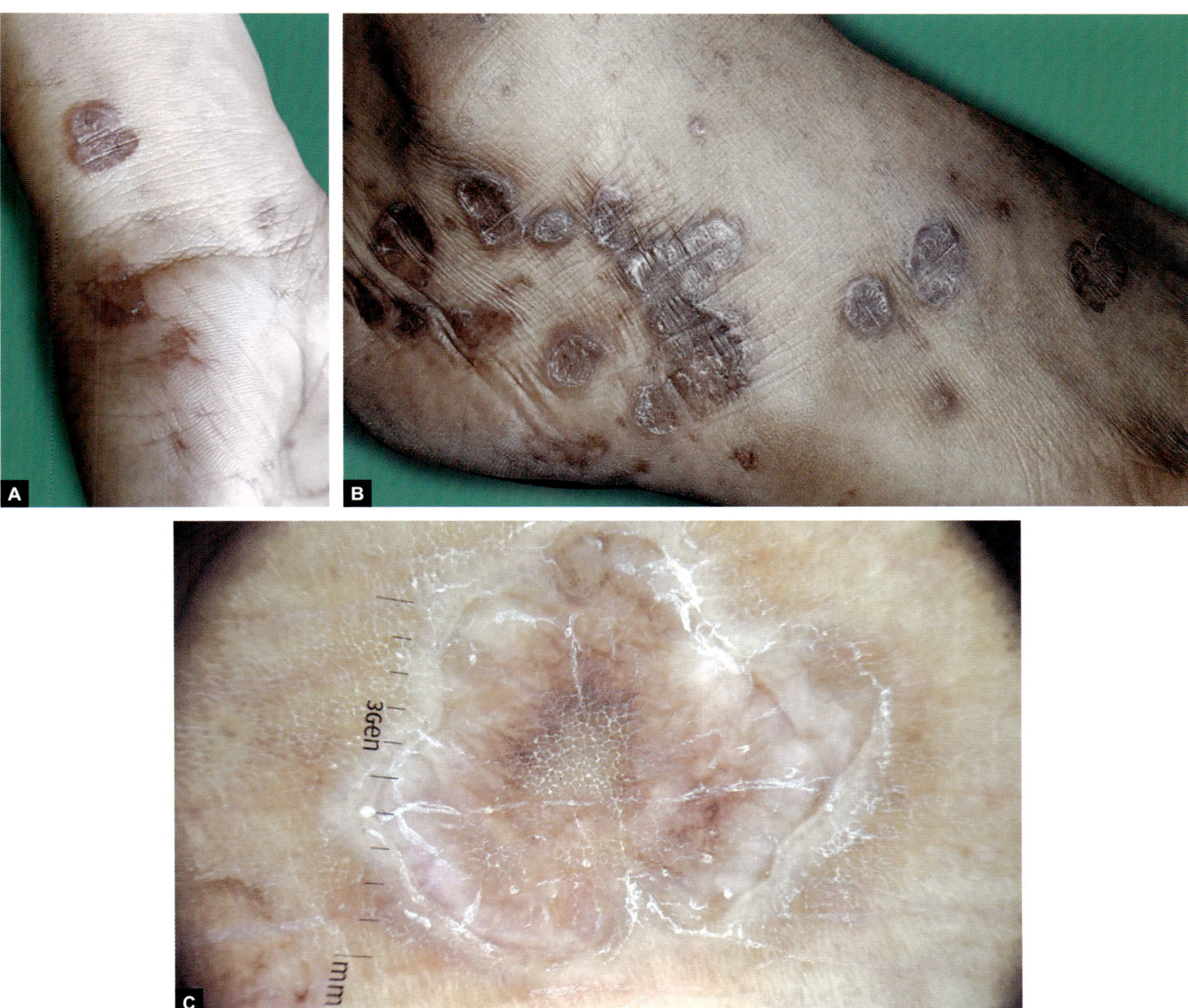

Figs. 20A to C: (A) Annular lichen planus (LP), a subtype of LP often occurs in the male genitalia. The lesions typically consist of a few localized lesions. Distal aspects of extremities may also be involved; (B) This patient presented with annular LP on both the upper and lower extremities; (C) Circular white peripheral Wickham's striae (WS), central homogeneous pigmentation, central and peripheral rippling is seen on dermoscopy.

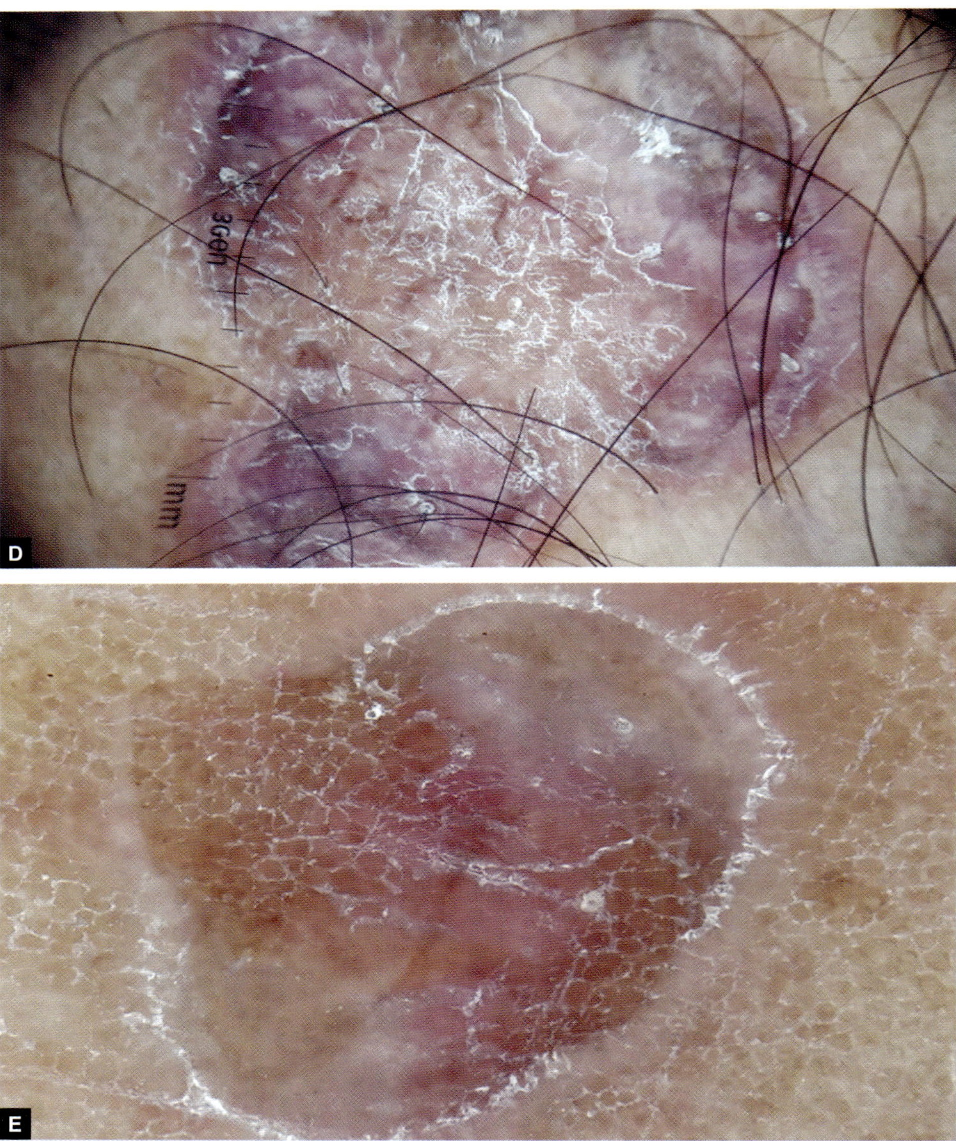

Figs. 20D and E: (D) Dermoscopy of another lesion of the same patient shows combination pattern WS consisting of globular, circular peripheral and radial streaming WS. Centrally there are rippled scales; (E) Different lesions of LP may be in different stages of evolution and remission. Consequently dermoscopic features also vary showing veil-like WS and starburst pattern in another lesion of annular LP.

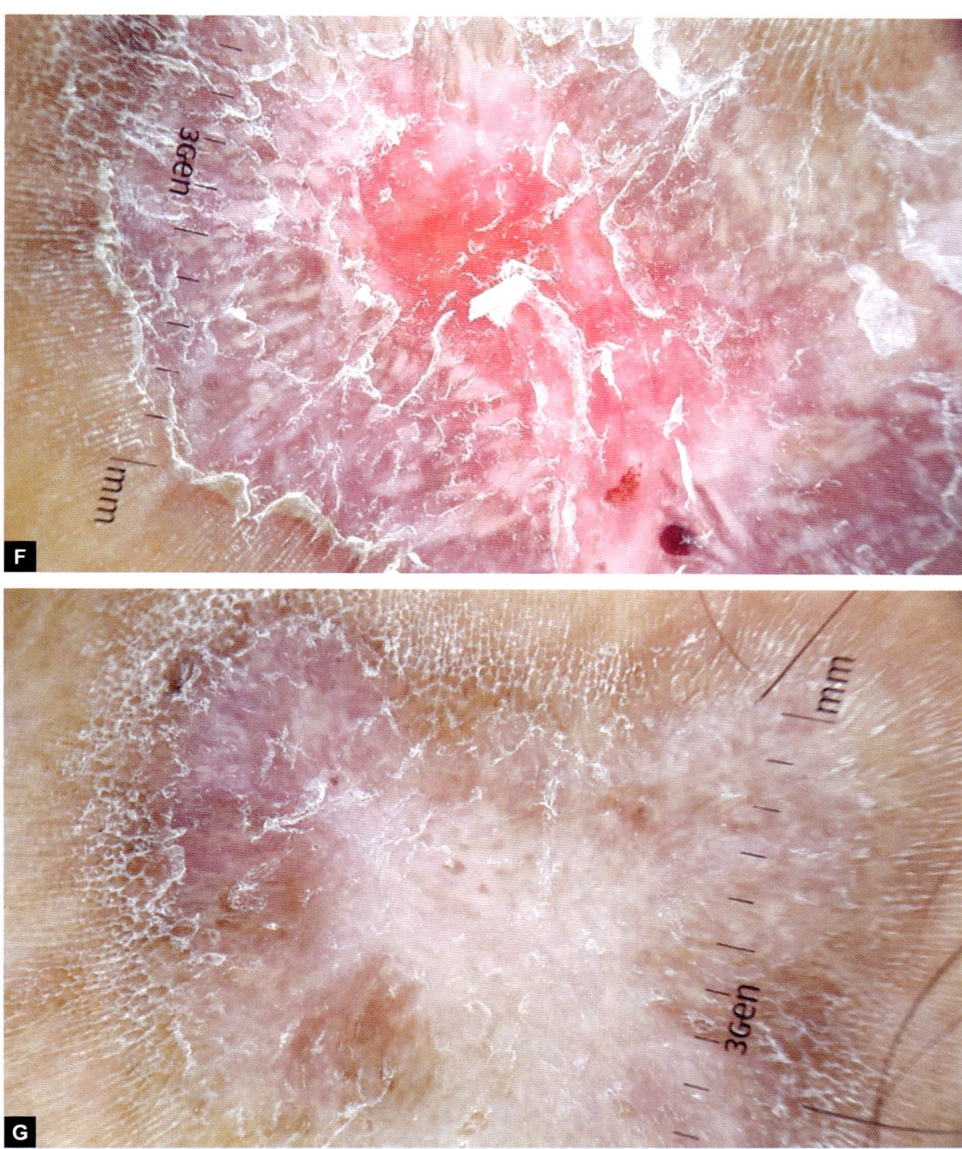

Figs 20F and G: (F) In another annular LP lesion, WS pattern is predominantly radial streaming. To the extreme right of this dermoscopic field, globular pattern admixed with few linear patterns of WS can be observed. The background is red while the special feature of starburst pattern is obvious; (G) The same lesion after 4 weeks of treatment shows remnant of WS in the upper left part of this field while background erythema has cleared completely. Remember WS is an activation marker in LP lesions.

CASE 19 (FIGS. 21 AND 22)[12-18]

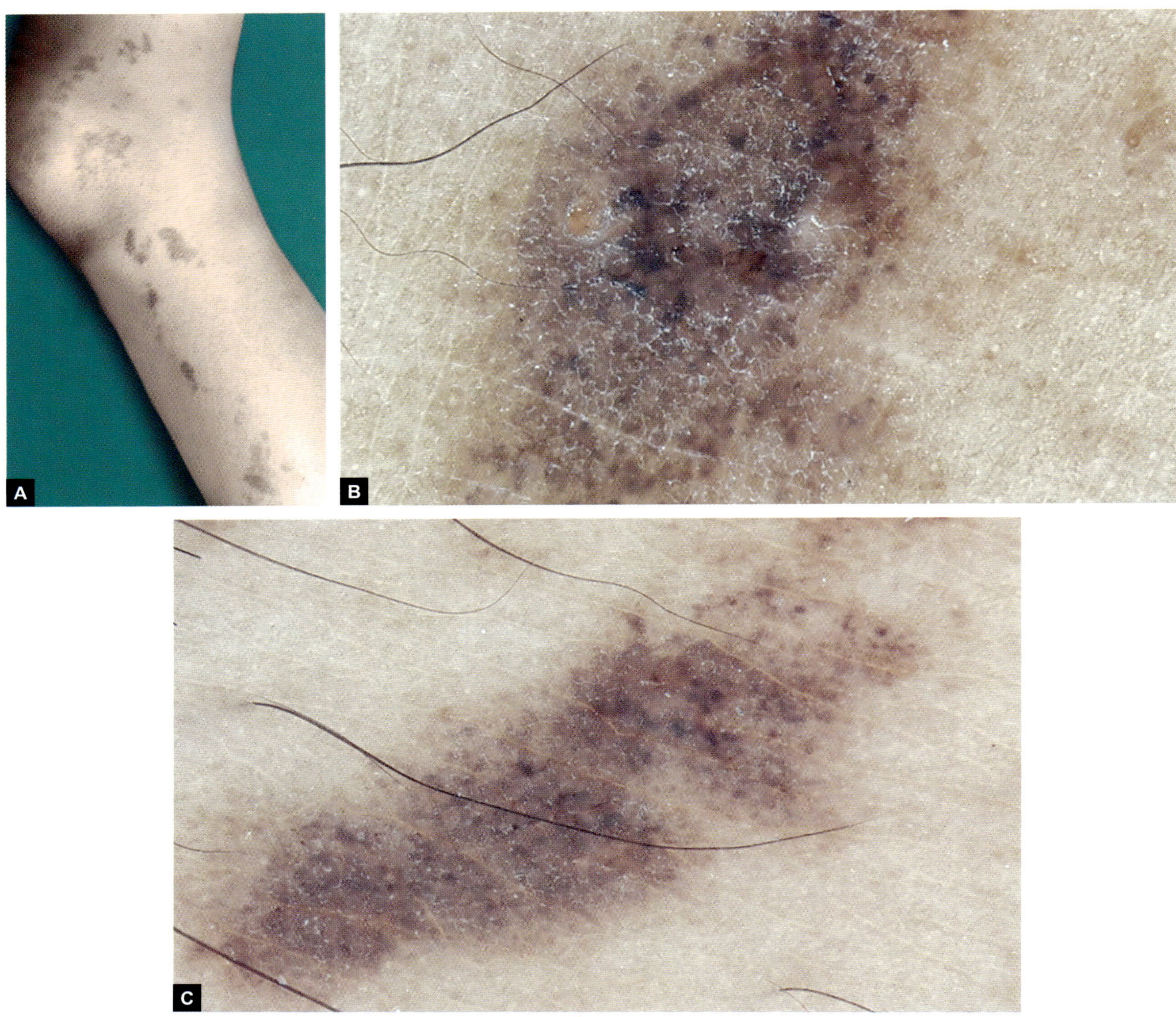

Figs. 21A to C: (A) Linear lichen planus (LLP). During the evolution of skin lesions, they may be randomly distributed or they may follow patterns that were laid down during embryologic development.[12] Individuals who have distinct cell populations within their skin (cutaneous mosaicism) are more likely to develop skin conditions with distinct patterns.[13] LLP is a model of this phenomenon that accounts for less than 0.2% of all patients with lichen planus (LP). There are few reports of LLP with isolated segmental distribution; following Blaschko lines, in a zosteriform distribution, or with segmental overlap where linear lesions may be seen along with other types of LP.[14-16] Linear distribution pattern of LP may occur simply as a result of the Koebner phenomenon; (B) Three dermoscopic patterns of LLP have been described; dots and globules, diffuse and mixed.[17] When granular deposits are intense, the course of the disease is slower and persistent. However, in diffuse pattern of pigmentation where dots and globules are absent, resolution is earlier.[17,18] This dermoscopic field reveals mixed pattern, i.e. dots and globules and diffuse; (C) Another dermoscopic field showing a mixed pattern of pigmentation.

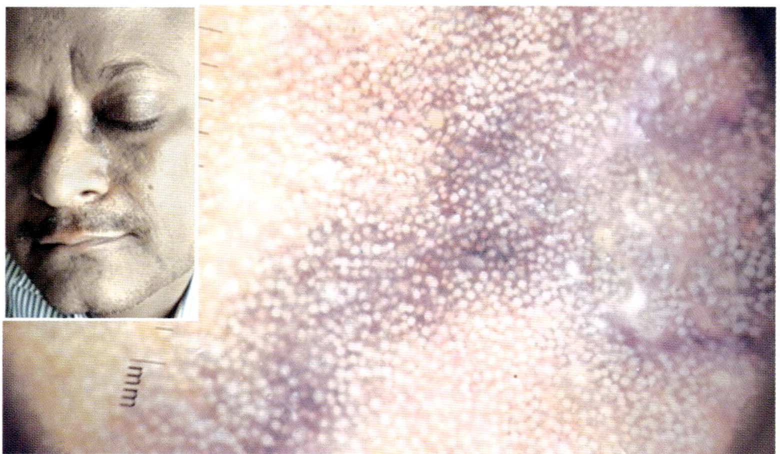

Fig. 22: A case of linear lichen planus (LLP) on face following Blaschkoid distribution. Perifollicular or annular pigmentation is revealed on dermoscopy.

CASE 20 (FIGS. 23A AND B)

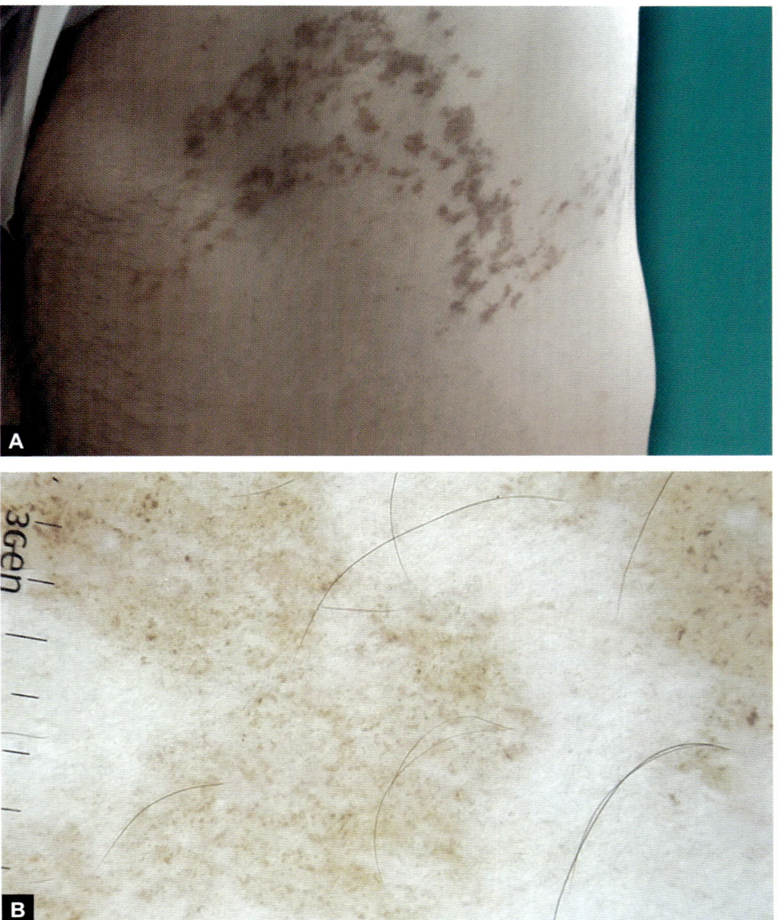

Figs. 23A and B: (A) case of zosteriform lichen planus (LP); (B) LP presents with diffuse peppering on dermoscopy.

CASE 21 (FIGS. 24A AND B)

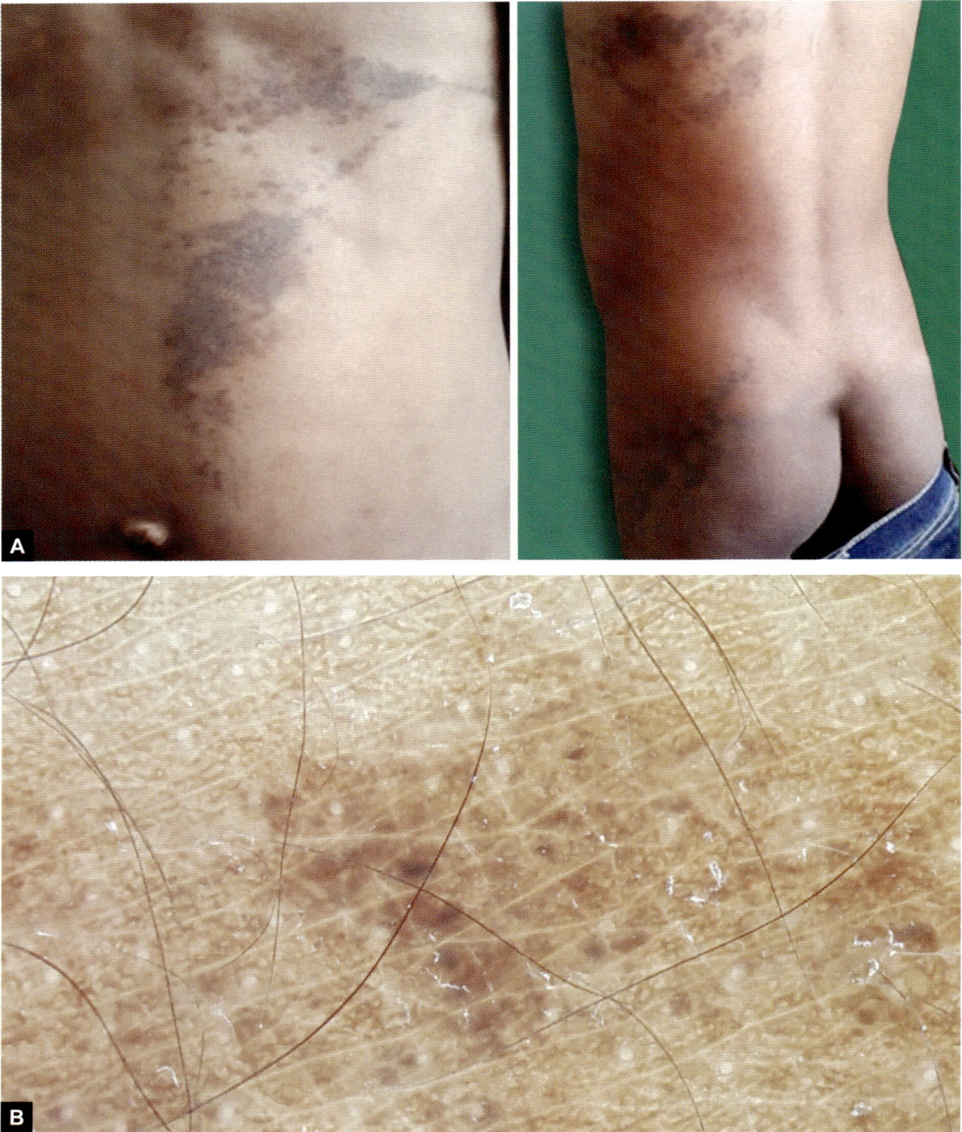

Figs. 24A and B: (A) Another case of zosteriform lichen planus (LP); (B) Dermoscopy demonstrates diffuse pigmentation and some globules.

CASE 22 (FIGS. 25A TO D)[2,19,20]

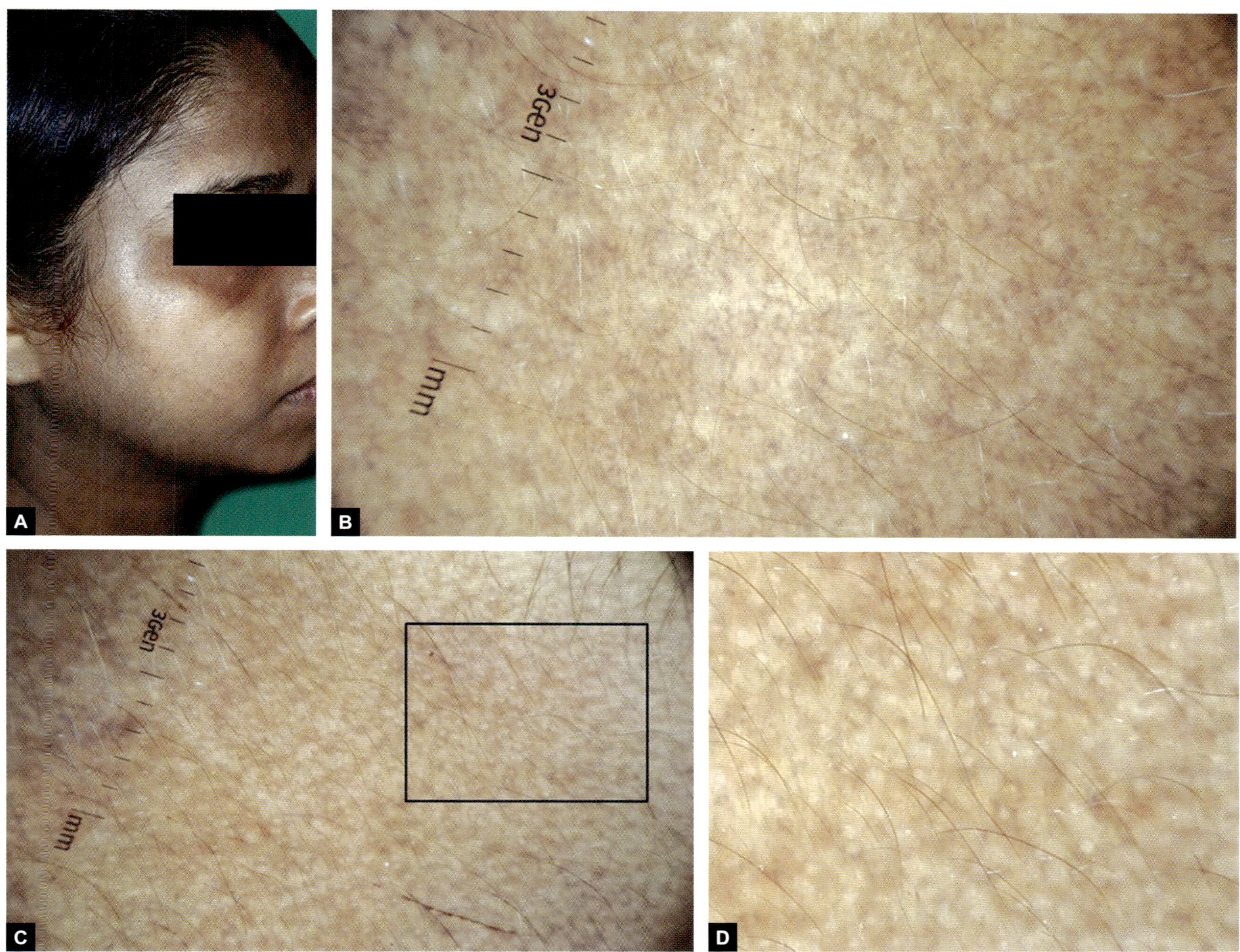

Figs. 25A to D: (A) In lichen planus pigmentosus (LPP), typical lichenoid papules with pruritus is an early feature. However, often the preceding lichenoid papules are scarcely present or missing completely. In late stage disease, diffuse or patchy macules of hyperpigmentation are the presentation. LPP usually affects the sun-exposed areas such as face neck and upper extremities;[19] (B) Dermoscopy of LPP shows diffuse brownish pigmentation, gray-blue or brown dots and globules and perifollicular or annular pigmentation. At times white dots are found;[2,20] (C) Besides diffuse brownish pigmentation, gray-blue or brown dots and globules are also seen. The rectangular area in the picture reveals perifollicular or annular pigmentation and has been magnified for better visualization in Figure 25D; (D) Perifollicular or annular pigmentation on dermoscopy in LPP.

CASE 23 (FIGS. 26A AND B)

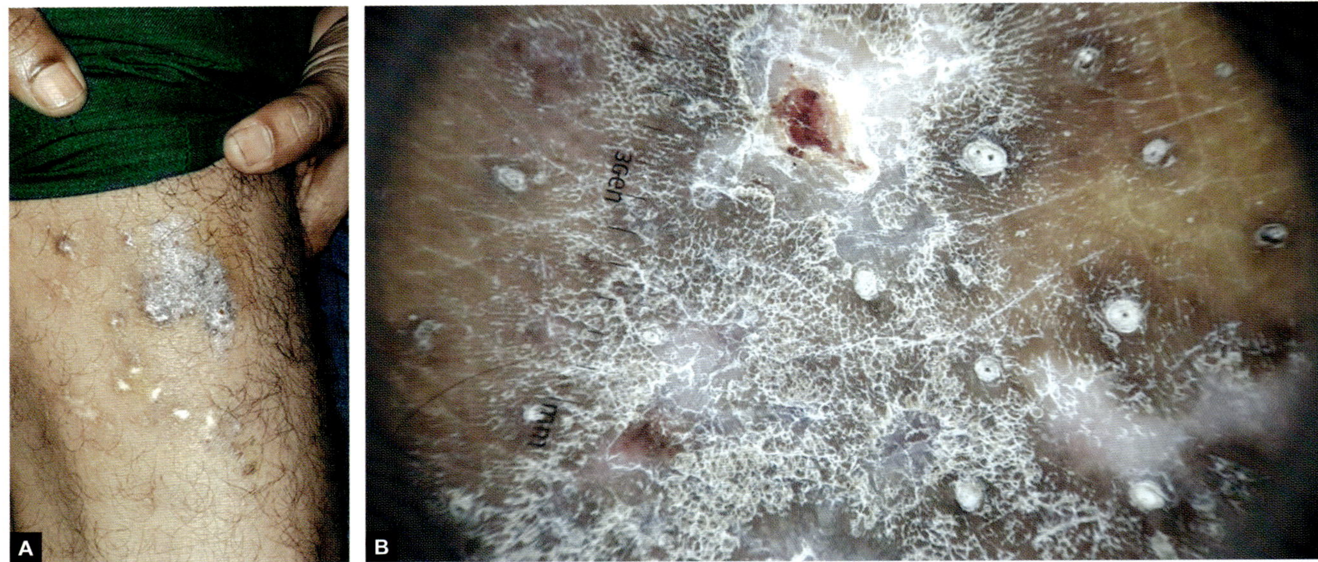

Figs. 26A and B: (A) An itchy plaque present on the right thigh since 5 months. Postinflammatory hypopigmentation and a papulonodule—both present adjacent to the plaque. Clinical differentials are lichen simplex, lichen planus, prurigo nodularis, etc. To confirm the diagnosis, histopathology is gold standard. We examined the lesion dermoscopically as a part of routine investigation before going for biopsy; (B) Rippled surface, comedo-like structures filled with keratinous plugs, veil-like Wickham's striae (WS) and violaceous background confirmed the case to be hypertrophic lichen planus (LP). Histopathology also was consistent with LP.

CASE 24 (FIGS. 27A TO G)

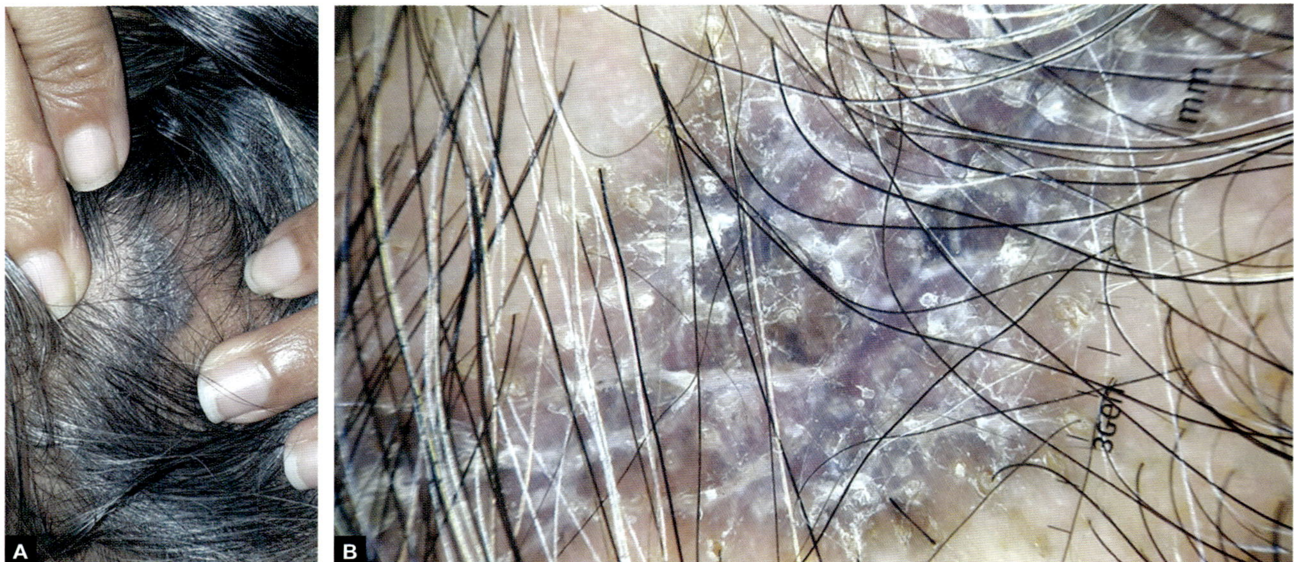

Figs. 27A and B: (A) A hyperkeratotic itchy plaque on occiput for last 3 months; (B) Dermoscopy reveals reticular Wickham's striae (WS), which was a surprise to us and we searched for other lesions of lichen planus (LP) elsewhere in the body.

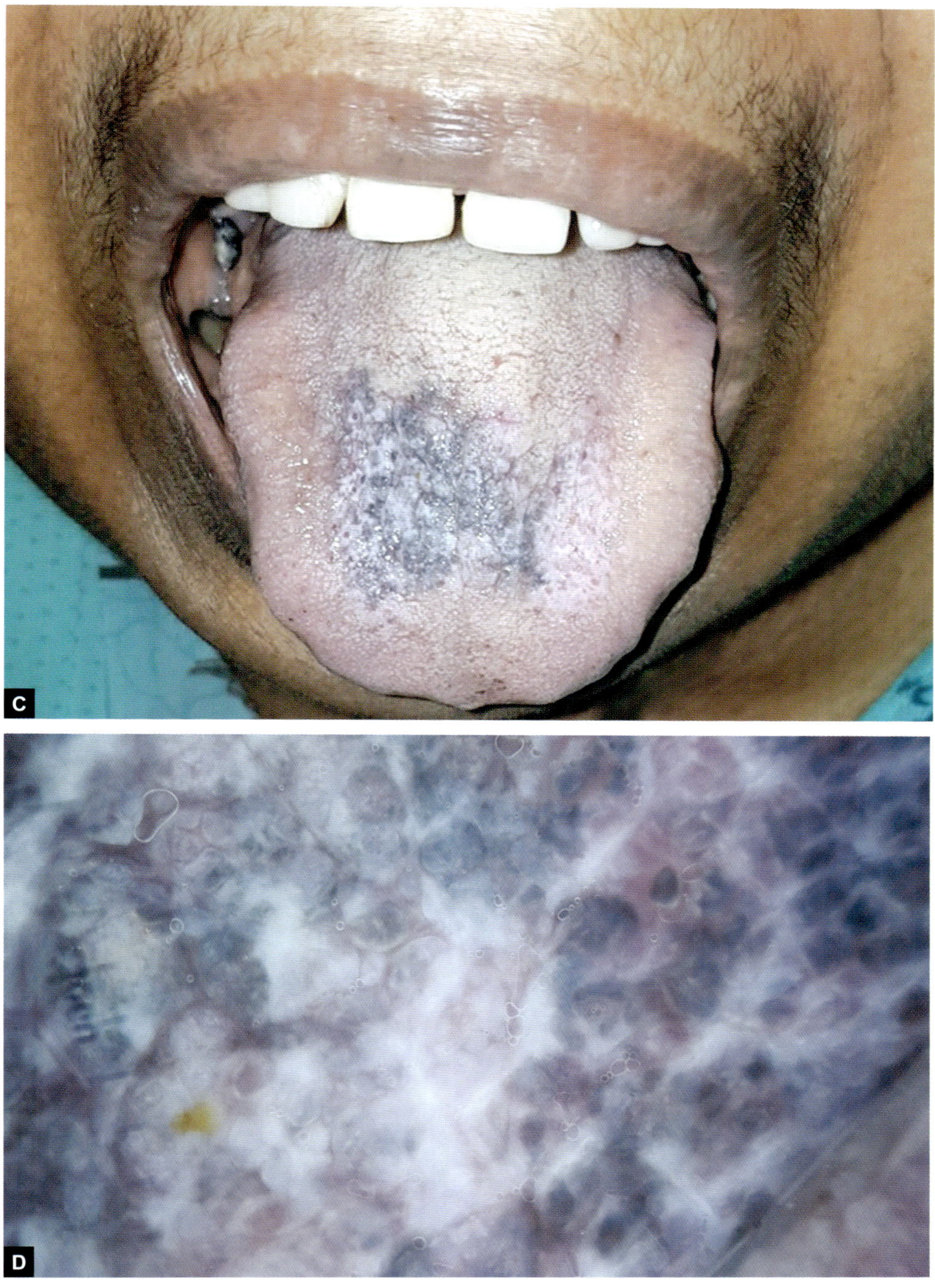

Figs. 27C and D: (C) Dorsum of the tongue of the same patient clinically shows a violaceous white plaque; (D) On dermoscopy of tongue, reticular WS is very obvious.

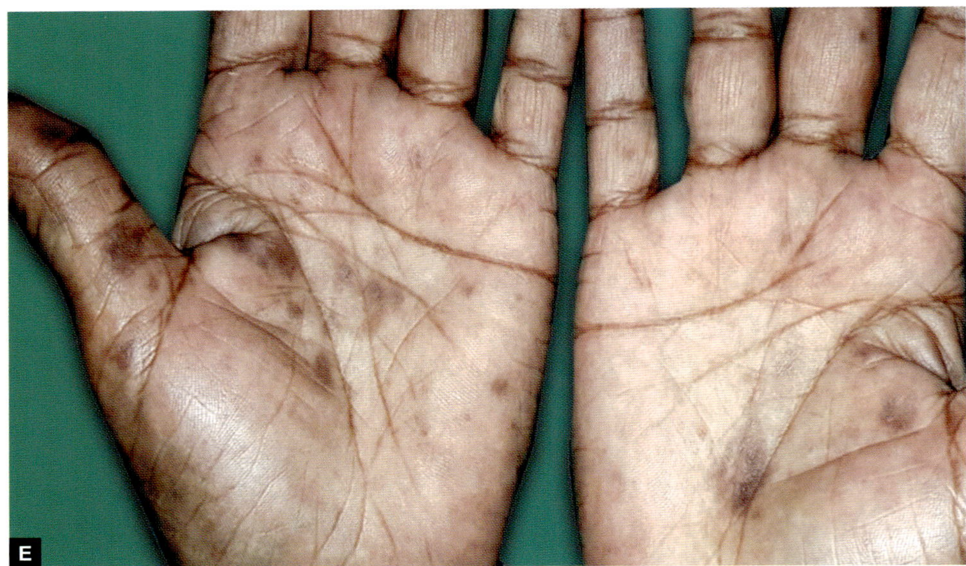

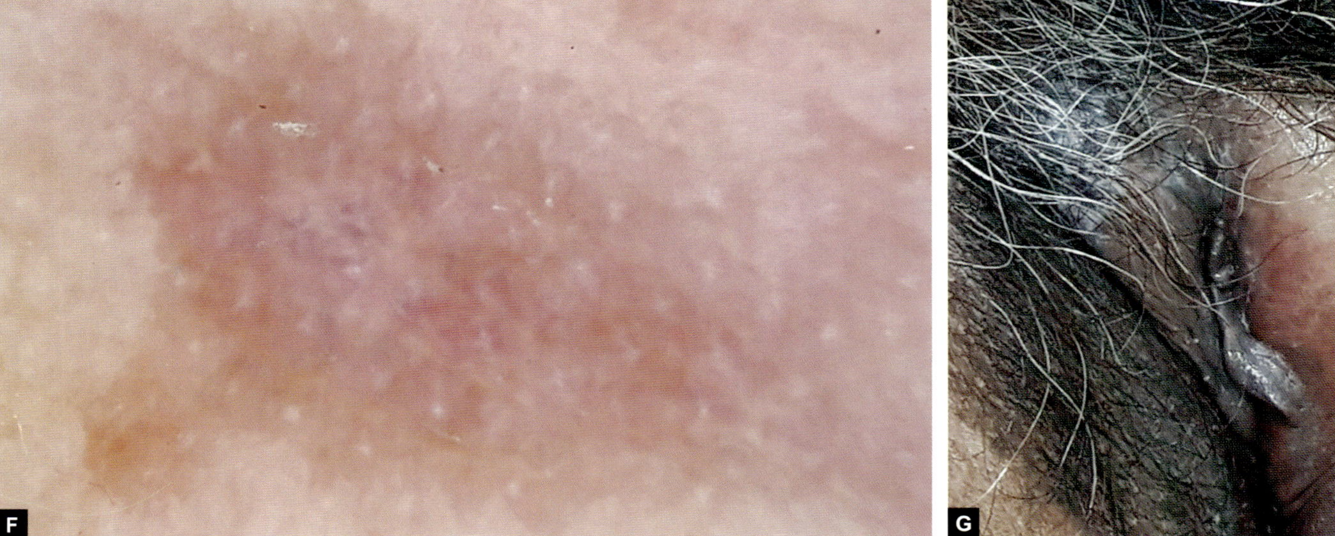

Figs. 27E to G: (E) We noticed scattered hyperpigmented patches on both the palms; (F) Dermoscopy of palm reveals violaceous background and invisible WS; (G) On inspection of the vulva, hyperkeratotic plaque of LP was seen in the upper left corner. Due to anatomical difficulty, we could not do dermoscopy of this area.

CASE 25 (FIGS. 28A TO G)[21]

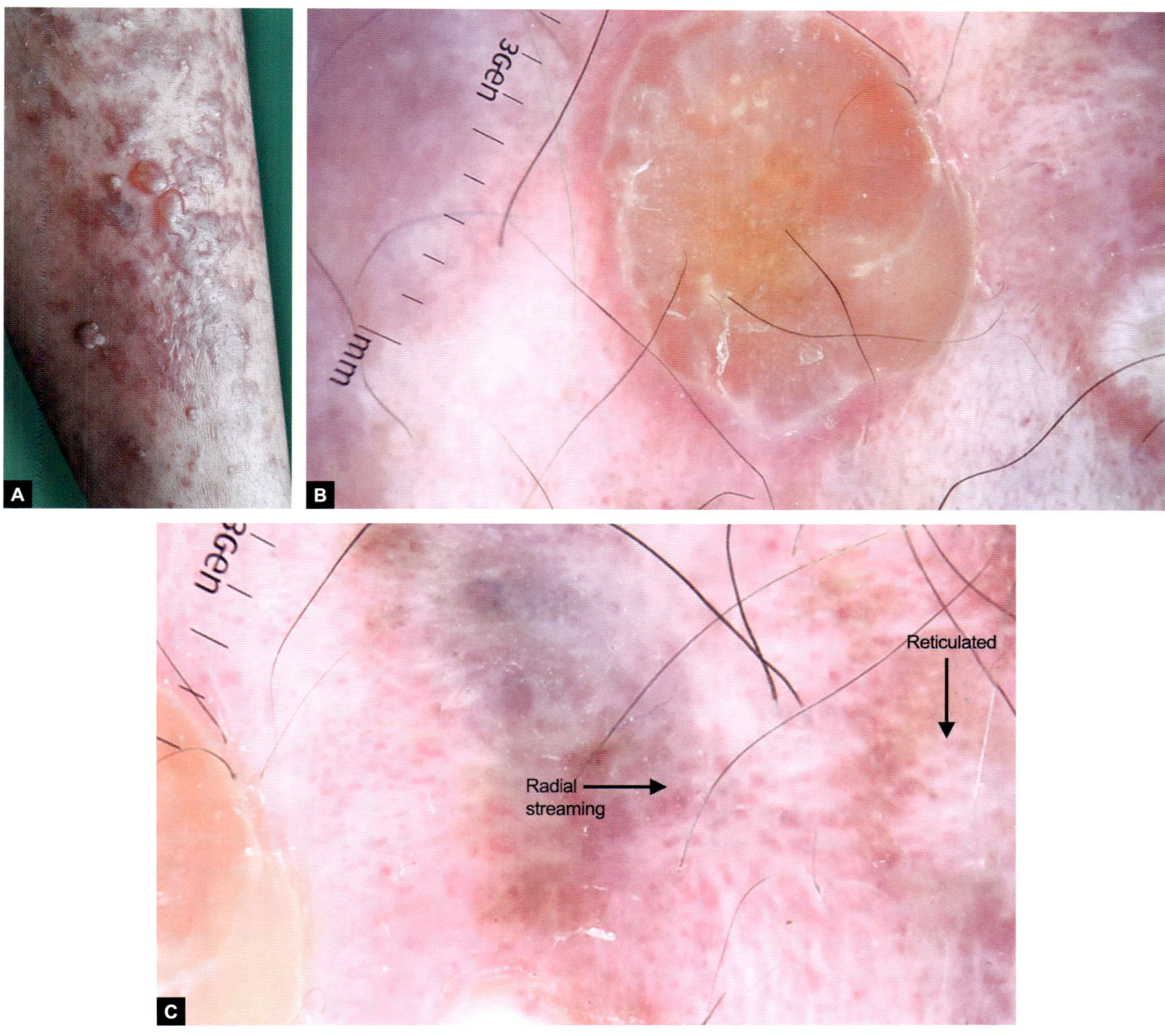

Figs. 28A to C: (A) Lichen planus pemphigoides (LPPG) has a rare incidence. The blisters develop atop lesions of lichen planus (LP). Bullous pemphigoid and bullous LP are very difficult to differentiate as they share common clinical, histopathological and immunological features; (B) Dermoscopy reveals an intact bulla with surrounding homogeneous erythema. Some whitish structures are visible on the right lower side of the bulla whereas a violaceous structure is seen in the right middle portion of the central bulla; (C) This dermoscopic field is to the right side of the bulla shown in the previous picture; note the bulla is partially visible in the extreme left. In this field, various patterns of Wickham's striae (WS) (radial streaming and reticulated) are present against an erythematous-violaceous background. Red globules and radial linear vessels are the main two vascular patterns present.

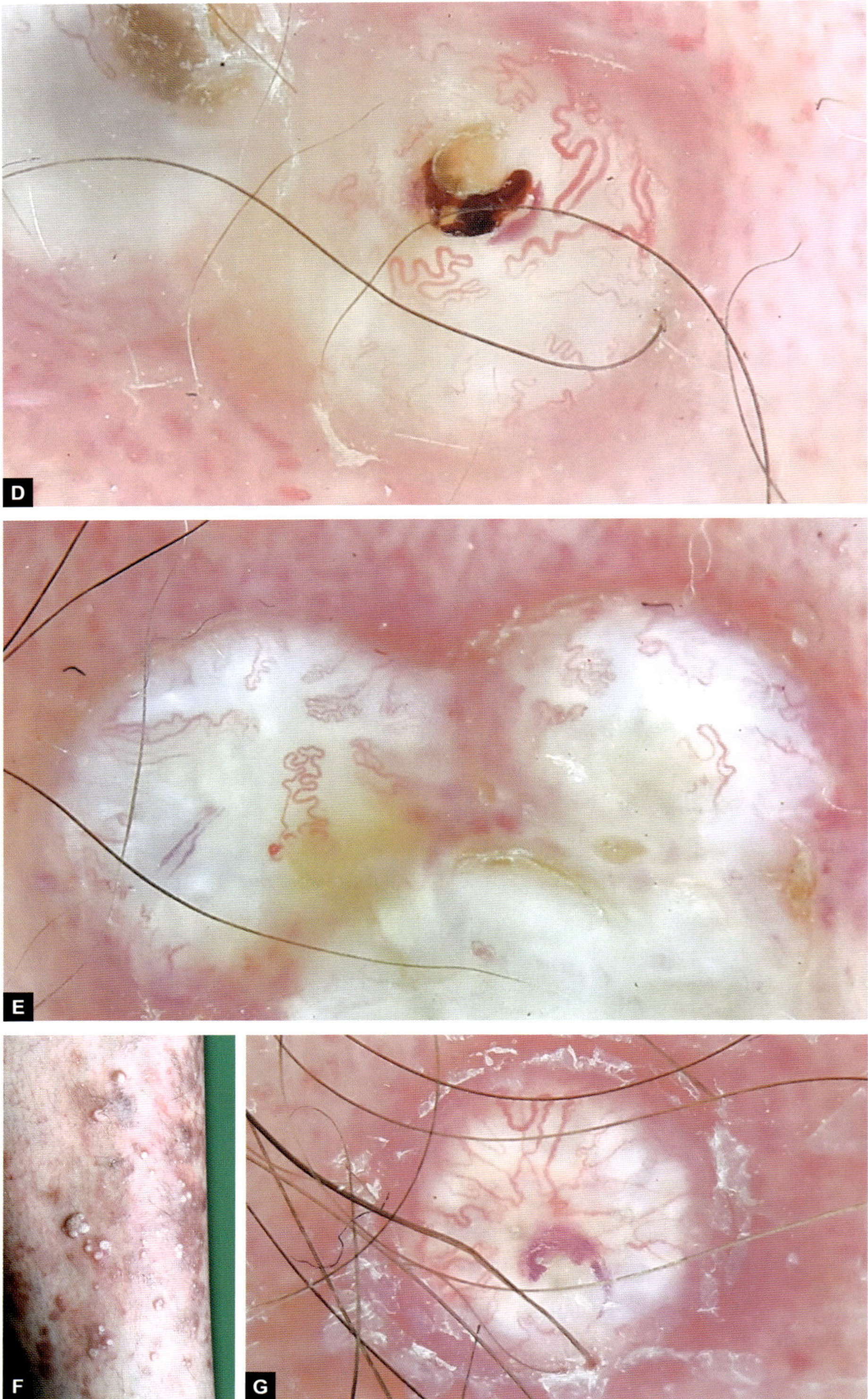

Figs. 28D to G: (D) Some lesions have healed with milia formation. A characteristic vascular pattern is observed on the surface of the milium. We describe the pattern as "corals and pearls" due to its resemblance to coral and pearls; (E) More milia with "corals and pearls" vascular pattern; (F) This patient of LP pemphigoides was resistant to most modalities of treatment but responded quite satisfactorily to cyclosporine as documented in the picture.[21] Milia were seen in the remission stage, a phenomenon seen in many subepidermal bullous disorders; (G) Remission stage is marked by desquamation and milia formation. On the surface of the milium, "corals and pearls" vascular pattern is obvious.

REFERENCES

1. Lallas A, Giacomel J, Argenziano G, et al. Dermoscopy in general dermatology: practical tips for the clinician. Br J Dermatol. 2014;170(3):514-26.
2. Gungor S, Topal IO, Goncu EK. Dermoscopic patterns in active and regressive lichen planus and lichen planus variants: a morphological study. Dermatol Pract Concept. 2015;5(2):6.
3. Lallas A, Kyrgidis A, Tzellos TG, et al. Accuracy of dermoscopic criteria for the diagnosis of psoriasis, dermatitis, lichen planus and pityriasis rosea. Br J Dermatol. 2012;166:1198-205.
4. Vasquez-Lopez F, Alvarez-Cuesta C, Hidalgo-Garcia Y, Perez-Oliva N. The handheld dermatoscope improves the recognition of Wickham striae and capillaries in lichen planus lesions. Arch Dermatol. 2001;137:1376.
5. Lallas A, Kyrgidis A, Tzellos TG, et al. Accuracy of dermoscopic criteria for the diagnosis of psoriasis, dermatitis, lichen planus and pityriasis rosea. Br J Dermatol. 2012;166(6):1198-205.
6. Zalaudek I, Argenziano G. Dermoscopy subpatterns of inflammatory skin disorders. Arch Dermatol. 2006;142(6):808.
7. Vazquez-Lopez F, Gomez-Diez S, Sanchez J, Perez-Oliva N. Dermoscopy of active lichen planus. Arch Dermatol. 2007;143(8):1092.
8. Vasquez-Lopez F, Manjon Haces JA, Maldonado-Seral C, et al. Dermoscopic features of plaque psoriasis and lichen planus: new observations. Dermatology. 2003;207:151-6.
9. Zalaudek I. Dermoscopy in general dermatology. In: Marghoob AA, Malvehy J, Braun RP (Eds). Atlas of Dermoscopy, 2nd edition. London: Informa Healthcare; 2012. p. 329.
10. Sachdeva S, Sachdeva S, Kapoor P. Wickham striae: etiopathogenesis and clinical significance. Indian J Dermatol. 2011; 56:442-3.
11. Knackstedt TJ, Collins LK, Li Z, et al. Squamous cell carcinoma arising in hypertrophic lichen planus: a review and analysis of 38 cases. Dermatol Surg. 2015;41(12):1411-8.
12. Chuong CM, Dhouailly D, Gilmore S, et al. What is the biological basis of pattern formation of skin lesions? Exp Dermatol. 2006;15:547-64.
13. Frank G, Happle R. Cutaneous mosaicism: right before our eyes. J Clin Invest. 2007;117:1216.
14. Gupta S, Thomas M, Mahendra A. Unilateral lichen planus along the lines of Blashko: a rare clinical presentation. Acta Med Indones. 2012;44:163-4.
15. Cho S, Whang KK. Lichen planus pigmentosus presenting in zosteriform pattern. J Dermatol. 1997;24:193-7.
16. Monteagudo B, Suarez-Armor O, Cabanillas M, et al. Superimposed lichen planus pigmentosus. Dermatol Online J. 20. doj_22639.2014;20:22639.
17. Vazquez F, Maldonado C, Lopez M, Perez N. Dermatoscopy of pigmented lichen planus lesions. Clin Exp Dermatol. 2003;28:554-5.
18. Vasquez F, Vidal AM, Zalaudek I. Dermoscopic subpatterns of ashy dermatosis related to lichen planus. Arch Dermatol. 2010;146:110.
19. Kanwar AJ, Dogra S, Handa S, et al. A study of 124 indian patients with lichen planus pigmentosus. Clin Exp Dermatol. 2003;28:481-5.
20. Friedman P, Sabban EC, Marcucci C, et al. Dermoscopic findings in different clinical variants of lichen planus. Is dermoscopy useful? Dermatol Pract Concept. 2015;5:51-5.
21. Malakar S, Saha A. Successful treatment of resistant lichen planus pemphigoides with cyclosporine: a new hope. Indian J Dermatol. 2016;61:112-4.

PITYRIASIS ROSEA

INTRODUCTION

Pityriasis rosea (PR) presents with round to oval erythematous scaly patches following the Blaschko's lines. It manifests as an acute, self-limiting, papulosquamous dermatosis with a duration of about 8–10 weeks. It usually begins with a solitary patch that heralds the eruption, referred to as "herald patch".

Approximately 20% of patients may have atypical presentations; their distribution pattern may vary, eg. inverse PR, localization in a single area like abdomen, distal extremities, palms, and soles, a unilateral variant, etc. sometimes herald patch may be absent.

It may mimic other dermatosis such as tinea corporis, secondary syphilis, guttate psoriasis, etc.[1-3]

In these circumstances dermoscopic examination may provide clues to exact diagnosis.

KEY DERMOSCOPIC FEATURES (FIGS. 29 TO 34)[4,5]

- Arrangement of peripheral scaling of annular lesion—may resemble collarette seen clinically, or scaling may be diffuse and irregular instead of collarette
- Peripheral annular brown patch
- Accentuation of central melanocytic network of the lesion (personal observation)
- Irregularly distributed dotted vessels
- Yellowish-orange structureless areas.

DISCUSSION

Dermoscopically both the secondary lesions and the herald patch may classically show "collarette sign" that consists of scale fragments at the border, which hang into the center of the lesion like a curtain. Scaling at the periphery may often not appear as a collarette but a diffuse irregular arrangement at the erythematous border.

Dotted vessels are distributed in an irregular or focal pattern in contrast to the regularly distributed dotted vessels in psoriasis; dotted vessels are found uncommonly in darker skin.

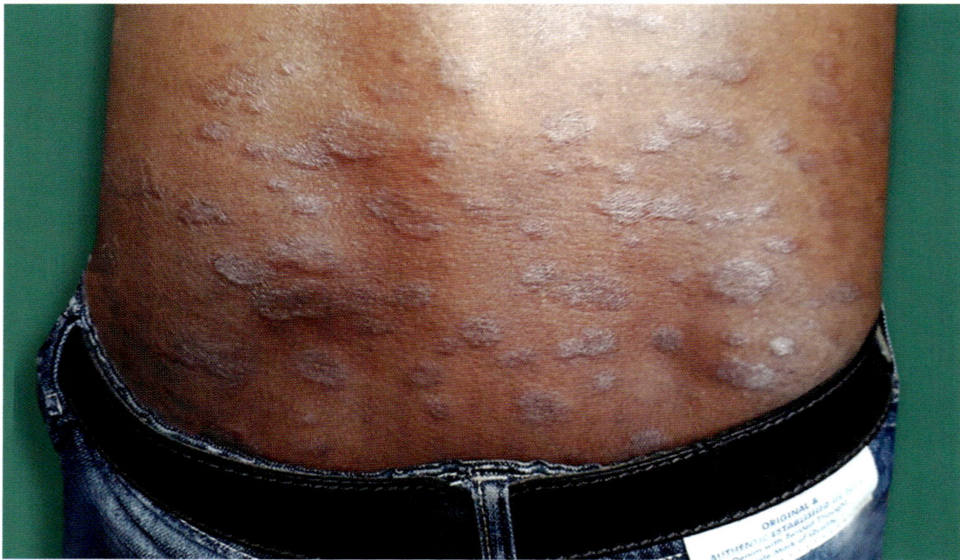

Fig. 29: A typical case of pityriasis rosea (PR).

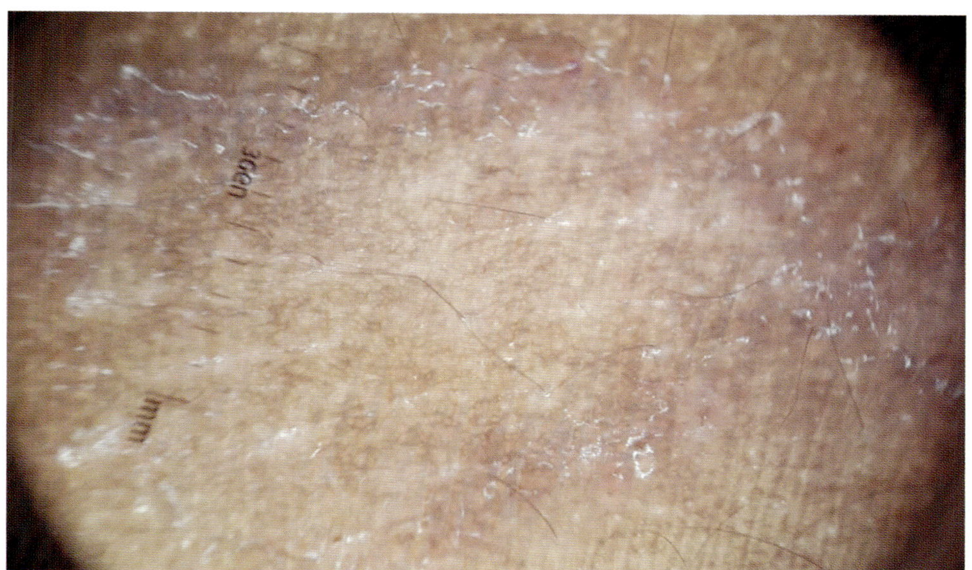

Fig. 30: Both the herald patches and the secondary lesions of pityriasis rosea (PR) present the peripheral scaling. The scaling may not always show typical collarette. This dermoscopic picture reveals a pattern of fine fragments of scales having no characteristic direction, or undefined direction.

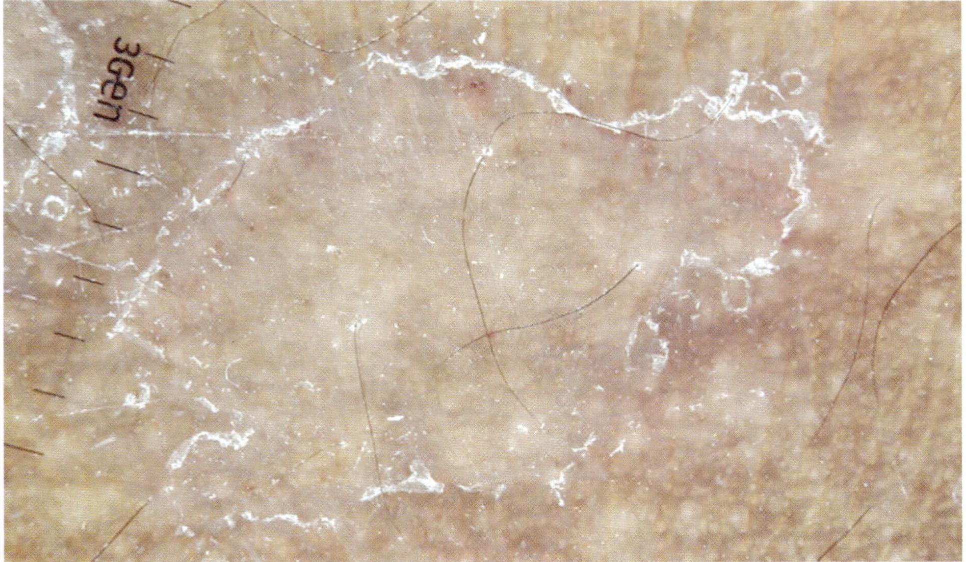

Fig. 31: Typical collarette scaling with peripheral brown pigmentation.

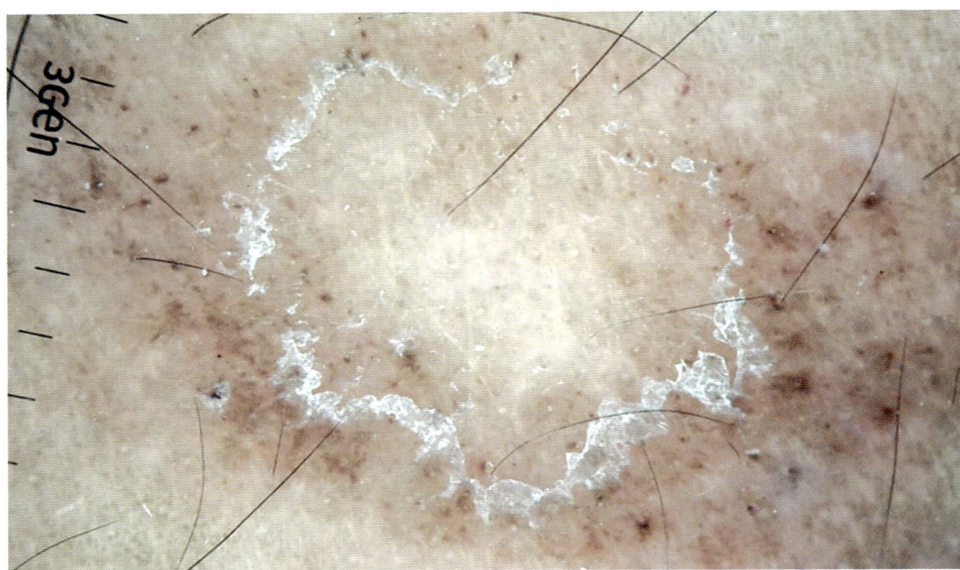

Fig. 32: A typical patch of pityriasis rosea (PR) showing collarette scale associated with brown patch peripherally; some erythema is visible outside the collarette.

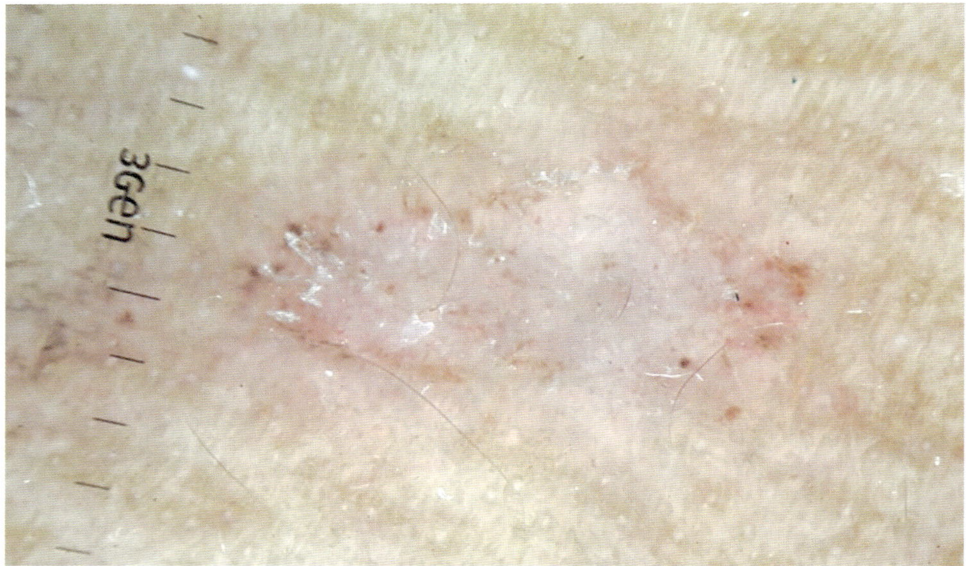

Fig. 33: Peripheral scaling with undefined direction of scales and few dotted vessels in patchy distribution. Red/orange color is seen peripherally.

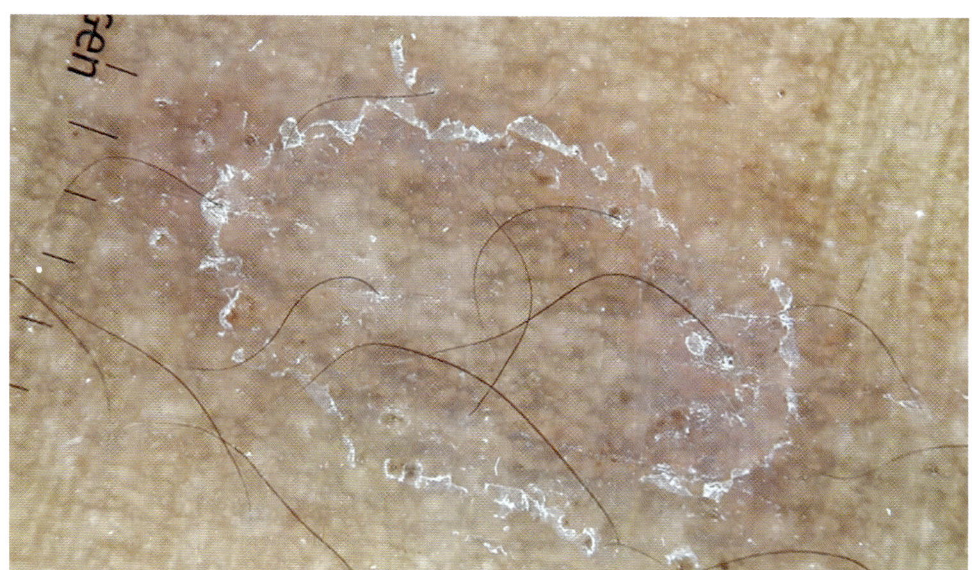

Fig. 34: Typical collarette scaling, peripheral annular brown pigmentation; note prominent melanocytic reticular network centrally.

Localized or diffuse yellowish-orange structureless areas may also be observed specially in Caucasians whereas in darker skin this dermoscopic structure is rarely visible. On the contrary, in darker skin, peripheral brown patch is frequently associated with the peripheral scale (personal observation).

KEYNOTE

Dermoscopy may be highly helpful to differentiate pityriasis from other annular dermatoses such as erythema annulare centrifugum, granuloma annulare, and porokeratosis; all of the other conditions have characteristic dermoscopic features.

REFERENCES

1. Allen RA, Janniger CK, Schwartz RA. Pityriasis rosea. Cutis. 1995;56(4):198-202.
2. González LM, Allen R, Janniger CK, et al. Pityriasis rosea: an important papulosquamous disorder. Int J Dermatol. 2005;44(9):757-64.
3. Browning JC. An update on pityriasis rosea and other similar childhood exanthems. Curr Opin Pediatr. 2009;21(4):481-5.
4. Tognetti L, Sbano P, Fimiani M, et al. Dermoscopy of Biett's sign and differential diagnosis with annular maculopapular rashes with scaling. Indian J Dermatol Venereol Leprol. 2017;83:270-3.
5. Lallas A, Kyrgidis A, Tzellos TG, et al. Accuracy of dermoscopic criteria for the diagnosis of psoriasis, dermatitis, lichen planus and pityriasis rosea. Br J Dermatol. 2012;166:1198-205.

PSORIASIS

INTRODUCTION

Usually the diagnosis of psoriasis is clinical, but atypical presentations such as a singular plaque or few plaques or guttate lesions may make the diagnosis of psoriasis very challenging and demand histopathology. Dermoscopy, in such cases can confirm diagnosis instantly thus avoiding the need for histopathology.

KEY DERMOSCOPIC FEATURES (FIGS. 35 TO 62)[1-3]

- Regularly distributed dotted vessels
- White scales
- Dermoscopic "Auspitz sign".

DISCUSSION

Dermoscopy of plaque psoriasis is characterized by regularly distributed dotted vessels against a pink background. Other vascular patterns such as "red globular rings" and convoluted loops also may be found. The "red globular ring" pattern is highly specific but rare whereas convoluted loops are visible under higher magnification (100–400). The convoluted loops correspond histopathologically to spiraled capillaries in the dermal papillae, associated with psoriasiform epidermal hyperplasia.

Dermoscopy of plaque psoriasis usually reveals diffuse white scales, simply highlighting the clinical picture.

In lesions with marked hyperkeratosis, removal of scales reveals a vascular pattern with blood droplets under dermoscopy and this is known as dermoscopic "Auspitz sign".

CASE 1 (FIGS. 35 AND 36)

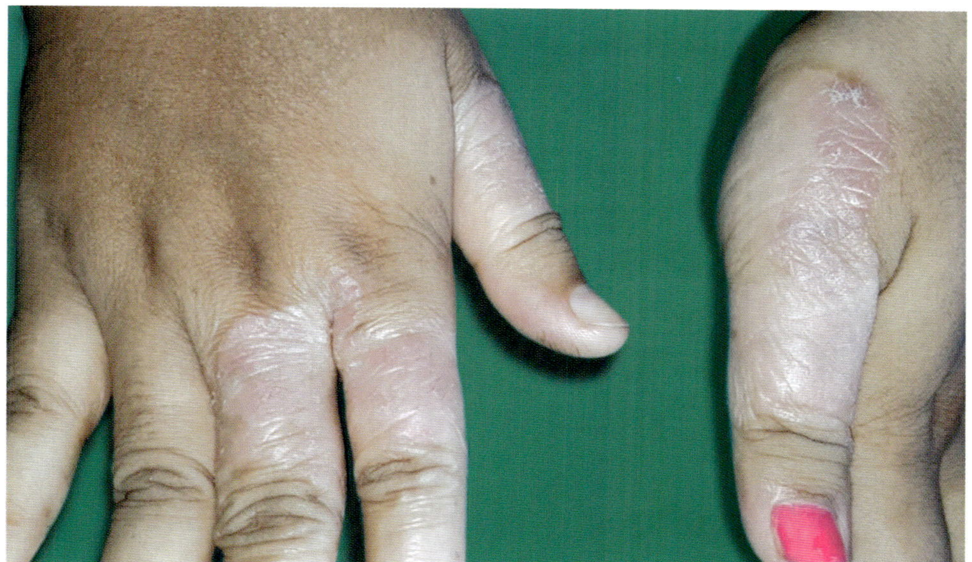

Fig. 35: Plaque psoriasis on extensor surfaces of fingers. It is covered with silvery white scales against an erythematous background. Scales may be scraped away to reveal the inflamed skin underneath, as in this case, where the patient is habituated to removing scales.

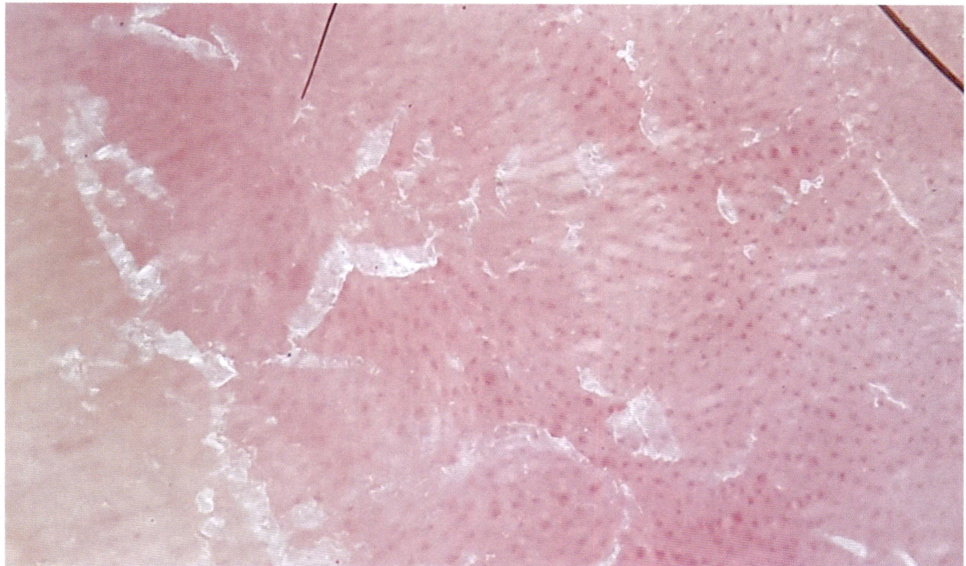

Fig. 36: Dermoscopy of plaque psoriasis reveals regularly distributed red dots and diffuse silvery white scales. Psoriasis has this characteristic vascular patterns due to dermal microcircular alterations, with larger and spiraled capillaries within dermal papillae associated with psoriasiform epidermal hyperplasia.

CASE 2 (FIGS. 37 AND 38)

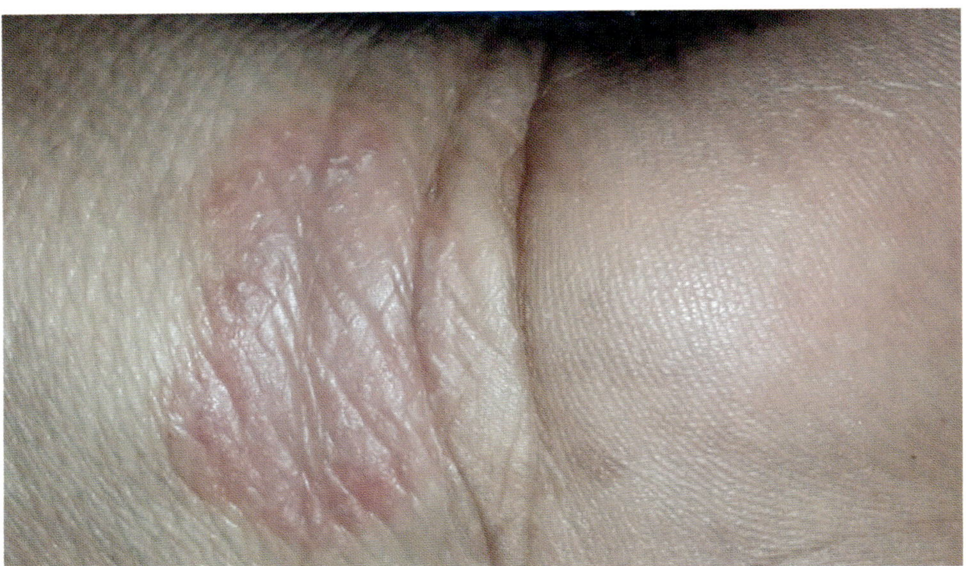

Fig. 37: Plaque psoriasis on wrist. Plaque psoriasis is frequent on the extensor surfaces of the knees, elbows, trunk, and scalp.

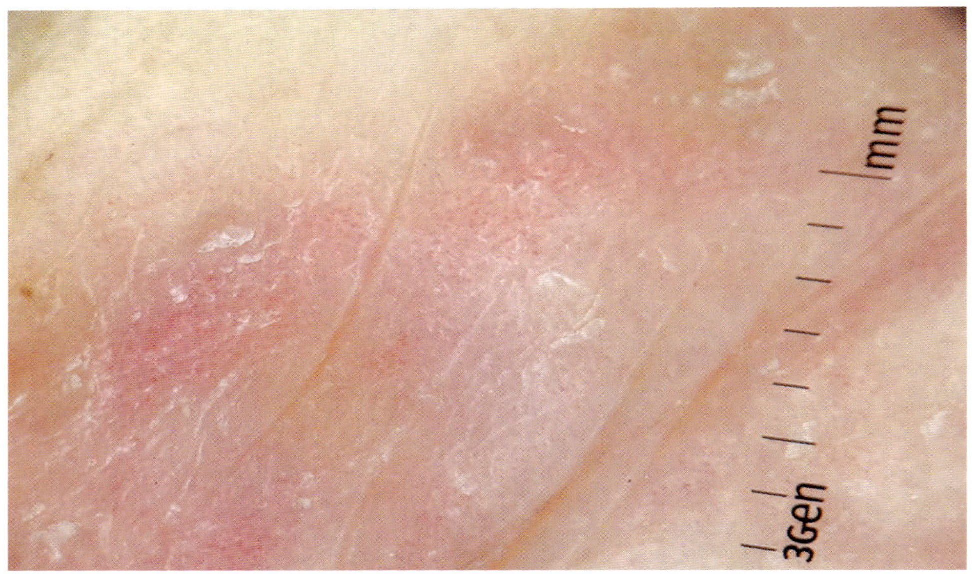

Fig. 38: Dermoscopy shows regular red dots on a pink background and white scales. The mere presence of red dots does not give a conclusive diagnosis, its regular and symmetric distribution is a must to label it as psoriasis.

CASE 3 (FIGS. 39 TO 42)

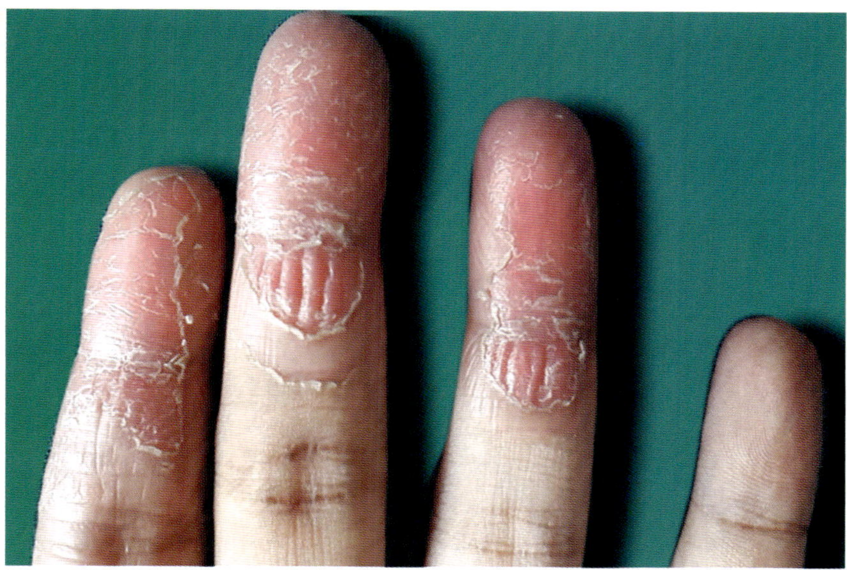

Fig. 39: Most common clinical presentation is erythematous plaque and scaling. Characteristically it begins with macules, which progress to maculopapules and ultimately evolve into silvery-white plaques on a glossy uniform erythema. Allergic contact dermatitis and hand eczema should be excluded.

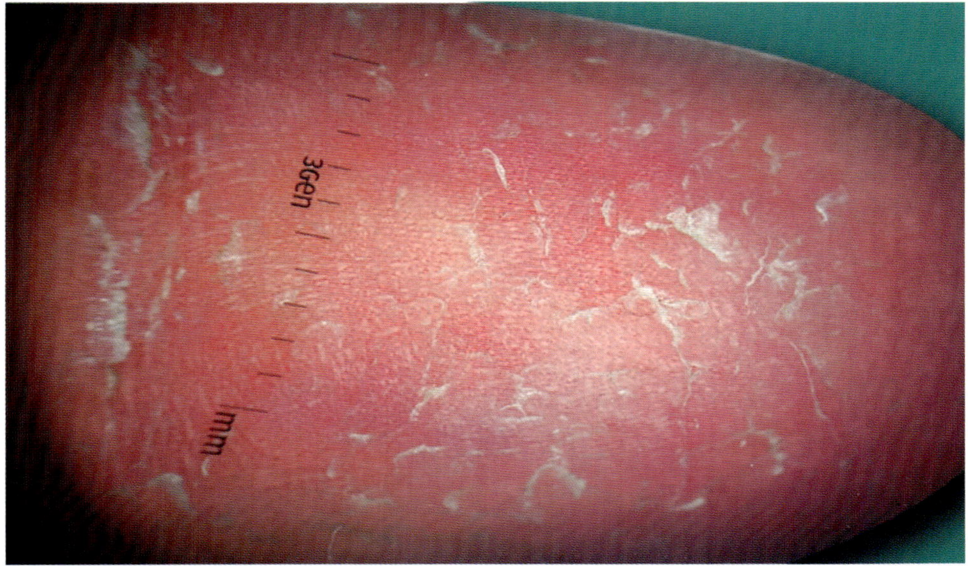

Fig. 40: White scales and regular red dots present throughout the lesion on the palmar aspect of the tip of the finger. Hand eczema and allergic contact dermatitis are common differentials in this case, but diagnosis of psoriasis can easily and instantly be made by finding the characteristic vascular pattern.

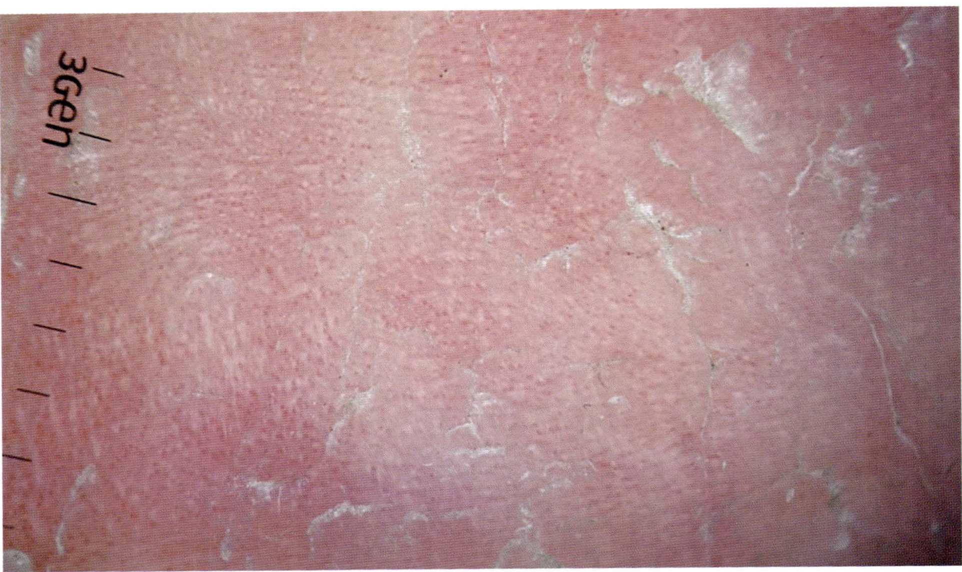

Fig. 41: Another finger of the same patient.

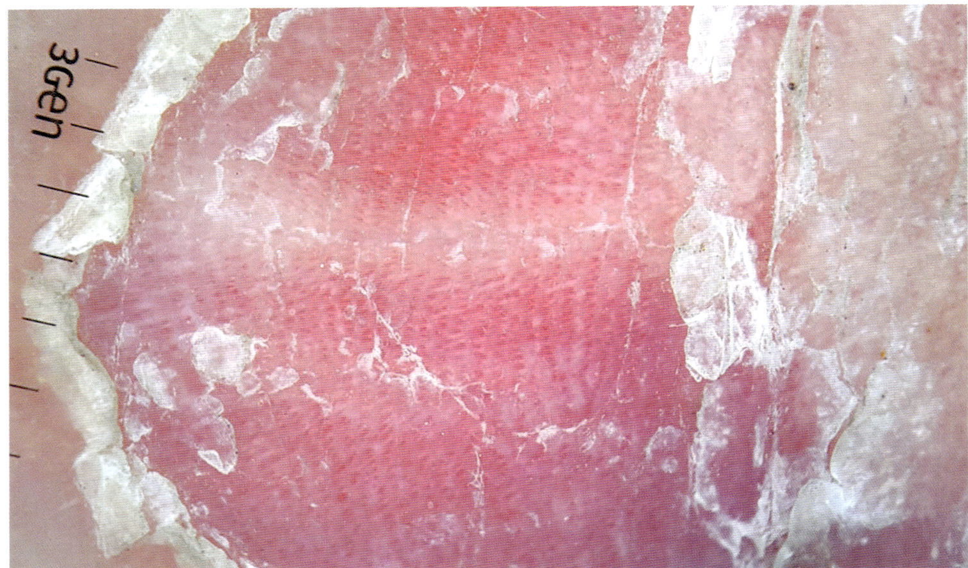

Fig. 42: Second finger of the same patient on magnification. Note the convoluted loops along with the red dots.

CASE 4 (FIGS. 43 AND 44)

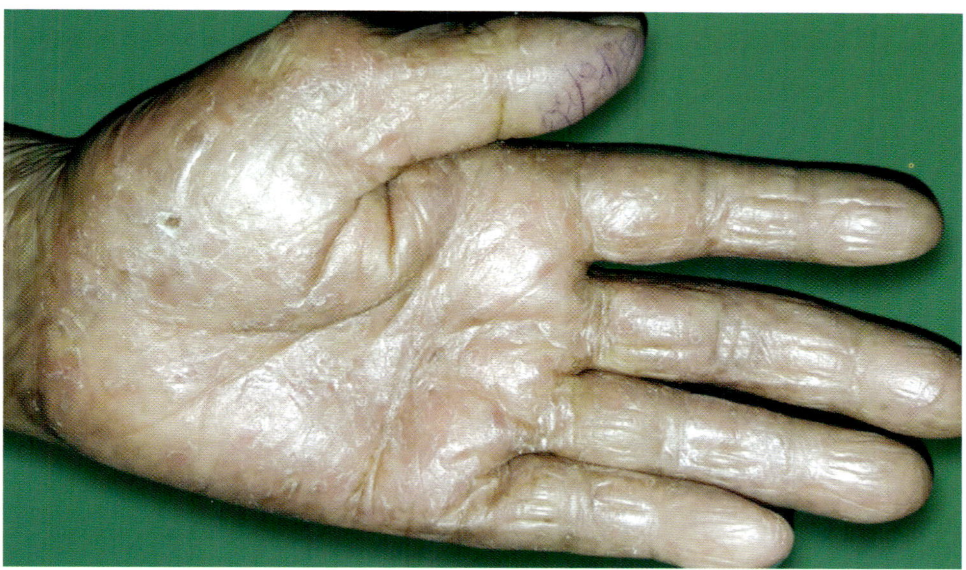

Fig. 43: Psoriasis may be localized on the palms and soles. Two main patterns are seen (a) well-circumscribed, red scaly plaques and (b) thickening and scaling of the whole of palms and soles. Often there are painful fissures. Sometimes acquired keratodermas and hand eczema may be difficult to differentiate from palmoplantar psoriasis.

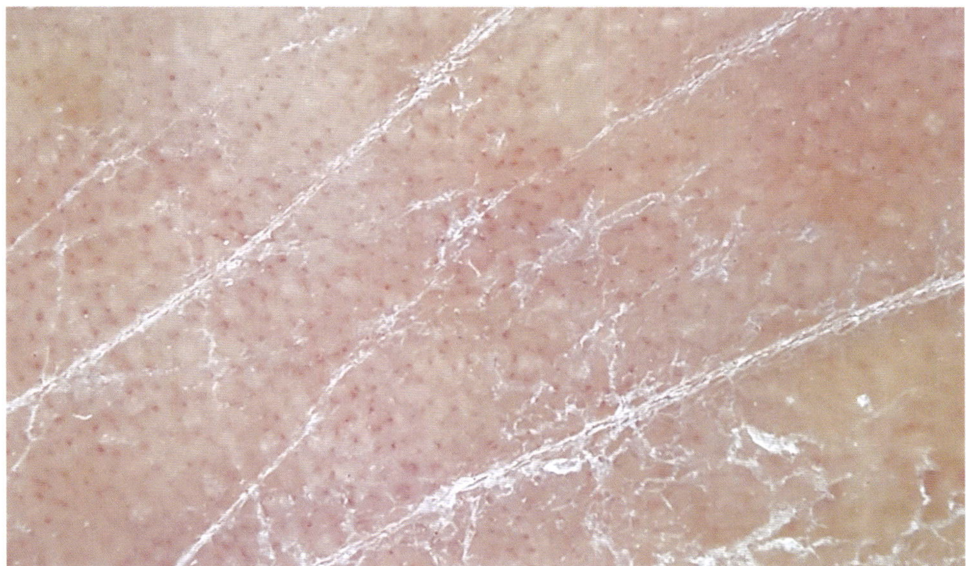

Fig. 44: Often dermoscopy is difficult in palmoplantar psoriasis due to the presence of thick scales. However, removal of scales in a particular area may help to reveal typical findings. In this patient of palmar psoriasis, red dots are seen to be distributed regularly and symmetrically on a dull red background; white scales are present over the palm and palmar creases are accentuated by the accumulation of scales.

CASE 5 (FIGS. 45 AND 46)

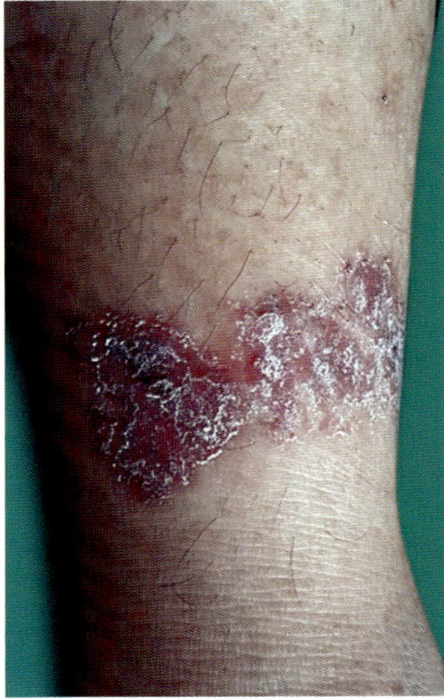

Fig. 45: Typically plaque psoriasis is raised, rough, and coated with thick silvery white scales. Fissures, a common finding of palmoplantar psoriasis, are seen in the upper left part of the lesion on the lower leg.

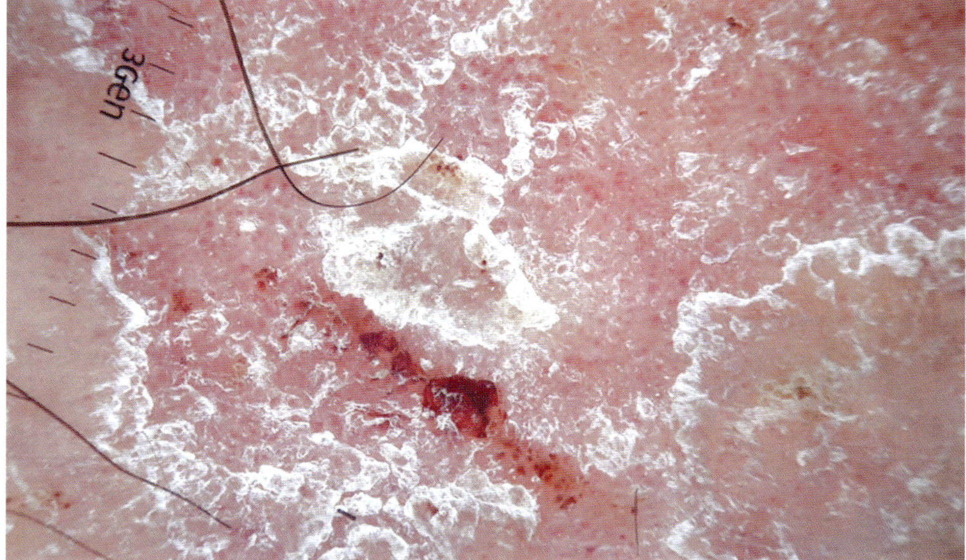

Fig. 46: Dermoscopic Auspitz sign (tiny red blood dots) is seen on dermoscopy in the region of the fissure. When a thick scale impedes the visualization of the underlying structure, scale removal may be followed by dermoscopic Auspitz sign. Typical findings of psoriasis such as regular red dots and diffuse white scales are also present.

CASE 6 (FIG. 47)

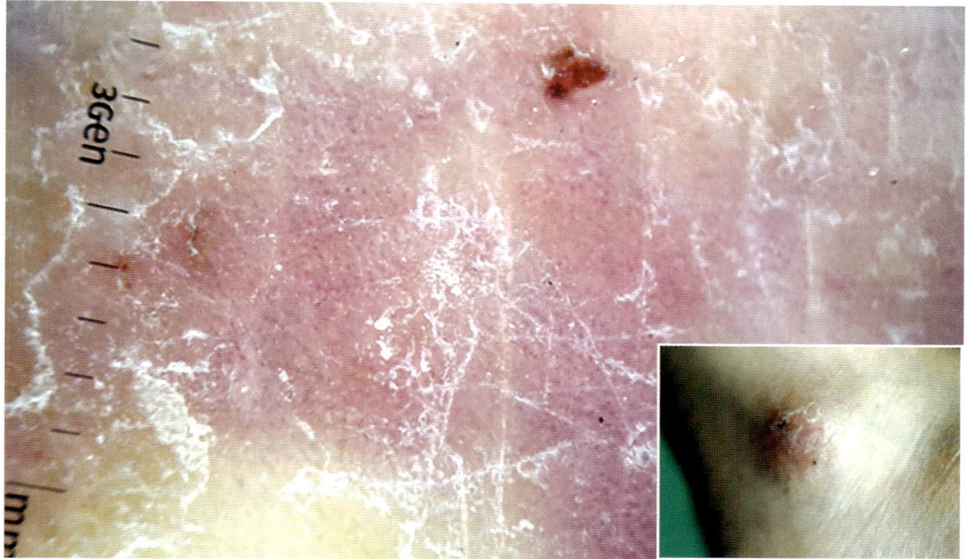

Fig. 47: Psoriasis may frequently be present over the skin of the lateral malleolus. Along with other typical features of psoriasis, dermoscopic Auspitz sign is also present.

CASE 7 (FIGS. 48 AND 49)

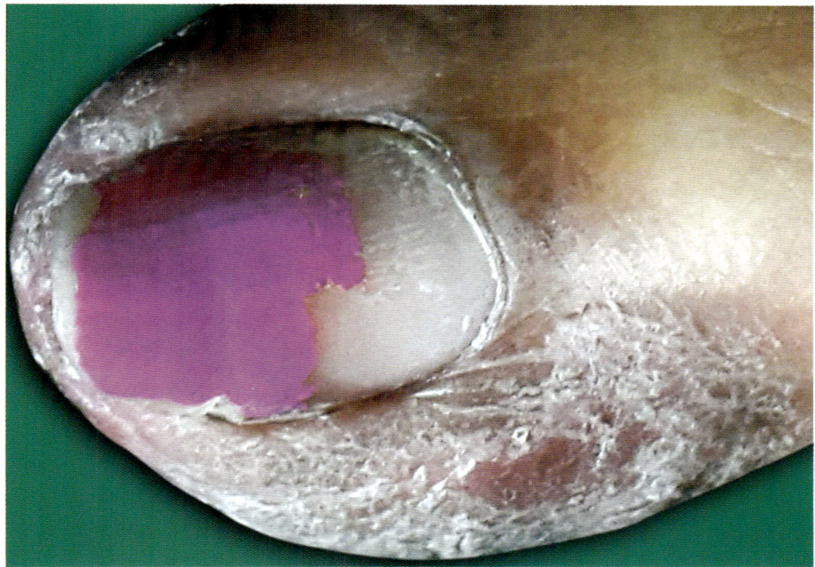

Fig. 48: Psoriasis of the distal toe may be localized or may occur as a part of generalized psoriasis.

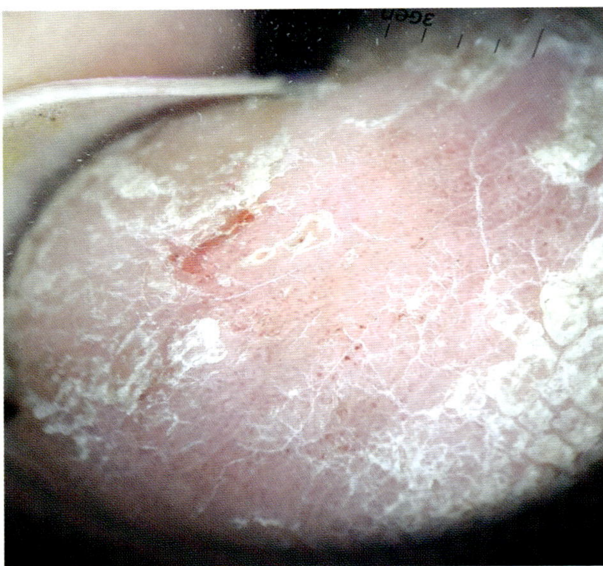

Fig. 49: Diffuse thick white silvery scales, homogeneous erythematous background, and clear visualization of regular red dots confirmed the diagnosis of psoriasis. Trauma is frequent in the region of toes due to habitual bare foot walking in village areas. The scales in the mid-area of the toe have been detached due to friction and trauma revealing the dermoscopic Auspitz sign.

CASE 8 (FIGS. 50 AND 51)

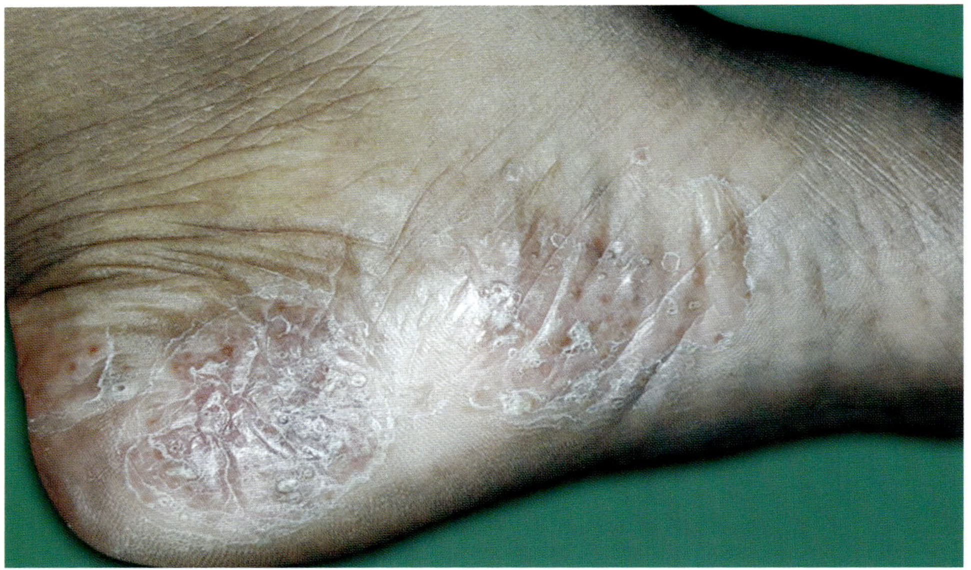

Fig. 50: Palmoplantar pustulosis presents as crops of sterile pustules and arises on one or both palms and or soles. Usually it is associated with thickened, scaly, and dull red skin. This category of psoriasis varies in severity and may persist for long. The discomfort may be minimum or at times considerable enough to interfere with day to day activities.

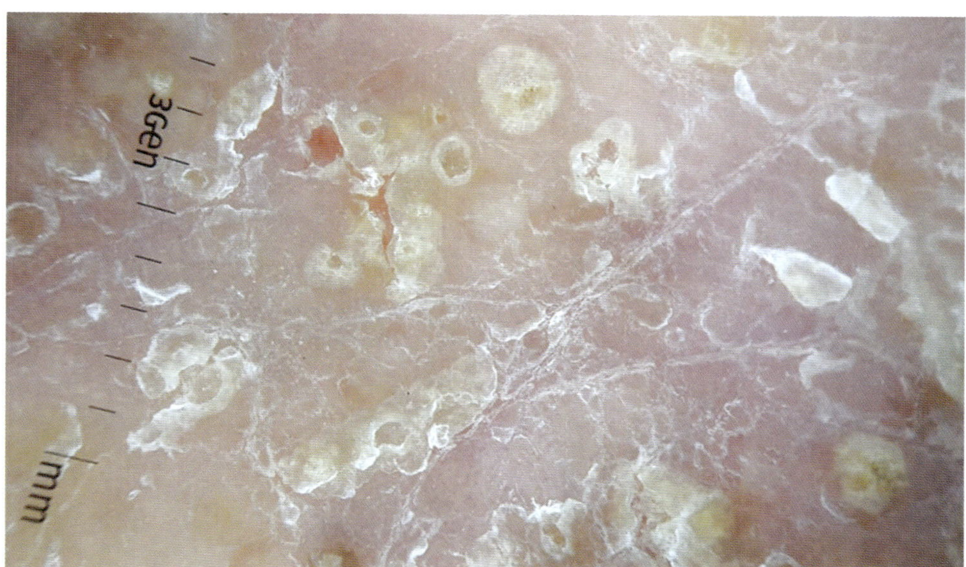

Fig. 51: On close inspection dermoscopically, red dots are interspersed with pustules. White scales are seen along with the yellow crusts of pustules. Some pustules are still intact whereas most of the pustules have ruptured with drainage of contents.

CASE 9 (FIGS. 52 AND 53)

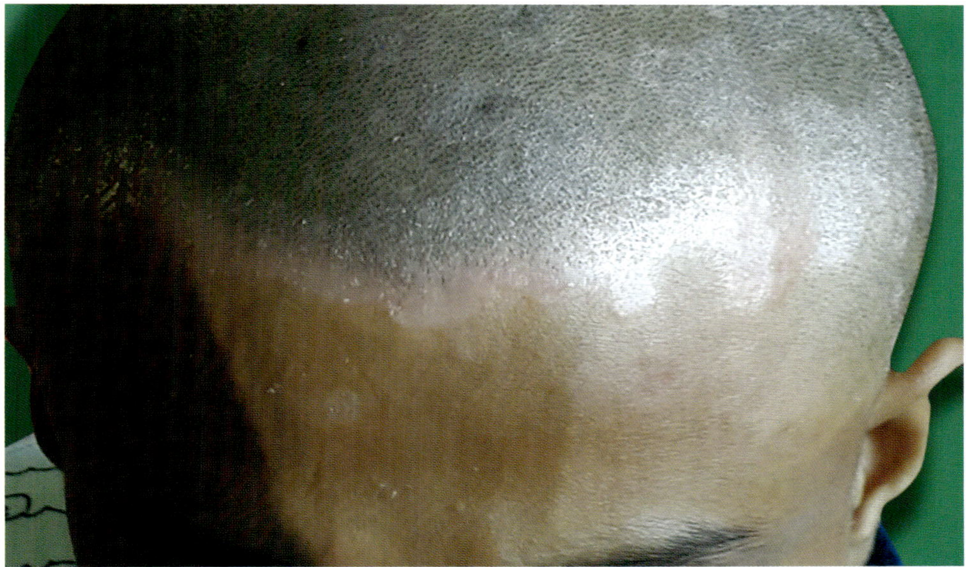

Fig. 52: Scalp psoriasis is characterized by sharply demarcated erythematous lesions covered with white scales which often spill onto the forehead.

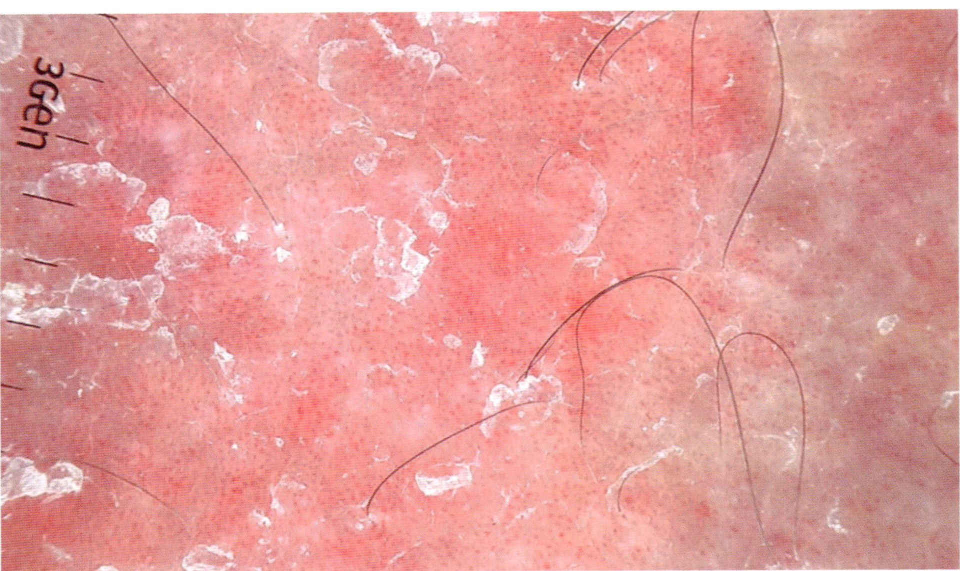

Fig. 53: Homogeneously distributed dotted vessels, entirely pink background, and diffusely disseminated white scales constitute a classical case of psoriasis on dermoscopy.

CASE 10 (FIGS. 54 AND 55)

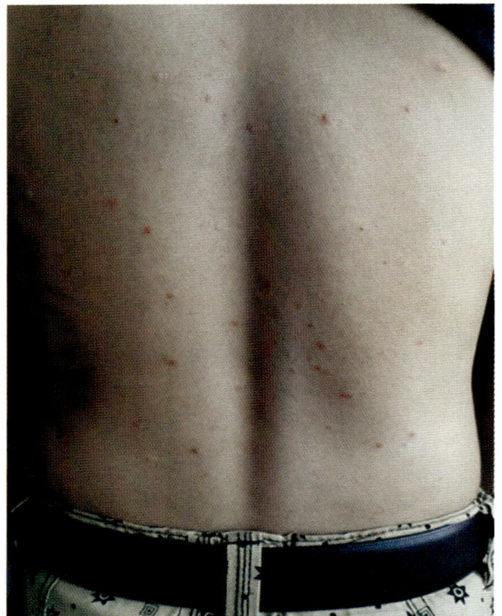

Fig. 54: Often the onset of guttate psoriasis is acute, follows a history of streptococcal infection of the upper throat and presents with multiple papules erupting on the trunk and extremities. Its common differentials are pityriasis lichenoides, pityriasis rosea, and secondary stage of syphilis.

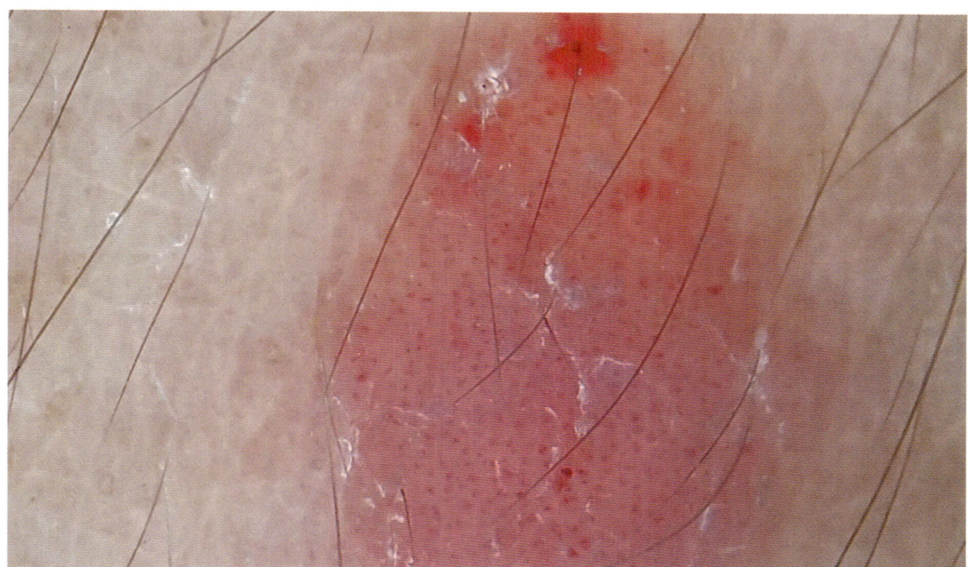

Fig. 55: Guttate psoriasis typically displays monomorphic dermoscopic pattern composed of regular red dots all throughout the lesion that are frequently associated with white scales; background erythema/orange-yellow structureless areas are also visible. These findings can easily differentiate guttate psoriasis from its close mimics.

CASE 11 (FIGS. 56 AND 57)

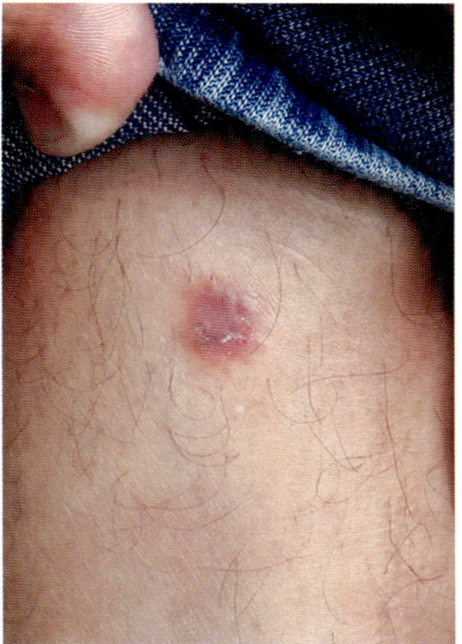

Fig. 56: Hyperpigmented, slightly lichenified, mildly itchy lesion just below the knee present since 6 weeks.

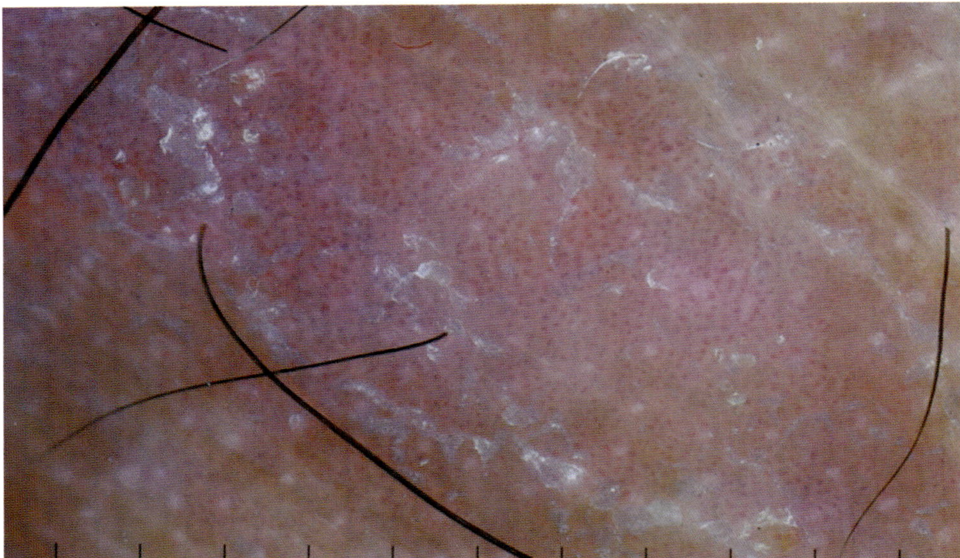

Fig. 57: On routine dermoscopy, red dots are distributed in a homogeneous fashion on a dull red backdrop; silvery white scales cover most of the surface of the lesion. A diagnosis of psoriasis is made and treatment is started. After a month the patient reports with improvement of the previous lesion but developed more lesions of psoriasis on trunk, elbows, and knees.

CASE 12 (FIGS. 58 TO 62)

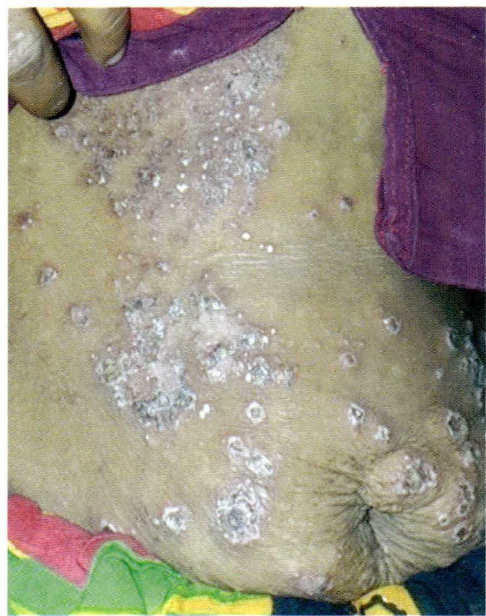

Fig. 58: Generalized pustular psoriasis presents with flares of widespread pustules on a red and tender skin. It is synonymous with acute generalized pustular psoriasis of Von Zumbusch. The most common differential diagnosis is subcorneal pustular dermatosis.

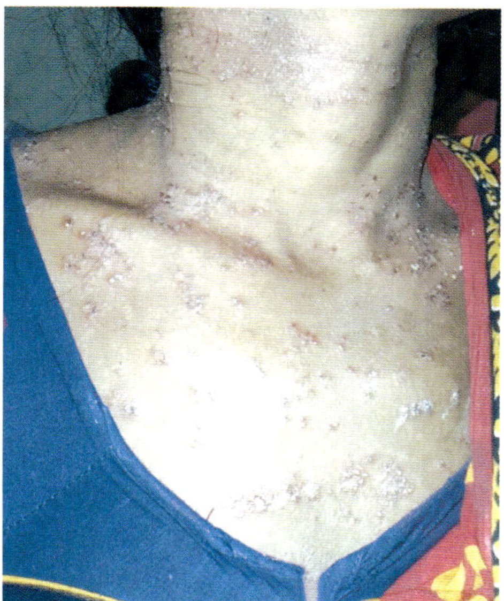

Fig. 59: Small pustules coalesce to form lakes of pus. They resolve and peel off to leave a smooth surface on which new crops of pustules appear. This cycle repeats itself every few days to weeks.

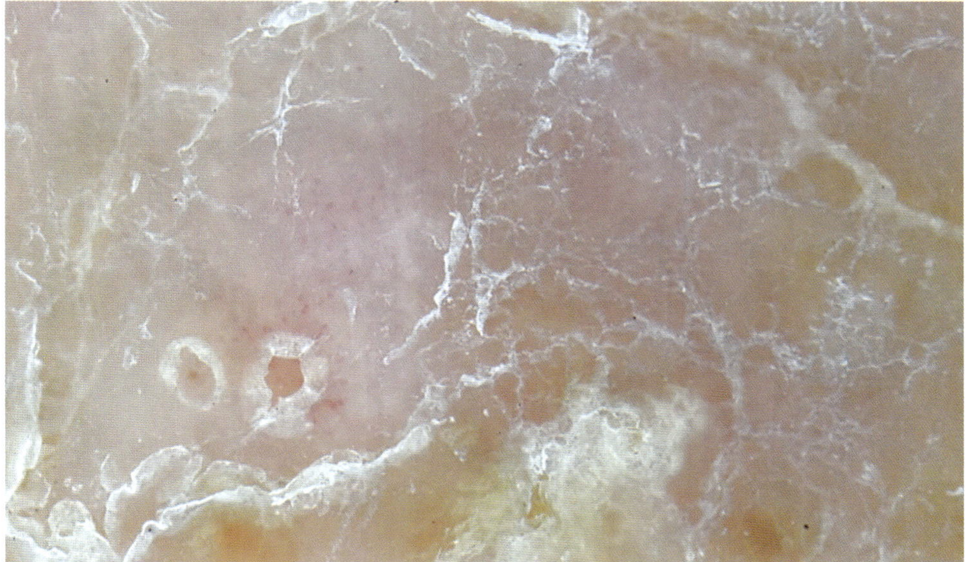

Fig. 60: Dermoscopy reveals red dots and pustules associated with white scales. The dried out pustules show yellowish scales.

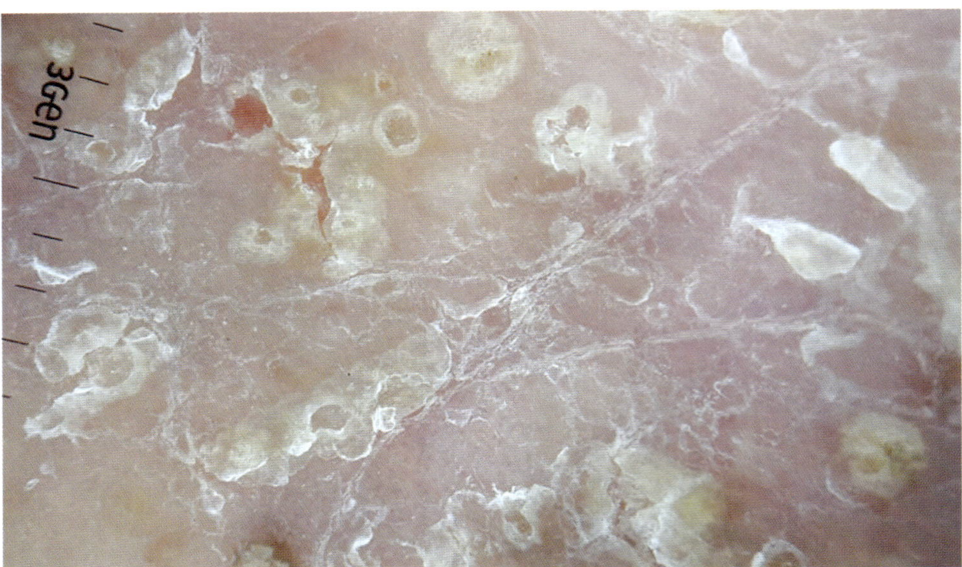

Fig. 61: Silvery white scales, erythematous background and red dots are observed in non-pustular areas. Both dried out and intact pustules are present in the field. Scales of pustules are yellowish in color.

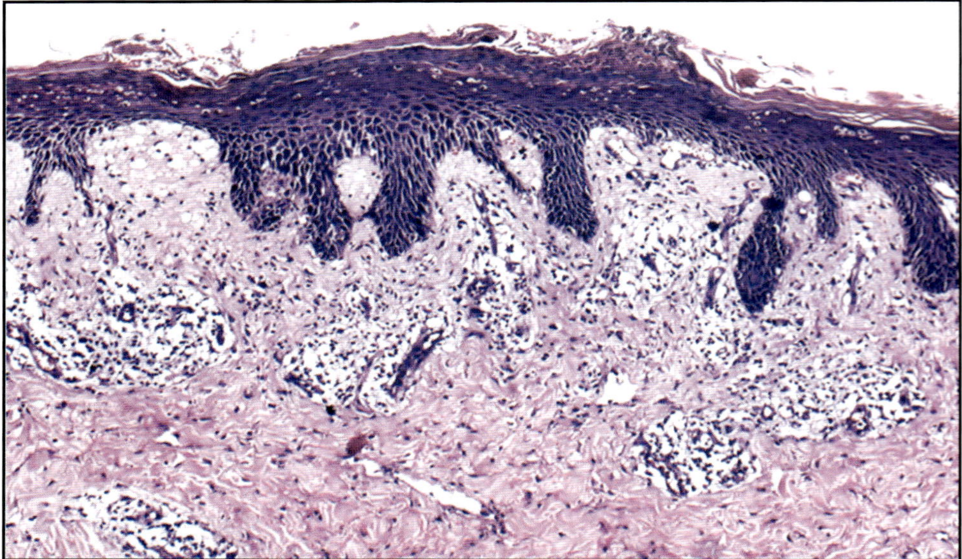

Fig. 62: Biopsy shows moderately dense superficial perivascular mixed infiltrate of lymphocytes, eosinophils, and neutrophils with papillary dermal edema and dilation of vessels. The epidermis shows large foci of spongiosis with a few neutrophils (neutrophilic spongiosis) with an upper epidermal spongiform pustule. The stratum corneum shows mounds of parakeratosis containing neutrophils.

KEYNOTE

Many erythematosquamous conditions share an almost similar clinical picture, thus differentiating them is difficult and may require an invasive investigating technique such as biopsy. Regularly distributed dotted vessels over a dull red background along with white scales are the dermoscopic key for diagnosis of psoriasis. Consequently, dermoscope is a useful tool for rapid diagnosis of psoriasis in case of a diagnostic dilemma.

REFERENCES

1. Lallas A, Kyrgidis A, Tzellos TG, et al. Accuracy of dermoscopic criteria for the diagnosis of psoriasis, dermatitis, lichen planus and pityriasis rosea. Br J Dermatol. 2012;166:1198-205.
2. Moscarella E, Longo C, Zalaudek I, et al. Dermoscopy and confocal microscopy clues in the diagnosis of psoriasis and porokeratosis. J Am Acad Dermatol. 2013;69:e231-3.
3. Vasquez Lopez F, Gonzalez-Lara L, Martin JS, et al. Dr K. Holubar (1936-2013). Teaching with dermoscopy: revealing the subsurface morphology of Auspitz 's sign and psoriasis. Int J Dermatol. 2014;53:e322-4.

CHAPTER 8

Infectious Dermatoses

Subrata Malakar, Anjali Pal

INTRODUCTION

The term entomodermoscopy has been introduced to describe the dermoscopic features in the diagnosis of infectious skin diseases. Dermoscopic patterns have been described and explained in various infectious dermatoses, such as bacterial, viral, fungal, and parasitic. On a number of occasions the dermoscopic patterns of several infectious dermatoses are highly specific and help in their instant and accurate diagnosis.

The use of new generation dermoscopes does not require direct contact with the lesion and hence minimizes the risk of cross infection among patients. For utmost precaution, one can use transparent cellophane sheet between the dermoscope and the lesion.

COMMON WARTS (VERRUCA VULGARIS)

INTRODUCTION

Verruca vulgaris although a clinical diagnosis may pose a diagnostic dilemma in children, or when present over the face where it may mimic other dermatological disorder like seborrheic keratosis, dermatosis papulosa nigra etc. Dermoscopy not only helps in diagnosing the condition but also in therapeutic monitoring after treatment to evaluate a possible recurrence.

KEY DERMOSCOPIC FEATURES (FIGS. 1 TO 3)[1-3]

- Multiple densely packed papillae, each containing a central red dot or loop
- Keratotic halo.

DISCUSSION

Dermoscopy displays numerous densely packed papillae each containing a central red or black dot or loop, surrounded by a whitish halo. This combination of features gives an appearance, which resembles frogspawn. The red dots and black dots correspond to normal and thrombosed vessels, respectively.

The central vessels are usually larger in comparison to plane warts and frequently associated with hemorrhages. This feature aids in doubtful diagnosis, such as in cases of irritated or periungual warts.[1]

The keratotic whitish halo represents papillomatosis on histopathology. The halo may not be visible in case of significant vascular occlusion.

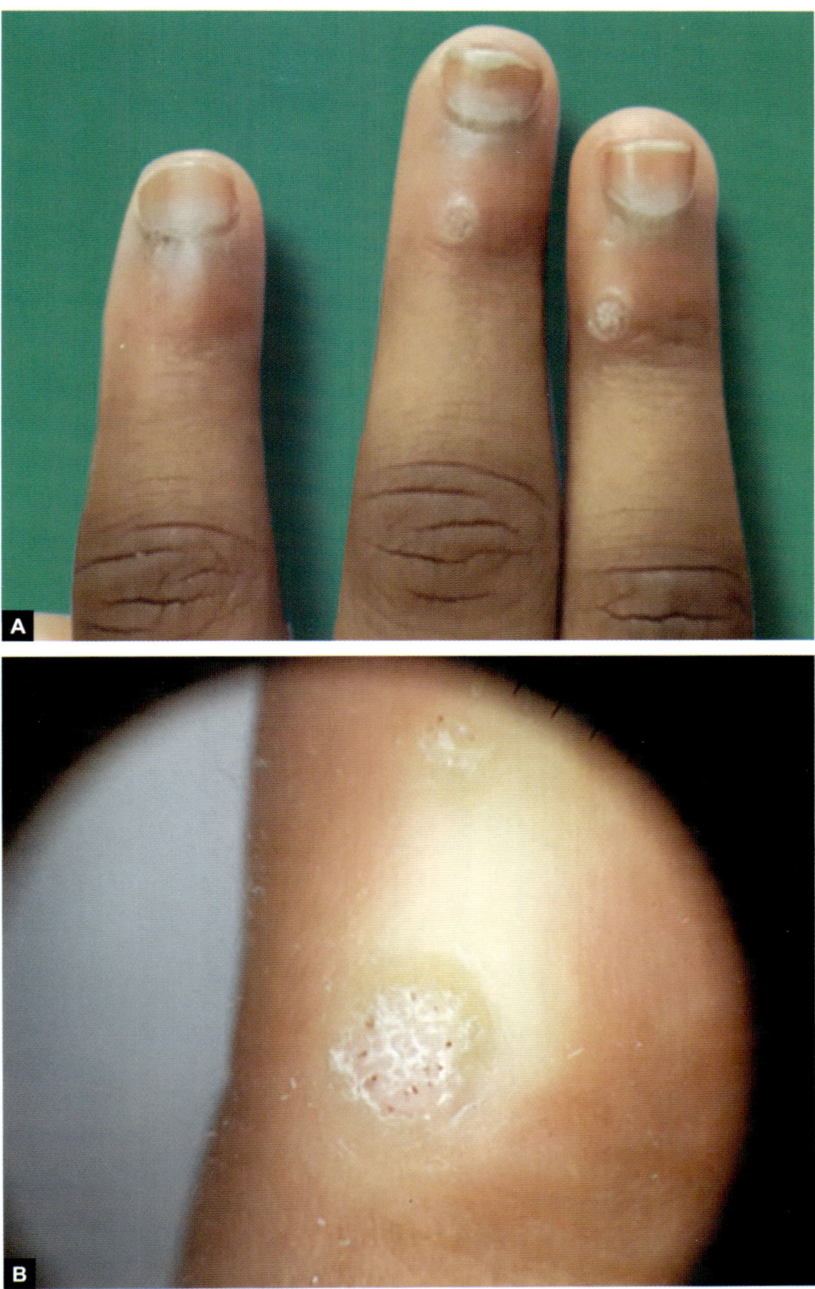

Figs. 1A and B: (A) Clinical picture of verruca vulgaris on the fingers (common in children with easy transmission through fomites/direct contact, therefore early diagnosis and treatment is imperative); (B) Dermoscopy reveals red dots and keratotic halos.

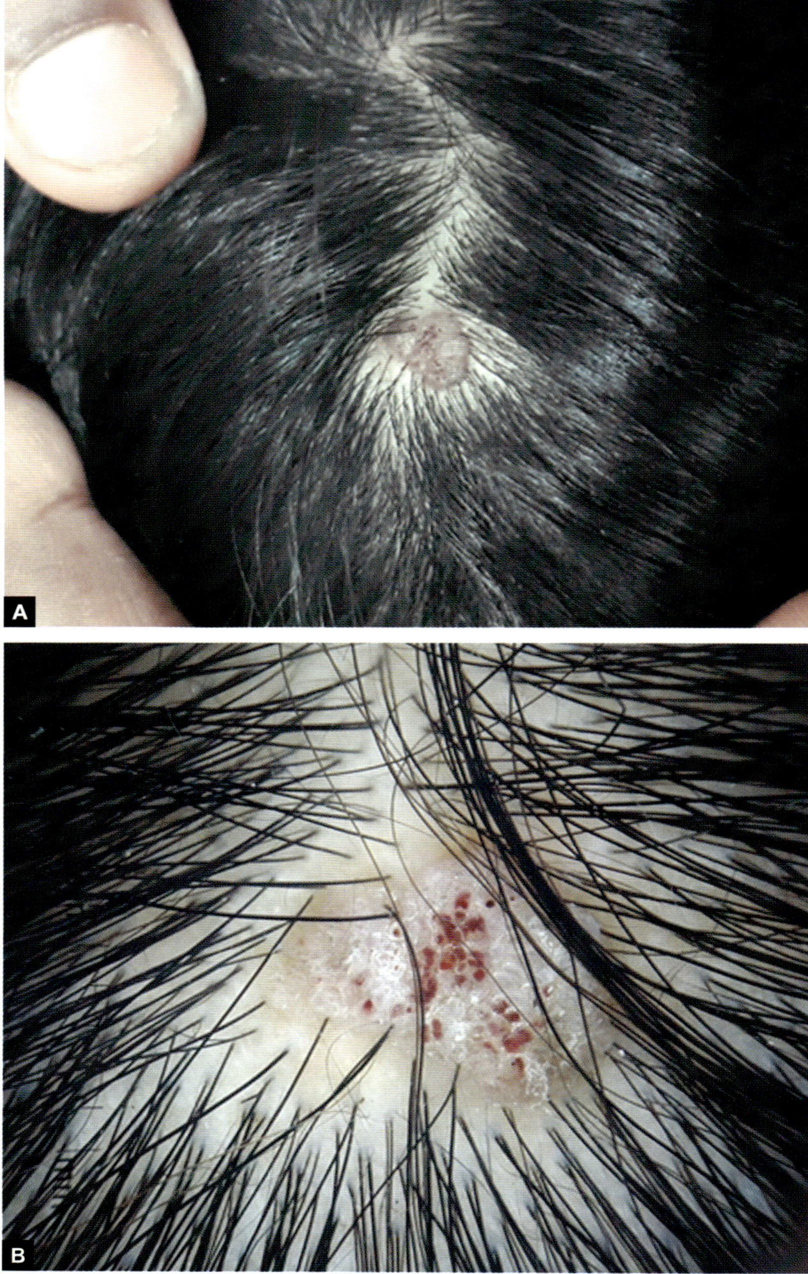

Figs. 2A and B: Verruca on the scalp (A); Dermoscopy revealing numerous red dots and keratotic halos (B).

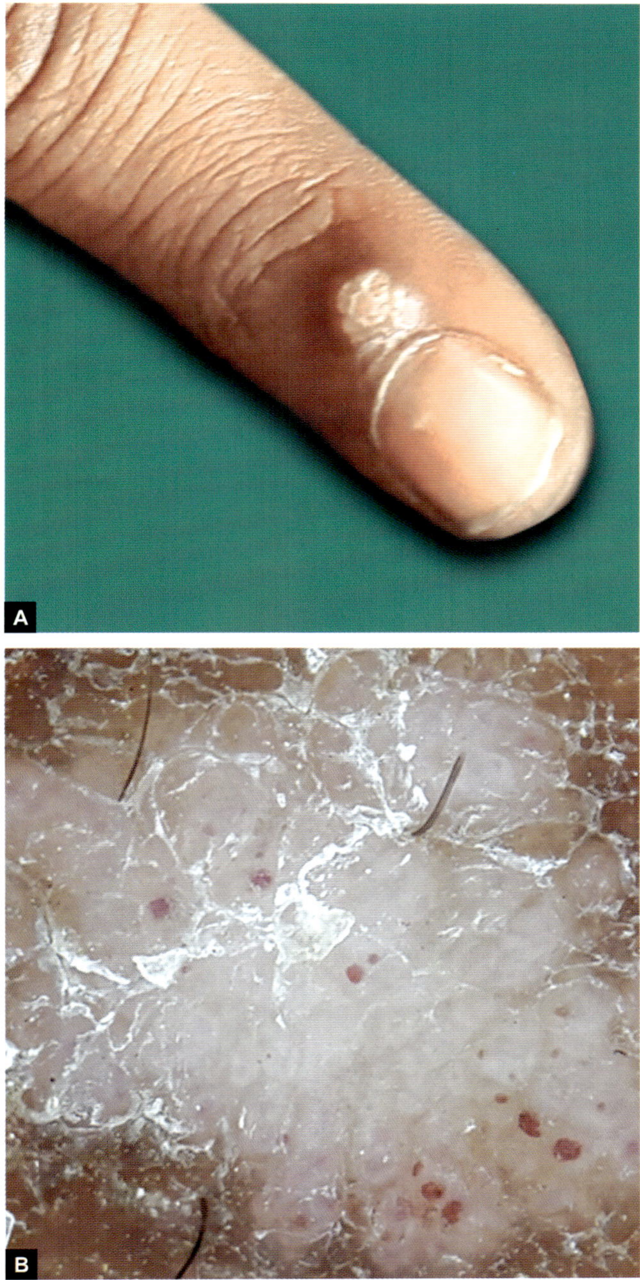

Figs. 3A and B: Periungual wart- (A) (Difficult to treat). Red dots with yellow white keratotic halos (B).

REFERENCES

1. Zalaudek I, Giacomel J, Cabo H, et al. Entodermoscopy: a new tool for diagnosing skin infections and infestations. Dermatology. 2008;216:14-23.
2. Tanioka M, Nakagawa Y, Maruta N, et al. Pigmented wart due to human papilloma virus type 60 showing parallel ridge pattern in dermoscopy. Eur J Dermatol. 2009;19:643-4.
3. Yoong C, Di Stefani A, Hofmann-Wellenhof R, et al. Unusual clinical and dermoscopic presentation of a wart. Australas J Dermatol. 2009;50:228-9.

FILIFORM WARTS (PERSONAL OBSERVATION)

INTRODUCTION

Filiform warts are lean growths commonly seen on the face, around the lips, and eyelids, and may occasionally develop on other parts of the body.

KEY DERMOSCOPIC FEATURES (FIGS. 4A AND B)

- Fingerlike projections
- Knoblike projections
- Hairpin vessels.

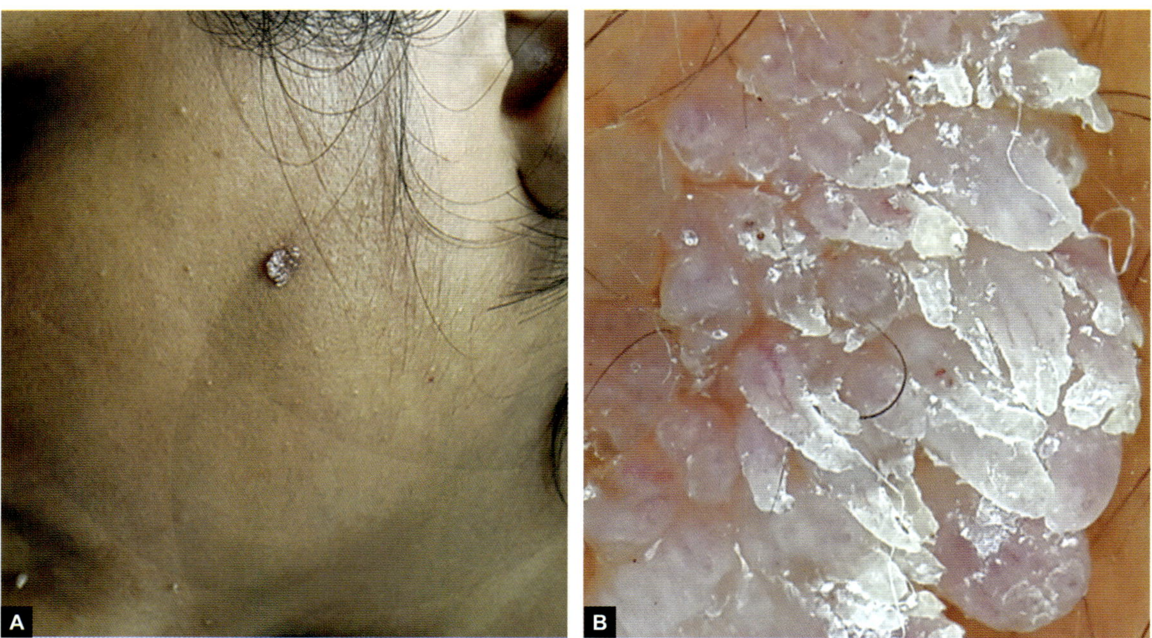

Figs. 4A and B: Filiform warts on the face (A); Fingerlike projections seen on dermoscopy (B).

GENITAL WARTS

INTRODUCTION

Genital warts can easily be diagnosed clinically. However, it can be difficult to rule out the early flat type without the acetowhite test.[1] Moreover, several other conditions in the anogenital area, such as condylomata lata, lichen planus, seborrheic keratosis, bowenoid papulosis, and erythroplasia of Queyrat also have to be differentiated from genital warts. Dermoscopy of genital warts reveals distinctive patterns and vascular features which not only helps diagnose the condition in the early stage of the disease, but also helps differentiate it from other conditions in the anogenital area.

KEY DERMOSCOPIC FEATURES (FIGS. 5 AND 6)

- Mosaic, knoblike, fingerlike, or in different combinations
- Vascular features, such as hairpin, glomerular, dotted, or in combinations
- Pigmentation
- Keratosis.

DISCUSSION

Genital warts display distinctive dermoscopic patterns and include mosaic, knoblike, fingerlike, or their different combinations.

"Mosaic" patterns are found in relatively flat genital warts and consist of a pattern of relatively flattened and rounded structures which appear as white reticular network. The "mosaics" are more or less similar in diameter and resemble a jigsaw puzzle.

"Knoblike" patterns reveal closely aggregated knoblike projections which are similar in both length and diameter.

A pattern with comparatively long and markedly separated fingerlike projections is called "fingerlike" pattern. These projections are similar in diameter but different in length. Fingerlike and knoblike patterns are most frequently seen in advanced, raised or papillomatous warts.

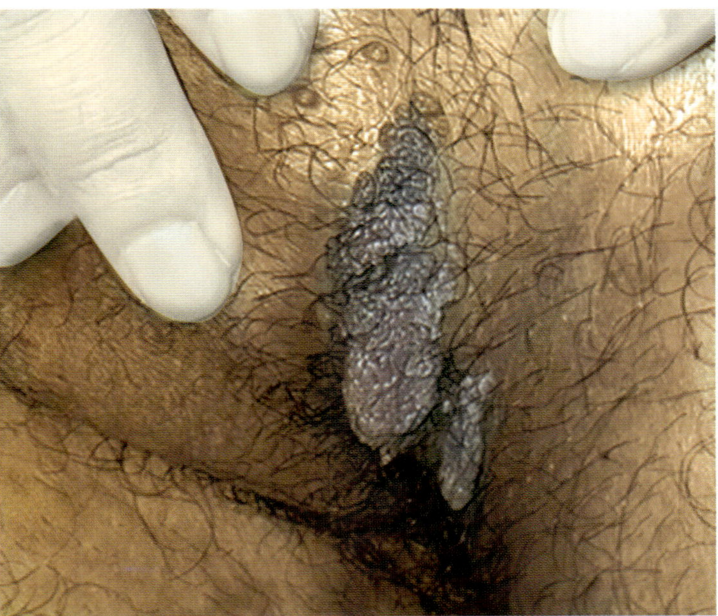

Fig. 5A: Papillomatous growth of genital warts in the groin.

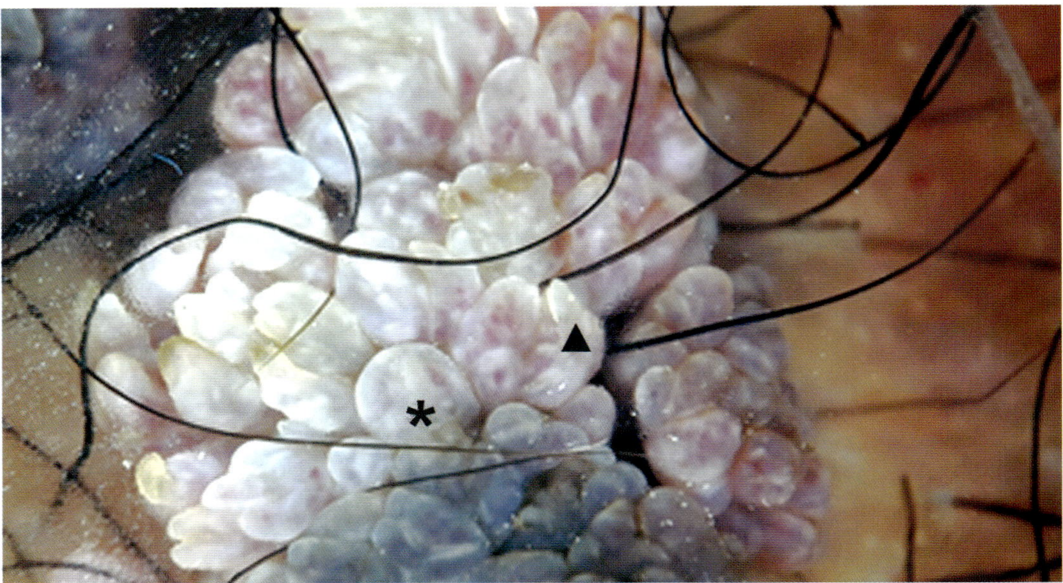

Fig. 5B: Knoblike (star) and fingerlike projections (triangle) on dermoscopy of genital warts.

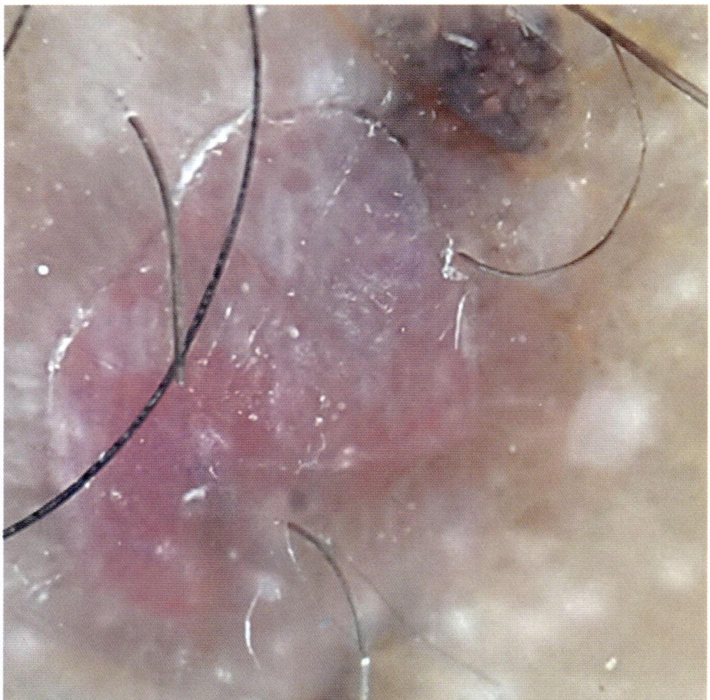

Fig. 6: Dermoscopy demonstrating reddish white areas of genital pyogenic granuloma. Thus, a dermoscope is very useful to differentiate warts from other genital lesions.

Dong et al. reported unspecified pattern, fingerlike and combinations of fingerlike/knoblike structures, which are the most frequent patterns seen dermoscopically.[2] Glomerular, glomerular/dotted, and hairpin/dotted vascular patterns are most common among vascular features. Dermoscopically pigmentation and keratosis are also observed but these features can also be seen with the naked eye.

KEYNOTE

Even in the early stage of genital wart, dermoscopy is highly helpful to diagnose the condition. Genital warts have distinctive dermoscopic patterns and can be utilized to differentiate it from other conditions in the anogenital area including lichen planus.

REFERENCES

1. Hunter H. Clinical presentation and natural course of anogenital warts. Am J Med. 1997;102:16-20.
2. Dong H, Shu D, Campbell TM, et al. Dermatoscopy of genital warts. J Am Acad Dermatol. 2011;64(5):859-64.

PLANE WARTS (VERRUCA PLANA)

KEY DERMOSCOPIC FEATURES[1]

- Regularly distributed tiny red dots intermingled with whitish lines
- Light brown or yellow background.

DISCUSSION

The hallmark dermoscopic sign of verruca plana is regularly distributed red dots on a light-brown or flesh-colored background. The red dots represent apices of capillaries in the papillary dermis (Figs. 7A and B).

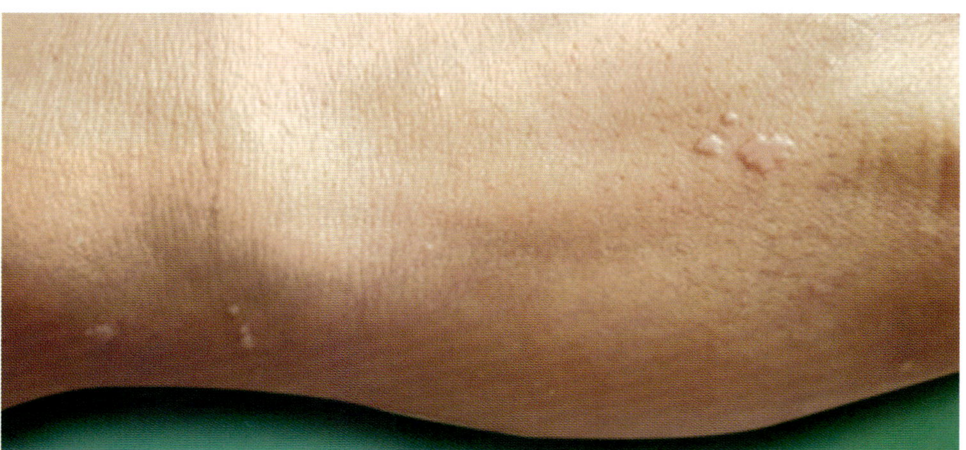

Fig. 7A: Fleshy skin-colored macules of verruca plana.

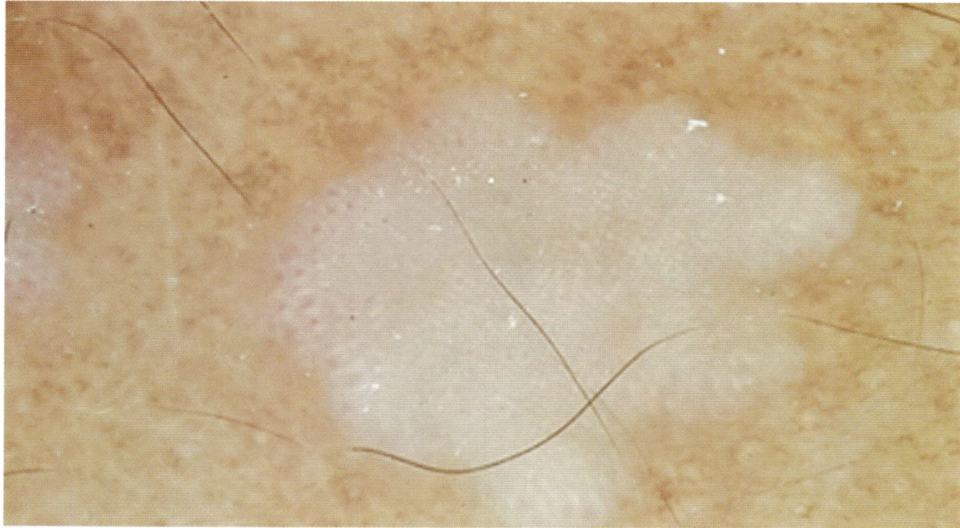

Fig. 7B: Dermoscopy shows tiny red dots with central homogeneous pattern.

REFERENCE

1. Zalaudek I, Giacomel J, Cabo H, et al. Entodermoscopy: a new tool for diagnosing skin infections and infestations. Dermatology. 2008;216(1):14-23.

PLANTAR WARTS

KEY DERMOSCOPIC FEATURES

- Irregularly distributed red/brown/black dots, loops or linear streaks
- Keratotic halo
- Verrucous yellowish structureless area
- Disruption of dermatoglyphics.

DISCUSSION (FIGS. 8 TO 12)

The dermoscopic picture of plantar wart is slightly modified in comparison to warts of other region, due to the pressure effect on vessels of the weight-bearing area.

On dermoscopy, they appear as verrucous yellowish structureless areas showing irregularly distributed red/brown/black dots, globules, loops or linear streaks representing hemorrhages; they are caused due to high pressure on plantar vasculature. The characteristic hemorrhages differentiate plantar warts from callus which is devoid of any hemorrhage.

The hemorrhagic dots are surrounded by keratotic halos which correspond to papillomatosis.[1]

Occasionally it is difficult to differentiate plantar warts from corns or calluses. Corns are painful localized hyperkeratosis that forms over interphalangeal joints due to pressure and friction. Calluses are hyperkeratotic lesions resulting from excess friction. Corns develop from localized forces whereas calluses develop from forces distributed over a broad area of skin.

KEYNOTE

Not uncommonly, it is difficult to differentiate plantar wart from corn or callus clinically. Dermoscopy can instantly solve this uncertainty. Corn shows a translucent central core that is more visible dermoscopically after trimming; whereas callus demonstrates homogeneous opacity.[2]

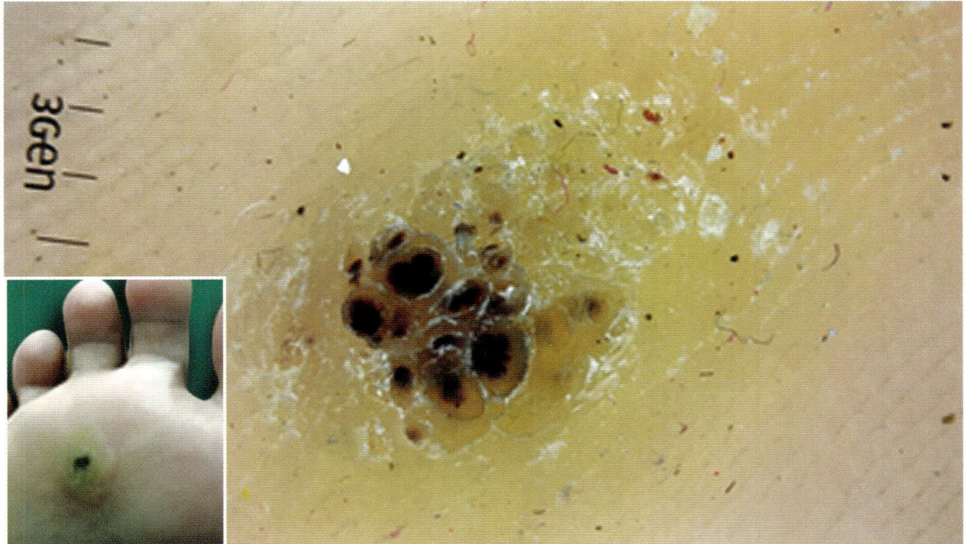

Fig. 8: A case of plantar wart dermoscopically showing red dots, black dots and keratotic halos. Note the disruption of dermatoglyphics.

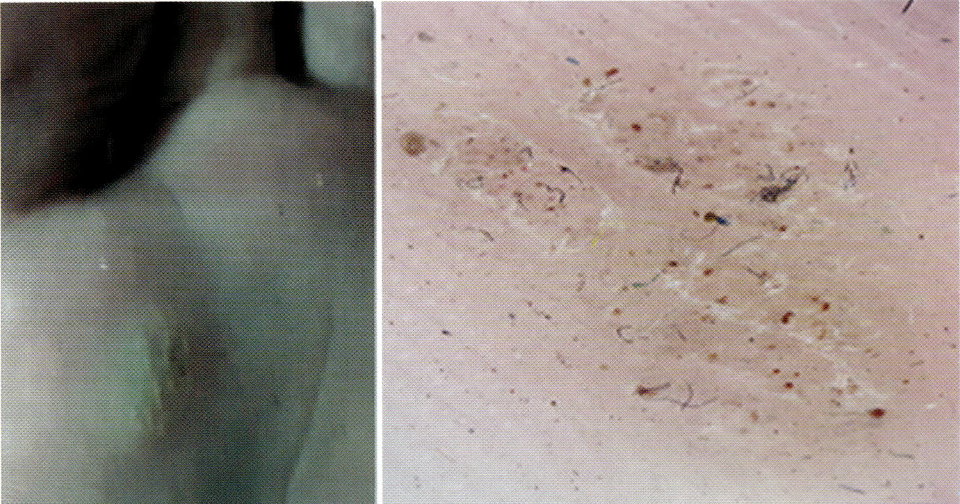

Fig. 9: Mosaic wart. A case of conglomeration of warts in a mosaic pattern showing extensive red dots, few black dots, and tiny keratotic halos.

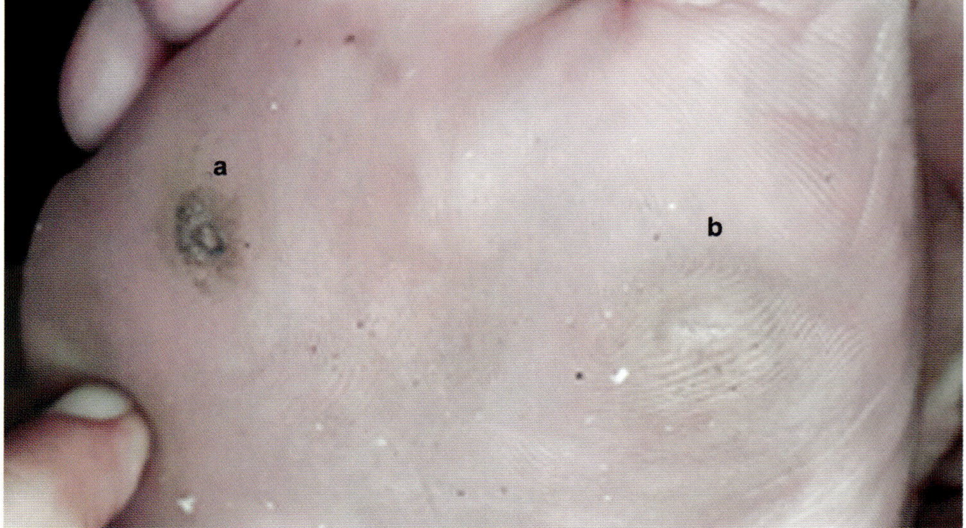

Fig. 10A: Figure showing both corn (a) and callus (b) which may at times be difficult to differentiate clinically.

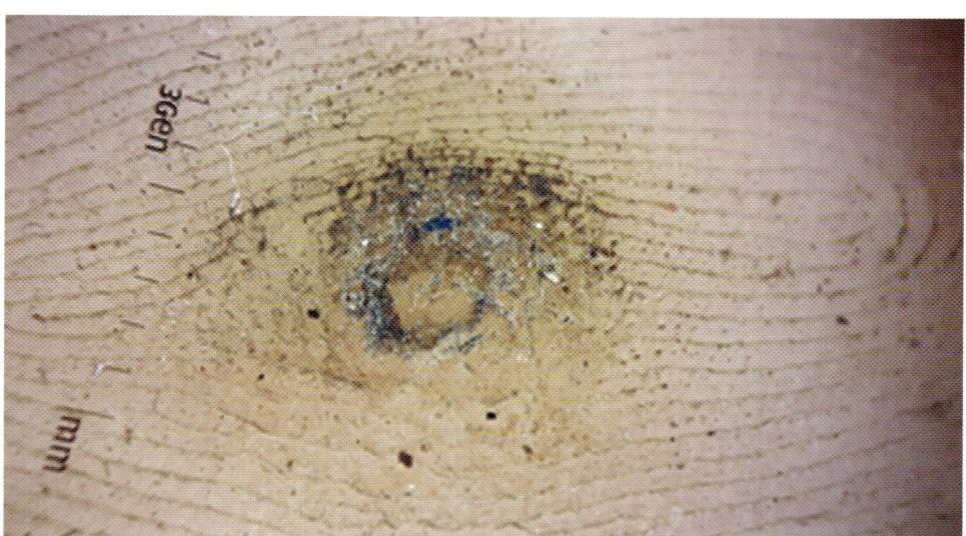

Fig. 10B: On dermoscopy, corn shows a central core with maintained dermatoglyphics.

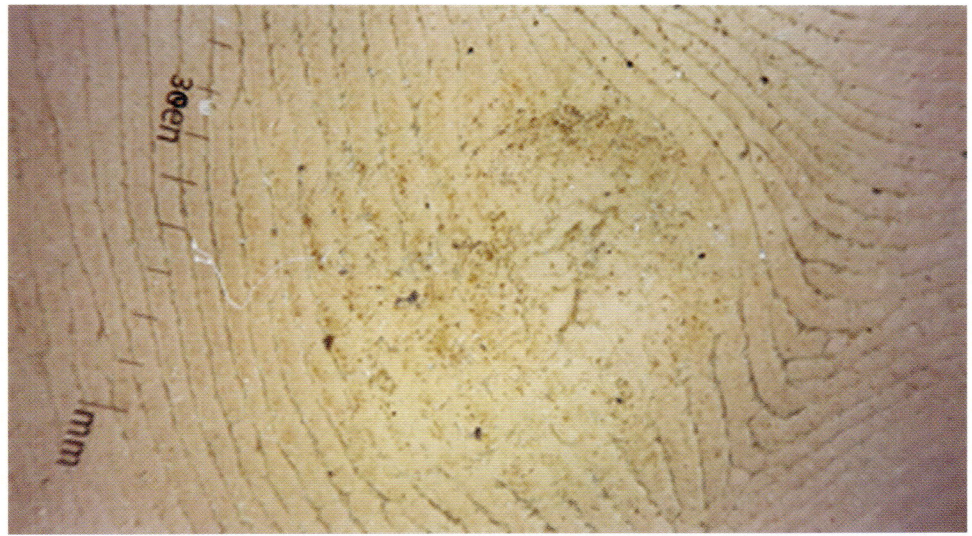

Fig. 10C: Dermoscopy of callus showing homogeneous opacity.

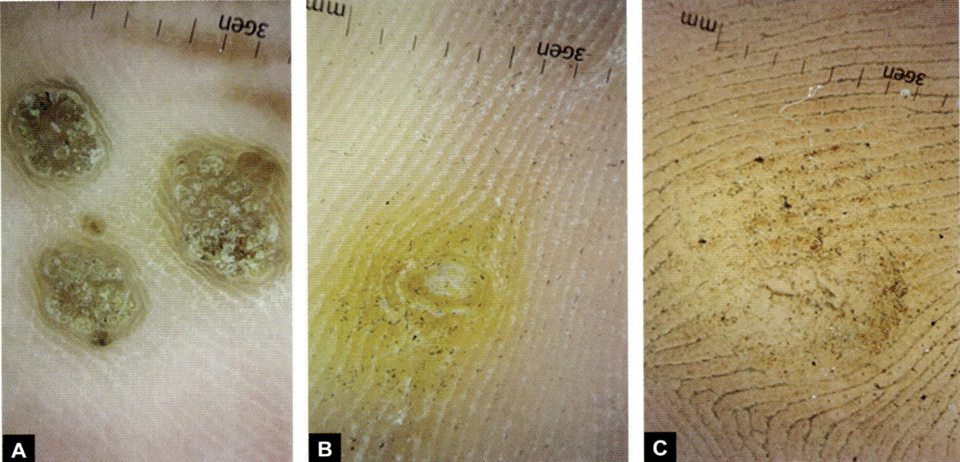

Figs. 11A to C: A comparative picture showing dermoscopic features of (A) Wart—red dots and black dots surrounded by keratotic halo along with disruption of dermatoglyphics; (B) Corn—central core with intact dermatoglyphics; and (C) Callus—homogeneous opacity.

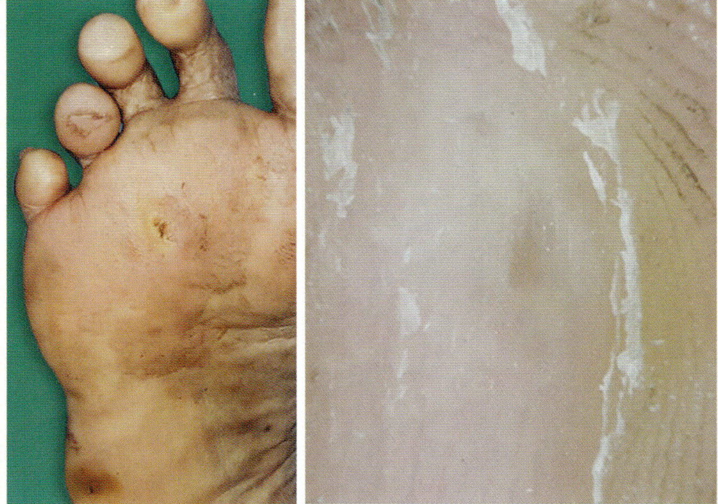

Fig. 12: Superficial paring of a corn revealed central core.

REFERENCES

1. Martín JM, Bella-Navarro R, Jordá E. Vascular patterns in dermoscopy. Actas Dermosifiliogr. 2012;103(5):357-75.
2. Bae JM, Kang H, Kim HO, Park YM. Differential diagnosis of plantar wart from corn, callus and healed wart with the aid of dermoscopy. Br J Dermatol. 2009;160(1):220-2

MOLLUSCUM CONTAGIOSUM

INTRODUCTION

Molluscum contagiosum (MC) viruses causes waxy papules, single or more commonly multiple, rounded and dome-shaped, that are umbilicated and contain a caseous plug.

KEY DERMOSCOPIC FEATURES

- Central pore or umbilication in association with white to yellow polylobular amorphous structure
- Crown vessels
- Rosettes.

DISCUSSION (FIGS. 13 TO 16)

In the center of the lesion, dermoscopy shows a pore or umbilication along with white-yellowish polylobular amorphous structure. The polylobulous structure corresponds histologically to inverted lobules of hyperplastic squamous epithelium occupied by molluscum bodies. The latter expands as the disease progresses, displacing the dermis to reveal dermal vessels at the periphery of the papule.[1,2]

The dermoscopic hallmark of MC consists of crown vessels at the periphery of the lesion with a radial distribution, thus resembling a crown. These vessels do not cross the center of the lesion.[3,4]

Rosettes are important additional features of MC; not infrequently, when other dermoscopic features are less evident rosettes may be highly valuable clue to the diagnosis.[5]

KEYNOTE

Molluscum contagiosum is usually a clinical diagnosis. Occasionally or in the very early stage when the lesions are tiny, diagnosis may be a dilemma. Here, dermoscopy comes to the rescue, with the classical and additional features diagnostic of the condition. Remember rosettes as an additional yet valuable a clue to the diagnosis of MC.

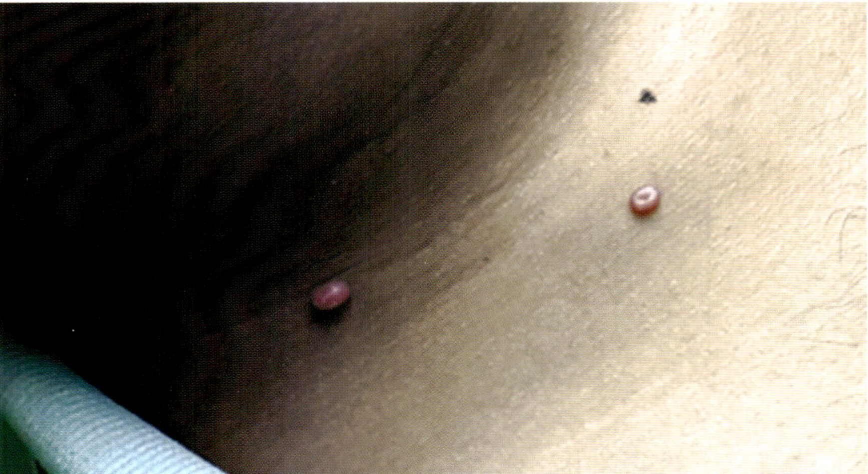

Fig. 13A: Molluscum contagiosum (MC) virus typically causes multiple, rounded, dome-shaped, skin-colored or pink papules; sometimes only a single papule is present. The papules are centrally umbilicated that contain caseous plug.

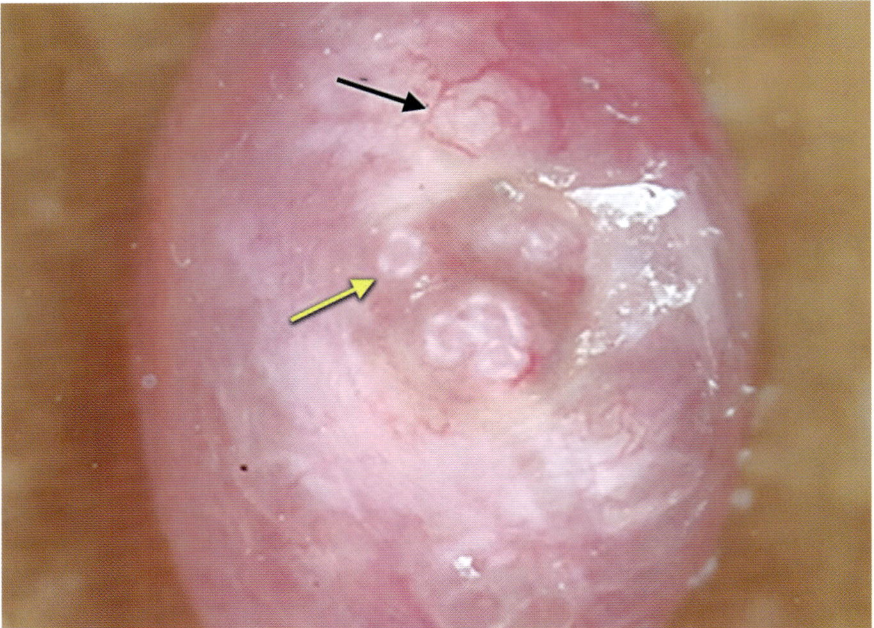

Fig. 13B: In the center of the lesion, dermoscopy shows a pore or umbilication along with white-yellowish polylobular amorphous structure. The dermoscopic hallmark of molluscum contagiosum (MC) consists of crown vessels (black arrow) at the periphery of the lesion with a radial distribution, thus resembling a crown. These vessels do not cross the center of the lesion. Rosettes (yellow arrow) are also observed.

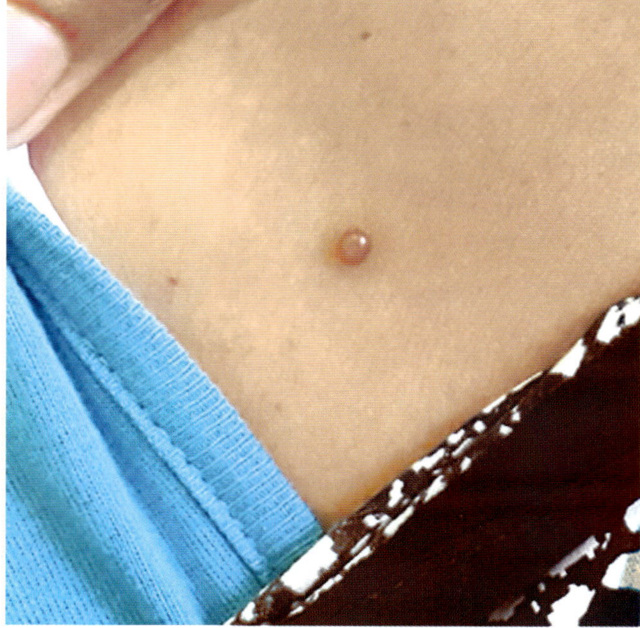

Fig. 14A: Larger molluscum contagiosum (MC) lesions may have multiple clumps of MC bodies rather than the single central umbilication. Diagnosis may be difficult in this situation.

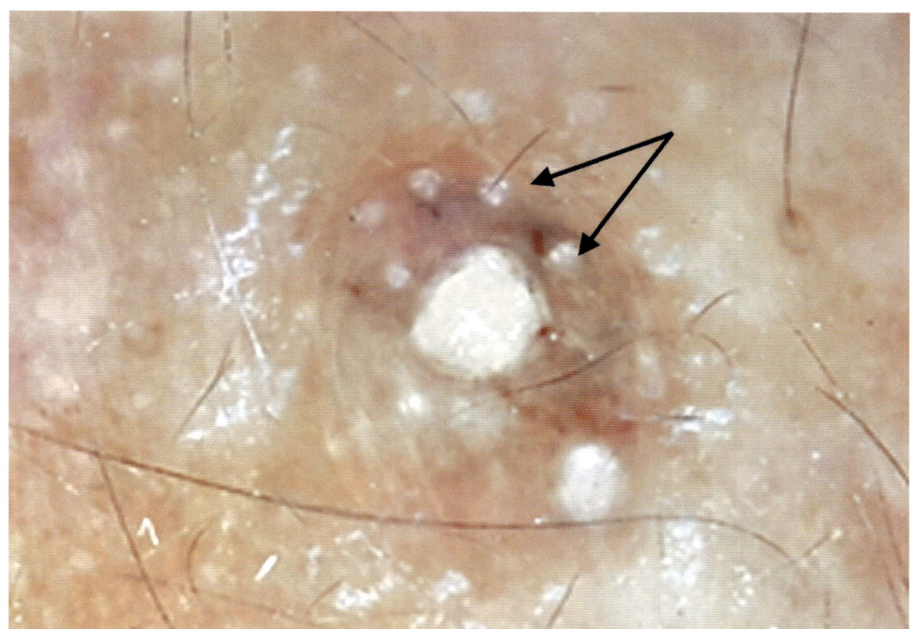

Fig. 14B: Rosettes are important additional features of molluscum contagiosum. When other dermoscopic features are less evident, rosettes may be highly valuable clue to the diagnosis. Multiple rosettes are seen (arrows).

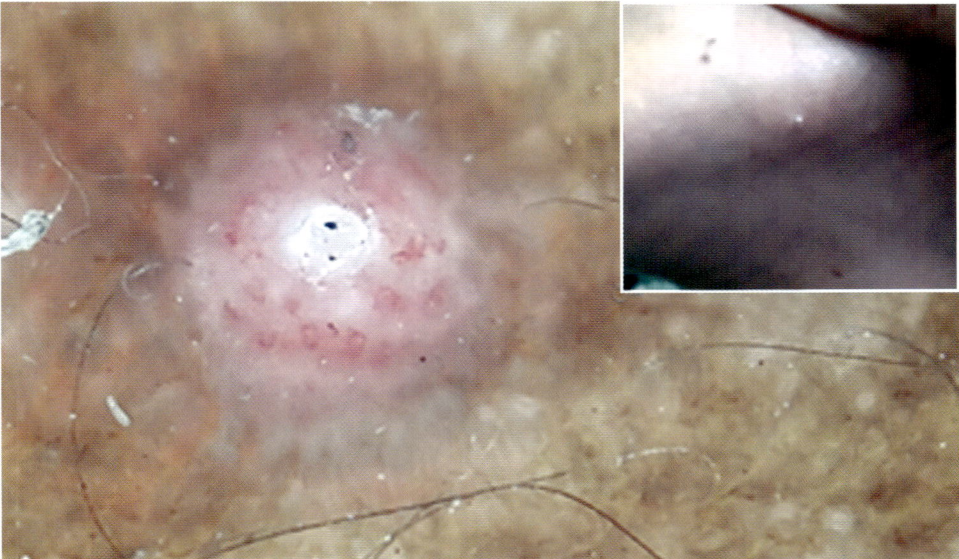

Fig. 15: Vascular pattern seen in this case is mixed vascular pattern instead of crown vessels described classically. However, the vessels do not cross the center of the lesion.

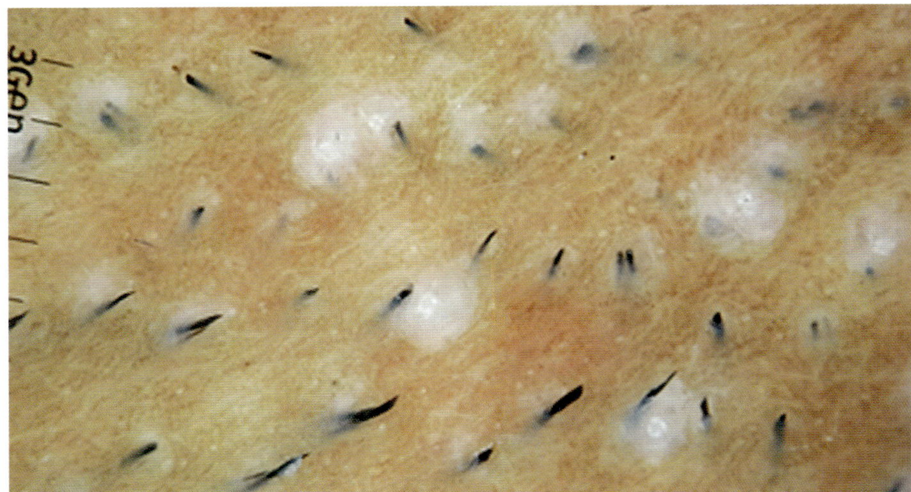

Fig. 16: In the absence of vascular features on dermoscopy, in some cases of molluscum contagiosum, the finding of rosettes is highly suggestive of the diagnosis.

REFERENCES

1. Morales A, Puig S, Malvehy J. Dermoscopy of molluscum contagiosum. Arch Dermatol. 2005;141(12):1644.
2. Zaballos P, Ara M, Puig S, Malvehy J. Dermoscopy of molluscum contagiosum: a useful tool for clinical diagnosis in adulthood. J Eur Acad Dermatol Venereol. 2006;20(4):482-3.
3. Malvehy J, Puig S. Principios de Dermatoscopia, 2nd edition. Barcelona: Cege Editores; 2010.
4. Zalaudek I, Kreusch J, Giacomel J, et al. How to diagnose nonpigmented skin tumors: a review of vascular structures seen with dermoscopy. Part II. Nonmelanocytic skin tumors. J Am Acad Dermatol. 2010;63:377-86.
5. Malakar S, Mukherjee SS. Rosette: an additional in vivo dermoscopic finding in molluscum contagiosum. Indian Journal of Pediatric Dermatology (Ahead of print).

PITYRIASIS VERSICOLOR

INTRODUCTION

- Pityriasis versicolor (PV)[1,2] is a superficial fungal infection of skin characterized by hypopigmented or hyperpigmented macules and patches on the chest, back, and/or arms.
- Pityriasis versicolor is usually asymptomatic, but in some people it is mildly itchy.
- Pityriasis versicolor is caused by mycelial growth of fungi of the genus *Malassezia*.

KEY DERMOSCOPIC FEATURES (FIGS. 17 TO 19)

- Fine scales localized in the skin furrows in an achromic/hypochromic lesion.
- Fine scaling overlying pigmentation in hyperpigmented lesion.
- Fine scales in net-like distribution (personal observation) in achromic hypochromic lesion.
- Net-like fine scales over erythematous background (personal observation) in erythematous PV.

KEYNOTES

Pityriasis versicolor is a clinical diagnosis, characterized by thin patches and fine scaling and can be confirmed by skin scraping and microscopy of KOH preparation which shows spaghetti and meatball appearance.

However, the fine scales on the affected lesion cannot always be easily observed; it becomes apparent only when the lesion is scratched or scraped. The fine scales with net-like distribution can easily be observed by dermoscope which prevents unnecessary invasive procedures such as biopsy, particularly in hyperpigmented and erythematous PV. Thus dermoscopy, in some cases, may be an essential tool for the diagnosis of PV.

Fig. 17: Net-like scaling confined to the skin furrows.

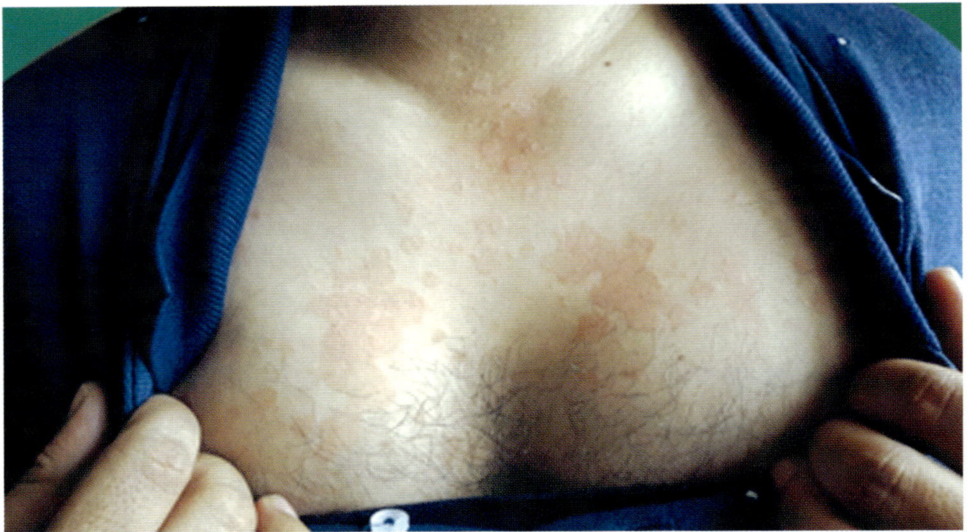

Fig. 18A: Erythematous variant of pityriasis versicolor.

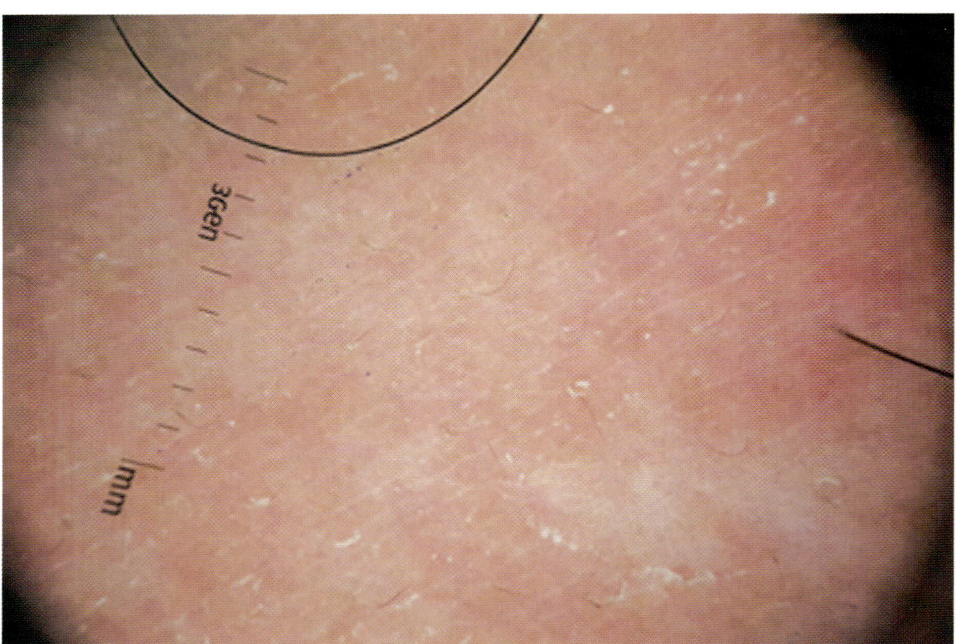

Fig. 18B: Dermoscopy of the above case revealing an erythematous background with net-like scaling.

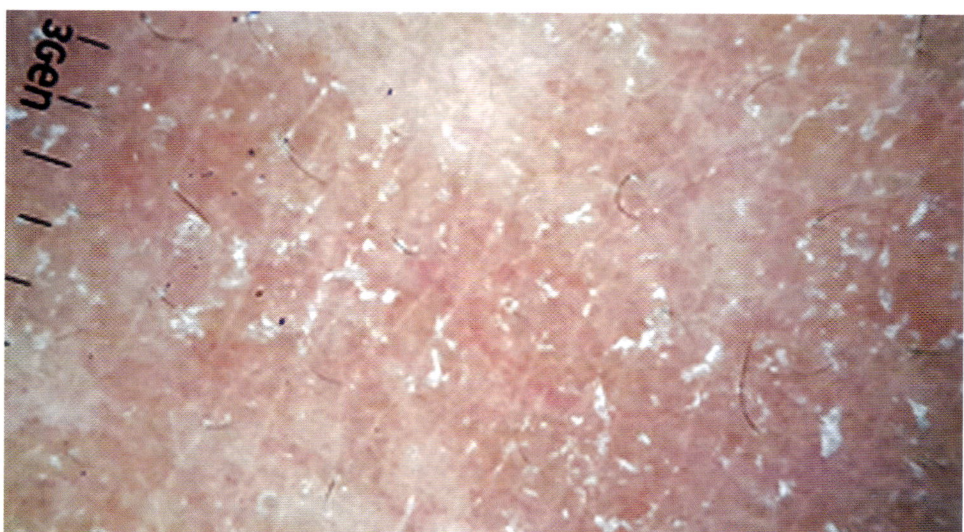

Fig. 18C: Close-up image of the same lesion after Grattage test (scraping of lesion with a glass slide). Note scales have become more prominent.

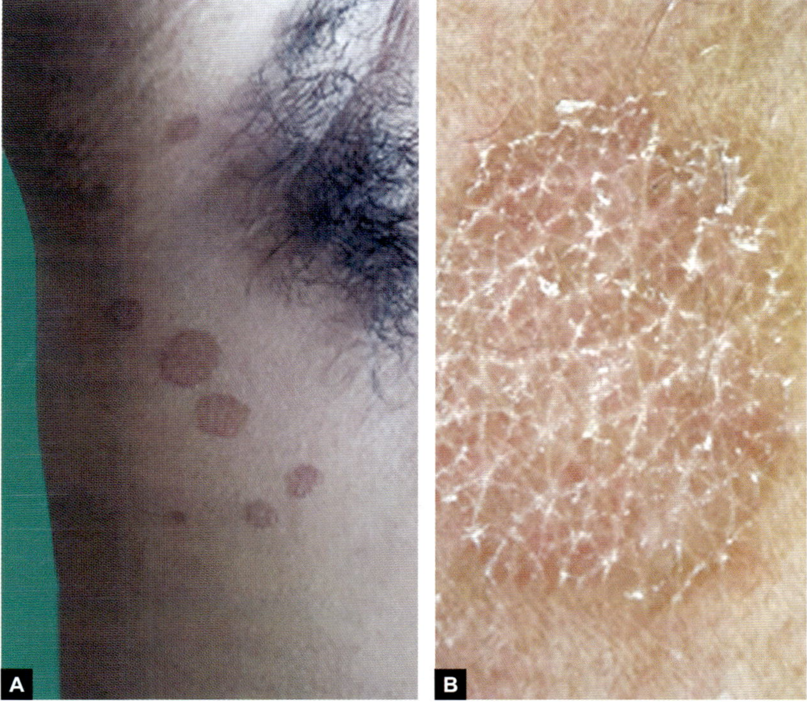

Figs. 19A and B: Clinical image showing hyperpigmented variant of pityriasis versicolor. Dermoscopy of the same lesion reveals a brownish background with net-like scales.

REFERENCES

1. Zhou H, Tang XH, De Han J, Chen MK. Dermoscopy as an ancillary tool for the diagnosis of pityriasis versicolor. J Am Acad Dermatol. 2015;73(6):e205-6.
2. Erichetti E, Stinco G. The practical usefulness of dermoscopy in general dermatology. G Ital Dermatol Venereol. 2015;150:533-46.

TINEA CAPITIS

INTRODUCTION

Tinea capitis is a fungal infection affecting the hair and scalp; most commonly seen in the pediatric age group.[1] It has been classified as—noninflammatory, inflammatory, and favus.[2,3] Tinea capitis in children is most commonly caused by Microsporum and Trichophyton species.[15] *Microsporum canis* causes ectothrix tinea capitis. Here, fungal hyphae and arthroconidia invade the outer part of hair shaft and may damage the hair cuticle.[2,3] Trichophyton causes endothrix tinea capitis. Fungal hyphae and arthroconidia in endothrix occupy the hair shaft from within and the whole hair shaft may be weakened.[2,3] *Trichophyton schoenleinii* is associated with formation of air spaces within the shaft.[2,3] Diagnosis is based on direct microscopic examination of infected hair and mycological cultures. Scalp scaling and patchy alopecia are the frequent clinical presentations. Pustular lesions are seen in inflammatory tinea capitis. Cervical lymph nodes are commonly enlarged in tinea capitis.

KEY DERMOSCOPIC FEATURES (FIGS. 20 TO 22)

- *Comma hairs:*[4] They are the dermoscopic markers of tinea capitis, hairs that appear as the punctuation mark "comma". The fungal elements infecting the hair shaft cause the hair to bend.
- *Corkscrew hairs:*[5] They are short hairs which are spiral in shape.
- *Broken hairs:*[5,6] Broken and dystrophic hairs are common but nonspecific findings.
- Black dots
- Hair casts
- Morse code (transverse white bands) hairs[7,8]
- i-hairs[9]
- Block hairs.[9]

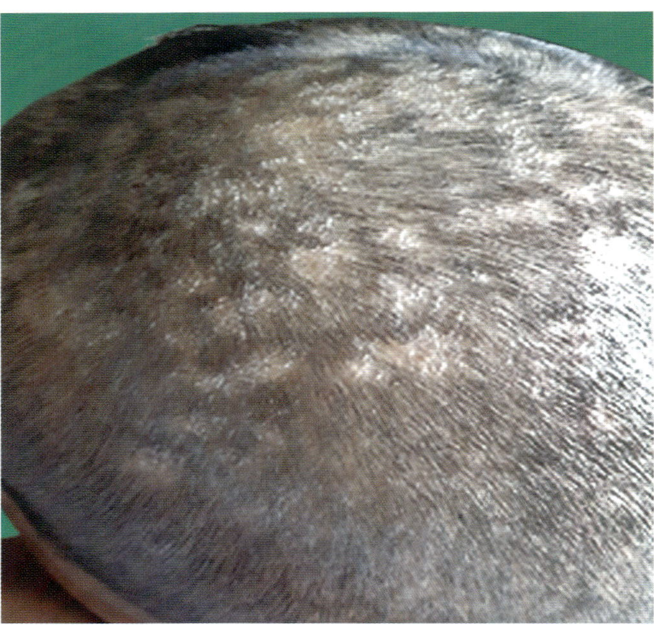

Fig. 20A: Patches of alopecia is a characteristic feature of tinea capitis. Hairs may be broken at the scalp level due to endothrix fungus infection whereas in ectothrix invasion the shafts are broken 1–3 mm away from scalp level. In all types of tinea capitis, scalp scaling is a common occurrence.

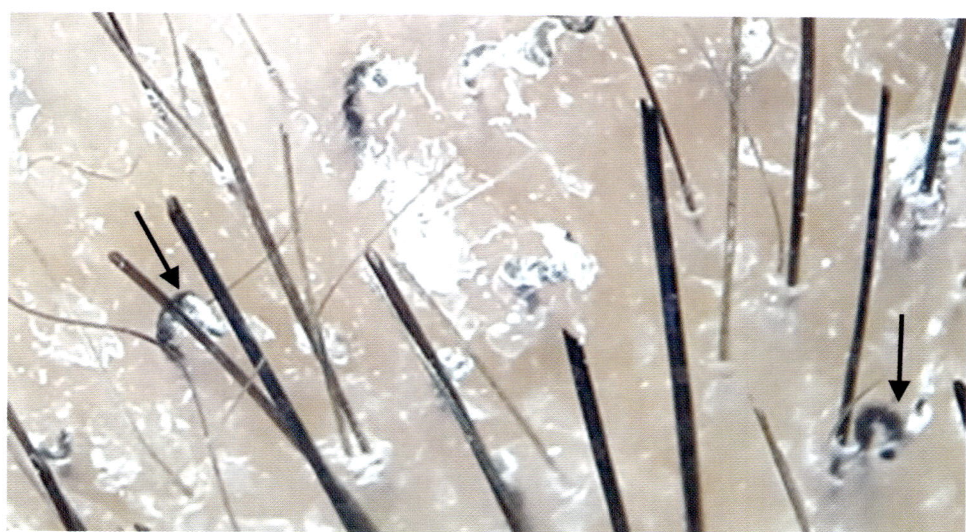

Fig. 20B: Patchy alopecia with multiple comma hairs is evident. Bending of the short hairs (comma hairs) is due to partial damage to hair shafts by ectothrix parasitization. Comma hairs (arrows) retain their normal thickness and color.

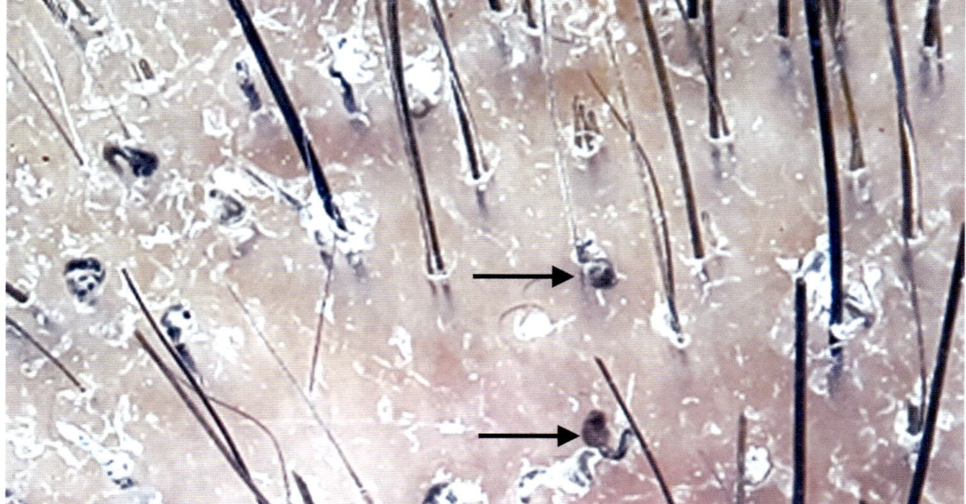

Fig. 21: Corkscrew hairs (arrows): They are short hairs, which appear spiral on trichoscopy. They can be distinguished from comma hairs by their multiple twists.

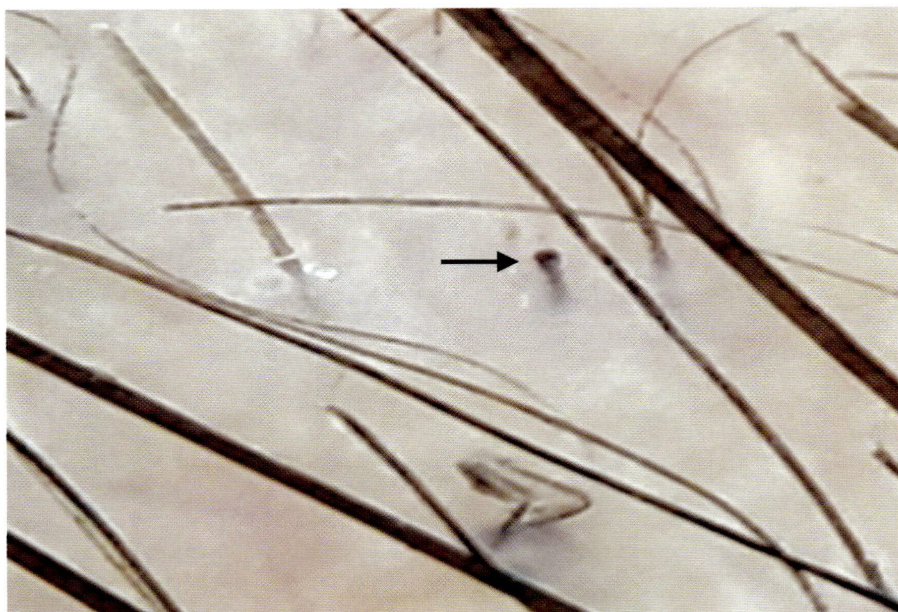

Fig. 22: "i-hair" in tinea capitis (arrow): i-hair is a short broken hair that looks like the alphabet 'i'.[9] A corkscrew hair is also present in the field.

Morse Code Hairs[7,8] (Figs. 23 and 24)

- They are a specific trichoscopic feature of fungal infection of scalp and eyebrow.
- *Polarized trichoscopy*: Horizontal white bands
- *Ultraviolet dermoscopy*: Fluorescence disappearing at the bands
- *Microscopy*: Numerous spores at the thinner fragment
- *Mechanism of formation of Morse code hairs*: Horizontal bands correspond to localized areas of fungal infection, which result in hair perforation.

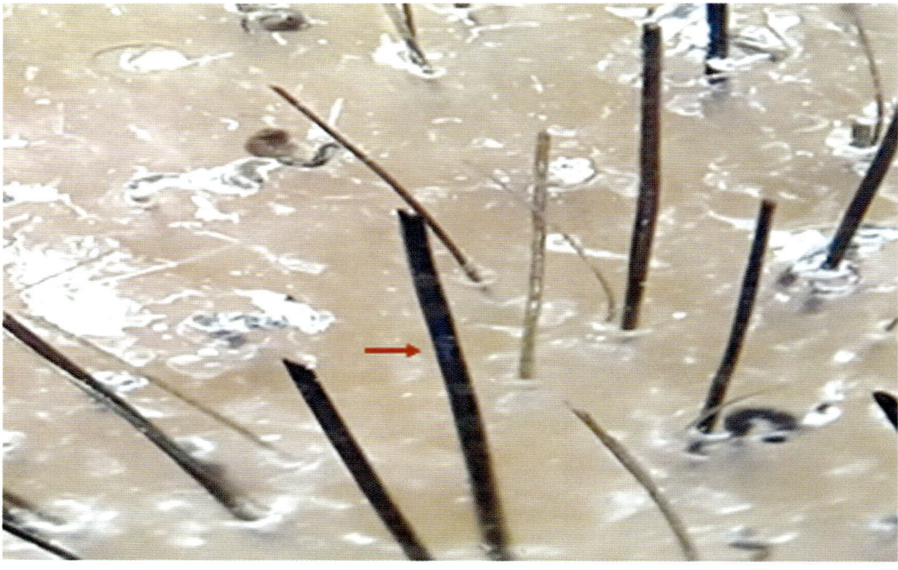

Fig. 23: "Morse code" hairs (arrow): horizontal white bands present in a regular distribution along the hair shaft.

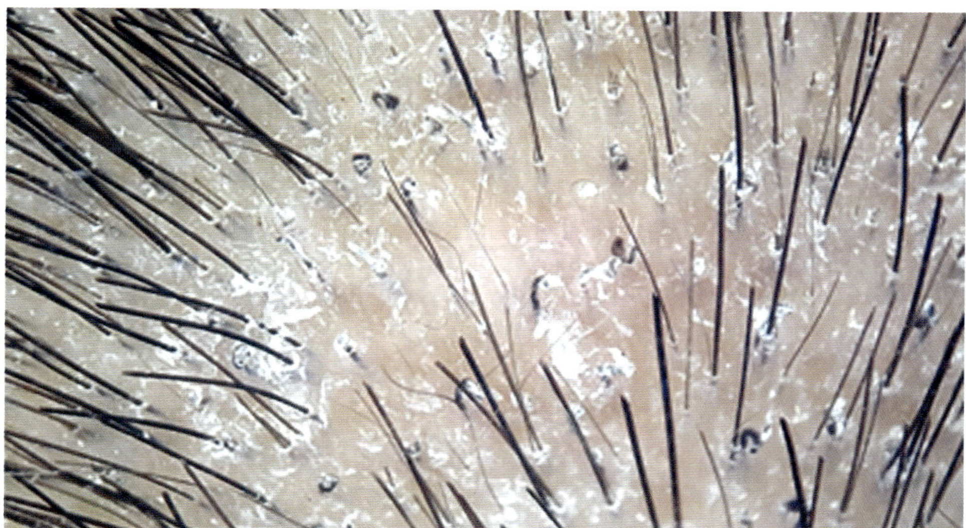

Fig. 24: Tinea capitis showing multiple comma and corkscrew hairs.

REFERENCES

1. Grimalt R. A practical guide to scalp disorders. J Investig Dermatol Symp Proc. 2007;12(2):10-4.
2. Mebazaa A, Oumari KE, Ghariani N, et al. Tinea capitis in adults in Tunisia. Int J Dermatol. 2010;49(5):513-6.
3. Ilkit M. Favus of the scalp: an overview and update. Mycopathologia. 2010;170(3):143-54.
4. Tangjaturonrusamee C, Piraccini BM, Vincenzi C, et al. Tinea capitis mimicking folliculitis decalvans. Mycoses. 2011;54:87-8.
5. Hughes R, Chiaverini C, Bahadoran P, Lacour JP. Corkscrew hair: a new dermoscopic sign for diagnosis of tinea capitis in black children. Arch Dermatol. 2011;147:355-6.
6. Slowinska M, Rudnicka L, Schwartz RA, et al. Comma hairs: a dermoscopic marker for tinea capitis; a rapid diagnostic method. J Am Acad Dermatol. 2008;59(suppl):S77-9.
7. Lin YT, Li YC. The dermoscopic comma, zigzag, and bar code-like hairs: markers of fungal infection of the hair follicles. Dermatologica Sinica. 2014;32(3):160-3.
8. Wang HH, Lin YT. Bar code-like hair: dermoscopic marker of tinea capitis and tinea of the eyebrow. J Am Acad Dermatol. 2015;72(1):S41-S42.
9. Rudnicka L, Szepietowski JC, Slowinska M, et al. Tinea capitis. In: Rudnicka L, Olszewska M, Rakowska A (Eds). Atlas of Trichoscopy. London: Springer; 2012. p. 367.

TINEA CORPORIS

It appears as coarse scales dermoscopically, which are oriented chaotically. The vascular pattern is mixed.[1]

REFERENCE

1. Vázquez-López F, Kreusch J, Marghoob AA. Dermoscopic semiology: further insights into vascular features by screening a large spectrum of nontumoral skin lesions. Br J Dermatol. 2004;150(2):226-31.

TINEA MANUUM

Tinea manuum dermoscopically displays white scaling distributed mostly in the physiological palmar creases.[1]

REFERENCE

1. Errichetti E, Stinco G. The practical usefulness of dermoscopy in general dermatology. G Ital Dermatol Venereol. 2015;150(5): 533-46.

DEMODICOSIS

INTRODUCTION

It results from infestation with the *Demodex* mite, an obligate human parasite having two species, *Demodex folliculorum* and *Demodex brevis*. *Demodex* can only live in the human hair follicle.[1] *Demodex* is an ecto-parasite of pilo-sebaceous follicle and sebaceous gland, typically found on the face including cheeks, nose, chin, forehead, temples, eye lashes, brows, and also on the balding scalp, neck, and ears. Clinically it may present as erythema, burning and stinging sensation or a nonspecific rash over the face. Demodicosis is diagnosed when there is high density of *Demodex* mites (>5/cm^2). Dermoscopy: white spicules protruding from the follicular openings. White spicules represent mite tails.[2]

KEY DERMOSCOPIC FEATURES (FIGS. 25 TO 28)

- *Demodex tails*: Appear as white spicules at the root of the hair follicle.
- *Demodex at follicular openings*: Appear as course follicular openings containing brownish/grayish plugs.
- Subtle erythema with reticular dilated vessels.
- Scaling and pustules.

KEYNOTE

Dermoscope provides clinical diagnosis instantly and noninvasively. Routine dermoscopy is a *must* in patients complaining of dry skin with facial erythematous rash, to rule out demodicidosis. A *Demodex* spicule is a protruding three-dimensional structure, whereas the scale is a flattened structure that does not protrude.

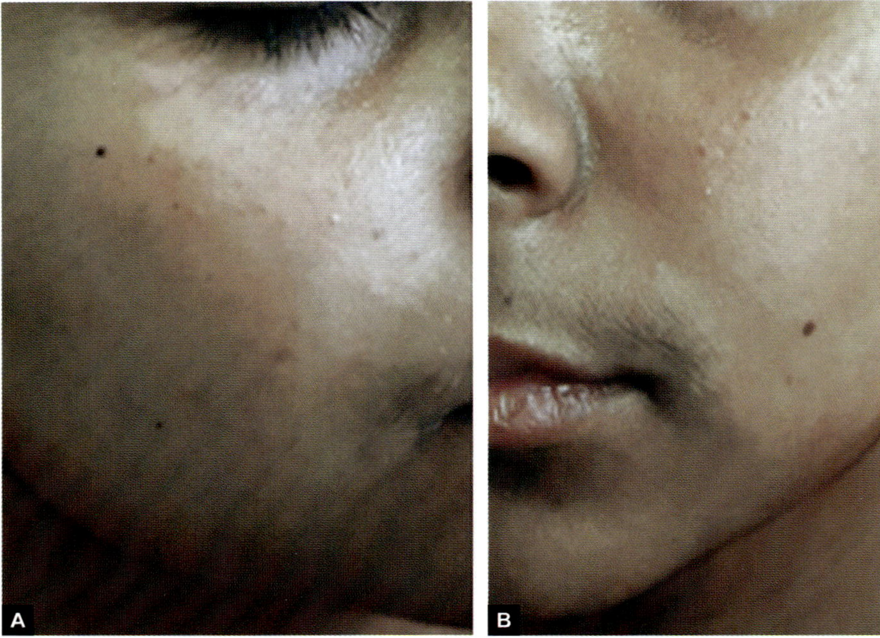

Figs. 25A and B: Mild erythematous rash and burning sensation over the face for 1 year which was not responding to topical steroid or calcineurin inhibitors.

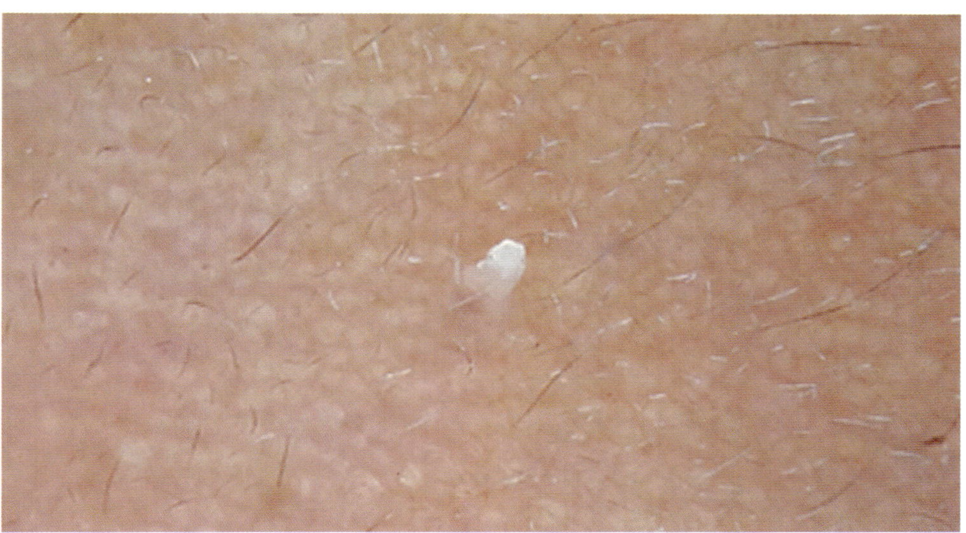

Fig. 25C: On trichoscopy of facial hairs, a white spicule is seen protruding from the follicular opening.

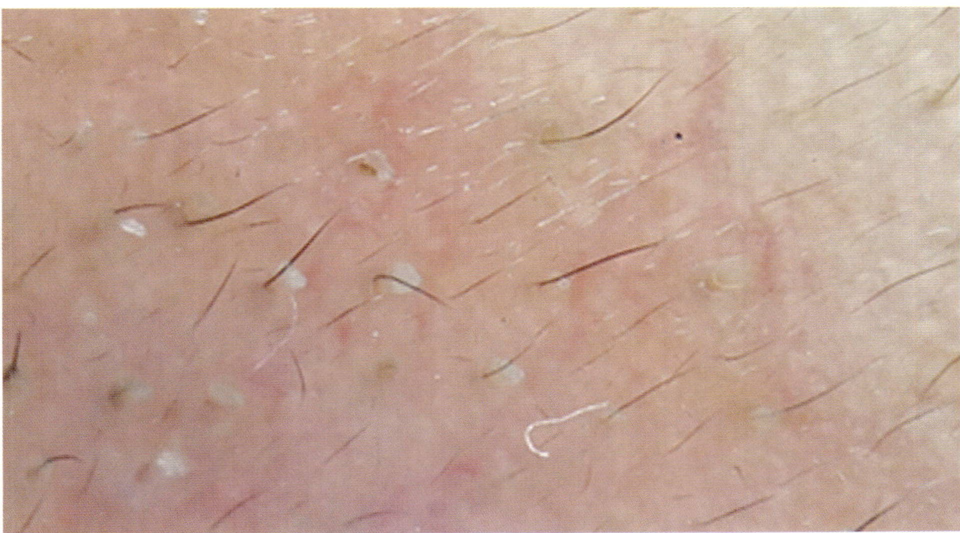

Fig. 25D: More white spicules in another field and subtle reticular dilated vessels forming a pink network.

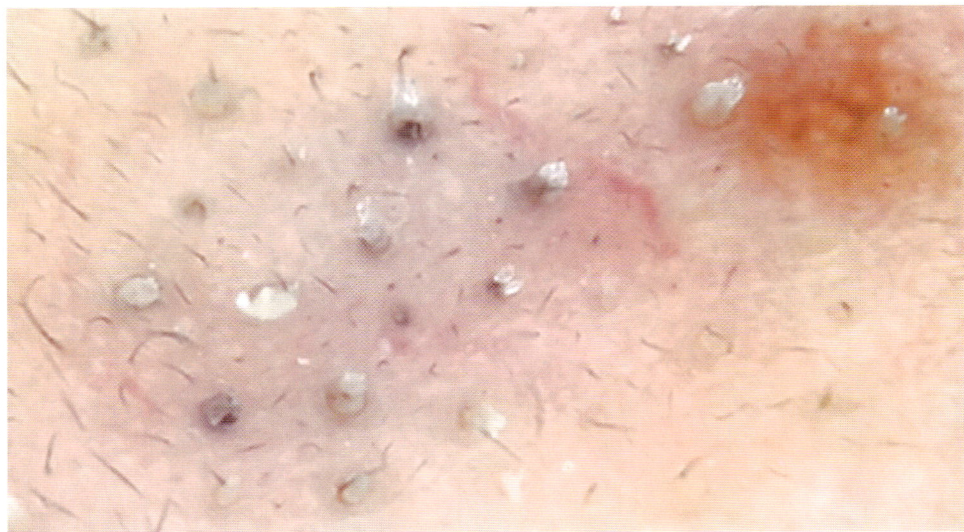

Fig. 26: Dilated pores containing amorphous brown/gray plugs can also be associated with this disorder.

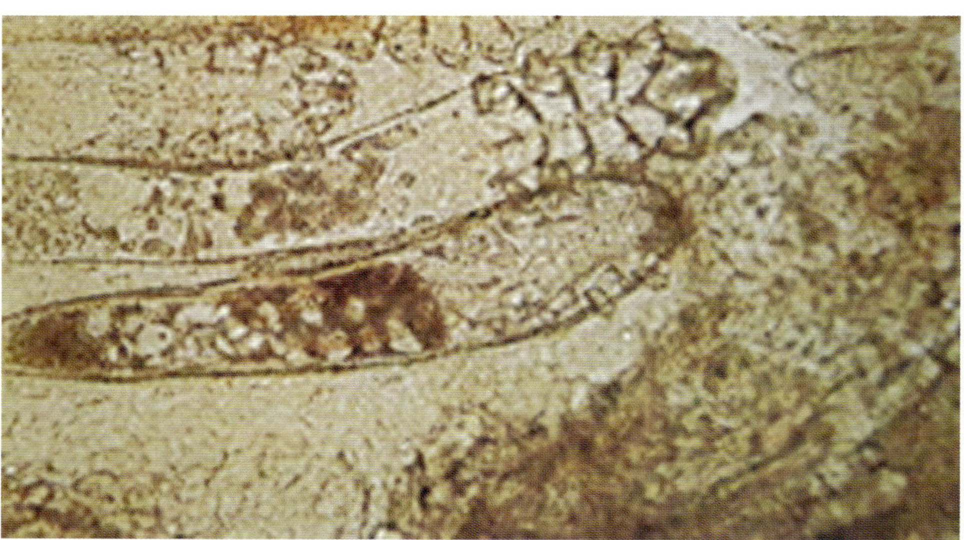

Fig. 27: Skin scrapings (KOH): live, cigar-shaped, actively moving ectoparasite.

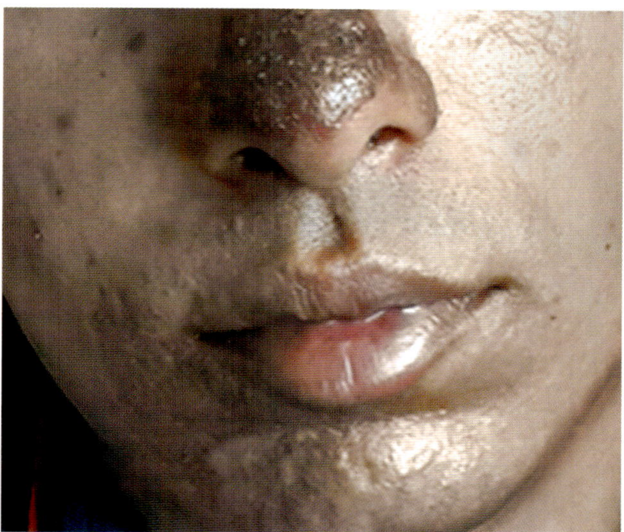

Fig. 28A: Asymptomatic dull erythematous rash over nose for the last 1 year.

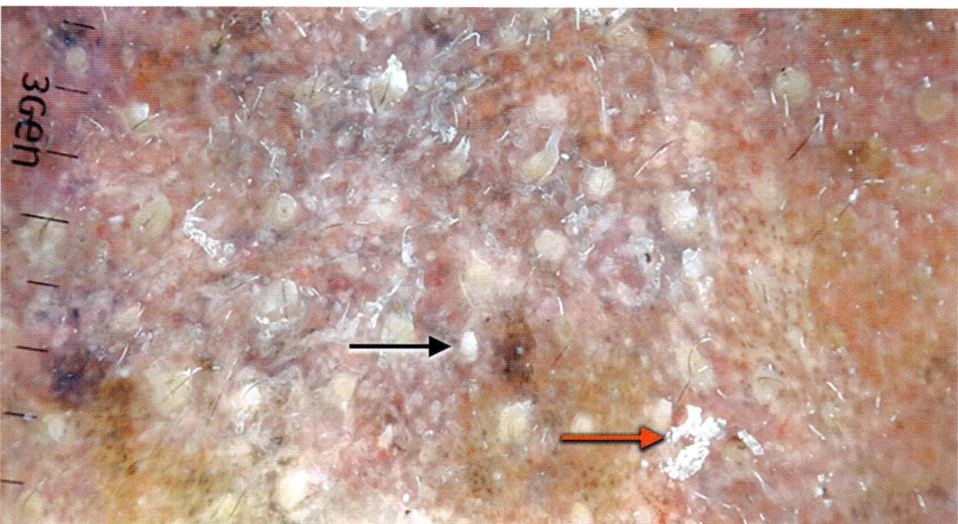

Fig. 28B: On trichoscopy of previous patient, the field is full of white spicules of *Demodex* (black arrow) on an erythematous background. Some scales are also present (red arrow).

REFERENCES

1. Forton F, Germaux MA, Brasseur T, et al. Democidosis and rosacea: epidemiology and significance in daily dermatologic practice. J Am Acad Dermatol. 2005;52(1):74-87.
2. Mangold A, Swanson DL. Dermoscopy in general dermatology. In: Johr RH, Stolz W (Eds). Dermoscopy, 2nd edition. McGraw-Hill; 2015. pp. 505-28.

PEDICULOSIS CAPITIS

INTRODUCTION

Infestation of pediculosis capitis *(pediculus humanus var capitis)* is common and can easily be diagnosed clinically by close examination. Diagnostic signs of head lice infestation are lice and/or nits. Nonetheless, it may be time consuming and nits may be confused with pseudonits (scales of different origin).[1] Trichoscopy allows straightforward identification of head lice and nits and also can differentiate the nit (louse egg) from the nit cast (empty egg). As trichoscopy can assess the viability of the contents of the nits, it can be used to monitor the treatment efficacy.[2,3]

KEY DERMOSCOPIC FEATURES (FIGS. 29 TO 31)

- *Nit:* Louse egg attached to hair shaft.
- *Nit cast*: Empty egg appearing as a translucent structure fixed to a hair shaft.
- Head louse.

KEYNOTE

Dermoscopy helps in diagnosing pediculosis capitis and differentiating nits from pseudonits. Pseudonits—they are scales of different origin. A pseudonit encircles the hair shaft, whereas a nit does not encircle the shaft but is attached to one side of the shaft. Single scales and yellowish background are clues to diagnosis of seborrheic capitis.

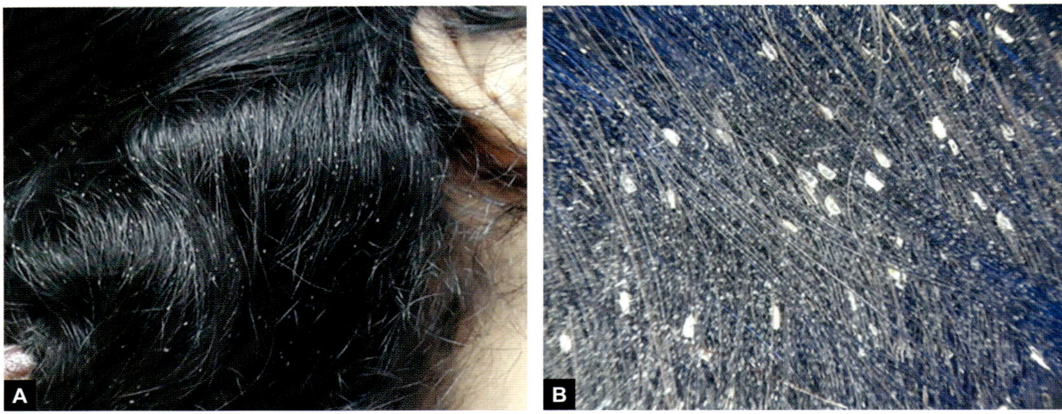

Figs. 29A and B: Multitude of nits on the hair shafts (A). Dermoscopy demonstrating live and dead nits (B).

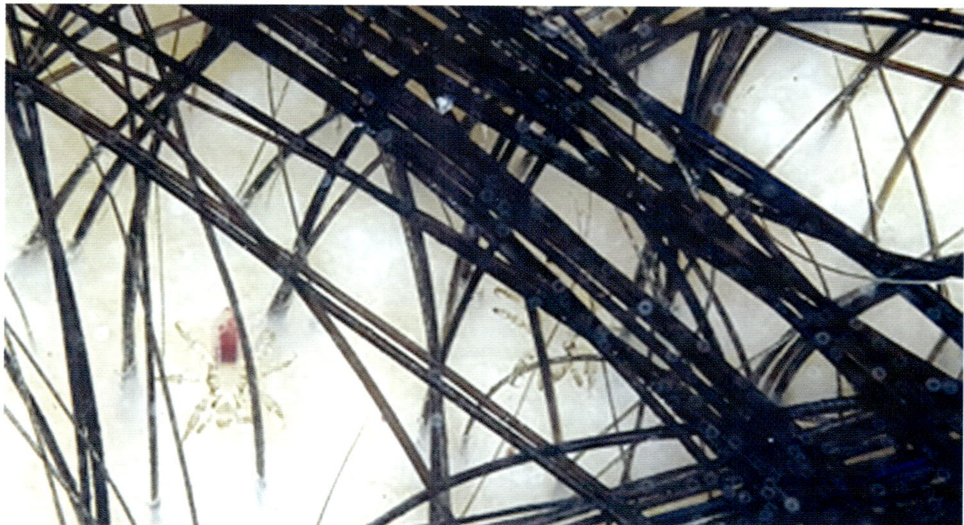

Fig. 30: Dermoscopy demonstrating head louse after blood meal.

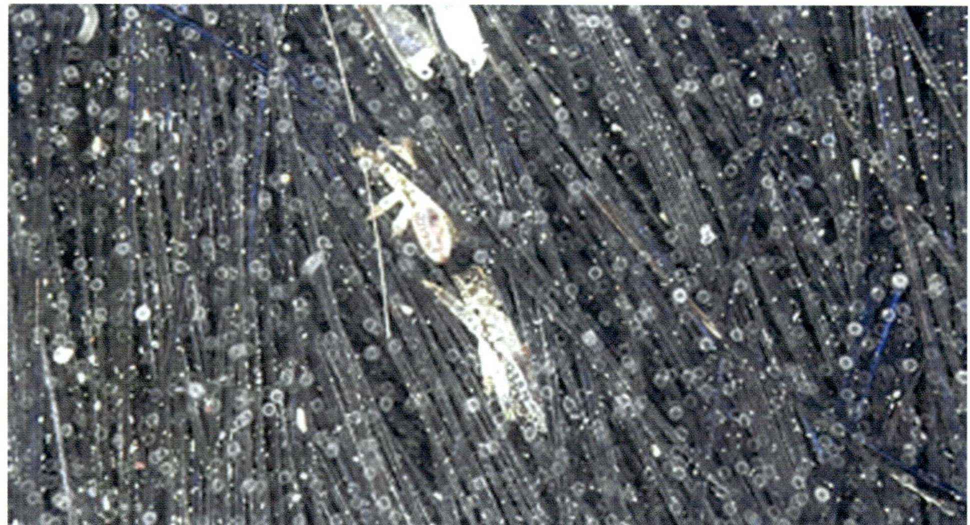

Fig. 31: Dermoscopy showing male and female head louse with nits.

REFERENCES

1. Micali G, Lacarrubba F, Massimino D, et al. Dermatoscopy: alternative uses in daily clinical practice. J Am Acad Dermatol. 2011;64:1135-46.
2. Bowling J. General dermatology. In: Bowling J (Ed). Diagnostic Dermoscopy. Oxford: Wiley; 2012. p. 123.
3. Lacarrubba F, Dinotta F, Micali G. Parasitic scalp infections. In: Rudnicka L, Olszewska M, Rakowska A (Eds). Atlas of Trichoscopy. London: Springer; 2012. p. 357.

DERMOSCOPY OF SCABIES

INTRODUCTION

Scabies is a contagious cutaneous condition where the mites are transferred by direct contact including sexual contact and indirect contact through fomites. Symptoms may be apparent after 2–6 weeks of acquiring infection. The rash is often most obvious in the interdigital web spaces, inner side of thighs, around the umbilicus, nipples, and genitals. The diagnosis can be confirmed by the microscopic examination of the contents of a burrow, however that may be cumbersome and time consuming. The modern gadget, dermoscopy provides instant diagnosis of the condition without a diagnostic dilemma.

Burrows are a pathognomonic sign and represents the intraepidermal tunnel created by the movement of the female mite.

KEY DERMOSCOPIC FEATURES (FIGS. 32 TO 36)[1]

- Burrows
- A black dot at the end of the burrow represents the mite
- Delta wing jet, translucent scabies body and scabious eggs.

KEYNOTE

Dermoscopy serves as an important tool with no down time in the diagnosis of dubious cases with nonspecific itching over the entire body, where the prime suspects for diagnosis are considered to be atopic dermatitis, scabies, and other nonspecific entities.

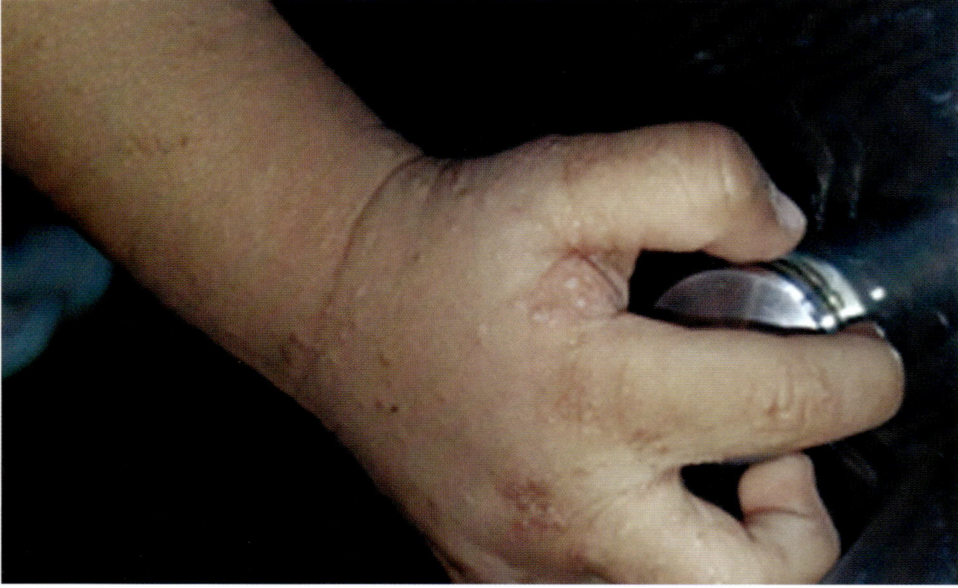

Fig. 32A: Multiple erythematous excoriated papules on the hands of a child involving the interdigital spaces.

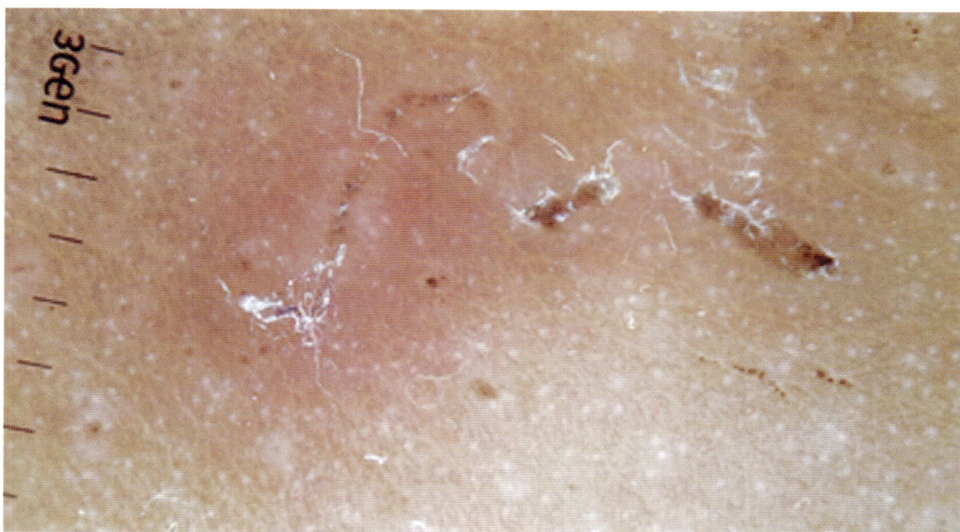

Fig. 32B: Dermoscopy demonstrating the tortuous full length burrow with a mite at the right end of the burrow represented by a triangular tip giving rise to the jet with contrail appearance. This triangular tip of the mite is the ventral view of the mite. In case of dorsal view of the mite, entire triangle will not be visible rather a partial triangle (dorsal view) is present.

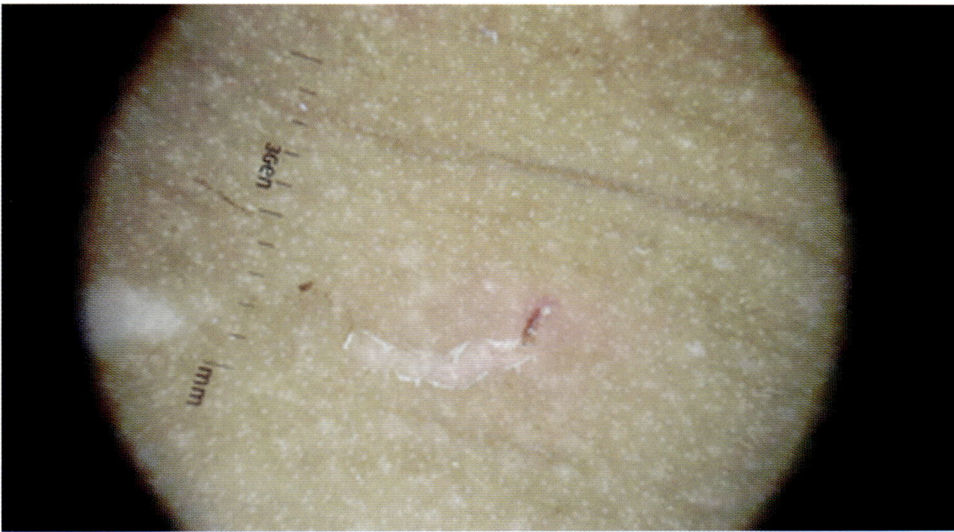

Fig. 33: Burrow on the palm.

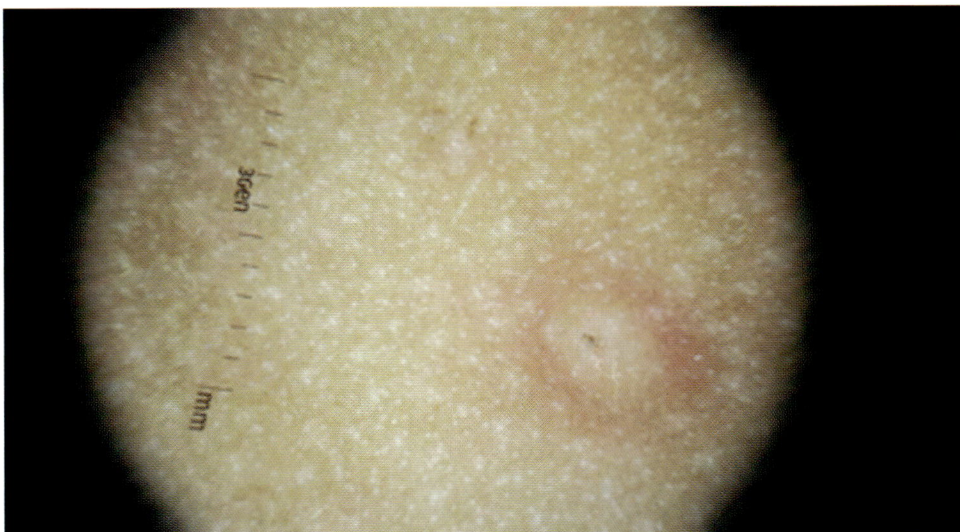

Fig. 34: Scabetic nodule showing central blackish brown representing the mite surrounded by yellow white structureless zone followed by a rim of erythema. In our experience almost all the nodules harbor scabetic mite.

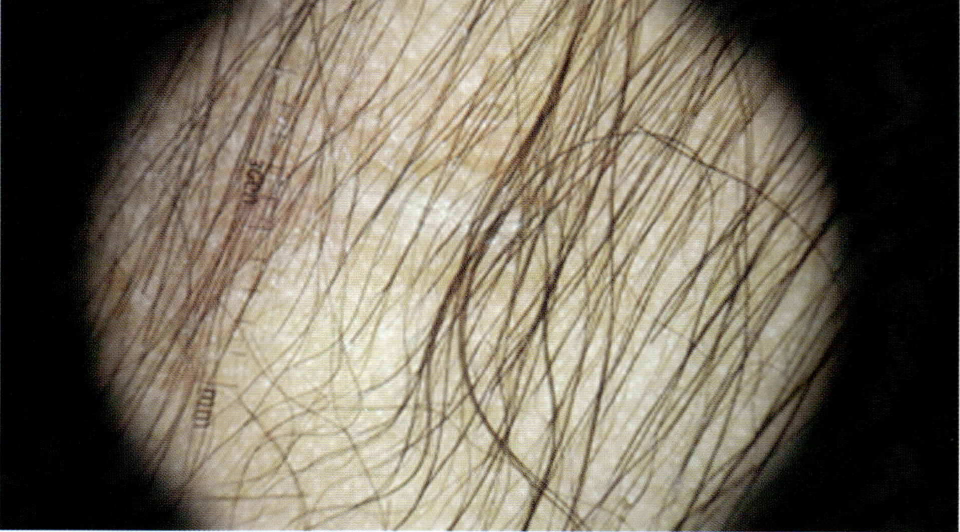

Fig. 35: Classical scabetic burrow on the scalp of a child.

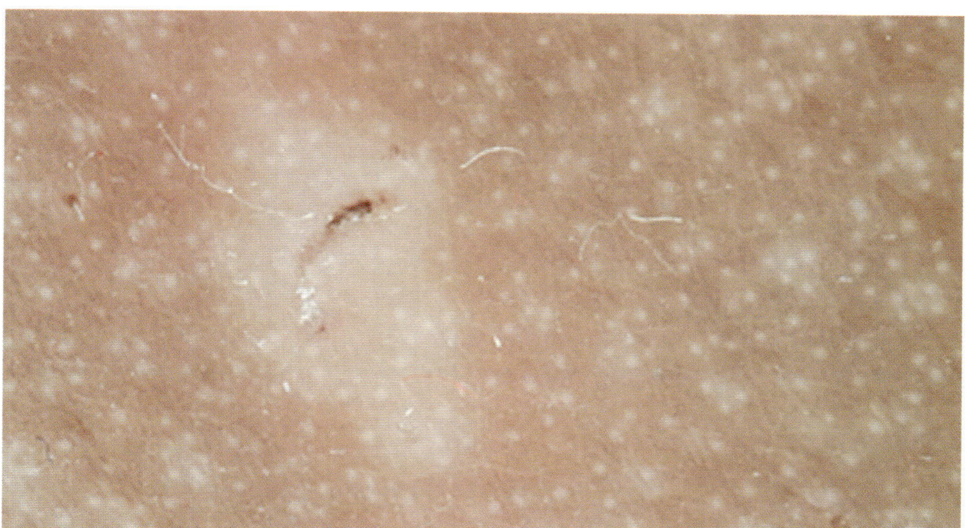

Fig. 36: Another image demonstrating the burrow.

REFERENCE

1. Park JH, Kim CW, Kim SS. The diagnostic accuracy of dermoscopy for scabies. Ann Dermatol. 2012;24:194-9.

CHAPTER 9

Skin Tumors

Subrata Malakar

BENIGN TUMORS OF SKIN

INTRODUCTION

Dermatoscopy has proven useful for studying benign skin tumors. The application of dermatoscope allows the assessment of important characteristics of tumor not evident on physical examination. The purpose of dermatoscopy is to provide additional information to the one already deduced by naked eyes.

BOWEN'S DISEASE

INTRODUCTION

It is an intraepidermal malignant dermatosis that presents as a slowly growing erythematous patch or plaque with irregular borders which has an overlying scale and crust (Fig. 1).

In a small percentage of cases, Bowen's disease (BD) progresses to SCC. Moreover, it is often misdiagnosed as various dermatoses like psoriasis, lichen planus, nummular eczema, etc. In these situations, dermoscopy serves as a very valuable investigative procedure because of its instant evaluation.

KEY DERMOSCOPIC FEATURES

- Patchy distribution of glomerular vessels
- Surface scale and/or crust.

DISCUSSION

Concomitant presence of clustered glomerular vessels and surface scale/and or crust is 98% predictive of BD (Fig. 2).[1]

Glomerular vessels are larger than dotted vessels and are tortuous capillaries, curled up into a ball, and distributed in regular clusters. Dotted vessels are also visible; in fact glomerular vessels are a variation of dotted vessels.

In pigmented BD, additional features are small brown globules in a patchy distribution and homogeneous brown to gray pigmentation (Fig. 3).[2]

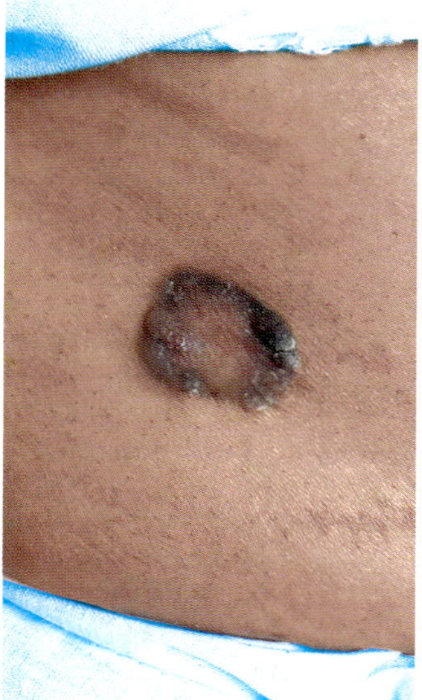

Fig. 1: Slowly growing erythematous plaque with irregular border on the abdomen of this 58 years old man for last 3 years. Histopathology confirmed Bowen's disease.

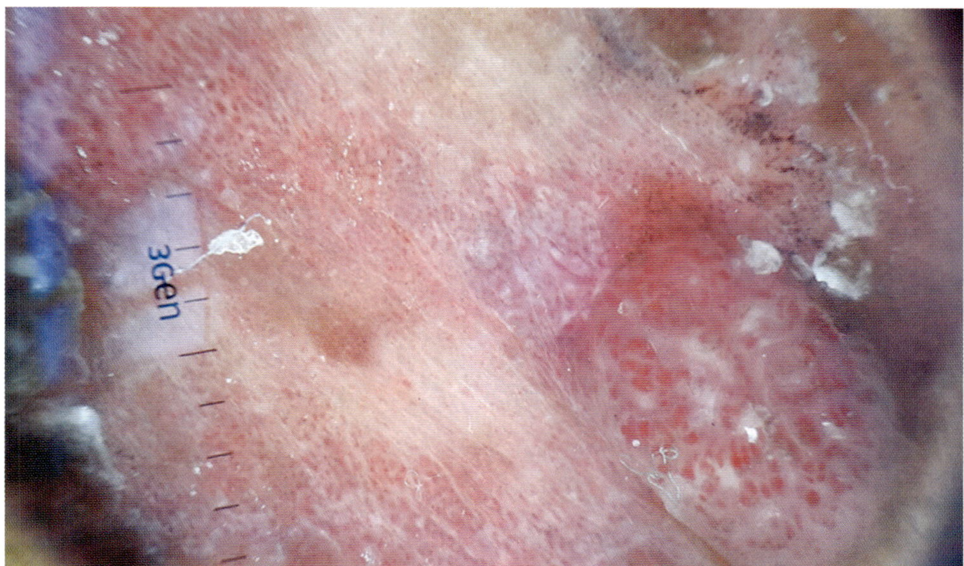

Fig. 2: Patchy distribution of glomerular vessels and few scales are also seen. In the extreme right upper corner brown dots and globules are visible.

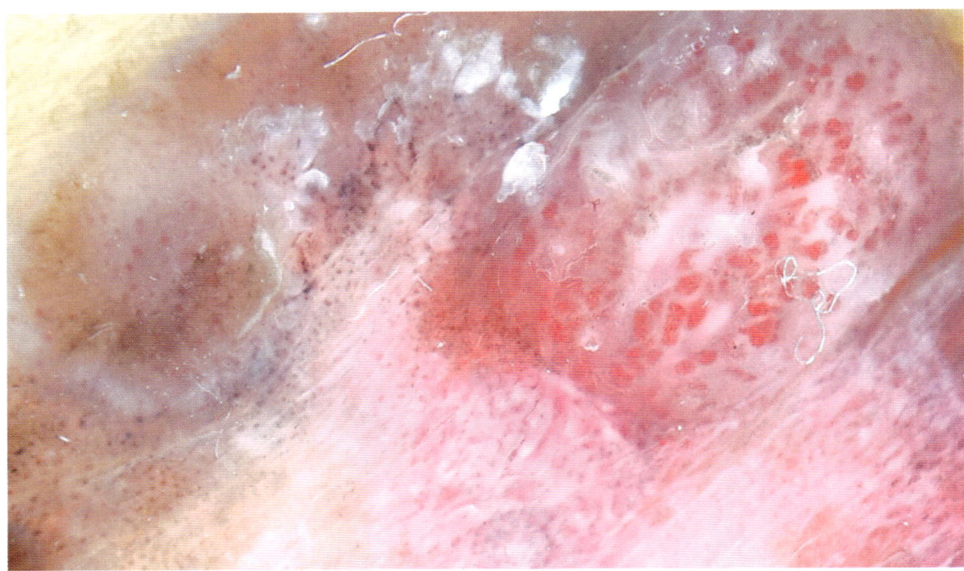

Fig. 3: Dermoscopy reveals small brown globules in patchy distribution and homogeneous brown-gray pigmentation is seen to the left of the field. Few scales and patchy glomerular vessels are also present.

REFERENCES

1. Pan Y, Chamberlain AJ, Bailey M, et al. Dermoscopy aids in the diagnosis of the solitary red scaly patch or plaque-features distinguishing superficial basal cell carcinoma, intraepidermal carcinoma, and psoriasis. J Am Acad Dermatol. 2008;59:268-74.
2. Hernandez-Gil J, Fernandez-Pugnaire MA, Serrano-Falcon C, et al. Clínica y dermatoscopia de la enfermedad de Bowen pigmentada. Actas Dermosifiliogr. 2008;99:419-20.

DERMATOFIBROMA

INTRODUCTION

Dermatofibroma is defined as benign fibrous histiocytoma and is characterized by: (a) an increased number of dermal fibrocytes, (b) coarse collagen bundles in haphazard array, (c) mixed inflammatory infiltrate, and (d) hyperplasia of adjacent structures such as epidermis, hair follicles, and/or melanocytes. DF represents one of the most common cutaneous tumors. A small raised cutaneous nodule with a red-brown color located on limbs, is a typical presentation of DF. Atypical cases may be difficult to diagnose clinically and consequently other investigative tools such as biopsy and dermoscopy is necessary. As dermoscope is noninvasive and gives instant report, it should serve as a routine in initial consultation.

KEY DERMOSCOPIC FEATURES (FIGS. 4 TO 33)

- Delicate pigment network at the periphery and central white scar-like patch is the most common type of dermoscopic presentation. Another nine types of DFs have also been described.
- Vascular patterns such as dotted, comma, and hairpin vessels may be seen; telangiectatic vessels and polymorphous atypical vessels are also observed.

DISCUSSION

The delicate pigment is usually light brown, fine, and delicate and gradually fades into the surrounding skin. It results from hyperpigmentation rather than from proliferation of melanocytes at the basal layer. In some types of DF, light to dark brown globule-like structures are present in place of delicate network. It can be explained by the gradual accumulation of melanin into the epidermis associated with the epidermal hyperplasia. These globule-like structures are formed because of the flattened rete ridges which are often flat and hyperpigmented. The small ring-like structures, seen in about 25% of DFs, are due to these flat and broad rete ridges.

Histologic correlation of central white scar-like patch is the pronounced fibrosis in the papillary dermis.

Sometimes scales and ulcerations are found, probably as a result of external injury.

In a small percentage of cases of DFs with pronounced epidermal hyperplasia, fissures and ridges are found.

A bluish/red-bluish homogeneous pigmentation is seen in hemosiderotic or aneurysmatic DFs. It represents prominent blood-filled spaces and intra and extracellular hemosiderin deposition.

- Dermoscopic patterns of DF described by Zaballos et al. (Table 1).[1]
- Rare and atypical patterns[2-4]—Many rare and atypical variants have been described which are beyond the scope of this book.
- Other patterns (personal observation) (Table 2).[5-7]

KEYNOTE

Dermatofibromas present with various dermoscopic patterns of which central white scar-like patch and peripheral delicate pigment is the most common type. In the atypical and rarer forms, histopathology should be done as a rule to detect malignancy and to diagnose uncommon DFs such as aneurysmal and hemosiderotic variants.

Table 1: Dermoscopic patterns of dermatofibroma (DF).

Pattern	*Description*
1	Complete delicate pigment network
2	Central white scar-like patch with peripheral delicate pigment network
3	Central white network with peripheral delicate pigment network
4	Central homogeneous pigmentation with peripheral delicate pigment network
5	Complete white network
6	Complete homogeneous pigmentation
7a	Complete white scar-like patch
7b	Multiple white scar-like patches
8	Central white scar-like patch with peripheral homogeneous area
9	Central white network with peripheral homogeneous area
10	Atypical pigment network/atypical scar-like patch/atypical homogeneous pigmentation or irregular distribution of these structures

Table 2: Other patterns of dermatofibroma (personal observation).

Pattern a	Central white scar-like structure with peripheral hyperpigmentation that in turn is further surrounded by delicate melanocytic network. Rosettes are present
Pattern b	Violaceous homogeneous pigmentation at the periphery and central star-shaped white scar associated with different vascular patterns
Pattern c	Dermatofibroma (DF) with peripheral seborrheic keratosis like structure and central reticular scar with brown holes
Pattern d	Peripheral homogeneous pigmentation and central seborrheic keratosis like DF
Pattern e	Complete pink-brown homogeneous DF with central white shiny streaks
Pattern f	Homogeneous pink with white streaks and globules
Pattern g	Central white scar-like structure with peripheral hyperpigmented parallel lines

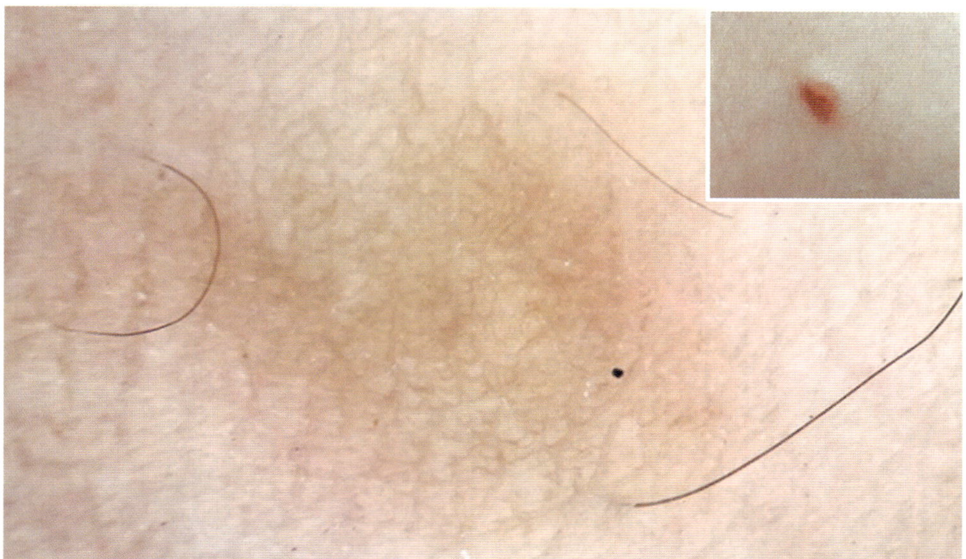

Fig. 4: Pattern 1: **Complete delicate pigment network**. This network is usually light to medium brown and gradually fades into the peripheral cutis. This network looks similar to network of melanocytic lesions but in dermatofibroma (DF), the network corresponds to hyperpigmentation of the basal layer in contrast to the increased rete ridge melanocytes in melanocytic network.

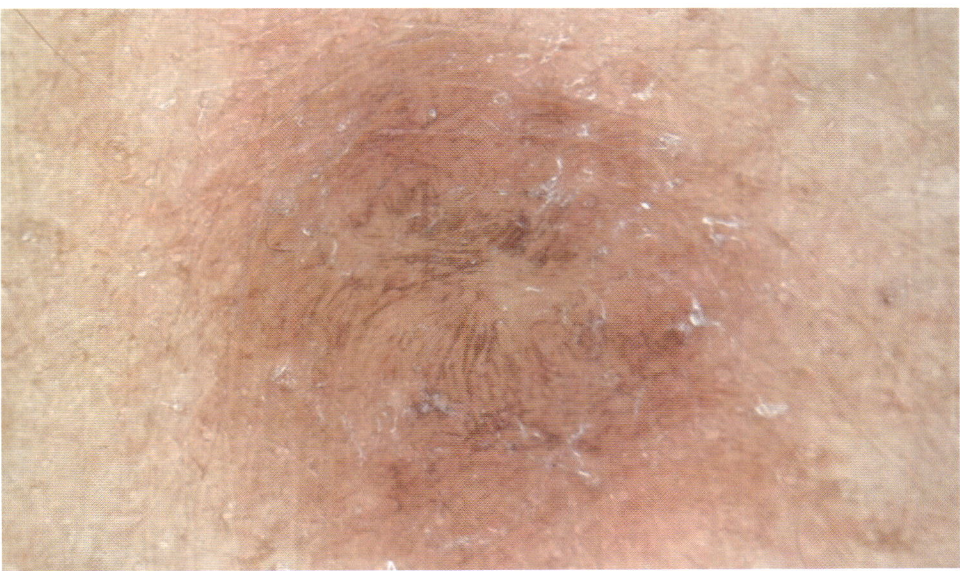

Fig. 5: Pattern 1: Complete delicate pigment network.

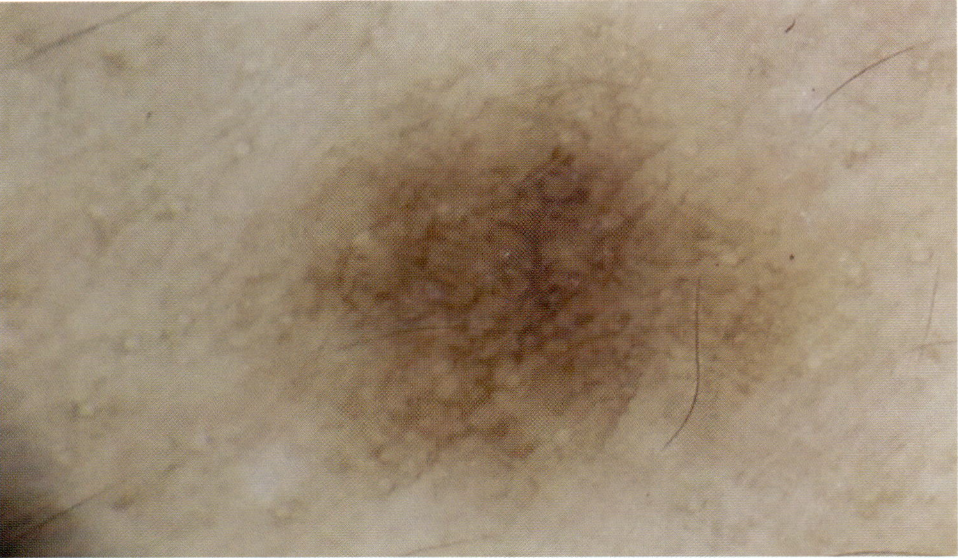

Fig. 6: Pattern 1: Another dermoscopic picture showing complete delicate pigment network.

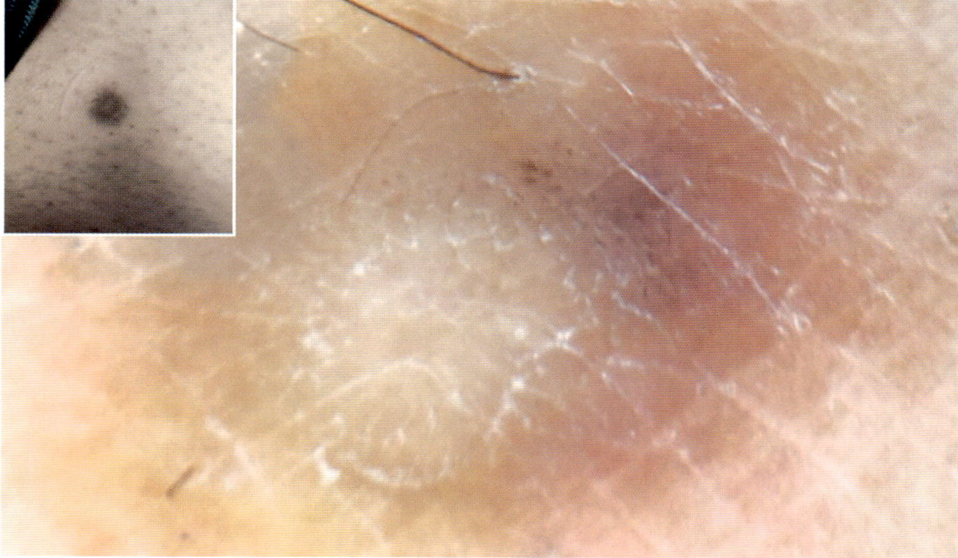

Fig. 7: Pattern 2: Delicate pigment network at the periphery and central white scar-like patch.

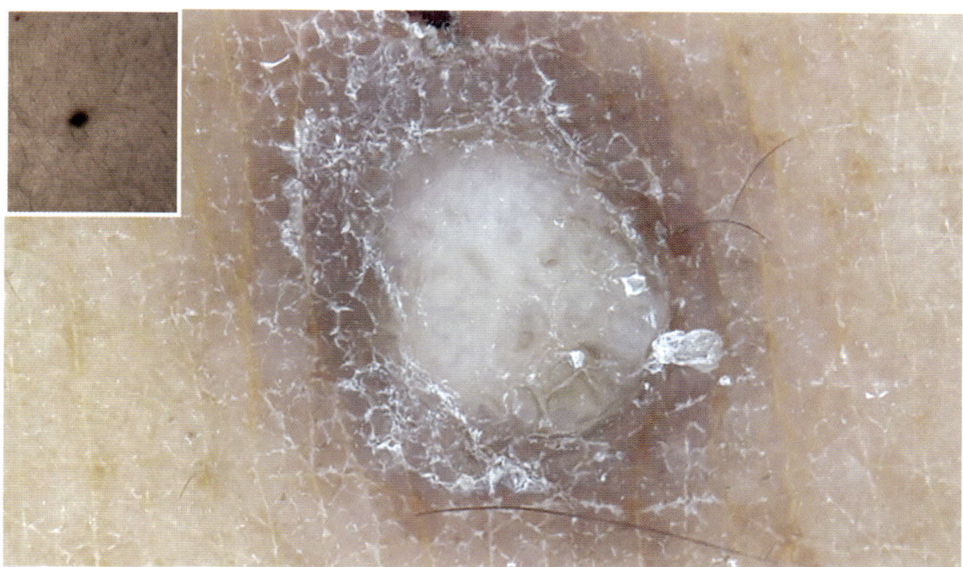

Fig. 8: Pattern 2: Central white scar-like patch with peripheral delicate pigment network.

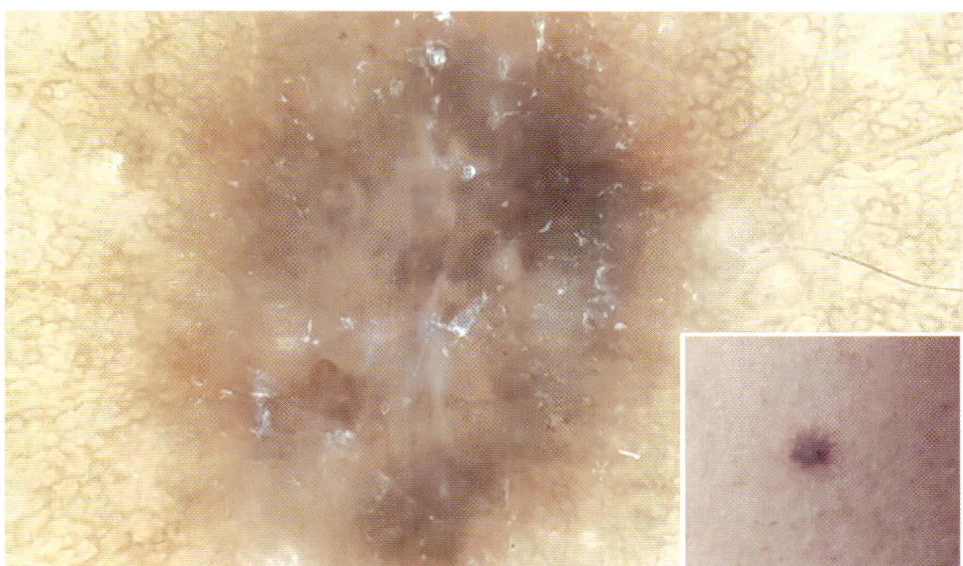

Fig. 9: Pattern 3: Delicate pigment network at the periphery and central white network.

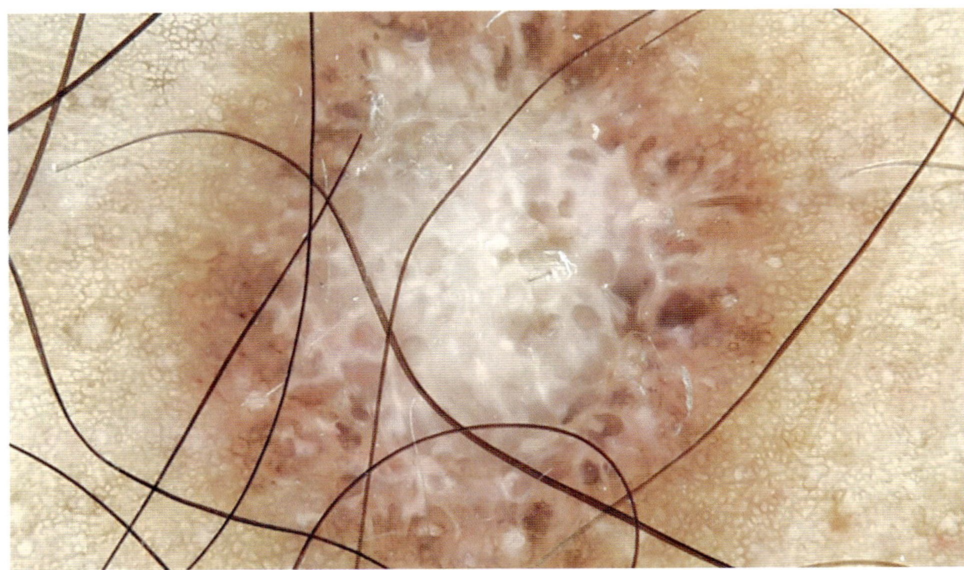

Fig. 10: Pattern 5: Complete white network pattern. Note the white line of scars and brown holes. It is considered a variation of the classic white scar-like patch with a similar histopathologic correlation.

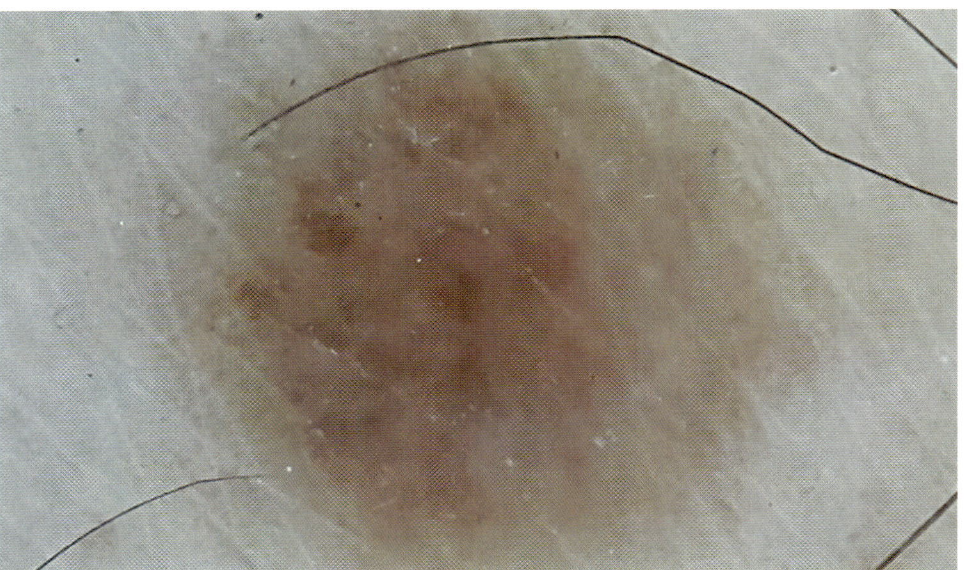

Fig. 11: Pattern 6: Complete homogeneous area. Note pink-brown hue of the dermatofibroma (DF) with a delicate brown pigment network at the periphery. Some brown globules are also present. The histopathologic diagnosis is aneurysmal DF.

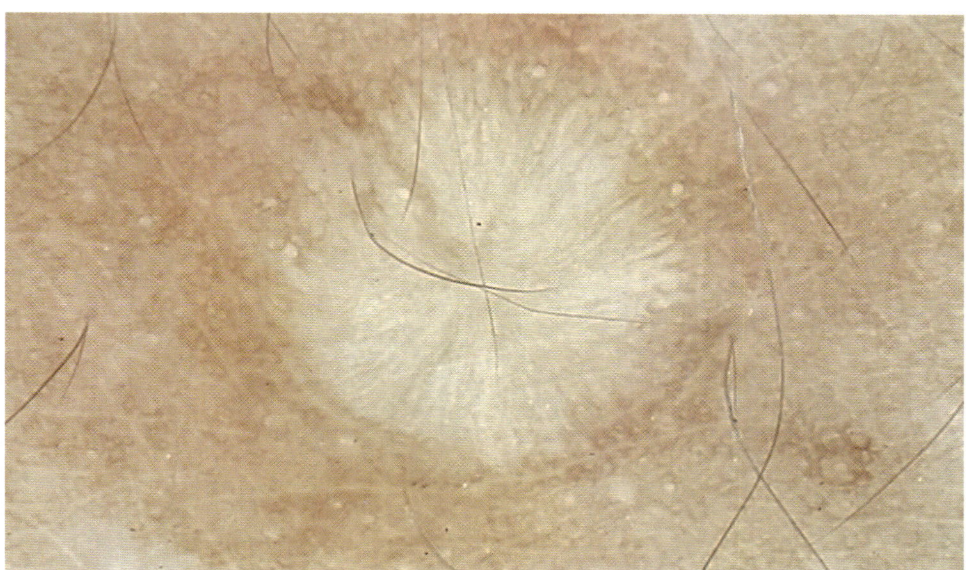

Fig. 12: Pattern 7a: Complete white scar-like patch. Histopathologically it corresponds to pronounced fibrosis in the papillary dermis.

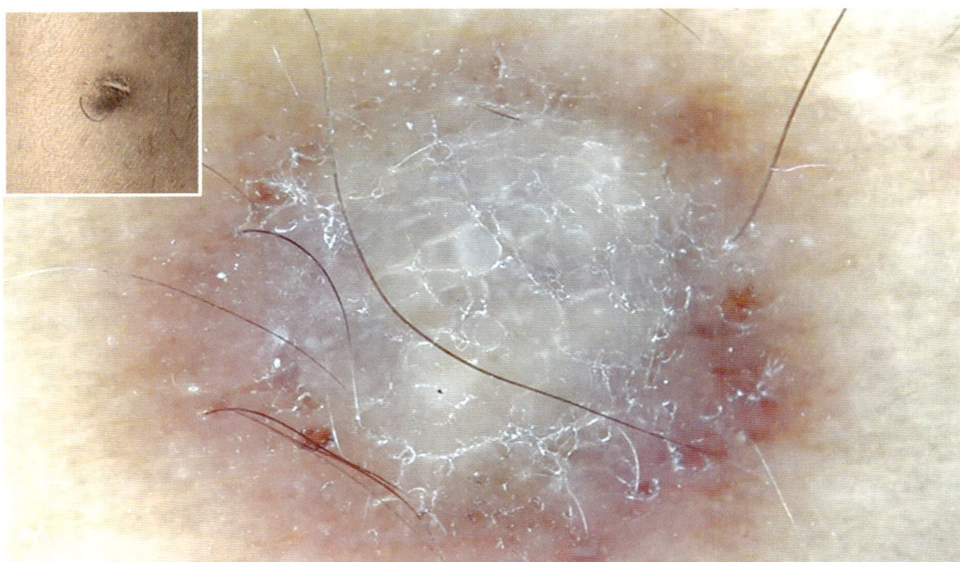

Fig. 13: Pattern 9: Peripheral homogeneous area and central white network. Blum and Bauer[5] reported a case of melanoma with peripheral delicate pigmentation network and central white scar-like patches. However, Zaballos could not find malignancy in four cases of dermatofibroma (DF) with multiple scar-like patches.[1] White network was reported recently in a case series where it occurred mostly in larger lesions of DF.[6,7]

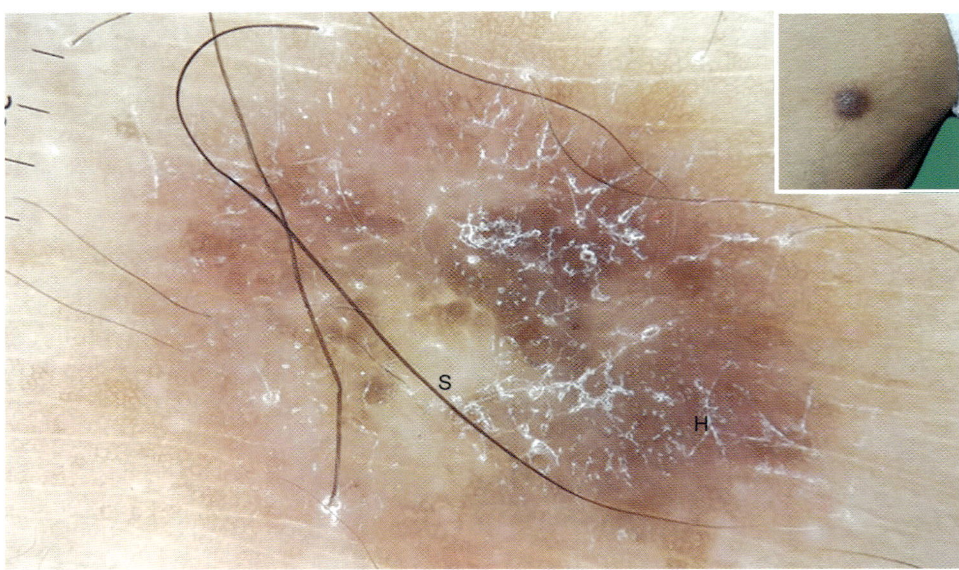

Fig. 14: Pattern 10: Atypical pattern. A multicomponent pattern of dermatofibroma (DF) composed of: (a) Atypical pigment network located in the center, (b) Atypical scar-like patch (S), (c) Atypical homogeneous pigmentation (H) of pink, grayish, and pink brown, or (d) Irregular distribution of these structures. In these atypical cases biopsy should be done to rule out malignancy.

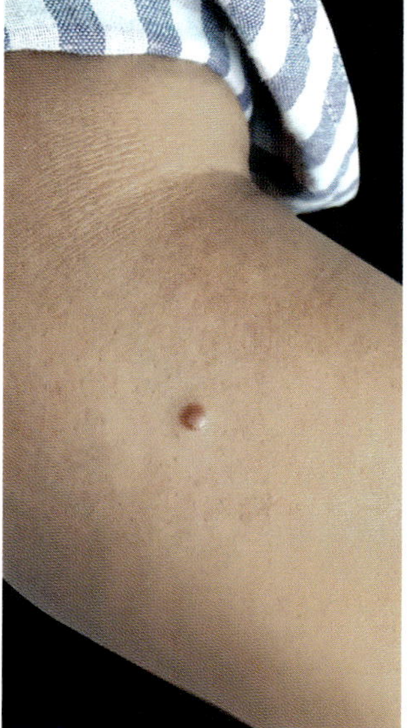

Fig. 15: Solitary dermatofibroma over forearm.

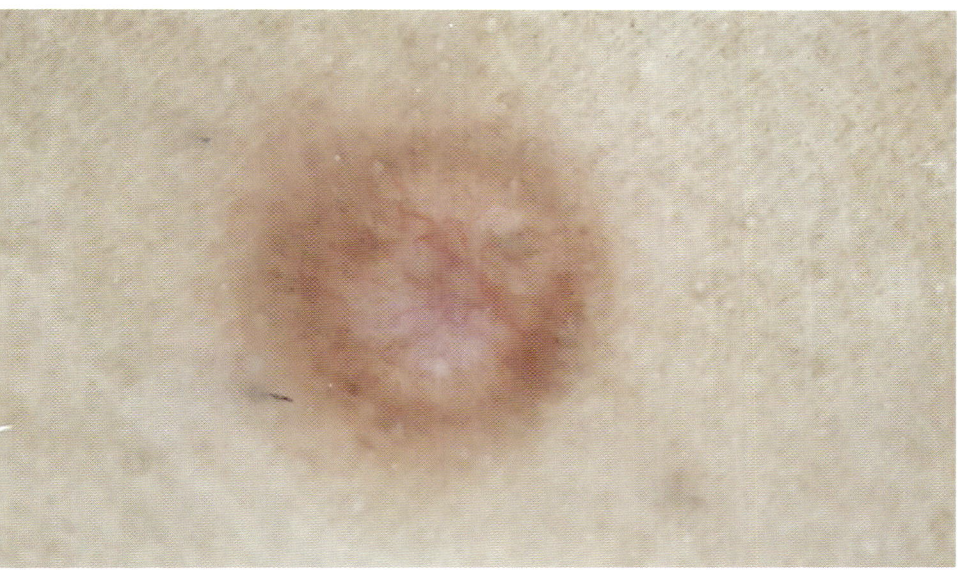

Fig. 16: Telangiectatic vessels are observed on dermoscopy in the previous patient.

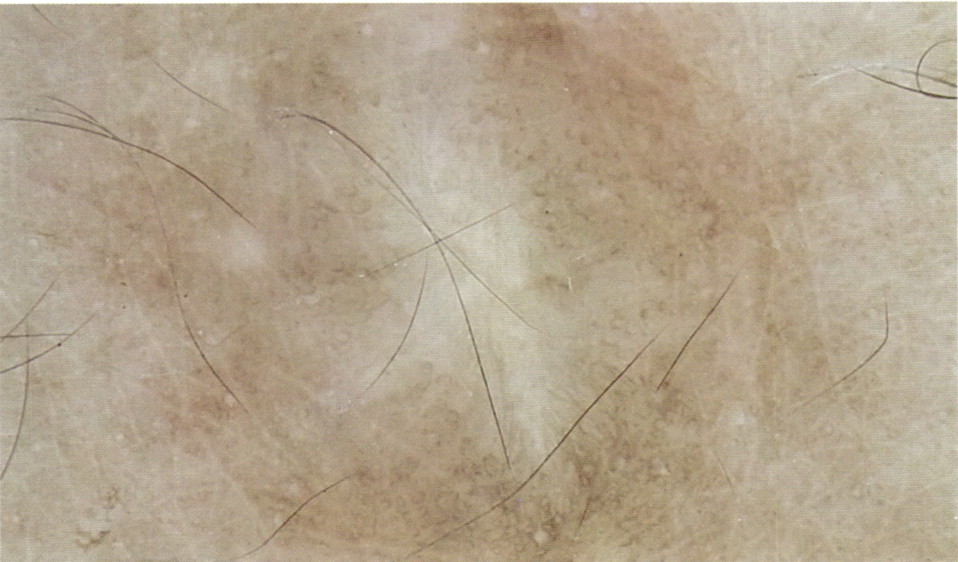

Fig. 17: Discrete peripheral network with central star-like white patch.

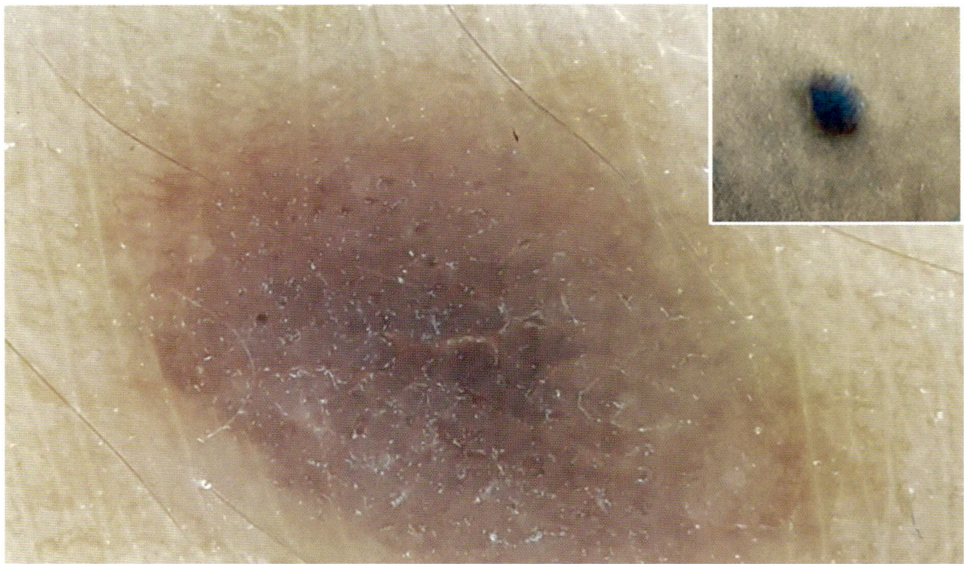

Fig. 18: Seborrheic keratosis like dermatofibroma (DF).

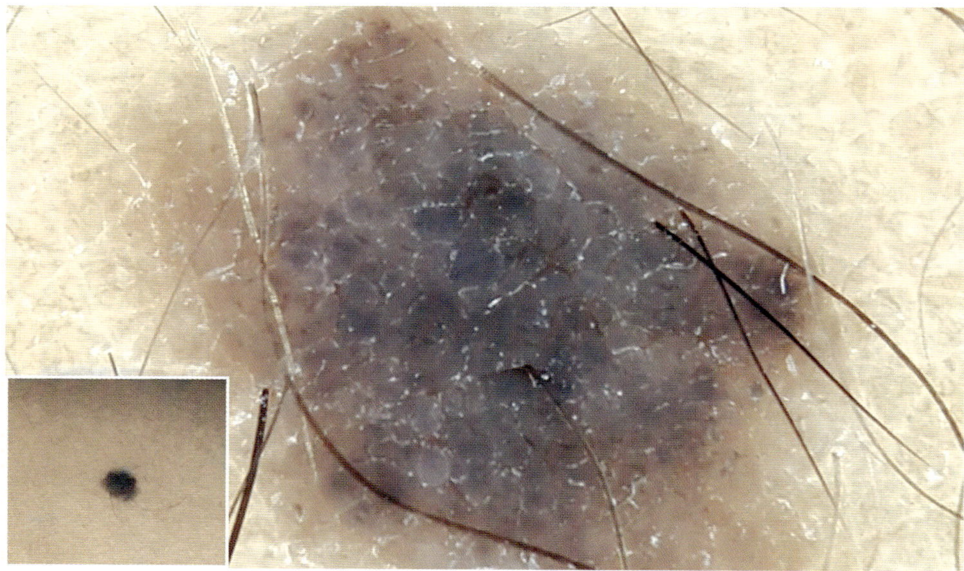

Fig. 19: Seborrheic keratosis like dermatofibroma (DF).

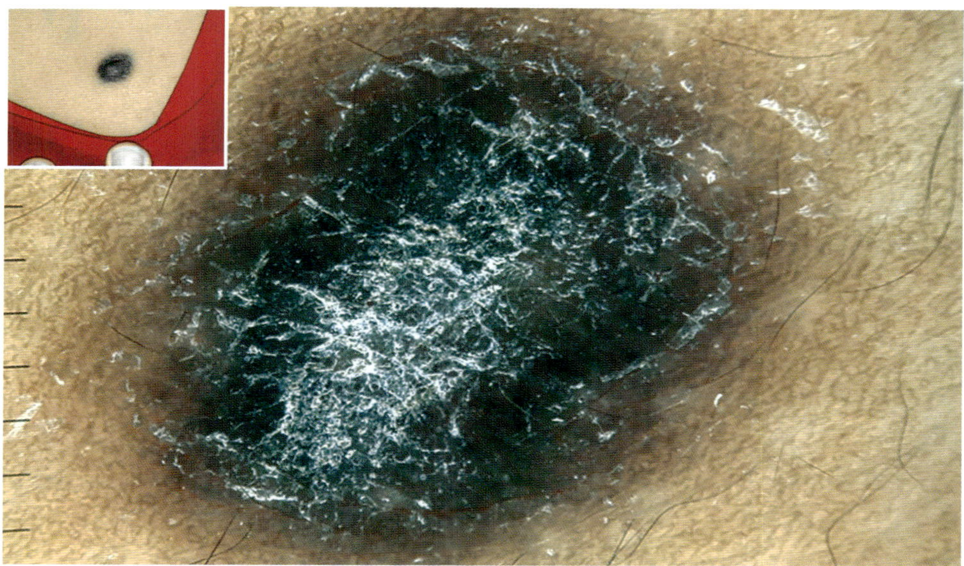

Fig. 20: Seborrheic keratosis like dermatofibroma (DF).

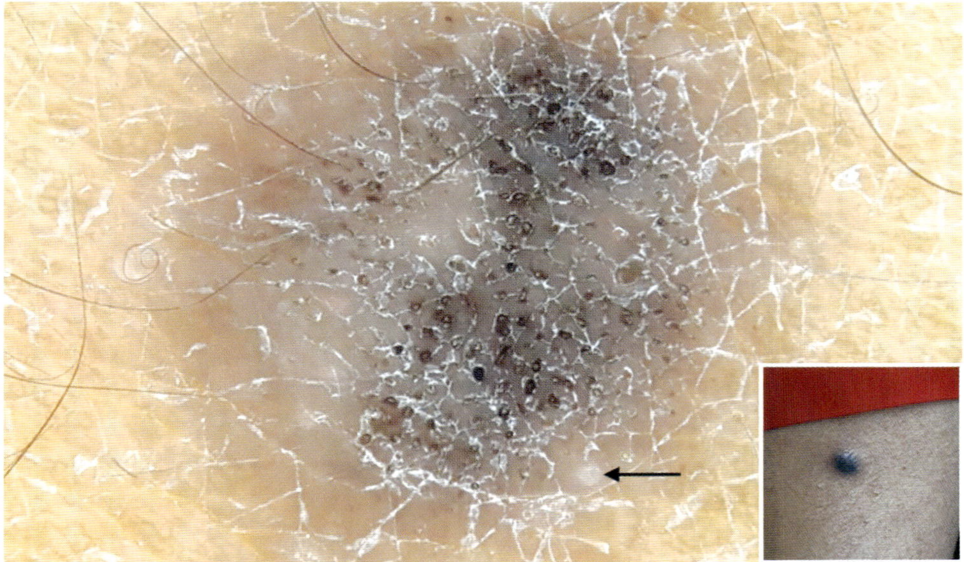

Fig. 21: Seborrheic keratosis like dermatofibroma (DF); Note the comedo-like structures. Milia-like cysts are also visible (arrow).

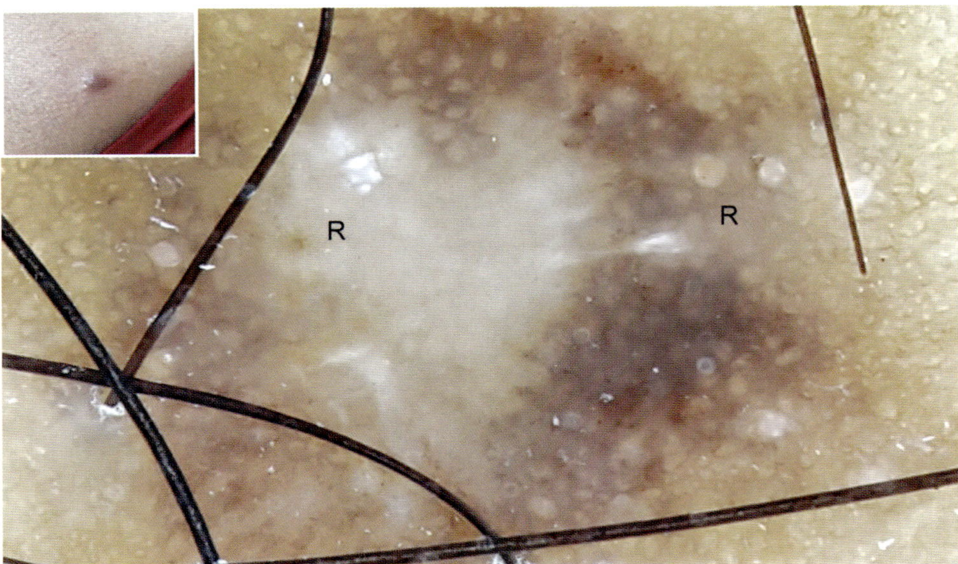

Fig. 22: Central white scar-like structure with peripheral hyperpigmentation that further is surrounded by delicate melanocytic network. Multiple rosettes (R) are seen both on the scars and peripherally.

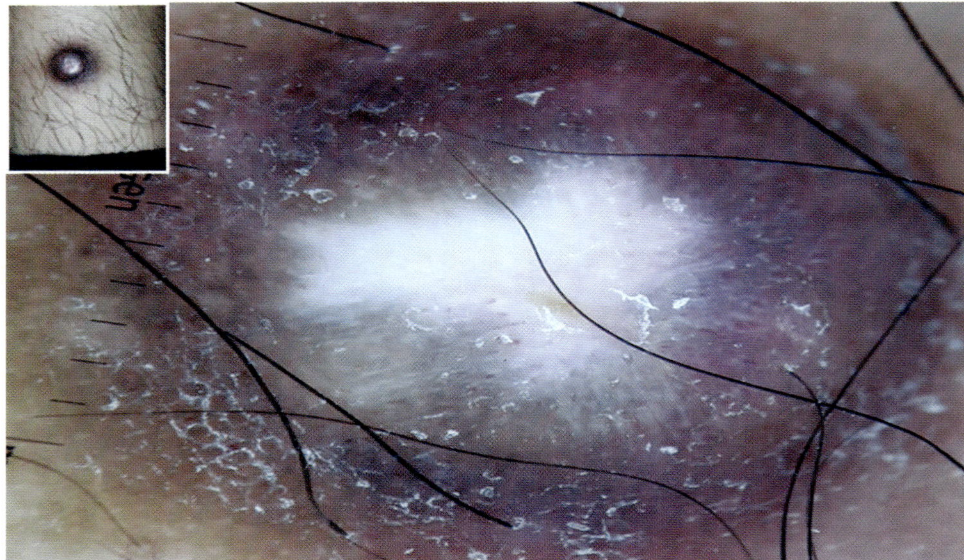

Fig. 23: Violaceous homogeneous pigmentation at the periphery and central star-shaped white scar associated with different vascular patterns. After histopathological examination there could be the presence of prominent blood-filled spaces and intra- and extracellular hemosiderin deposition. Histopathology confirmed this type of dermatofibroma (DF) as hemosiderotic.

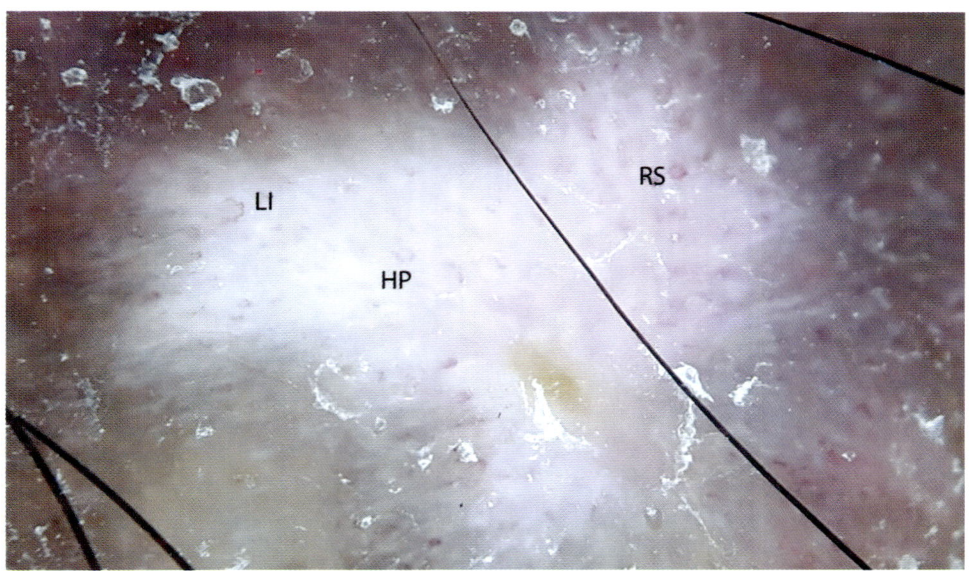

Fig. 24: The previous picture has been magnified to show details of the central area with various vascular structures. Central scar is star-shaped with scales and a yellow structure probably of keratinous origin. Different vascular structures are observed such as hairpin (HP), linear irregular (LI), and ring shaped (RS).

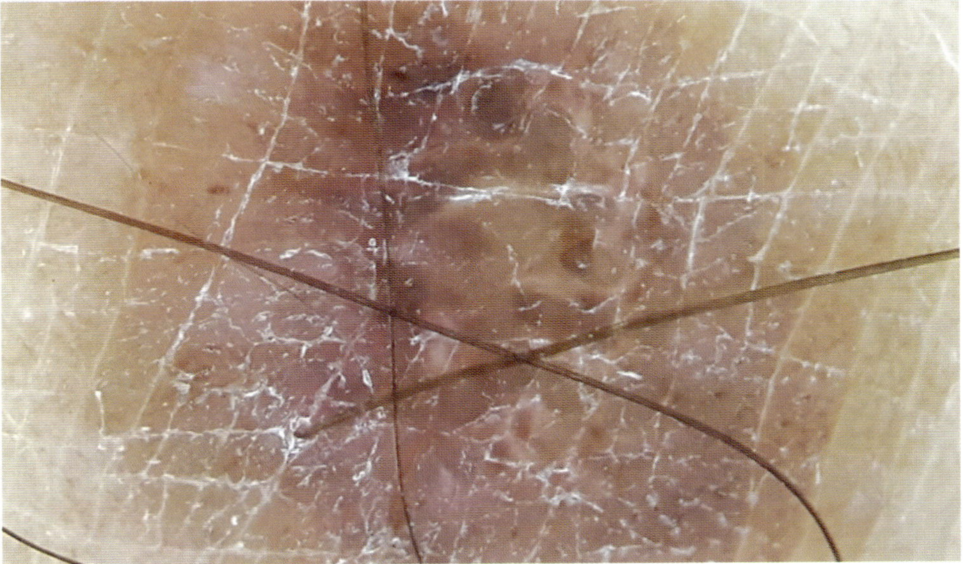

Fig. 25: Dermatofibroma (DF) with peripheral seborrheic keratosis like structure and central reticular scar with brown holes.

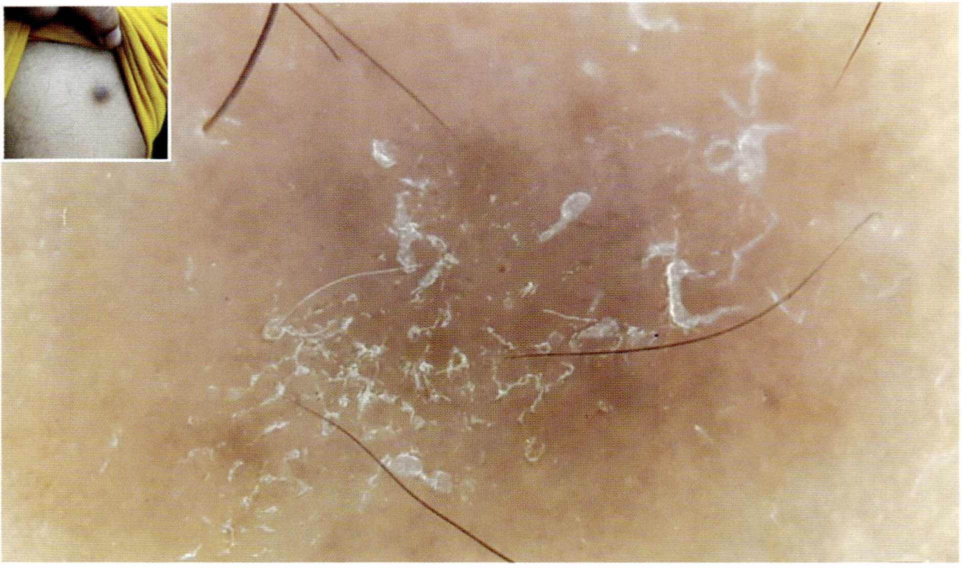

Fig. 26: Peripheral homogeneous pigmentation and central seborrheic keratosis like dermatofibroma (DF).

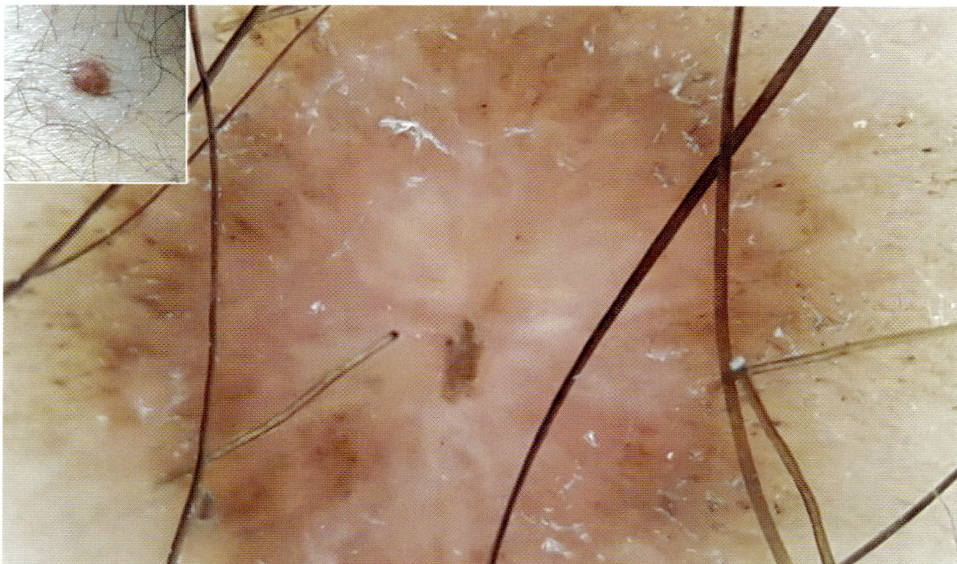

Fig. 27: Complete pink-brown homogeneous dermatofibroma (DF) with central white shiny streaks. Histopathology showed aneurysmal DF.

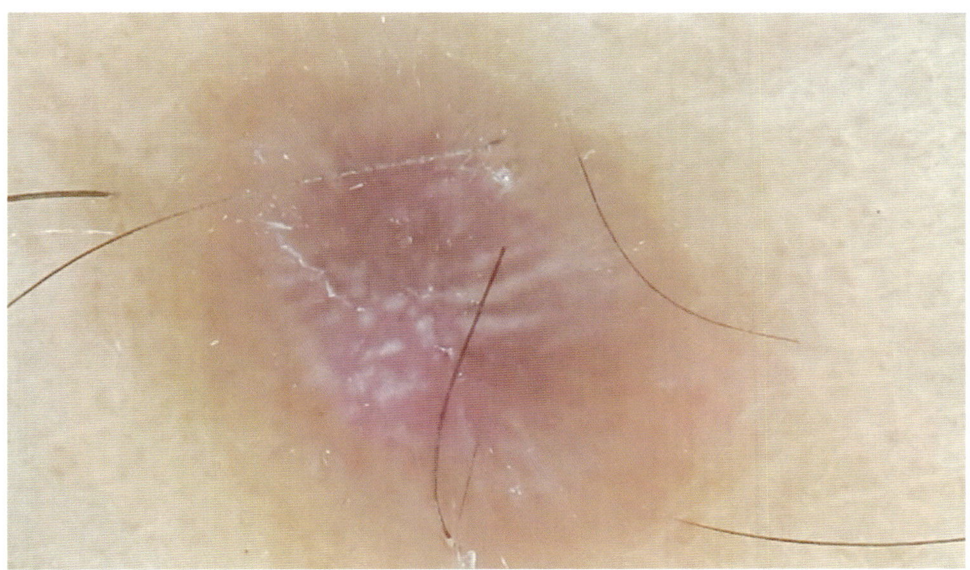

Fig. 28: Homogeneous pink color with white streaks and globules.

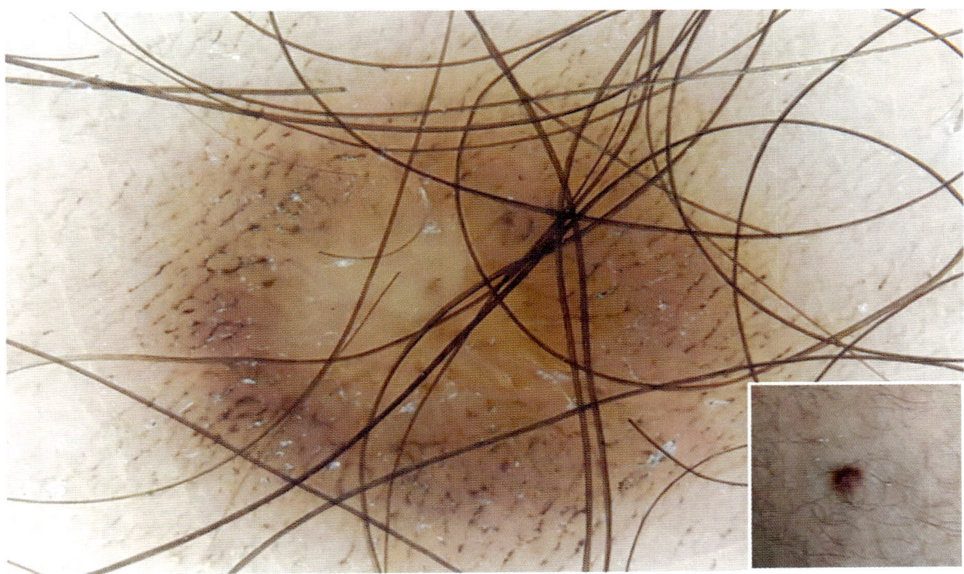

Fig. 29: Central white scar-like structure with peripheral hyperpigmented parallel lines.

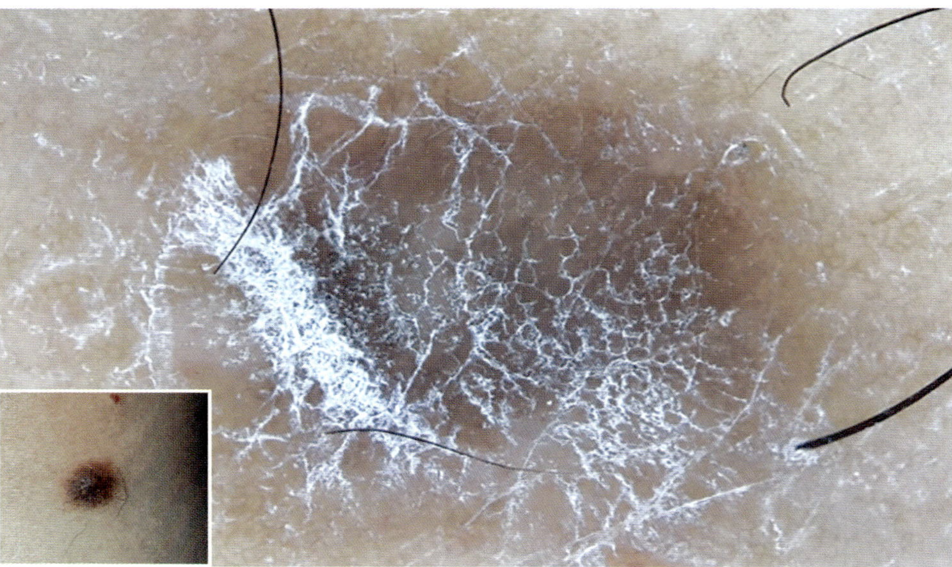

Fig. 30: Reticular pattern of scales over homogeneous brown background.

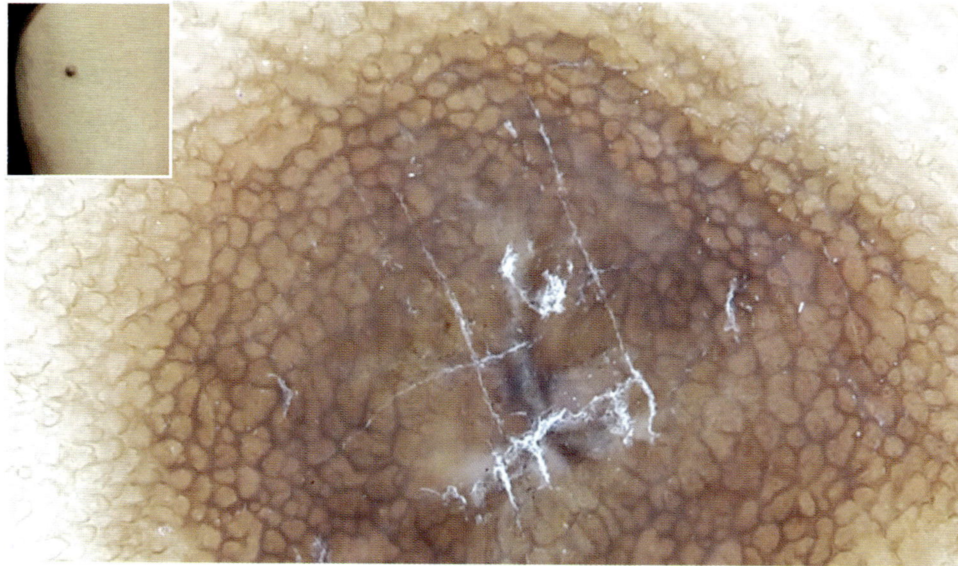

Fig. 31: Dermatofibroma (DF) with pronounced melanocytic network and central scar-like structure.

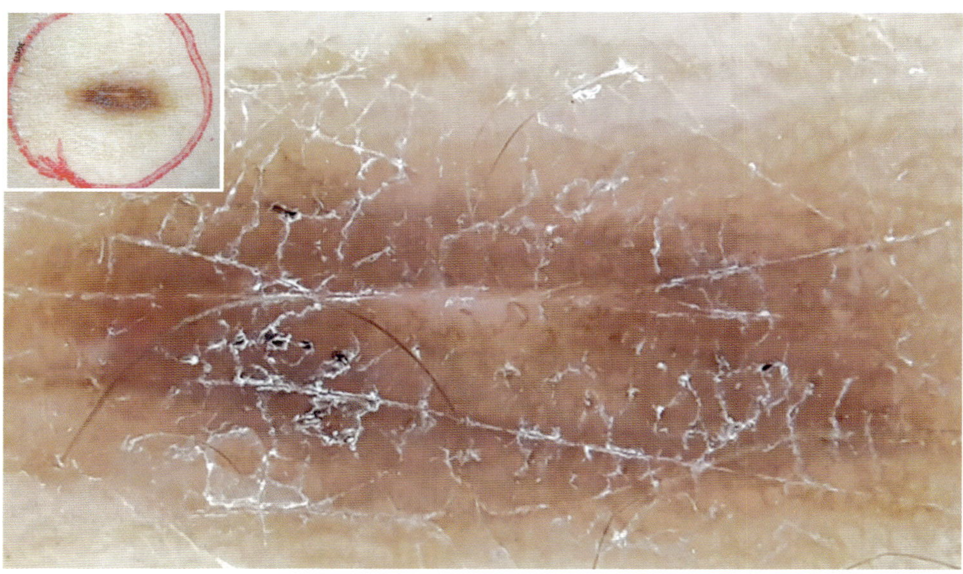

Fig. 32: Peripheral seborrheic keratosis like structure and centrally a band-like scar.

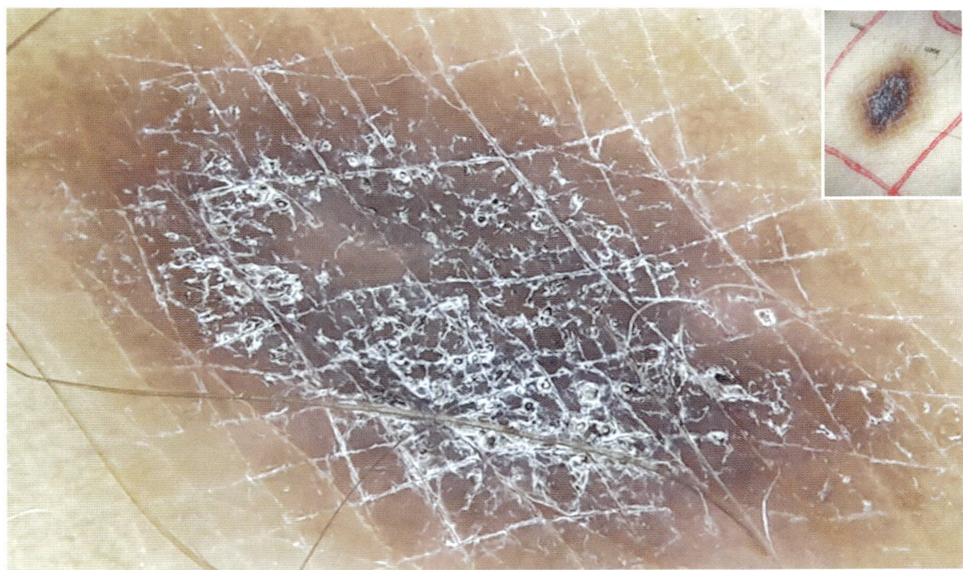

Fig. 33: Seborrheic keratosis like dermatofibroma (DF) with two brown homogeneous scars and peripheral delicate pigment.

REFERENCES

1. Zaballos P, Puig S, Llambrich A, et al. Dermoscopy of dermatofibromas: a prospective morphological study of 412 cases. Arch Dermatol. 2008;144(1):75-83.
2. Ferrari A, Argenziano G, Buccini P, et al. Typical and atypical dermoscopic presentations of dermatofibroma. J Eur Acad Dermatol Venereol. 2013;27(11):1375-80.
3. Agero AL, Taliercio S, Dusza SW, et al. Conventional and polarized dermoscopy features of dermatofibroma. Arch Dermatol. 2006;142(11):1431-7.
4. Kilinc Karaarslan I, Gencoglan G, Akalin T, et al. Different dermoscopic faces of dermatofibromas. J Am Acad Dermatol. 2007;57(3):401-6.
5. Argenziano G, Soyer H, Chimenti S, et al. Dermoscopy of Pigmented Skin Lesions: An Atlas Based on the Consensus Net Meeting on Dermoscopy. Italy: EDRA Medical Publishing and New Media; 2001.
6. Zaballos P, Guionnet N, Puig S, et al. Central white network: an additional dermoscopic feature for the diagnosis of dermatofibroma. Dermatol Surg. 2005;31(8 Pt 1):960-2.
7. Zaballos P, Puig S, Malvehy J. Dermoscopy of atypical dermatofibroma: central white network. Arch Dermatol. 2006;142(1):126.

KERATOACANTHOMA

INTRODUCTION

Keratoacanthoma (KA) originates in the pilosebaceous gland that mimics squamous cell carcinoma (SCC). It is characterized by rapid growth for a few weeks to months followed by spontaneous resolution. In most of the cases, KA occurs on sun-exposed areas. Typically it is solitary round, skin colored, or pinkish papule with a smooth shiny surface and a central keratin plug that may ulcerate.

KEY DERMOSCOPIC FEATURES[1,2]

- Central keratin
- Hairpin/looped vessels at the periphery
- White structureless zone at the periphery.

DISCUSSION

Dermoscopically KA reveals central mass of keratin typically surrounded by hairpin vessels along with a whitish halo.[2] Vessels have a radial distribution and may be accompanied by atypical linear or glomerular vessels. The peripheral arrangement of hairpin vessels distinguishes KA from seborrheic keratosis (SK) where the vessels are distributed throughout the lesion.[3]

A central plug is an architectural criterion for the diagnosis of KA which correlates well with histopathology.[1] The other features, which may be present, are white structureless zone, blood spots, ulceration, and some vascular structures.

KEYNOTE

Though keratin is a clue to the diagnosis of KA and SCC, central keratin is the only dermoscopic parameter that differentiates KA from SCC.

CASE STUDY (FIG. 34 TO 37)

- A 40-year-old male presented to us with a lesion on the upper lip since a few years.
- The lesion was asymptomatic and static in nature.
- On cutaneous examination, there was a singular, firm, sessile, and skin-colored papular lesion measuring 0.5 × 0.5 cm in size, with two to three hair protruding from it.

- A 35-year-old female patient presented to us with a lesion on the nose since a couple of years. The lesion was asymptomatic in nature and static in size. Cutaneous examination revealed a single, firm, pea sized, and brown to black-colored sessile papule on the nose.
- Considering the clinical appearance of the lesion, we thought of seborrheic keratosis, compound nevus, verruca vulgaris, and solitary fibrous papule of the nose as differential diagnosis. To confirm our clinical suspicion we used a dermoscope.

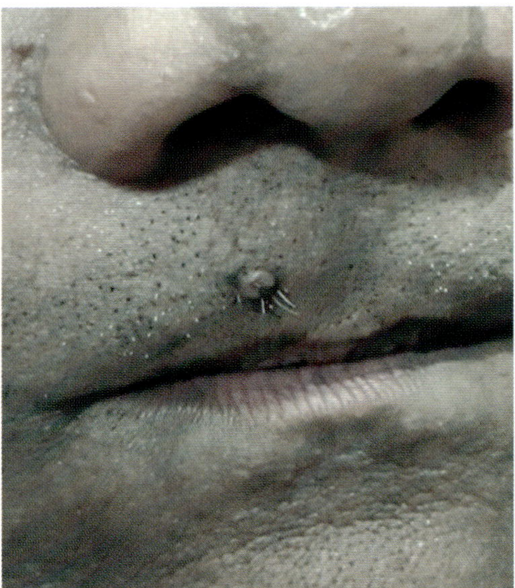

Fig. 34: Clinical diagnosis in this case is tough and hence biopsy is necessary. However, dermoscopy can clinch the diagnosis.

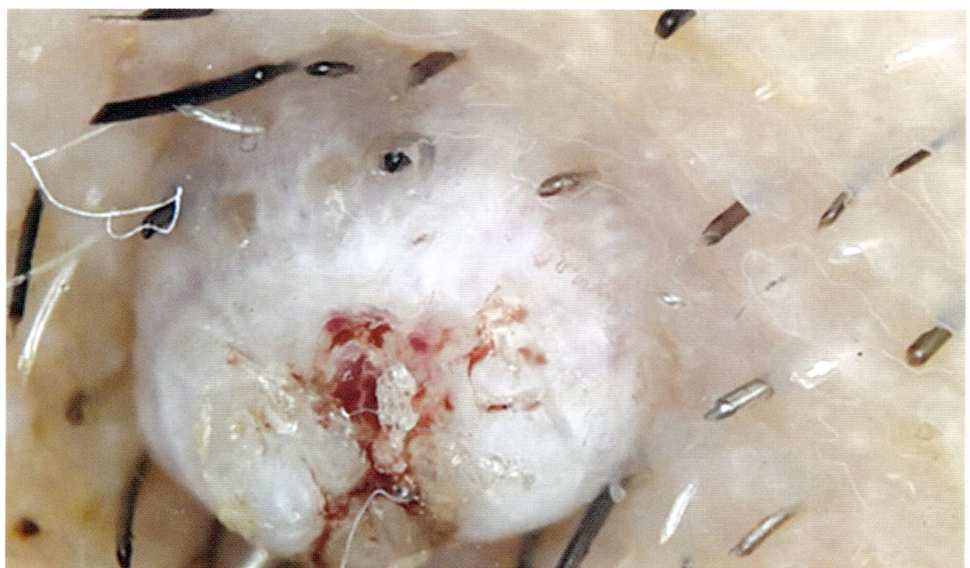

Fig. 35: On dermoscopy: (a) Central crater, (b) White structureless area, and (c) Peripheral hairpin vessels almost confirming the diagnosis of keratoacanthoma.

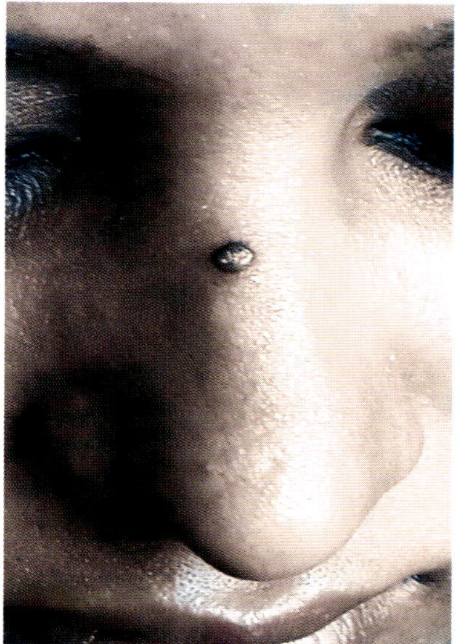

Fig. 36: A 35-year-old female patient having a papular lesion on the nose.

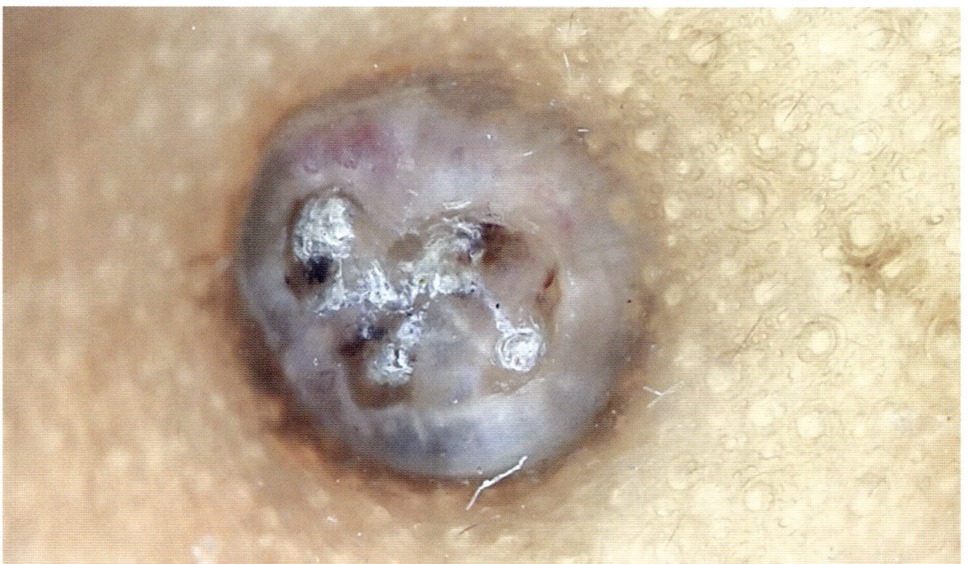

Fig. 37: At the center of the mass, there was a keratin plug which was surrounded by a white structureless zone. At the periphery of the mass, we observed hairpin blood vessels. These features are highly suggestive of keratoacanthoma.

REFERENCES

1. Rosendahl C, Cameron A, Argenziano G, et al. Dermoscopy of squamous cell carcinoma and keratoacanthoma. Arch Dermatol. 2012;148(12):1386-92.
2. Martína JM, Bella-Navarroa R, Jordá E. Vascular patterns in dermoscopy. Actas Dermosifiliogr. 2012;103(5):357-75.
3. Zalaudek I, Kreusch J, Giacomel J, et al. How to diagnose nonpigmented skin tumors: a review of vascular structures seen with dermoscopy. Part I. Melanocytic skin tumors. J Am Acad Dermatol. 2010;63:361-74.

SEBORRHEIC KERATOSIS

INTRODUCTION

Seborrheic keratosis (SK) is a common benign epithelial tumor. A number of conditions that clinically mimic SK are melanocytic nevus, basal cell carcinoma, Bowen's disease (BD), verruca vulgaris, and melanoma; thus leading to diagnostic dilemmas. Dermoscopy being an in vivo, noninvasive investigative method, can almost instantly diagnose SK.

KEY DERMOSCOPIC FEATURES (FIGS. 38 TO 69)[1]

- Cerebriform pattern
- Fingerprint structures
- Comedo-like openings
- Milia-like cysts
- Moth-eaten border
- Hairpin vessels.

DISCUSSION

Cerebriform pattern or brain-like appearance dermoscopically appears as multiple fissures and ridges where fissures correspond to the sulci of the brain and the ridges to the gyri. This pattern often is the sole feature of SK. "Fat fingers" are described as linear and wide dermoscopic structures corresponding to ridges. The length of fat fingers can vary from very short sausage-like structures to as long as the half of the diameter of the lesion. They have a spectrum of colors which range from tan/brown to blue to hypopigmented. They may have multiple shapes such as linear, curvilinear and branched such as "W" or "V".

Fingerprint-like structures appear as fine parallel lines of light brown to dark brown colors resembling a fingerprint.[2,3] As the solar lentigo matures (SK may arise within solar lentigo), the fingerprint-like structures are more easily seen and may develop a reticulated appearance. This reticulated appearance or net-like structures differ from the melanocytic network because they do not correspond to melanin pigment of lower epidermis or rete ridge melanocytes. The holes/grids here have much wider diameter than those in the typical melanocytic network, and the holes do not correlate with the tips of dermal papillae.[2] A solar lentigo can evolve into an SK.[4]

Comedo-like openings are round to ovoid follicular openings that have brown or black keratin plugs. They represent keratin-filled invaginations on histology. Sometimes comedo-like openings may be the dominant dermoscopic features of SK.

Milia-like cysts are keratin cysts in the epidermis and appear as white to yellow, round, bright bodies on dermoscopy. They are less conspicuous and often difficult to visualize with polarized dermoscopy; hence turn your dermoscope on to nonpolarized mode to observe them easily.

Often, in some places, the borders of SK are scalloped, giving rise to moth-eaten border.

Hairpin vessels in SK are an occasional finding. They usually have a whitish halo corresponding to neighboring keratin. In melanomas, the surrounding halo of hairpin vessels is pink in color instead of white; however, in case of irritated SK, pink halo is seen surrounding hairpin vessels.[5,6]

KEYNOTE

Dermoscopy is a highly valuable tool to diagnose SK by differentiating it from other similar conditions. However, irritated SK may look like SCC or melanoma; moreover skin cancer can develop within an SK, thus, a biopsy and histopathology cannot be avoided in such situations.

Fifteen dermoscopic criteria have been identified (Box 1).
Twelve patterns of SKs are described (Box 2).

Box 1: Fifteen dermoscopic criteria.

- Milia-like cysts
- Comedo-like openings
- Brain-like structures (fissures and ridges)
- Fingerprint-like structures
- Moth-eaten border
- Hairpin vessels
- Mica-like structures
- Coral-like structures
- Yellowish color
- Network-like structures
- Grape-like vessels
- Globule-like structure
- Focal hemorrhage
- Opaque brown pigmentation
- Vascular structure.

Box 2: Twelve patterns of seborrheic keratosis (SKs).

- Fissures/ridges
- Exophytic papillary
- Mica like
- Coral
- Crypts
- Cobblestone like
- Multicomponent
- Structureless
- Globule like
- Network like
- Vascular
- Unspecific.

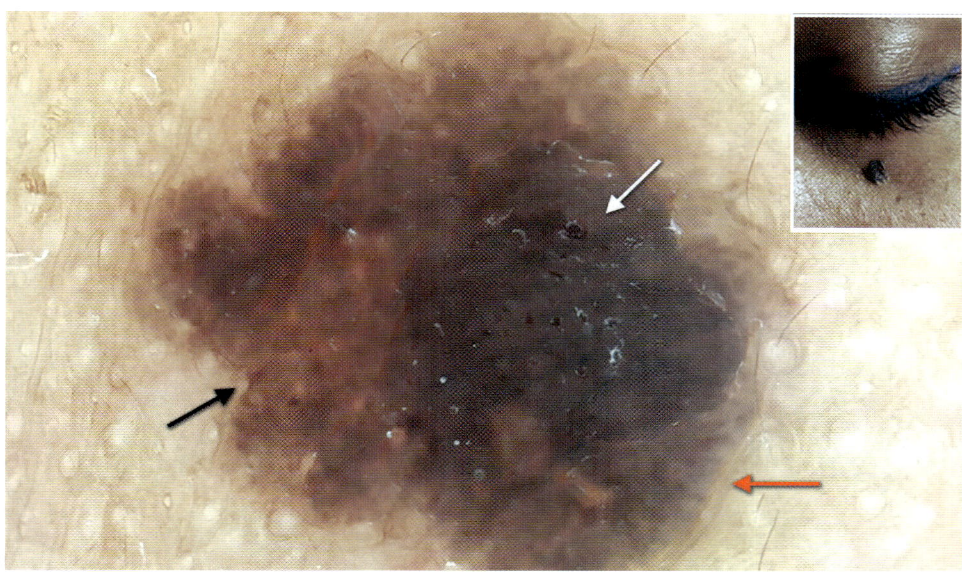

Fig. 38: Comedo-like openings (CLOs—white arrow), fat fingers (red arrow), and moth-eaten border (black arrow).

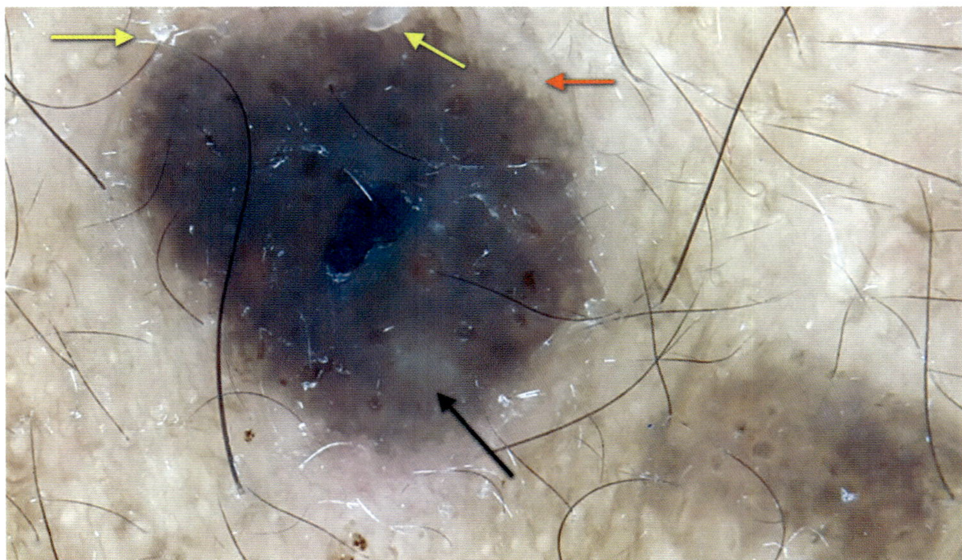

Fig. 39: Comedo-like openings (CLOs), a large milia-like cyst (black arrow), fat fingers (red arrow), and Demodex is revealed on dermoscopy. Demodex is not associated with seborrheic keratosis (SK) but a commensal on the face and resides in the hair follicles. The white spicule (yellow arrows) that is visible in this field is the tail of *Demodex folliculorum*.

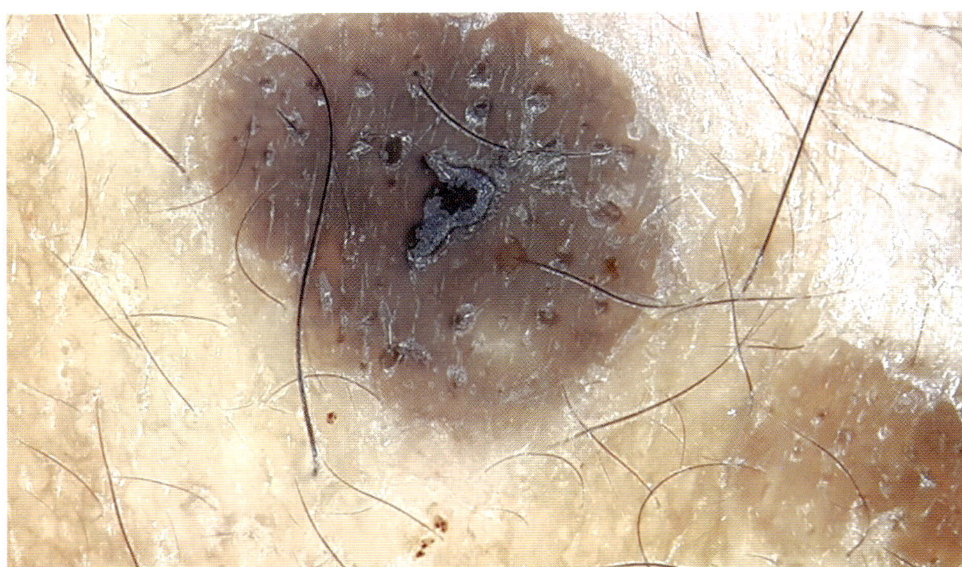

Fig. 40: Nonpolarized view of the previous field. Keratotic plugs of the comedo-like opening (CLO) are revealed. The milia-like cyst has become more prominent.

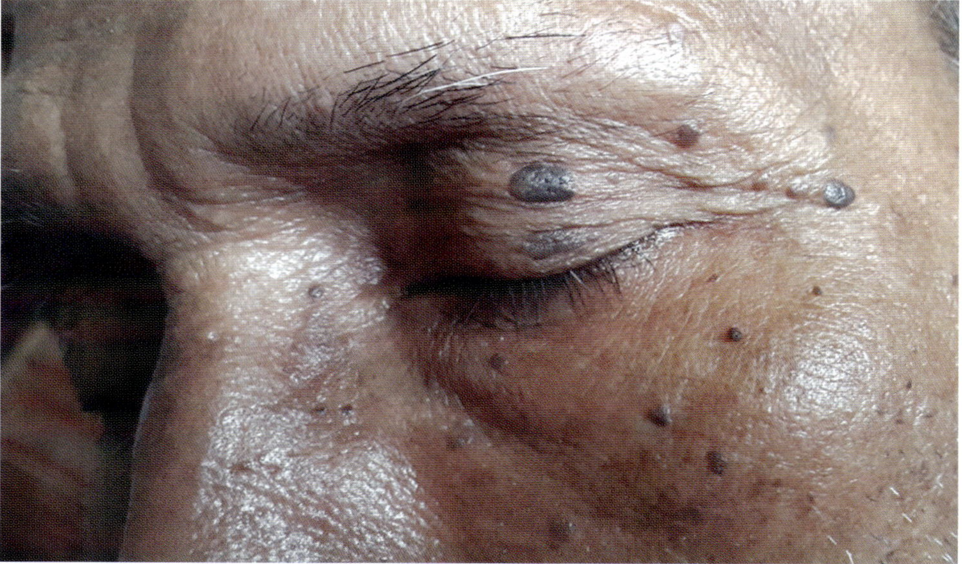

Fig. 41: In one of the largest series of dermoscopy of seborrheic keratosis (SK), it was most often found on the face and the trunk, followed by the extremities, the neck, and the scalp.

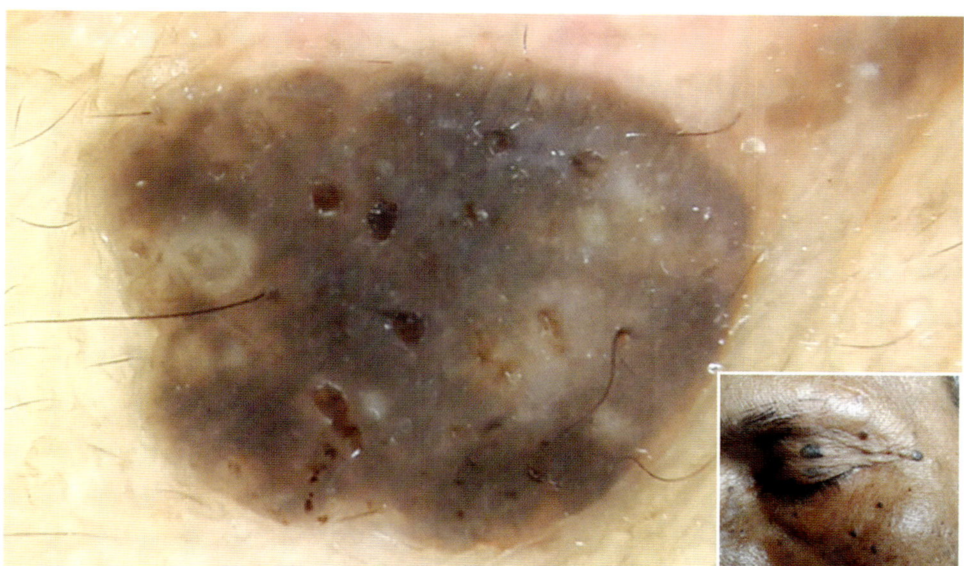

Fig. 42: Many large and small milia-like cysts and comedo-like openings (CLOs).

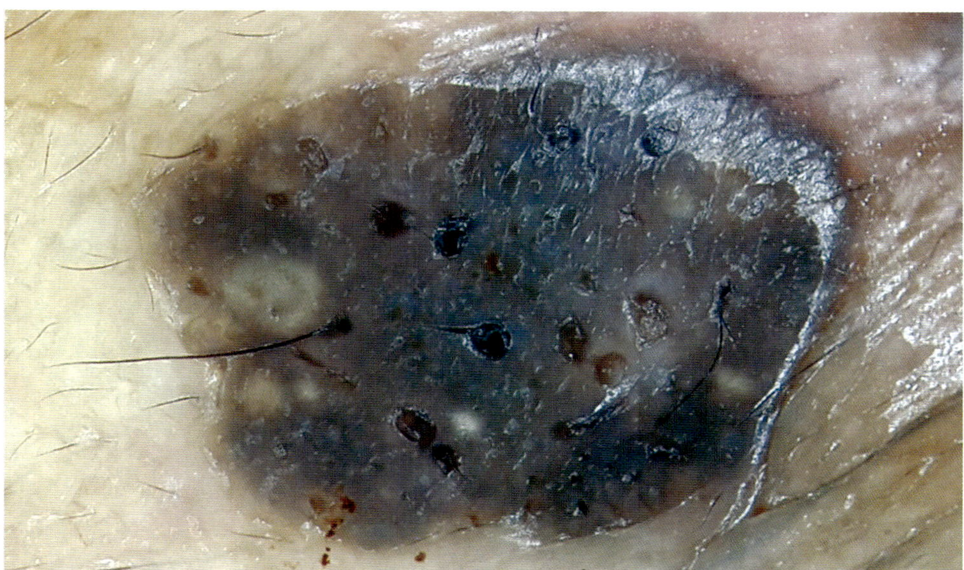

Fig. 43: Nonpolarized mode of the previous picture. More obvious milia-like cysts and prominent keratin plugs in comedo-like openings (CLOs).

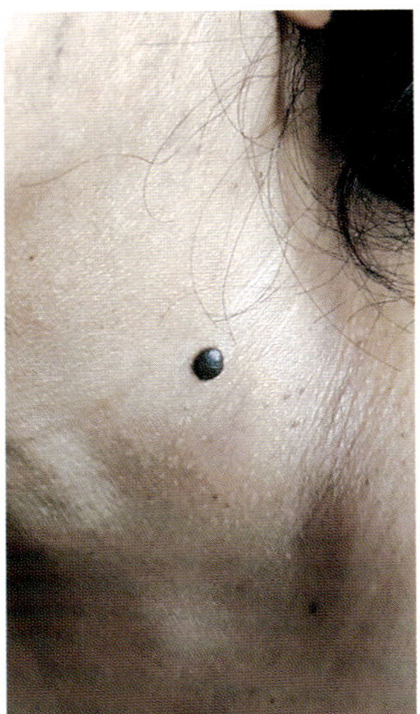

Fig. 44: Sometimes melanocytic nevus and seborrheic keratosis are close mimics clinically. The clinical diagnosis of the lesion on the neck is more in favor of melanocytic nevus.

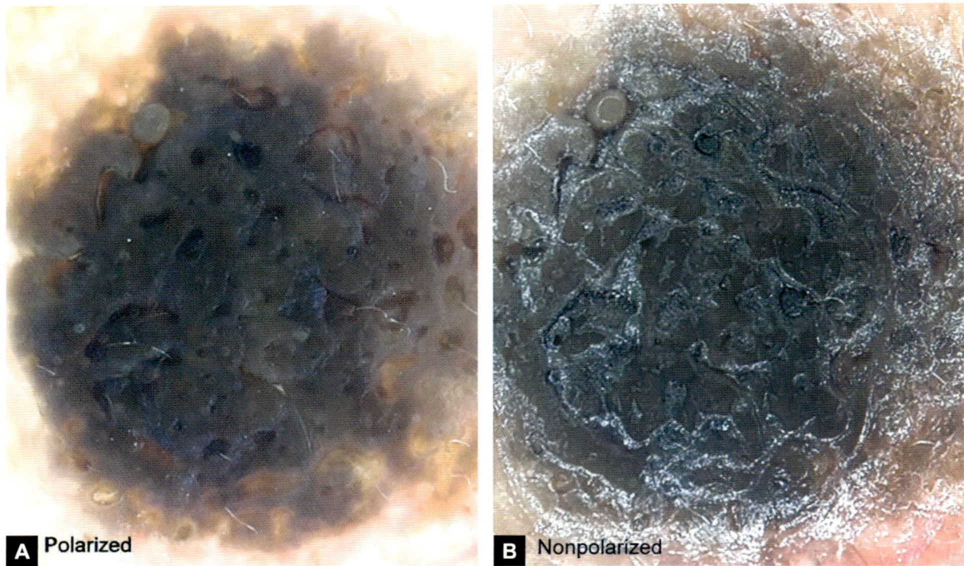

Figs. 45A and B: Dermoscopy of the previous lesion revealed SK. Appreciate the difference of dermoscopic appearance of the same SK lesion due to application of different modes of dermoscope. It reveals a milium at the top left corner, CLOs; moreover brain-like appearance is the main feature of this SK lesion. (CLOs: Comedo-like openings; SK: Seborrheic keratosis).

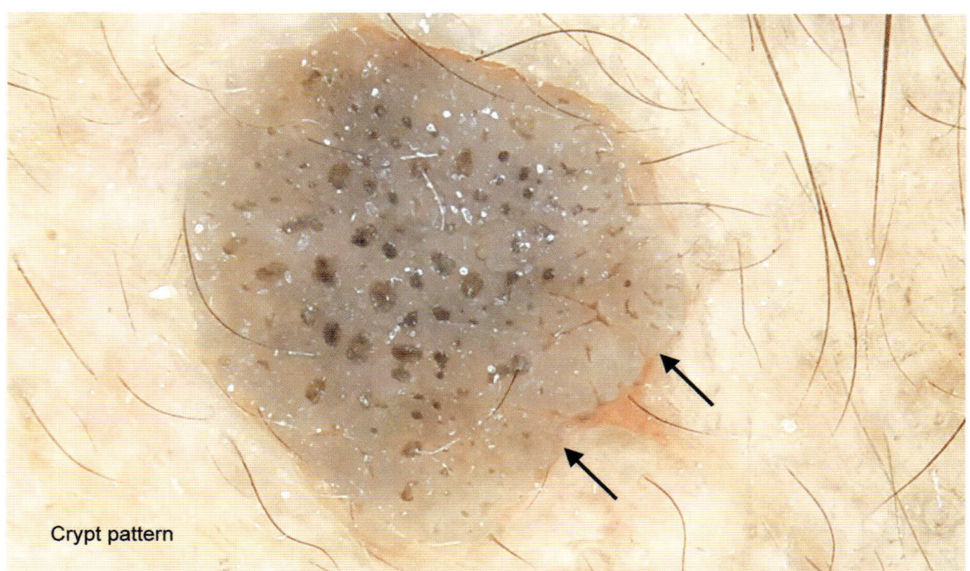

Fig. 46: Crypt pattern of SK is characterized by multiple CLOs. In addition to the CLOs, brain-like structures (arrows) are found at the lower right side of the periphery. Note the sharp demarcation. (CLOs: Comedo-like openings; SK: Seborrheic keratosis).

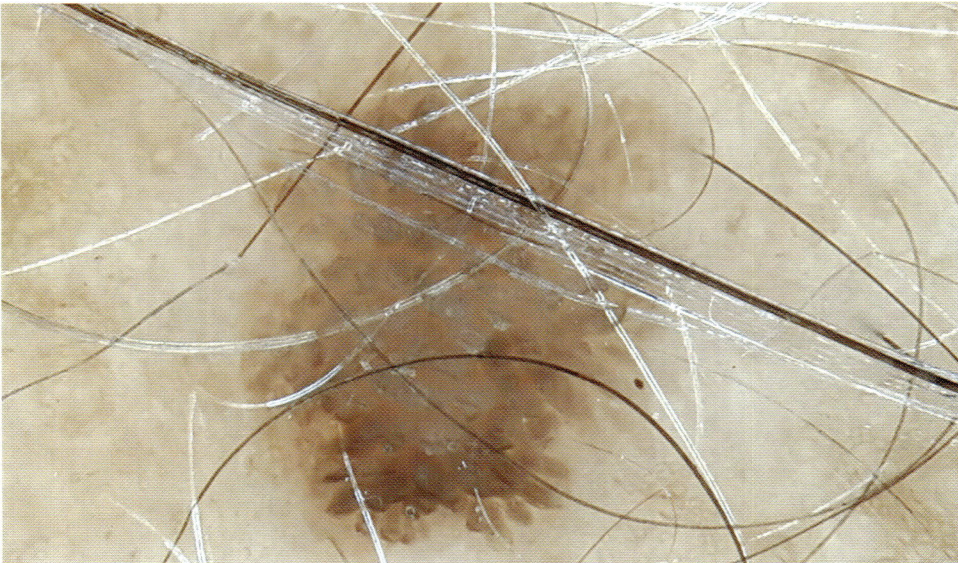

Fig. 47: Fat fingers-like structures. "Fat fingers" are described as linear and wide dermoscopic structures corresponding to ridges. They may have multiple shapes such as linear, curvilinear and branched: "W" or "V".

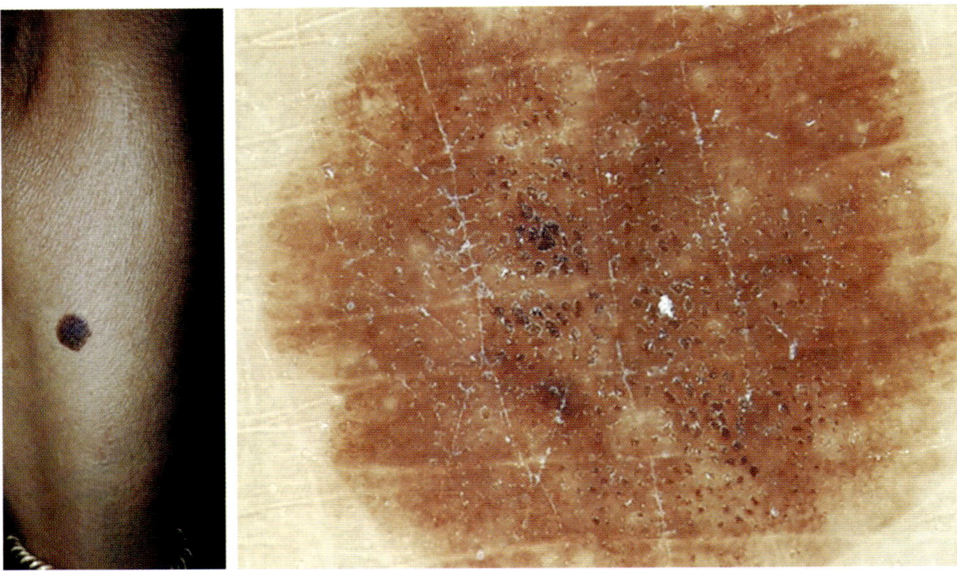

Fig. 48: Seborrheic keratosis (SK) on the forearm. Comedo-like openings and fingerprint-like structures are seen (probably it started initially as solar lentigo and later converted into SK).

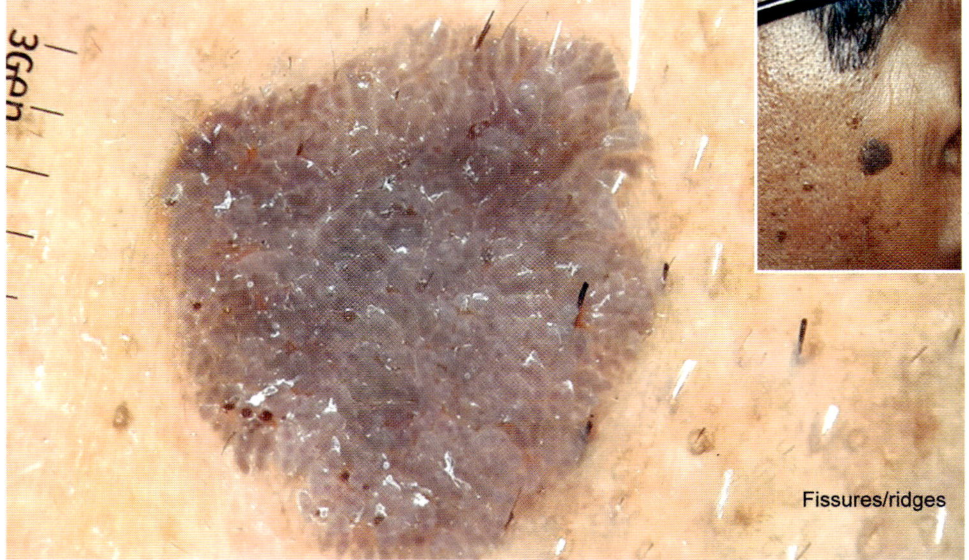

Fig. 49: Fat fingers-like structures.

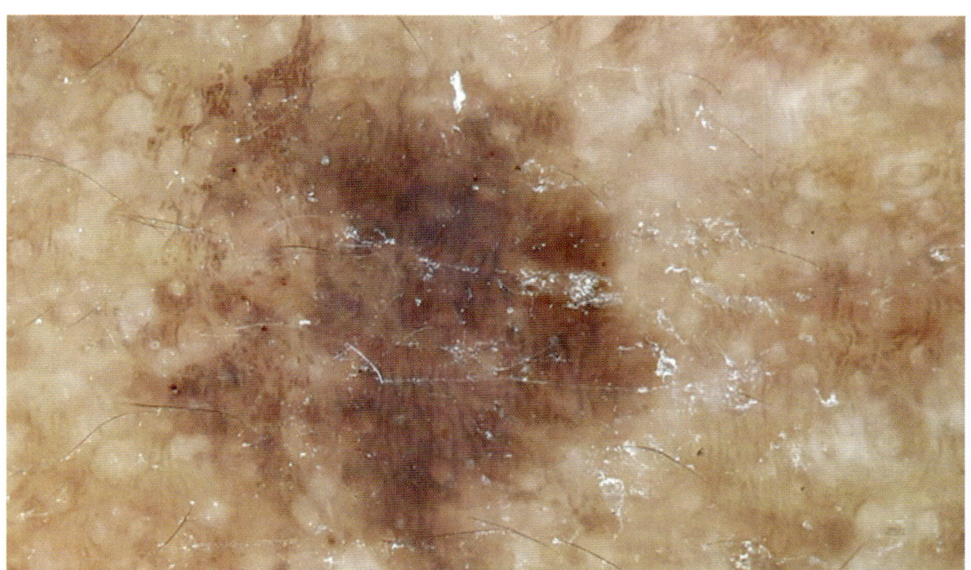

Fig. 50: Fingerprint-like structures. They are seen in early seborrheic keratosis (SKs) (patch type). Fingerprint-like structures appear as fine parallel lines of light brown to dark brown colors resembling a fingerprint.

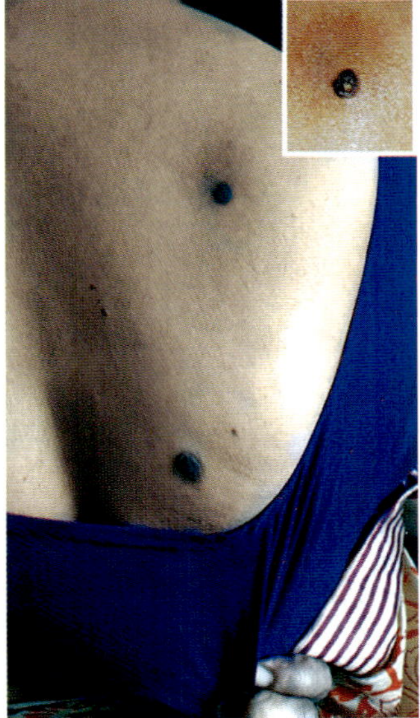

Fig. 51: Two lesions on the back of this lady. Histopathology of the upper lesion was done that showed seborrheic keratosis (SK).

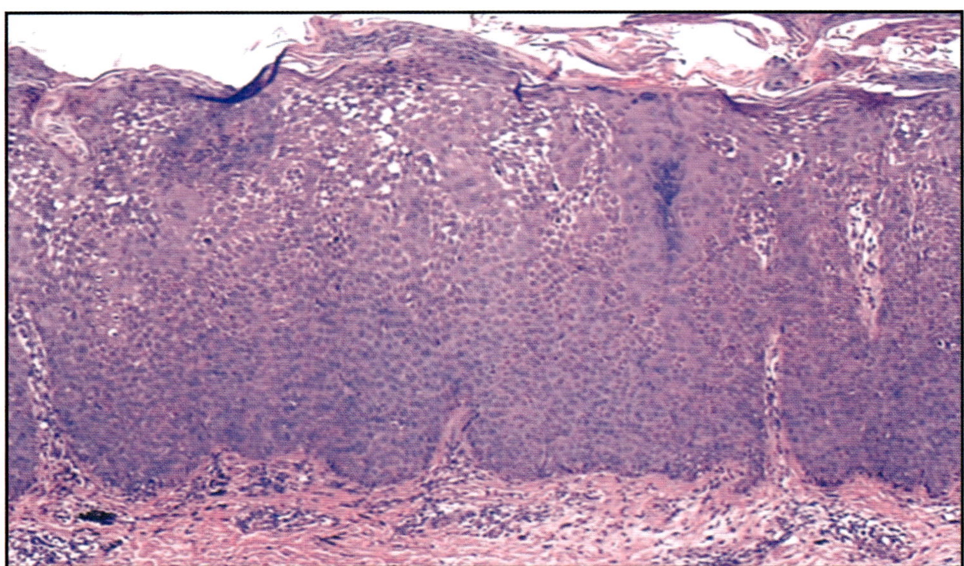

Fig. 52: Biopsy shows mild epidermal hyperplasia with marked lamellated and basket weave orthohyperkeratosis as well as moderate papillomatosis with several horn pseudocysts. Sparse superficial perivascular lymphohistiocytic infiltrate is present. There is no interface change or lichenoid pattern to the infiltrate. The dermis shows moderately dense perivascular infiltrate of lymphocytes and histiocytes. The infiltrate spills into or encroaches on the hyperplastic epidermis. The surface shows parakeratosis.

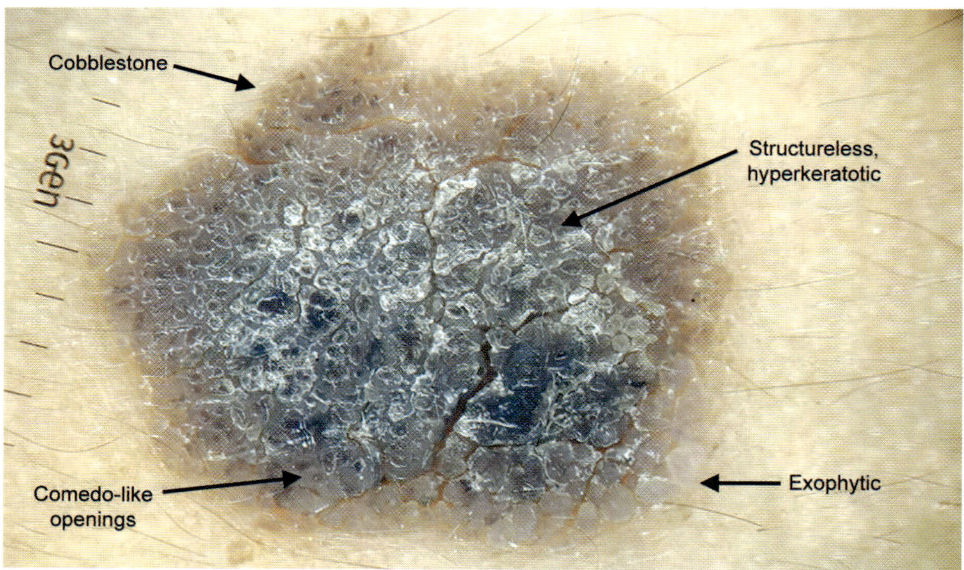

Fig. 53: Dermoscopy revealed combination of seborrheic keratosis (SK) patterns which consist of cobblestone, exophytic, and structureless patterns. The structureless area shows hyperkeratosis. Note: The comedo-like openings are important diagnostic criteria of SK. Hyperkeratosis and fissures can be correlated with the histopathological findings.

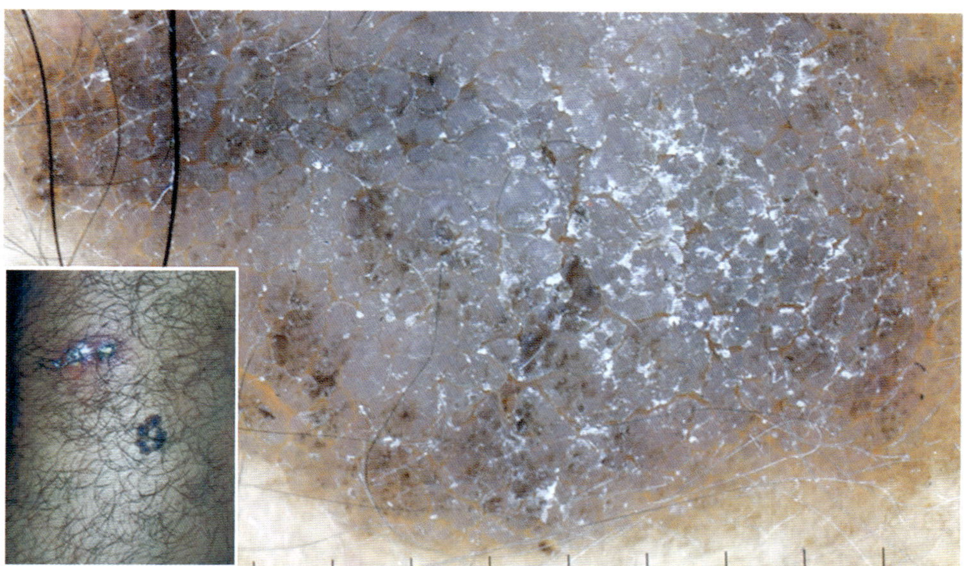

Fig. 54: Brain-like pattern (fissures and ridges) and some CLOs are also seen. Two similar lesions were present over left leg. Biopsy of the upper lesion was done which confirms SK. (CLOs: Comedo-like openings; SK: Seborrheic keratosis).

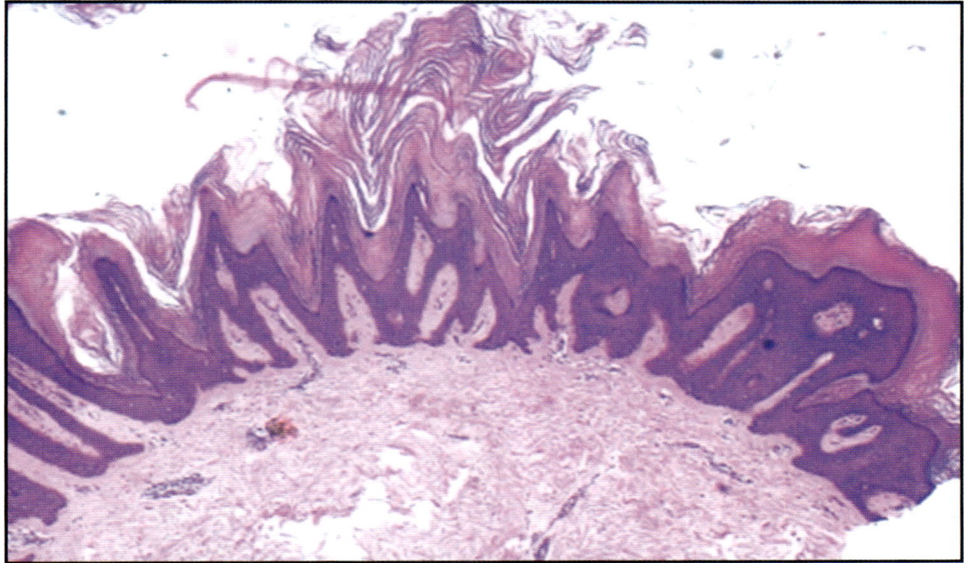

Fig. 55: Biopsy shows marked epidermal hyperplasia with orthokeratotic lamellated hyperkeratosis, marked papillomatosis along with few pseudoho·n cysts. There is mild superficial perivascular infiltrate seen in the dermis.

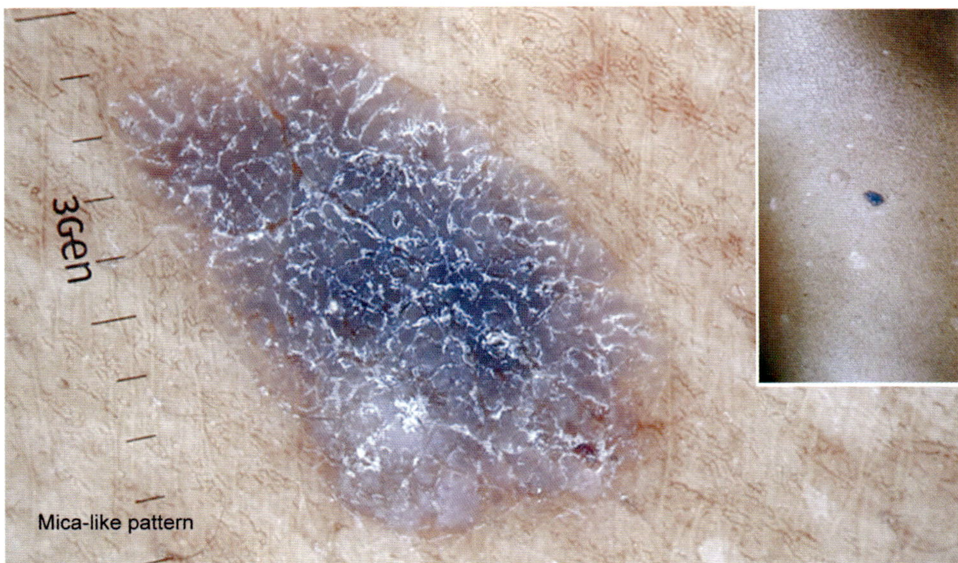

Fig. 56: The mica-like pattern is characterized by mica-like structures that cover the surface of the lesion. Dermoscopy reveals the mica-like structure that is characterized by thick rough scales with mica-like lustre, covering the entire surface of the seborrheic keratosis (SK).

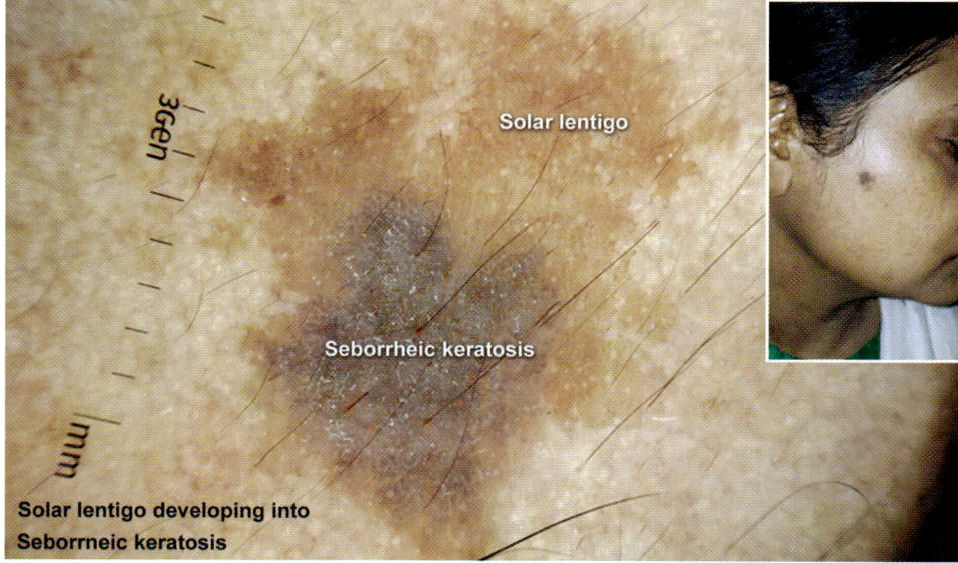

Fig. 57: Solar lentigo (SL) and seborrheic keratosis (SK). SL, SK, and lichen planus-like keratosis represent a spectrum of benign neoplasms with common clinical, dermoscopic, and histopathologic findings. SK and SL are benign neoplasms of keratinocytes consisting of macules, papules, and plaques which are distributed on sun-exposed areas. SK represents a late stage of SL.

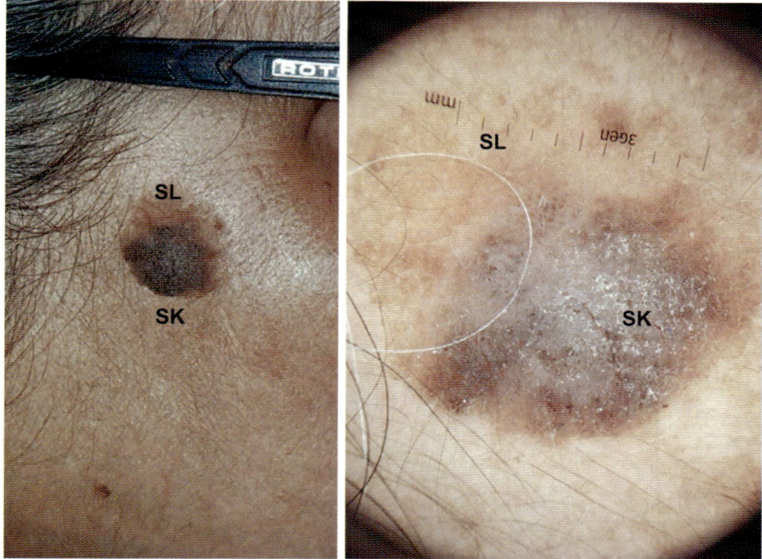

Fig. 58: Clinicodermoscopic picture showing solar lentigo (SL) developing into seborrheic keratosis (SK).

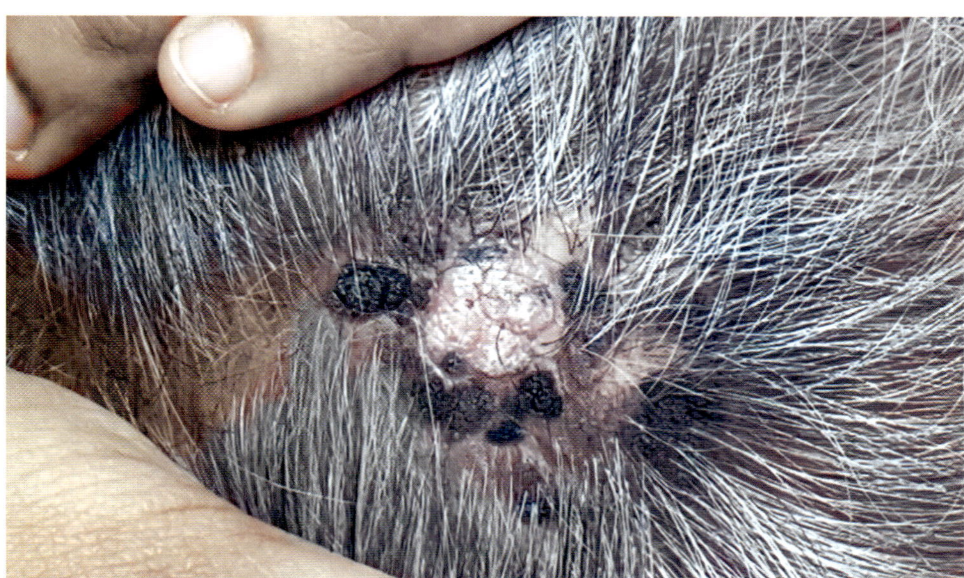

Fig. 59: Irritated seborrheic keratosis (SK). Clinically most commonly SK is hyperpigmented, but hypopigmented and nonpigmented SKs have also been reported.

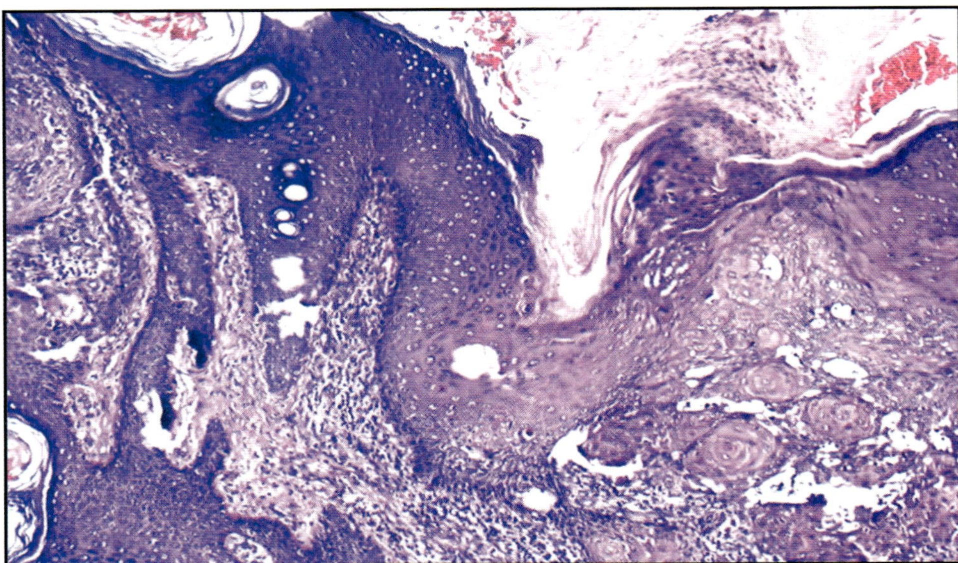

Fig. 60: Histopathology of the previous clinical picture showing features of irritated seborrheic keratosis (SK): epidermal hyperplasia with superficial erosion along with focal interface change of the epidermis with polymorphonuclear lymphocytic infiltrate.

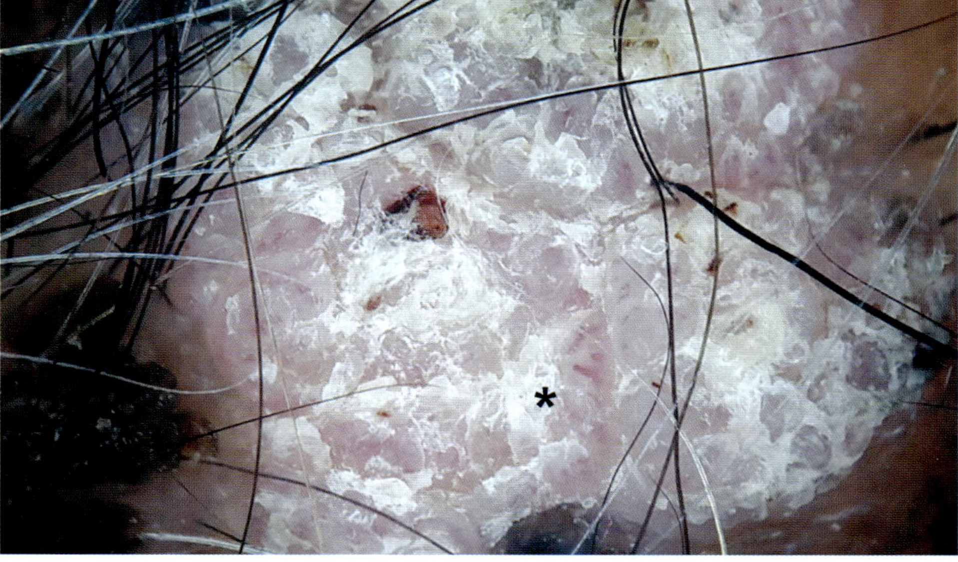

Fig. 61: Hairpin-like vessels (star).

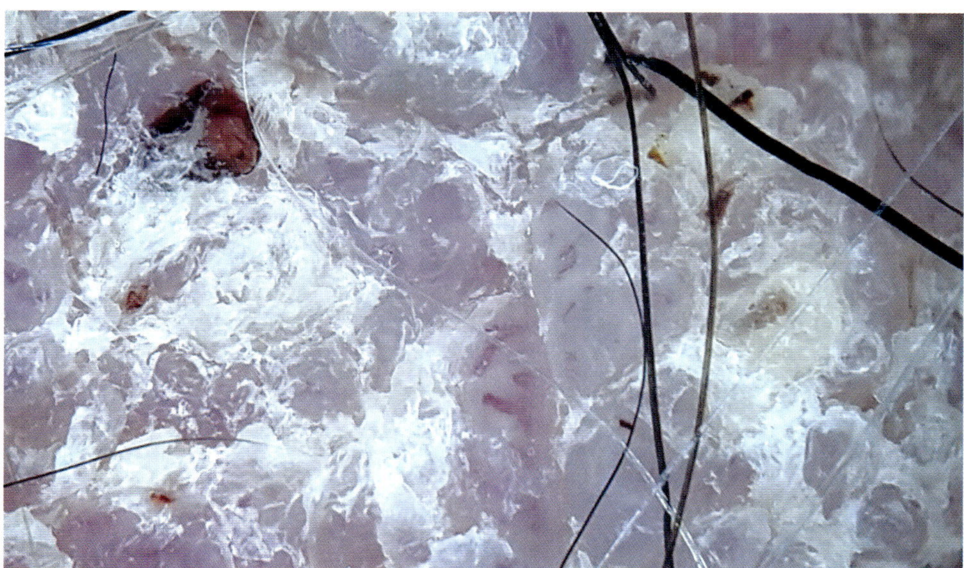

Fig. 62: Close-up view of the previous dermoscopic field to highlight the hairpin vessels.

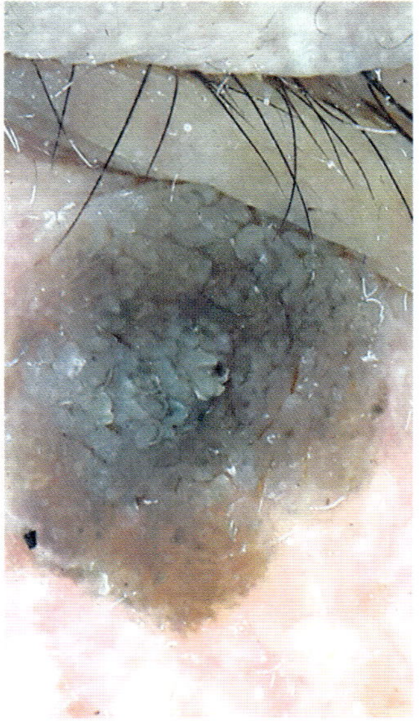

Fig. 63: Exophytic papillary pattern of seborrheic keratosis (SK).

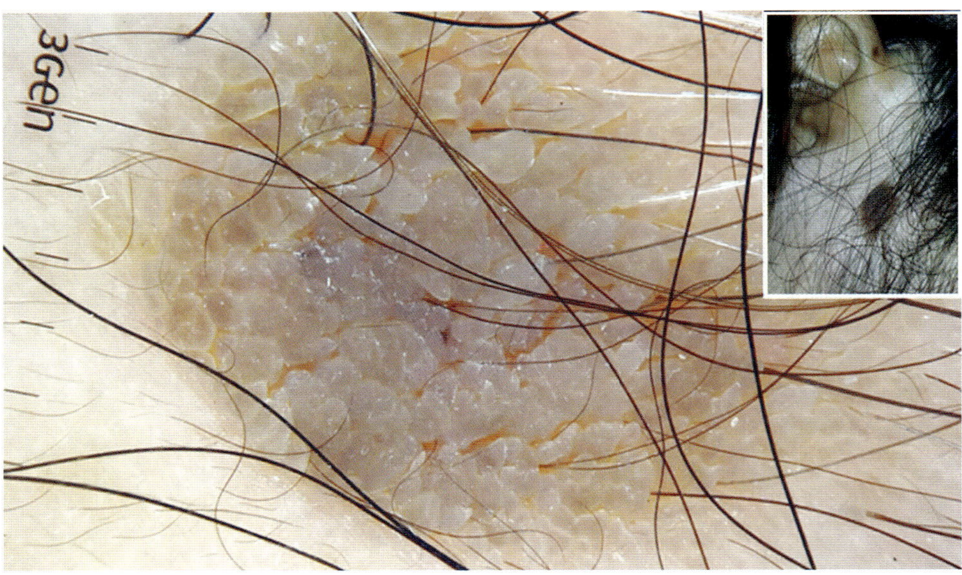

Fig. 64: Exophytic pattern.

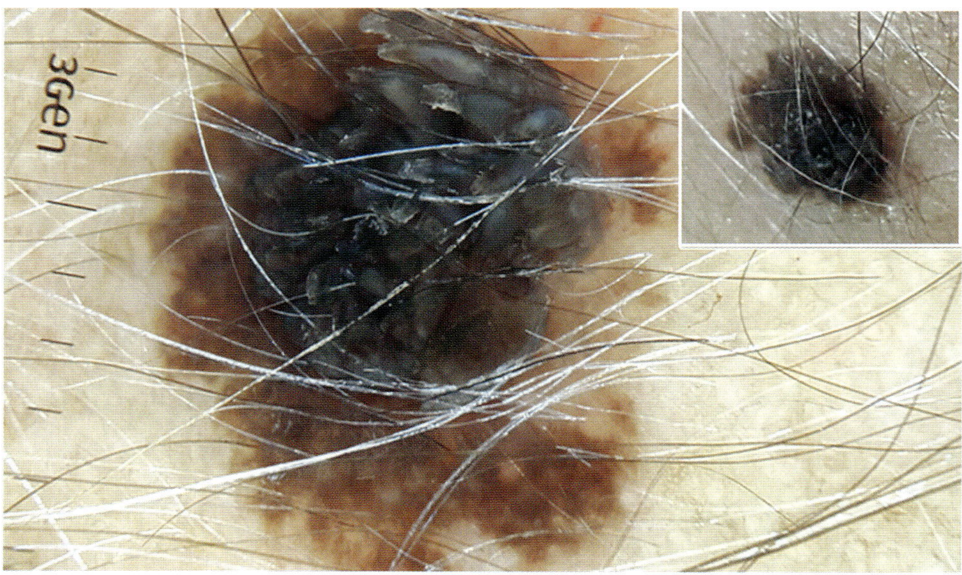

Fig. 65: Exophytic papillary pattern.

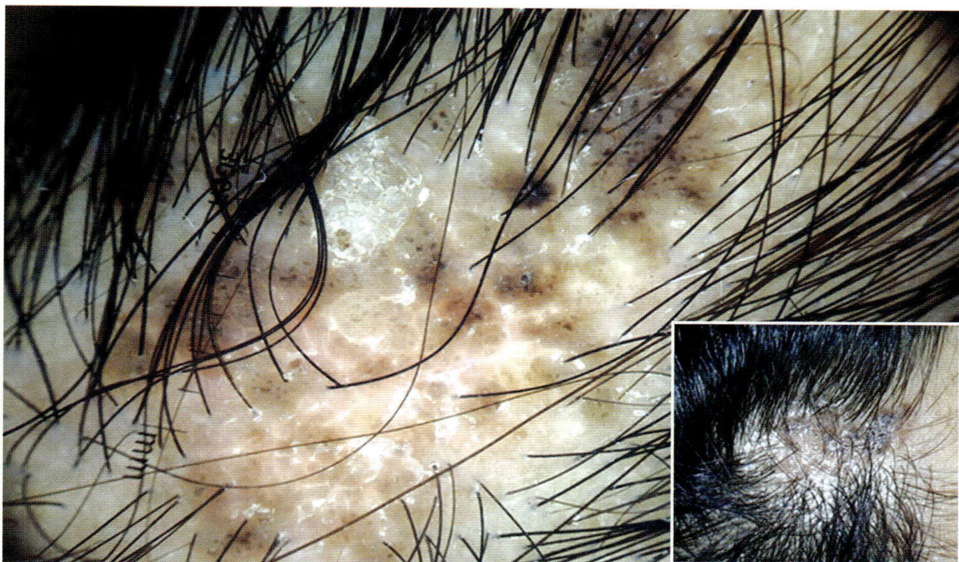

Fig. 66: Cobblestone-like pattern.

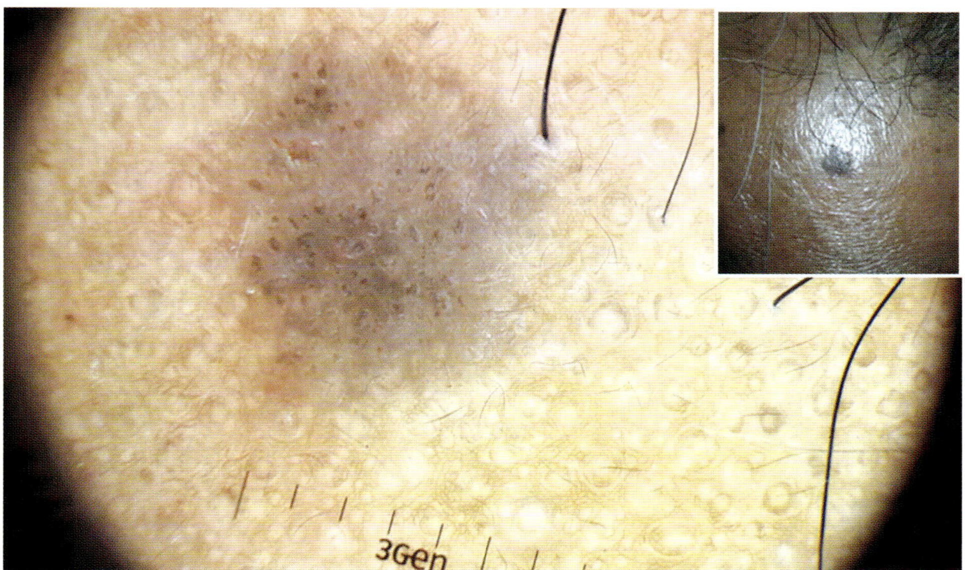

Fig. 67: Cobblestone pattern.

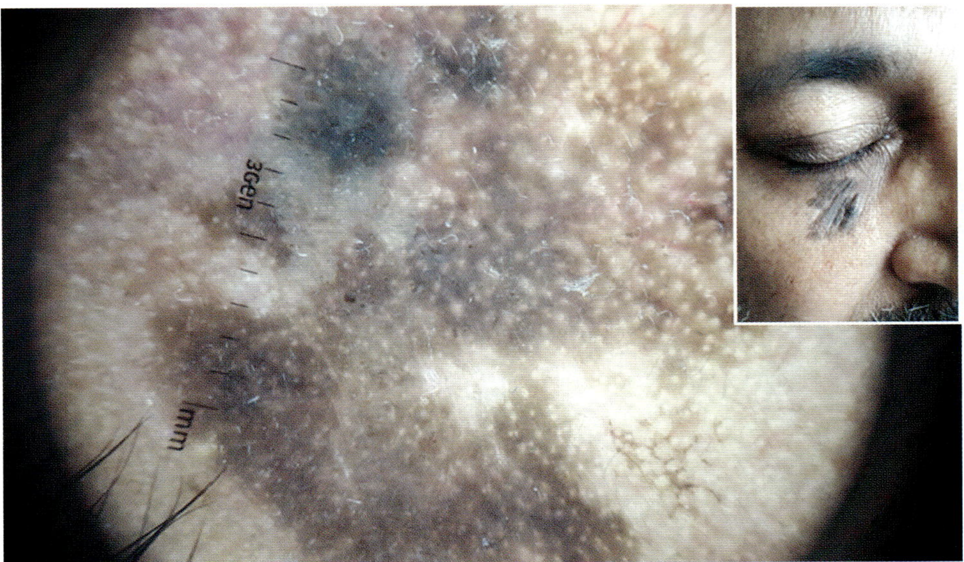

Fig. 68: Multicomponent pattern of seborrheic keratosis (SK).

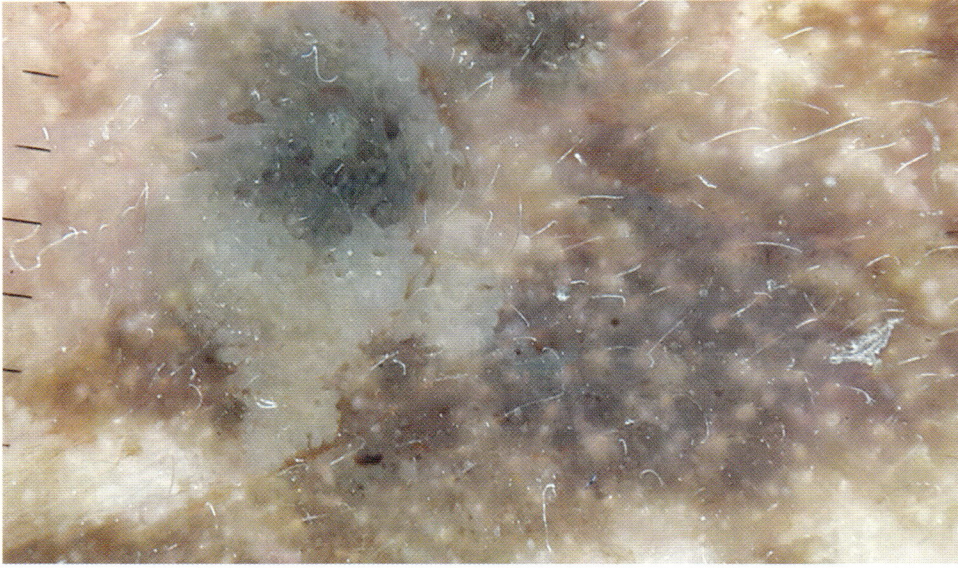

Fig. 69: Multicomponent pattern, magnification of the previous image.

REFERENCES

1. Wang SQ, Rabinovitz HS, Oliviero MC. Solar lentigens, seborrheic keratosis and lichen planus-like keratosis. In: Marghoob AA, Malvehy J, Braun RP (Eds). Atlas of Dermoscopy, 2nd edition. New York: Informa Healthcare; 2012. p. 58.
2. Kopf AW, Rabinovitz H, Marghoob A, et al. Fat fingers: a clue in the dermoscopic diagnosis of seborrheic keratoses. J Am Acad Dermatol. 2006;55(6):1089-91.
3. Schiffner R, Schiffner-Rohe J, Vogt T, et al. Improvement of early recognition of lentigo maligna using dermatoscopy. J Am Acad Dermatol. 2000;42(1 Pt 1):25-32.
4. Zaballos P, Blazquez S, Puig S, et al. Dermoscopic pattern of intermediate stage in seborrheic keratosis regressing to lichenoid keratosis: report of 24 cases. Br J Dermatol. 2007;157(2):266-72.
5. Braun RP, Rabinovitz HS, Krischer J, et al. Dermoscopy of pigmented seborrheic keratosis: a morphological study. Arch Dermatol. 2002;138(12):1556-60.
6. Marghoob AA, Braun RP, Kopf AW. Re: Differentiating vessels from globules on dermoscopy. Dermatol Surg. 2005;31(1):120.

APOCRINE HIDROCYSTOMA

INTRODUCTION

Apocrine hidrocystomas (AHs) are rare, commonly solitary, benign, and cystic lesion of apocrine glands frequently occur on the cheeks or eyelids. AH typically present as an asymptomatic, intradermal, dome shaped, and translucent flesh-colored to blue-black nodule with a smooth surface in middle-aged persons. Histologically, AH is a large unilocular or multilocular dermal cyst typically lined by a double layer of epithelial cells. Decapitation secretion is usually present and is the hallmark of apocrine glands.[1]

Apocrine hidrocystoma may be confused with basal cell carcinoma, blue nevus, and melanoma.[2]

Dermoscopy shows specific patterns in skin conditions corresponding to histopathological changes.[3] Thus, the lesion can be screened by dermoscopy for specific patterns of the condition to avoid histopathological investigation and consequent scarring over the face.

KEY DERMOSCOPIC FEATURES[4,5]

- Brown pigment globules arranged in a haphazard pattern
- Homogeneous area; the color of the homogeneous area is uniform in the whole lesion and varies from skin-colored to pink, yellow, or blue in different lesions
- Arborizing telangiectasia
- Whitish structures traversing across the tumor.

DISCUSSION

The brown globules are not arranged in any specific patterns but follow a haphazard pattern. Ankad et al.[4] opined that irregular pattern of globules in AH is possible due to stretching of epidermis as a consequence of cystic dilatation of tumor. Homogeneous area corresponds to the presence of a large unilocular or multilocular cysts situated within the dermis; the color of the homogeneous area is uniform in the whole lesion and varies from skin colored to pink, yellow, or blue in different lesions. Zaballos et al.[5] did not find any cause of the blue coloration of the homogeneous area. Whitish structures are believed to be due to increase in fibrosis/collagen but Zaballos et al. did not find an increased amount of collagen and opined that the changes in the orientation of collagen due to the pressure of the large dermal cysts could be the explanation for the whitish structures. They found arborizing vessels in 68.2% of AHs and they were indistinguishable from those found in basal cell carcinomas.

REFERENCES

1. Brenn T, McKee PH. Tumors of the sweat glands. In: Mckee PH, Calonje E, Granter SR (Eds). Pathology of the Skin with Clinical Correlations. London: Elsevier; 2005. pp. 1599-602.
2. Anzai S, Goto M, Fujiwara S, et al. Apocrine hidrocystoma: a case report and analysis of 167 Japanese cases. Int J Dermatol. 2005;44:702-3.
3. Micali G. Introduction. In: Micali G, Lacarubbba F (Eds). Dermatoscopy in Clinical Practice: Beyond Pigmented Lesions, 1st edition. London: Informa Healthcare; 2010. pp. 1-2.
4. Ankad BS, Domble V, Sujana L. Dermoscopy of apocrine hydrocystoma: a first case report. Our Dermatol Online. 2015;6(3): 334-6.
5. Zaballos P, Banuls J, Medina C, et al. Dermoscopy of apocrine hidrocystomas: a morphological study. J Eur Acad Dermatol Venereol. 2014;28:378-81.

ECCRINE HIDROCYSTOMA

INTRODUCTION

They are cystic dilatations of the eccrine sweat duct and usually present as multiple skin colored to bluish cystic papules typically seen in middle-aged women. They are benign tumors and most commonly occurs over the central part of the face.[1] Histopathological examination shows dermal cysts containing clear fluid, lined by two layers of cuboidal epithelium.

Though histopathology is the gold standard in diagnosing eccrine hidrocystomas, dermoscopy can be utilized to diagnose the condition correctly, and thus biopsy that may produce a scar on face can be avoided.

KEY DERMOSCOPIC FEATURES

- Homogeneous blue-purple central area surrounded by a pale halo.[2]
- Arborizing vessels.[3]
- Vessel-free cystic lesions.[1]

DISCUSSION

The common clinical differentials of eccrine hidrocystomas on face[4,5] are comedonal acne, eruptive syringomas, multiple pilomatricomas, basal cell carcinomas, and eruptive vellus hair cysts. All of them have characteristic dermoscopic findings and thus can be easily differentiated. Dermoscopy of vellus hair cysts show light yellow-white center and erythematous halo and few radiating capillaries in the periphery[4] whereas comedonal acne reveals brown homogeneous areas with keratin plugs;[6] eruptive syringomas represent yellow-brown structureless areas and fine linear vessels on dermoscopy;[5] pilomatricomas show irregular white-yellow structures, whitish streaks, linear vessels, and reddish homogeneous areas;[7] dermoscopic features of basal cell carcinomas vary according to the pigment and nonpigment varieties. Arborizing vessels on dermoscopy is the most characteristic feature, other features are leaf-like areas, spoke wheel appearance, blue-gray globules, and nests, etc.[8]

KEYNOTE

To avoid biopsy and possible scar on face, dermoscopy should be mastered to correctly diagnose eccrine hidrocystomas on face.

REFERENCES

1. Correia O, Duarte AF, Barros AM, et al. Multiple eccrine hidrocystomas—from diagnosis to treatment: the role of dermatoscopy and botulinum toxin. Dermatology. 2009;219:77-9.
2. Duman N, Duman D, Sahim S. Pale halo surrounding a homogeneous bluish-purplish central area: dermoscopic clue for eccrine hidrocystoma. Dermatol Pract Concept. 2015;5(4):43-4.
3. Zaballos P, Bañuls J, Medina C, et al. Dermoscopy of apocrine hidrocystomas: a morphological study. J Eur Acad Dermatol Venereol. 2014;28:378-81.
4. Alfaro-Castellón P, Mejía-Rodríguez SA, Valencia-Herrera A, et al. Dermoscopy distinction of eruptive vellus hair cysts with molluscum contagiosum and acne lesions. Pediatr Dermatol. 2012;29:772-3.
5. Lallas A, Moscarella E, Argenziano G, et al. Dermoscopy of uncommon skin tumours. Australas J Dermatol. 2014;55:53-62.
6. Kamińska-Winciorek G, Spiewak R. Dermoscopy on nevus comedonicus: a case report and review of the literature. Postepy Dermatol Alergol. 2013;30:252-4.
7. Zaballos P, Llambrich A, Puig S, et al. Dermoscopic findings of pilomatricomas. Dermatology. 2008;217:225-30.
8. Altamura D, Menzies SW, Argenziano G, et al. Dermatoscopy of basal cell carcinoma: morphologic variability of global and local features and accuracy of diagnosis. J Am Acad Dermatol. 2010;62:67-75.

SEBACEOUS HYPERPLASIA

INTRODUCTION

Sebaceous hyperplasia (SH) presents as yellowish small soft papules on the face in the middle age and the elderly people. It is a common benign condition of the sebaceous gland. The common differentials are angiofibroma, various adnexal tumors, and intradermal nevus. Dermoscopic examination can readily identify SH from its close mimics.

KEY DERMOSCOPIC FEATURES (FIGS. 70 TO 72)[1-3]

- Aggregated yellow-white lobules
- A small crater at the center of the lobules
- Crown vessels.

DISCUSSION

Dermoscopy of SH reveals polylobulated yellow-white structure which corresponds to hyperplastic sebaceous glands. Sometimes the ostium of the gland is visible at the center of the polylobulated structure as a small crater. The gland is surrounded by scarcely branching vessels that may extend to the center but characteristically never cross it. The vessels are tortuous yet not arborizing and are described dermoscopically by the term "crown vessels".

KEYNOTE

Dermoscopy may be of great value in distinguishing SH and nodular basal cell carcinoma by finding the crown vessels in the former and arborizing vessels in the latter, avoiding unnecessary excision.

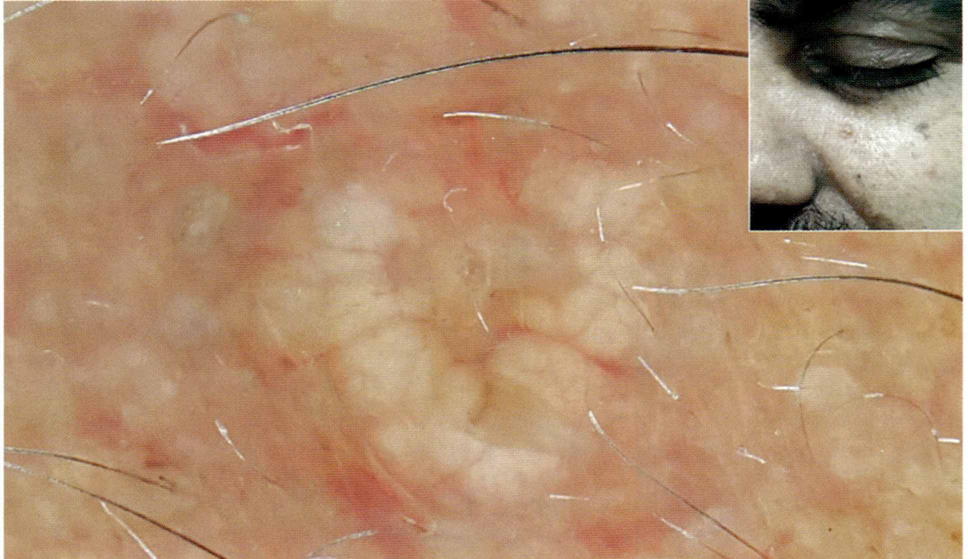

Fig. 70: Dermoscopy reveals yellow-white lobules which correspond to hyperplastic sebaceous gland. Crown vessels are seen at the periphery which do not cross the center of the lesion. Central crater is also visible.

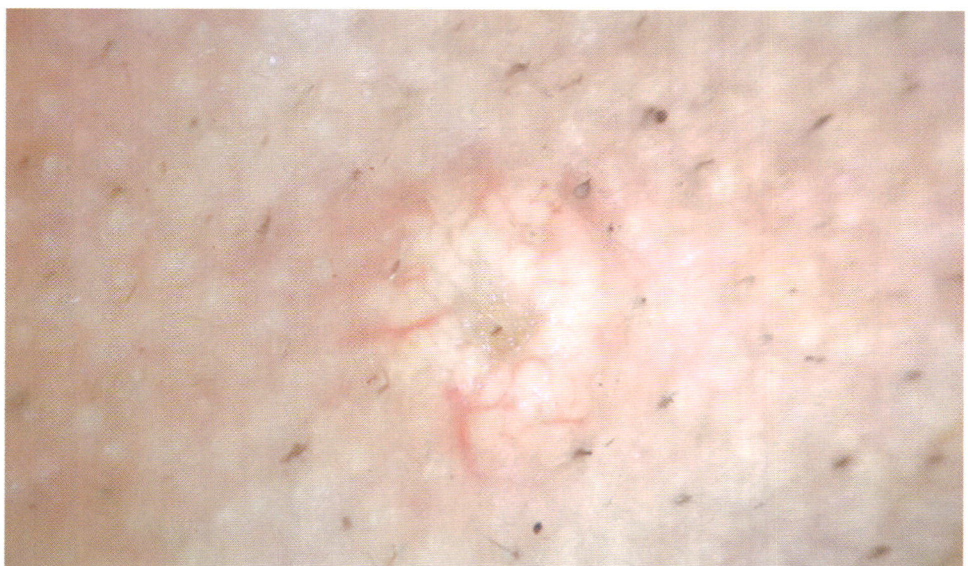

Fig. 71: Crown vessels rarely branch in contrast to arborizing vessels. Polylobulated yellowish sebaceous gland and crown vessels are the dermoscopic hallmark of sebaceous hyperplasia.

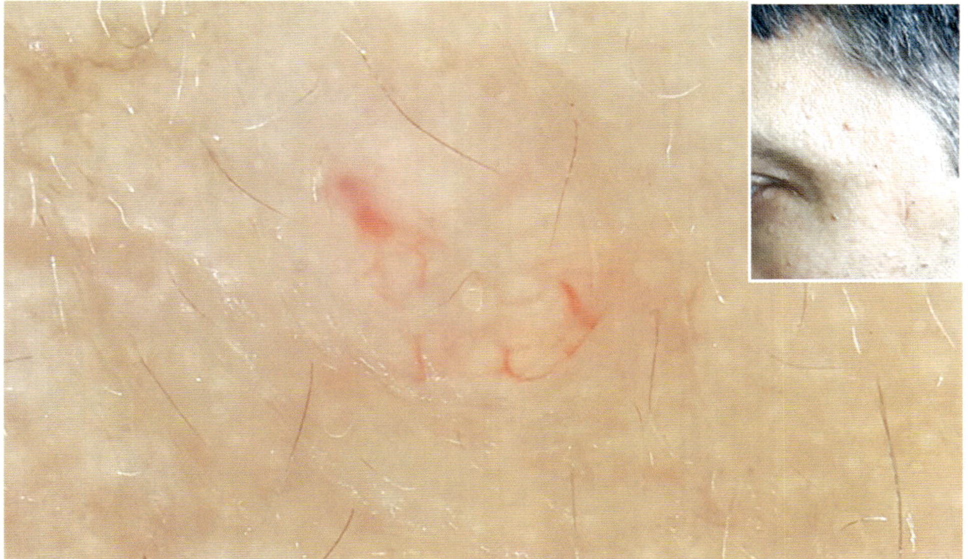

Fig. 72: All the three dermoscopic features (central crater, crown vessels, and yellow-white lobules) of sebaceous hyperplasia are visible.

REFERENCES

1. Kim NH, Zell DS, Kolm I, et al. The dermoscopic differential diagnosis of yellow lobular-like structures. Arch Dermatol. 2008;144:962.
2. Zaballos P, Ara M, Puig S, et al. Dermoscopy of sebaceous hyperplasia. Arch Dermatol. 2005;141:808.
3. Bryden AM, Dawe RS, Fleming C. Dermoscopic features of benign sebaceous proliferation. Clin Exp Dermatol. 2004;29:676-7.

SYRINGOMA

INTRODUCTION

Syringomas are sweat duct tumors and present as skin-colored or yellowish, small, and dermal papules. They are most often found in clusters on the eyelids but may also arise elsewhere on the face, in the armpits, umbilicus, upper chest, and vulva. The surface of syringomas can be rounded or flat. Syringomas are usually smaller than 3 mm in diameter. Eruptive syringomas typically appear as hyperpigmented papules on the chest, penile shaft, or vulva.

KEY DERMOSCOPIC FEATURES (FIGS. 73 TO 81)

- Ivory white/white homogeneous areas (cloudy sky pattern).

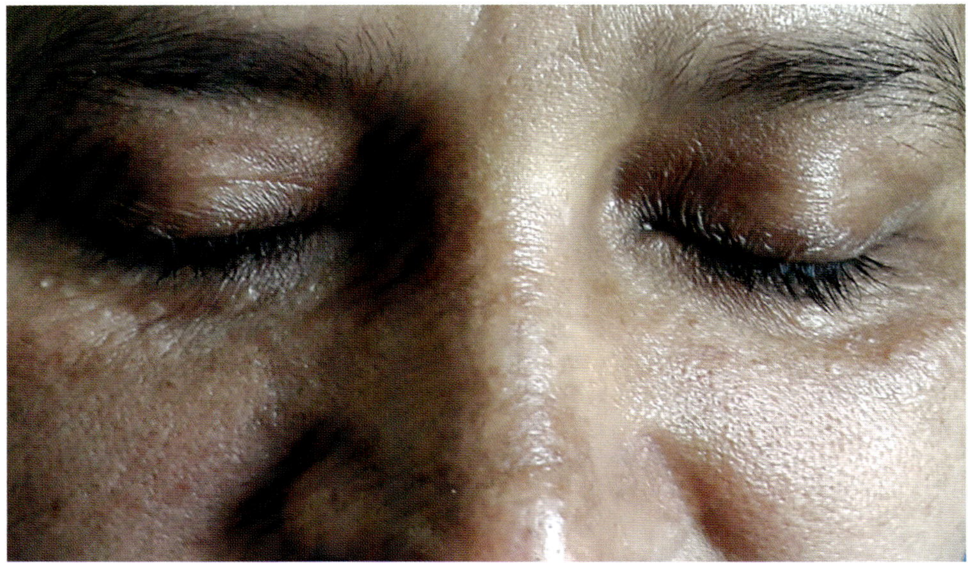

Fig. 73: A lady of 50 years of age presenting with multiple, small, and yellowish papules on both the eyelids that correspond to syringomas.

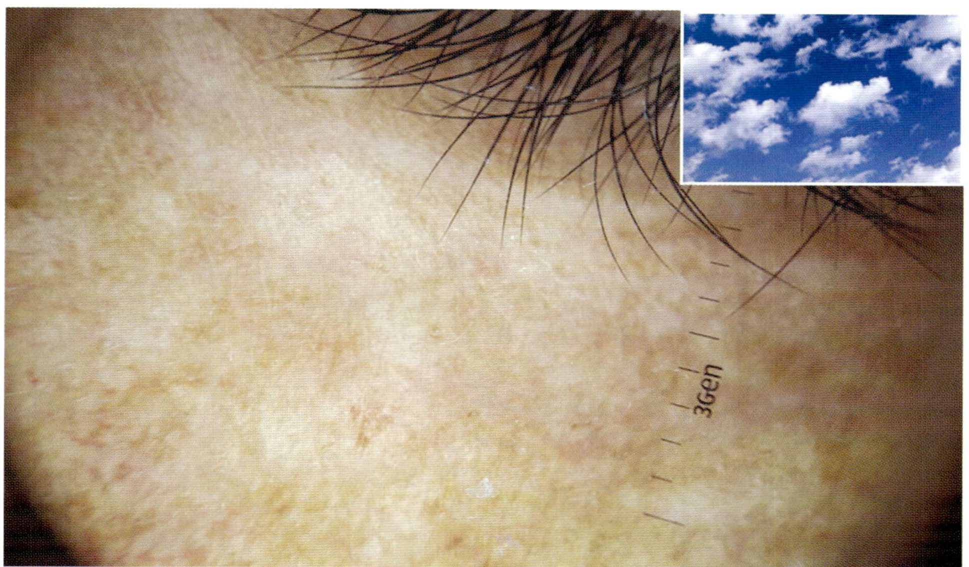

Fig. 74: On dermoscopy multiple white homogeneous areas, described as "cloudy sky" pattern is visible which is highly suggestive of syringomas.

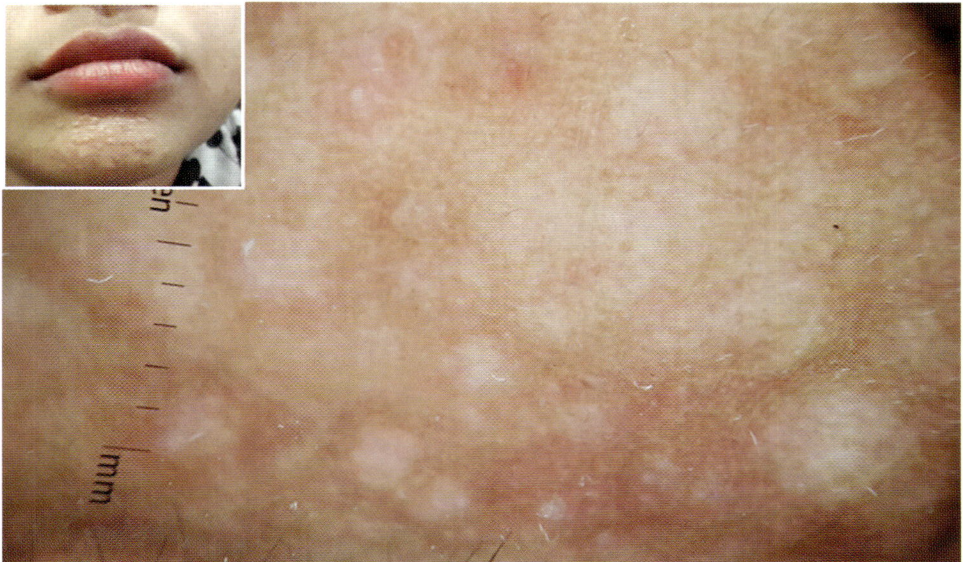

Fig. 75: Syringomas are most often found in clusters on the eyelids but may also arise elsewhere on the face. In our experience syringomas are not uncommon over the chin but are underdiagnosed. Dermoscopy reveals the characteristic homogeneous white appearance. Probably the homogeneous white areas can be correlated with the fibrous and sclerotic stroma around the eccrine ducts.

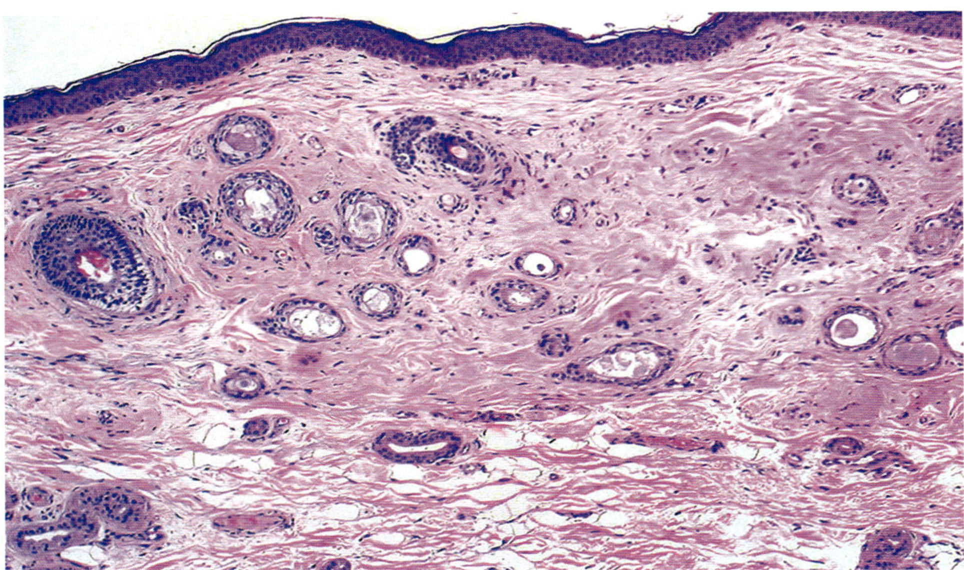

Fig. 76: Histopathology of previous patient demonstrates numerous small ducts in a sclerotic stroma. Note: The tadpole-shaped ducts. Usually the walls of these ducts are lined by two rows of cuboidal epithelial cells and the lumen contains PAS—positive eosinophilic amorphous debris.

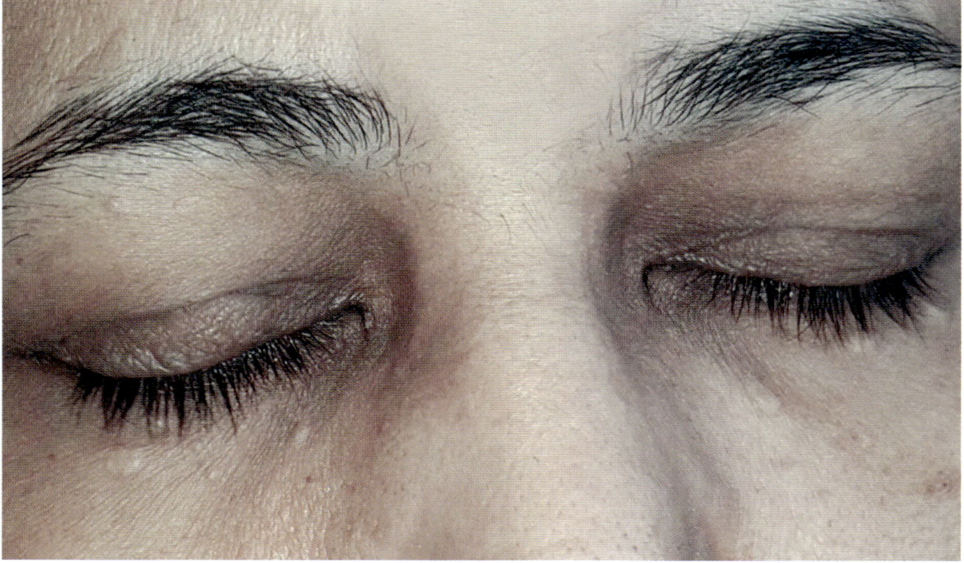

Fig. 77: Syringomas are usually multiple and symmetrically distributed.

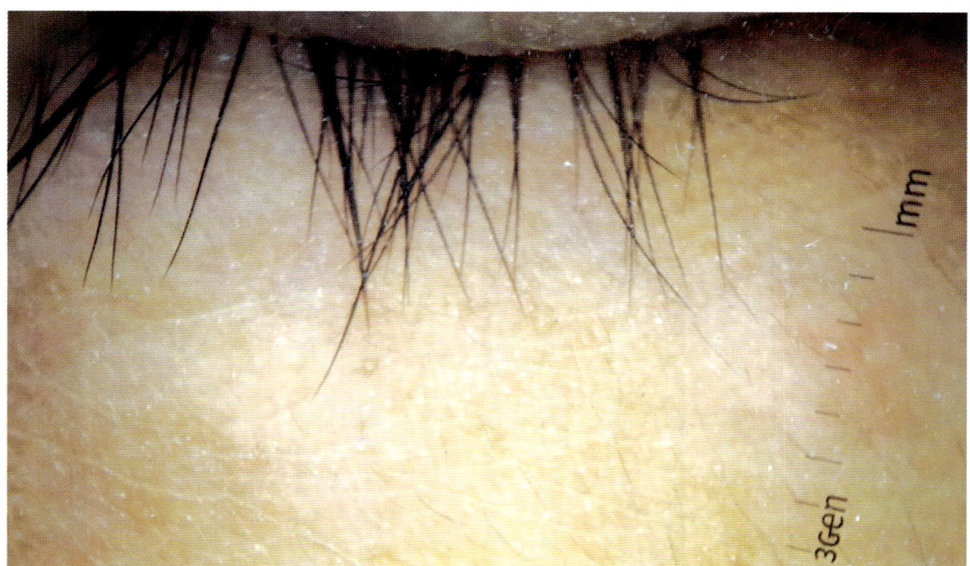

Fig. 78: Faint white homogeneous areas are visible on dermoscopy of the previous patient.

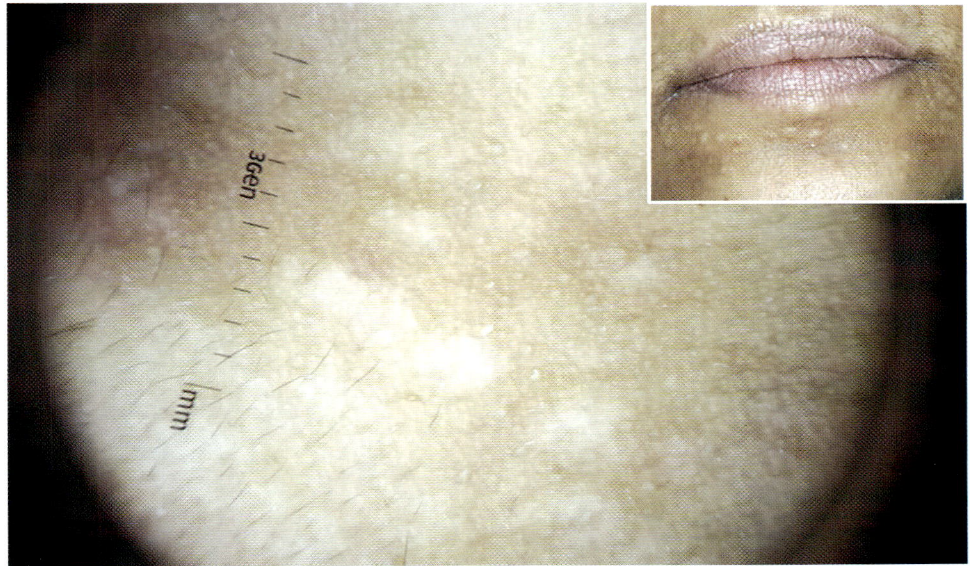

Fig. 79: Another case of syringomas over chin demonstrates "cloudy sky" pattern dermoscopically.

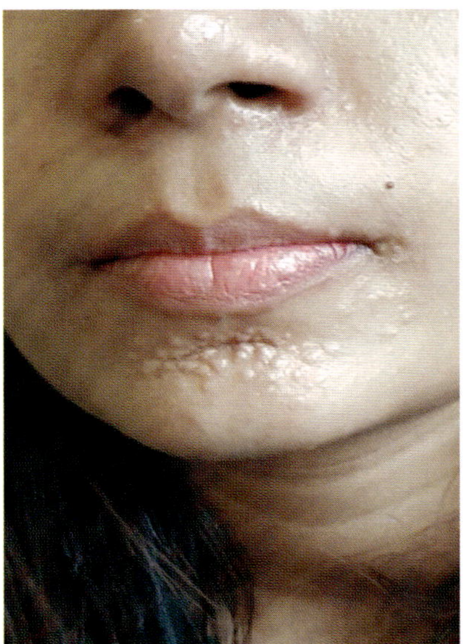

Fig. 80: Clustered syringomas on the chin of this young lady since last 3 years. Usually the condition either is unnoticed or underdiagnosed. Biopsy shows tadpole-shaped ducts in sclerotic stroma.

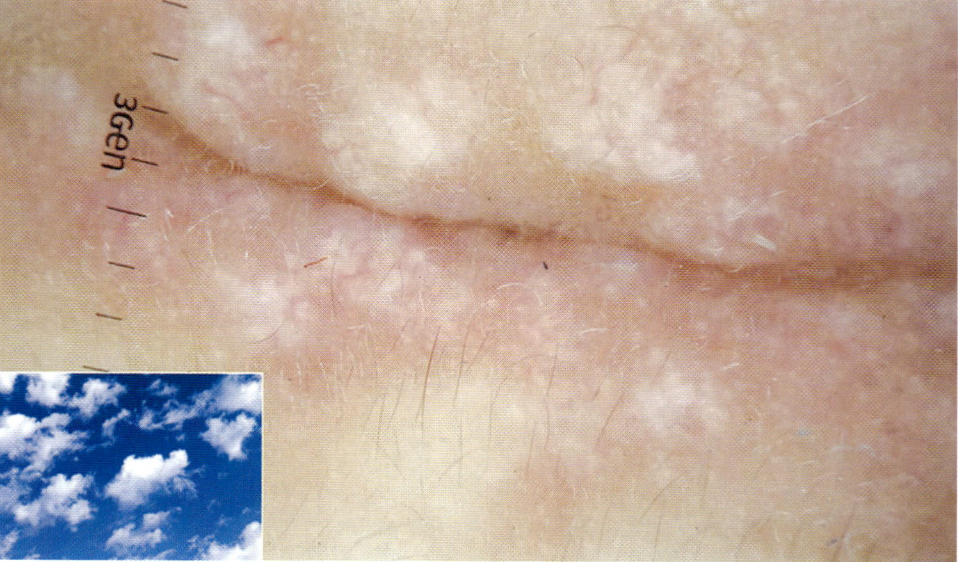

Fig. 81: Dermoscopy demonstrates ivory-white homogeneous areas which are classically described as "cloudy sky" pattern.

TRICHOEPITHELIOMA

INTRODUCTION

Skin colored flat topped lesions on the face more often than not pose a diagnostic dilemma to the treating physician. Establishing the diagnosis in such a case depends generally on the clinical presentation history and invasive diagnostic techniques like histopathology, which however, is not very popular on the face owing to the risk of scarring. In recent years, dermoscopy is gaining appreciation in the diagnosis of various skin diseases where diagnosis is made by better visualization of the surface and subsurface structures, the permutation and combination of which leads to specific diagnosis.

KEY DERMOSCOPIC FEATURES (FIGS. 82 TO 86)[1]

- Arborizing vessels
- Milia-like cysts
- Rosettes.

DISCUSSION

Dermoscopic examination of the lesions revealed a whitish background, in focus arborizing vessels, few lesions in addition demonstrated milia-like cysts while others showed rosettes.

Histopathological examination shows well-circumscribed dermal tumor with branched nests of basaloid cells, small keratin cysts, and a dense collagenous stroma with fibroblasts.

Vascular pattern depicting arborizing vessels or linear vessels suggest the lifting up of overlying skin with vascular proliferation. The background color whether erythematous or whitish will depend on proliferation of fibroblasts and presence of collagenous material or an underlying inflammatory pathology. The milia-like cysts on dermoscopy correspond to the keratinous cysts on histopathology.[2] Rosettes are peculiar structures only observed with polarized dermoscopy and are defined as four white points, arranged as a four leaf clover.[3] Another view suggests that they arise from interaction of the polarized light with narrowed or keratin filled adnexal openings.[4] Others suggested that rosettes correspond to an alternating focal hyperkeratosis and normal corneal layer and keratin-filled openings.[4] Haspeslagh et al. in their study stated that rosettes are an optical effect of crossed polarization by concentric fibrosis or horny material and hence are not lesion-specific.[5] Also these structures are more commonly seen in actinic skin. This probably explains the demonstration of rosettes in our case of trichoepithelioma where concentric fibrosis was seen on histopathology and also that the lesions were located in the actinic area of face.

KEYNOTE

Although clinical diagnosis is usually straightforward by naked-eye examination, dermoscopy may aid in its confirmation.

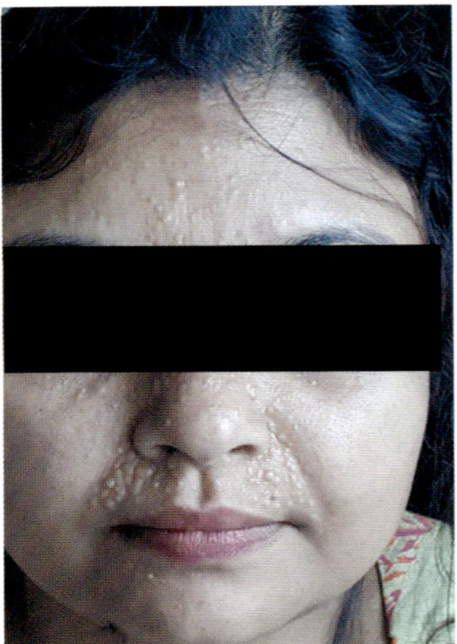

Fig. 82: Multiple flat topped skin-colored papules on the face of a middle-aged female.

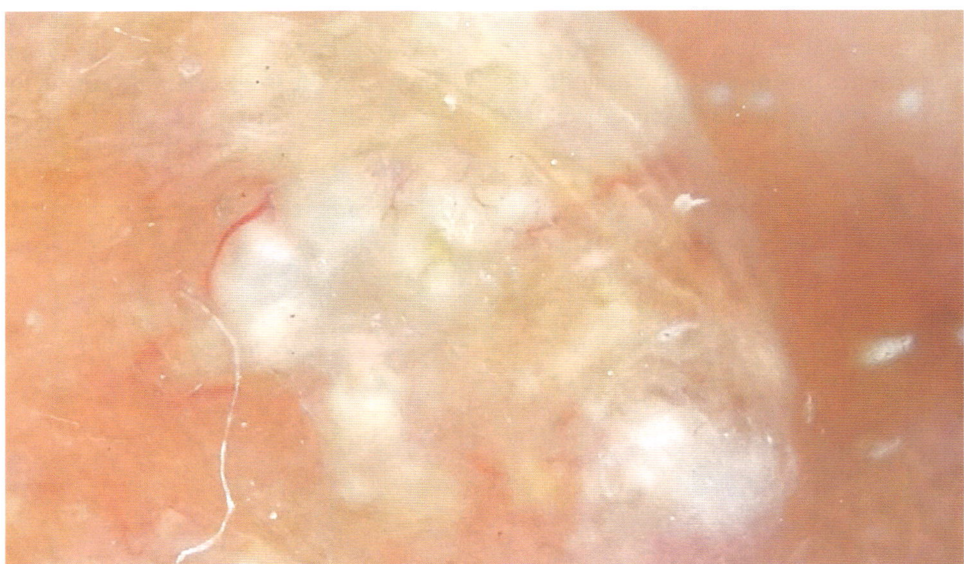

Fig. 83: In-focus arborizing vessels, multiple milia-like cysts.

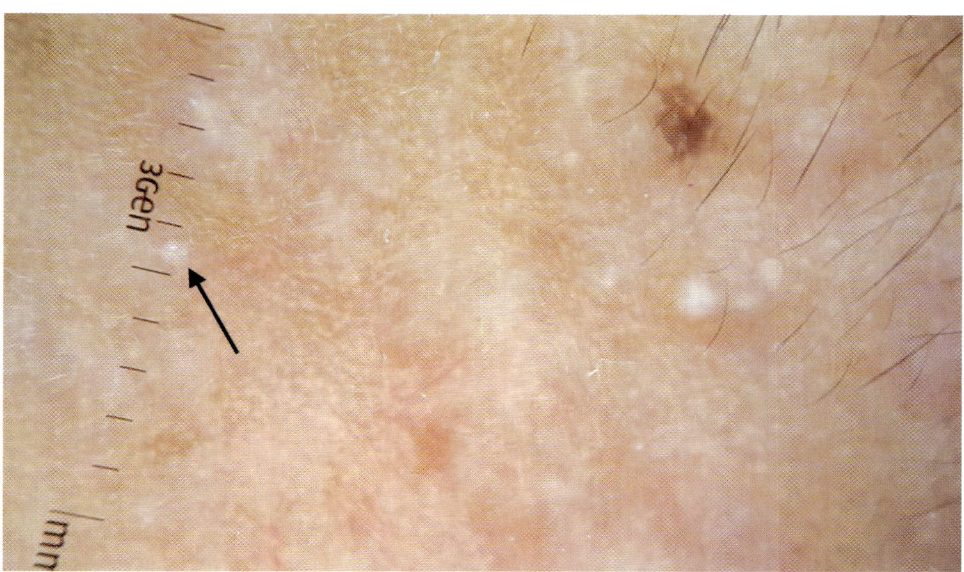

Fig. 84: Milia-like cysts correspond to keratin cysts in the histopathology. Rosette is also visible in the left side of the field (arrow).

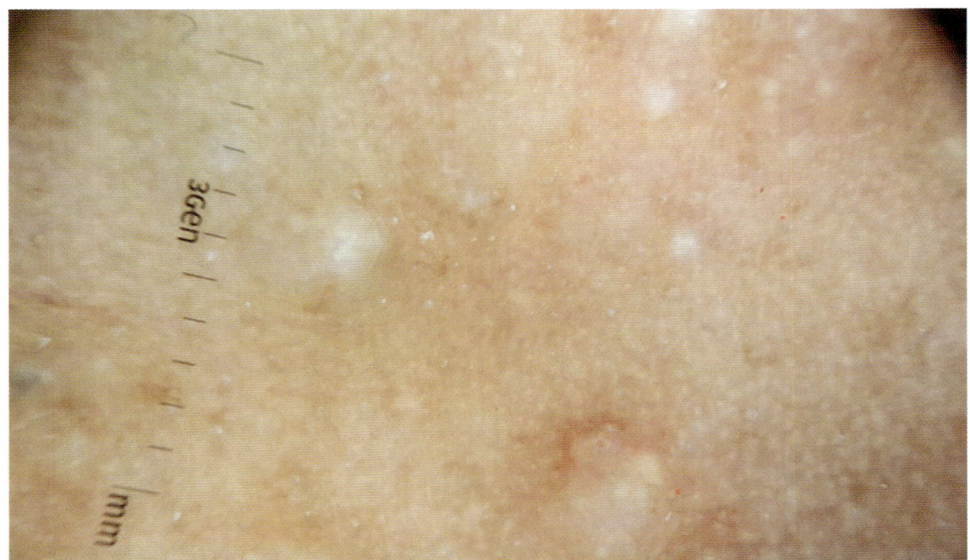

Fig. 85: Milia-like cysts against a whitish background.

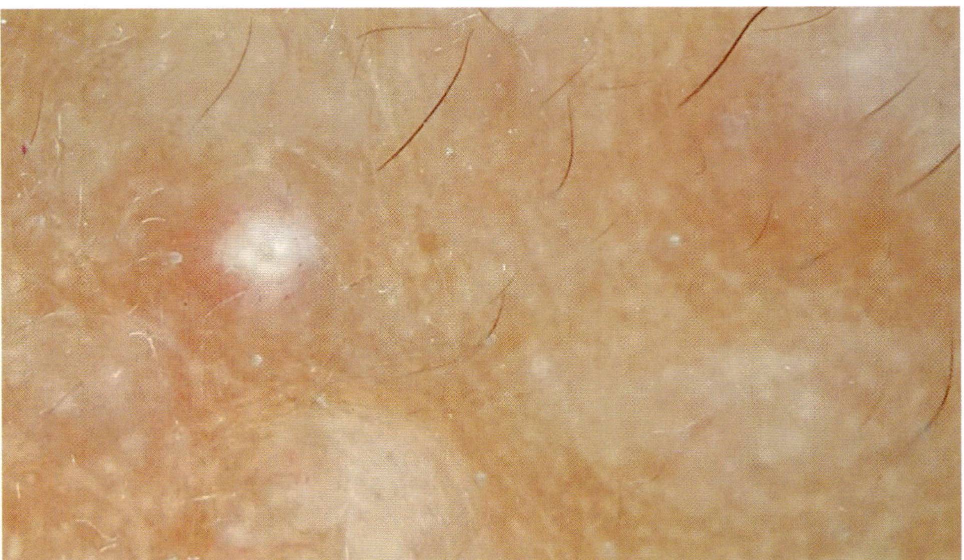

Fig. 86: The picture demonstrates a classical rosette. Rosettes are peculiar structures only observed with polarized dermoscopy and are defined as four white points, arranged as a four leaf clover. Whitish ill-defined areas denote trichoepitheliomas.

REFERENCES

1. Navarrete-Dechent C, Bajaj S, Marghoob AA, et al. Multiple familial trichoepithelioma: confirmation via dermoscopy. Dermatol Pract Concept. 2016;6(3):51-4.
2. Stricklin SM, Stoecker WV, Oliviero MC, et al. Cloudy and starry milia-like cysts: how well do they distinguish seborrheic keratoses from malignant melanomas? J Eur Acad Dermatol Venereol. 2011;25(10):1222-4.
3. Cuellar F, Vilalta A, Puig S, et al. New dermoscopic pattern in actinic keratosis and related conditions. Arch Dermatol. 2009;145:732.
4. Liebman TN, Rabinovitz HS, Balagula Y, et al. White shiny structures: dermoscopic features revealed under polarized light. J Eur Acad Dermatol Venereol. 2012;26:1493-7.
5. Haspeslagh M, Noë M, De Wispelaere I, et al. Rosettes and other white shiny structures in polarized dermoscopy: histological correlate and optical explanation. J Eur Acad Dermatol Venereol. 2016;30(2):311-3.

MALIGNANT TUMORS OF SKIN

BASAL CELL CARCINOMA

INTRODUCTION

Basal cell carcinoma (BCC) is a keratinocytic cutaneous malignancy that is locally invasive. It presents with a skin-colored, pink, or pigmented slowly growing plaque or nodule, the size of which varies from a few mm to several cm in diameter. It may ulcerate or there may be spontaneous bleeding. A small percentage of BCCs invade deeply or metastasize. There are many types of BCCs of which nodular variety is most common.

PIGMENTED BASAL CELL CARCINOMA

KEY DERMOSCOPIC FEATURES[1,2]

In addition to the dermoscopic features described for nonpigmented BCC, the other key dermoscopic features of pigmented BCC may have one or more of the following:

- Blue-gray ovoid nests
- Blue-gray dots/globules
- Maple leaf-like structures
- Spoke wheel structures
- Concentric structures.

DISCUSSION

Blue-gray ovoid nests appear dermoscopically as well circumscribed, almost confluent ovoid, or elongated pigmented structures, not closely connected to the pigmented tumor mass. They correlate histologically to the large tumor nests with aggregates of pigment.

Blue-gray dots/globules dermoscopically represent multiple oval to round well-demarcated structures; they are smaller than the blue-gray ovoid nests. They correspond to small round tumor nests with central pigmentation present in the papillary and/or reticular dermis.

Dermoscopically, maple leaf-like structures look like peripheral bulbous extensions having brown/gray/blue color. They do not arise from the pigmented network or from the pigmented areas. The maple leaf-like structures are highly specific for BCC. These structures should be differentiated from streaks seen in melanoma and Spitz nevi. The extensions of the maple leaf-like areas tend to be broader and almost always appear fuzzy. They correspond histologically to multifocal tumor nests having pigment aggregates which are connected together by lobular extensions. Their principal location is in the epidermis but rarely may be present in the upper dermis.

Dermoscopy of spoke wheel areas show well-demarcated radial projections which meet at a dark central axis; the projections may have tan or blue or gray color. It histopathologically correlates with the epidermally-associated tumor mass that has finger-like projections and central pigmentation.

The concentric structures probably represent variations or precursors of the spoke wheel structures. Dermoscopy shows irregular globular structures with different colors ranging from brown to black to blue or gray; these globular structures have a central dark area. They correspond to epidermally-associated small tumor nests with central pigmentation.

CASE 1 (FIGS. 1 TO 4)

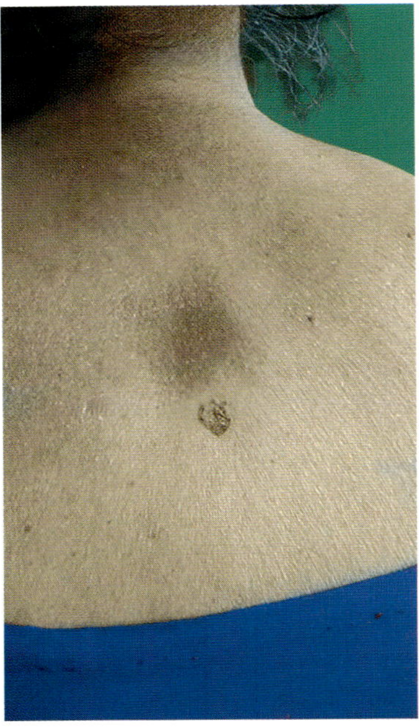

Fig. 1: Asymptomatic plaque on the back of a middle-aged lady of 1 year duration.

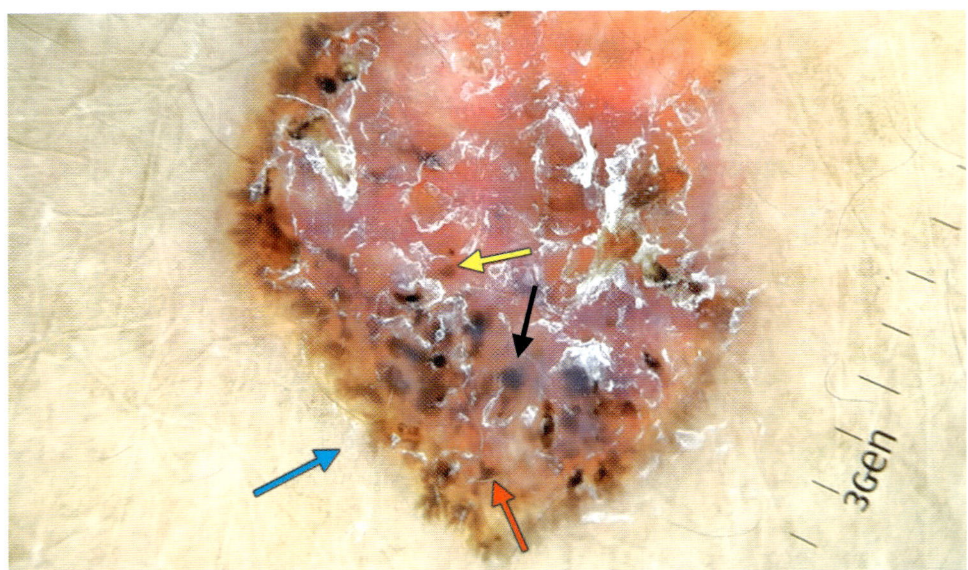

Fig. 2: Dermoscopy reveals maple leaf-like structure (blue arrow), blue-gray ovoid nests (black arrow), spoke wheel structures (red arrow), and concentric structures (yellow arrow).

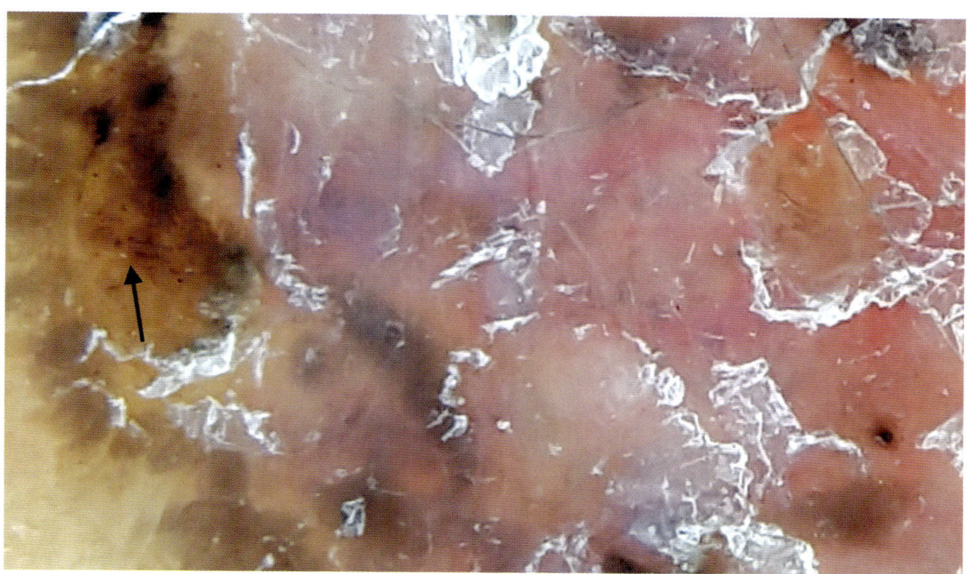

Fig. 3: Blue-gray dots and globules (arrow).

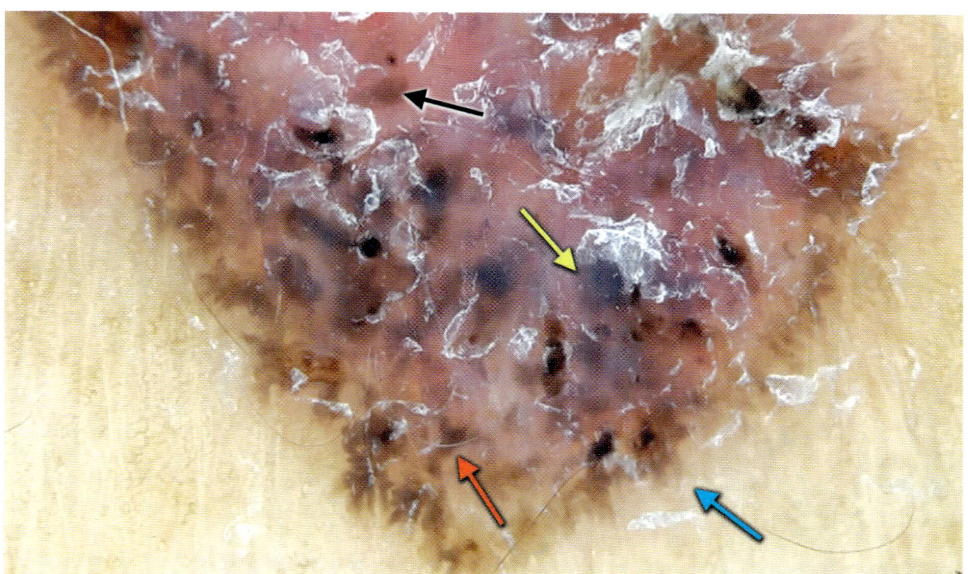

Fig. 4: Maple leaf-like structure (blue arrow), blue-gray ovoid nests (yellow arrow), spoke wheel structures (red arrow), and concentric structures (black arrow).

CASE 2 (FIGS. 5 TO 8)

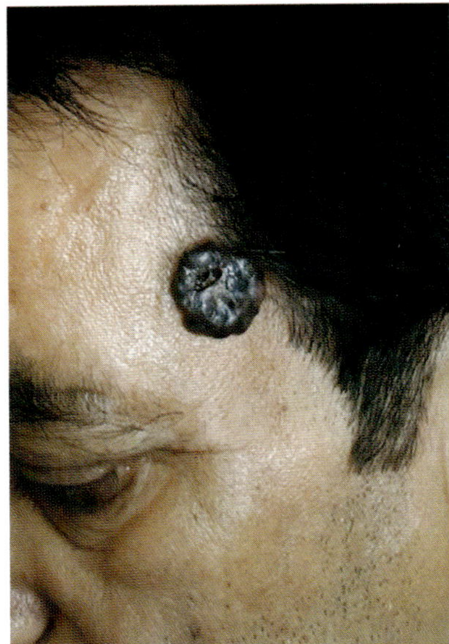

Fig. 5: Hyperpigmented nodule on the forehead of 9 months duration.

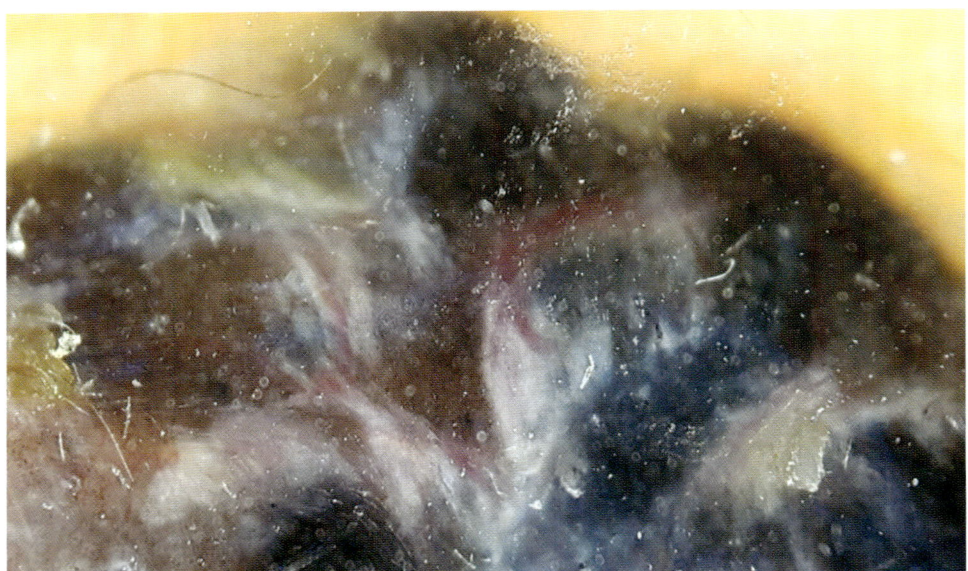

Fig. 6: Often in our case series of pigmented basal cell carcinoma (BCC), especially in the noduloulcerative variety, we have encountered dermoscopically a combination of blue, black, red, yellow, and white color giving a kaleidoscopic appearance that can be correlated well with histopathological findings.

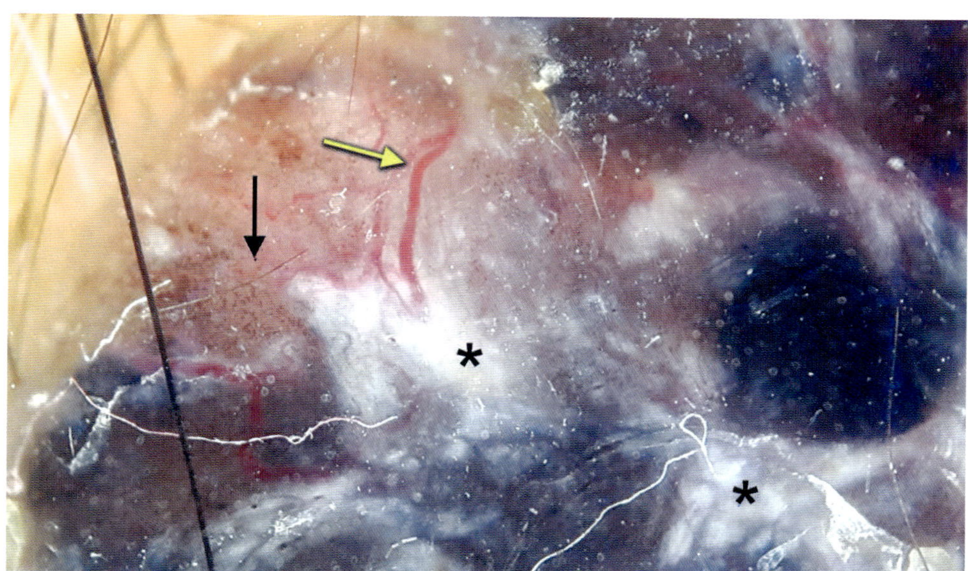

Fig. 7: In another field, dermoscopy also reveals combination of blue, black, red, yellow, and white colors. The field presents blue-gray dots and globules (black arrow), arborizing vessels (yellow arrow), and white shiny streaks (stars).

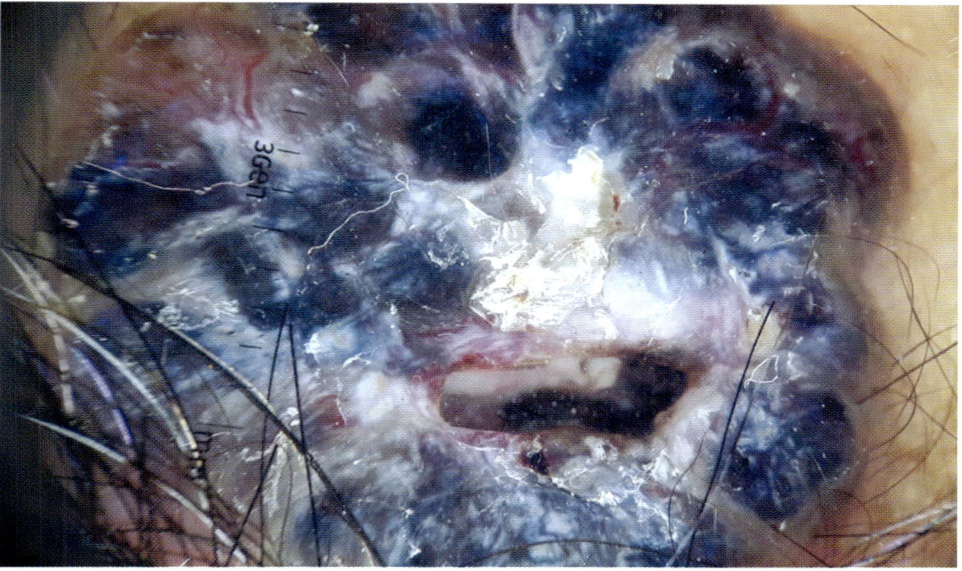

Fig. 8: Almost every field presents the same combination of color, in addition to blue, black, red, yellow, and white, this field also shows violet color (V).

CASE 3 (FIGS. 9 TO 11)

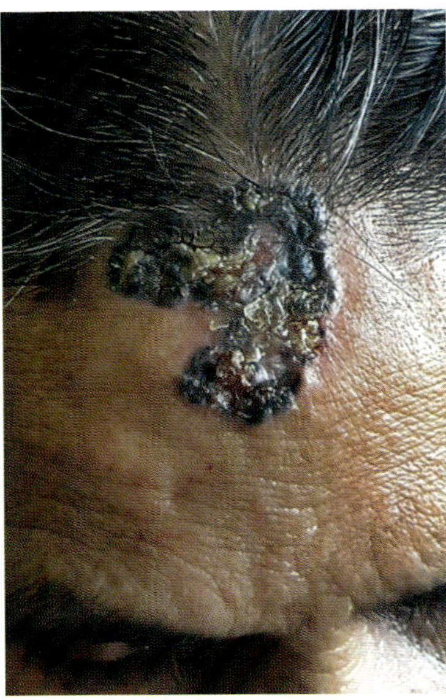

Fig. 9: An ulcerative plaque present over the forehead of an elderly female patient since 4 years.

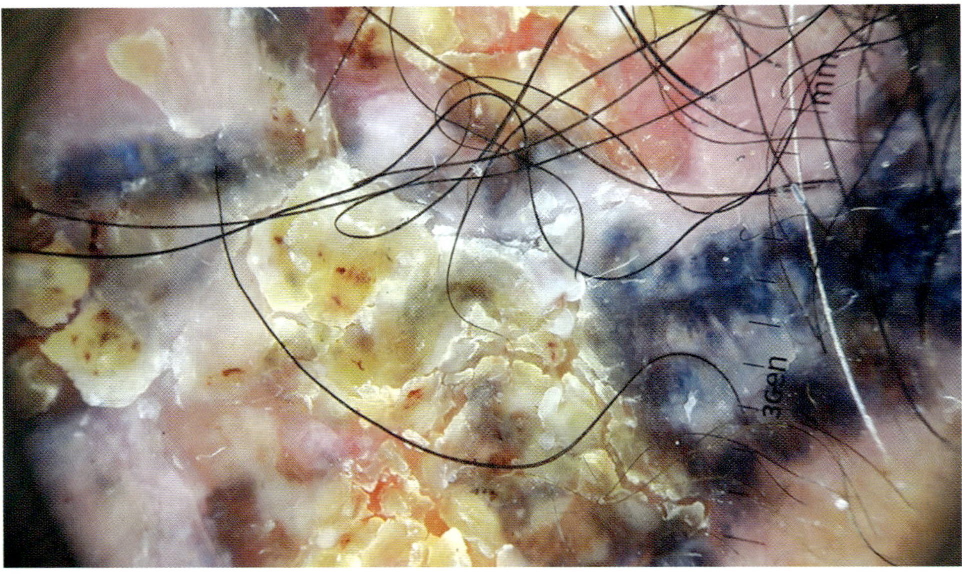

Fig. 10: Same combination of colors; blue, black, red, yellow, and white constitute the overview of the dermoscopic criteria of noduloulcerative pigmented basal cell carcinoma (BCC). Yellow color corresponds to keratin, blue and black to melanin aggregates in papillary and reticular dermis and also to melanin in the epidermis, white to collagen and fibrosis both in the dermis and in the tumor mass and red to arborizing vessels or erosions and ulcerations.

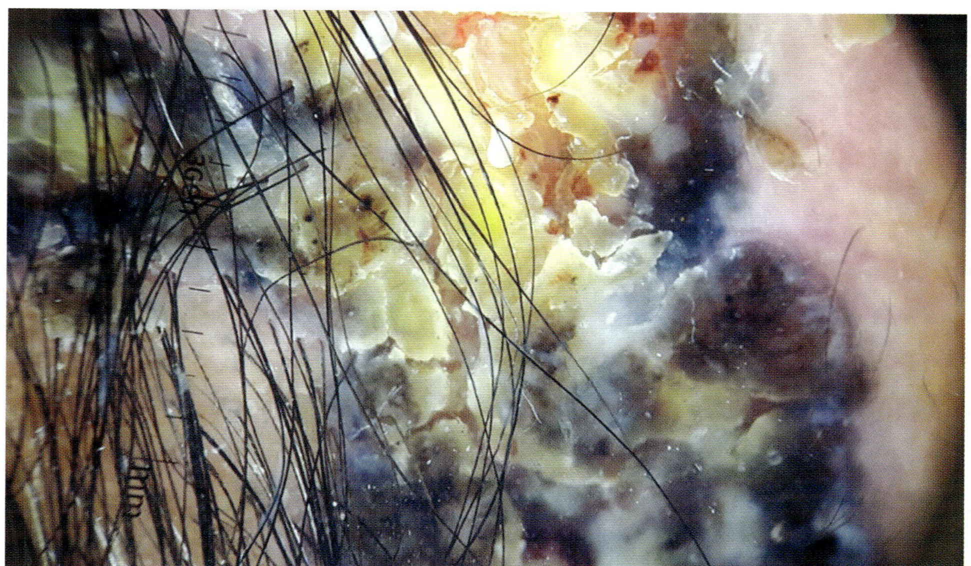

Fig. 11: Sometimes an additional color can be visible such as violet (V).

CASE 4 (FIGS. 12 TO 16)

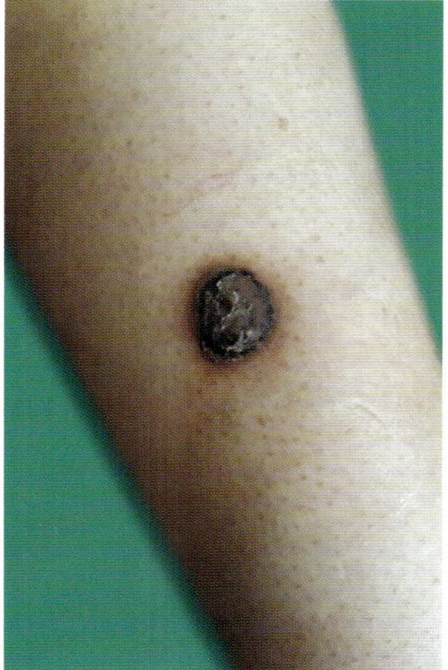

Fig. 12: Atypical presentation of basal cell carcinoma (BCC) on the legs.

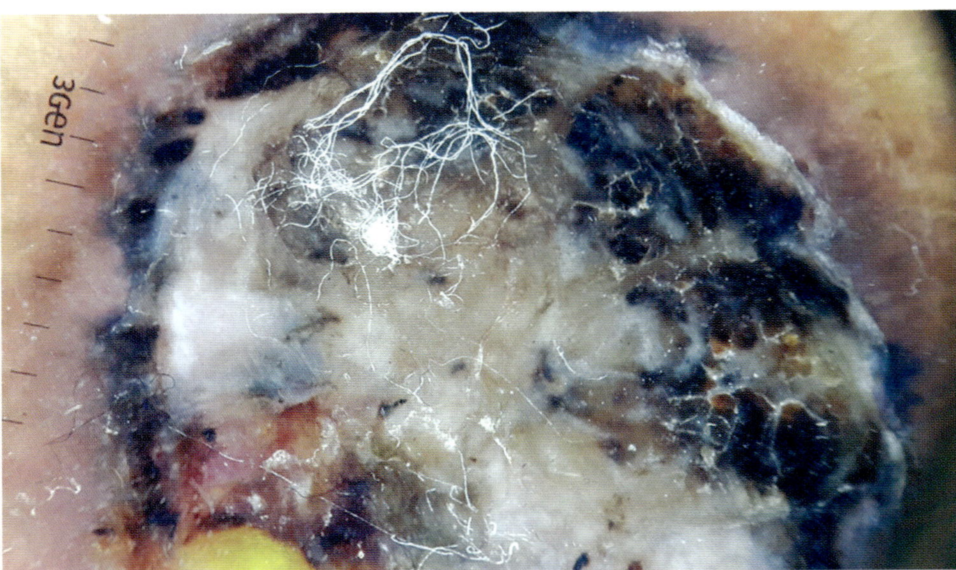

Fig. 13: In a third consecutive case of BCC, we found the characteristic combination, of blue, black, red, yellow, and white. The classical features of blue-gray ovoid nests, spoke wheel, concentric structures, maple leaf-like structures, and white shiny structures are prominently visible in this dermoscopic field.

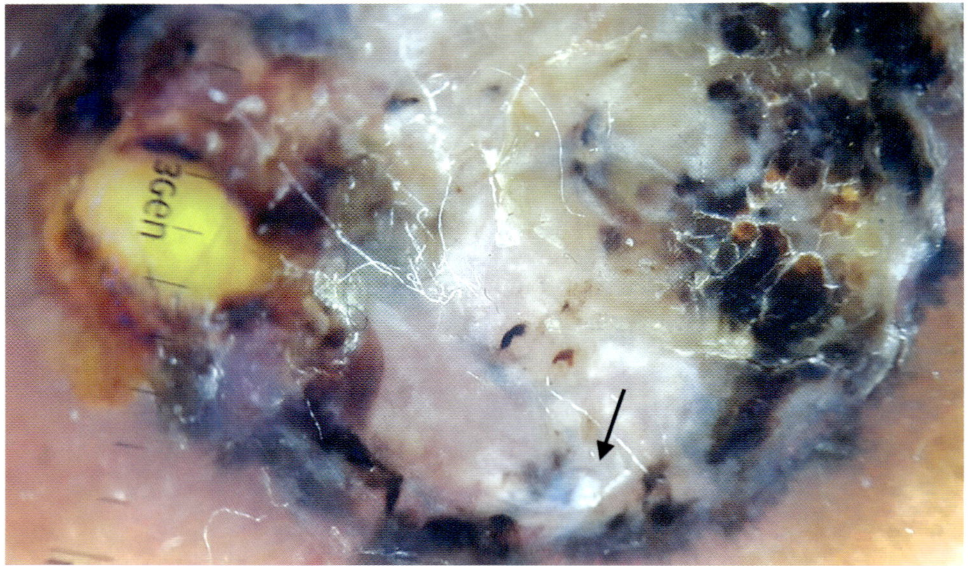

Fig. 14: Rosette (arrow).

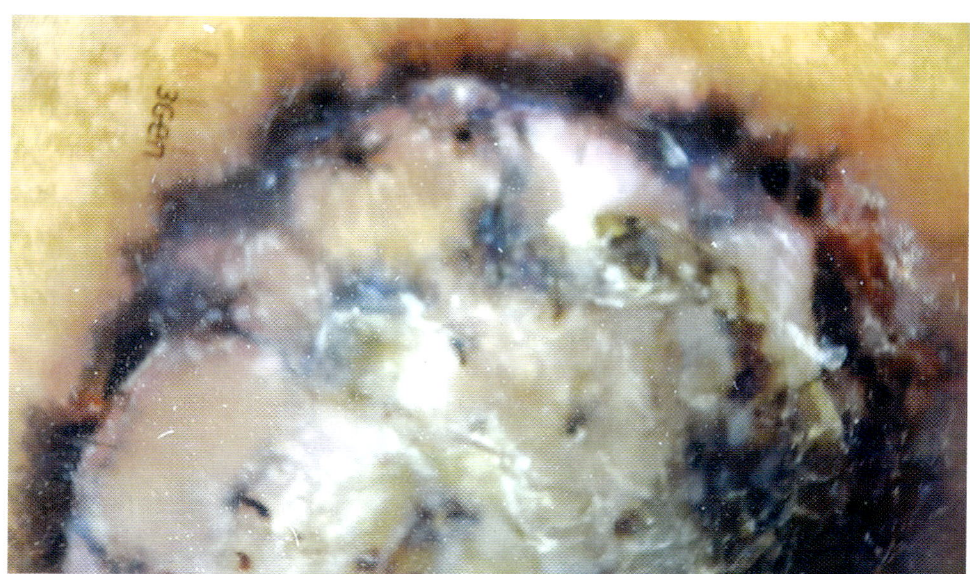

Fig. 15: Maple leaf structures seen.

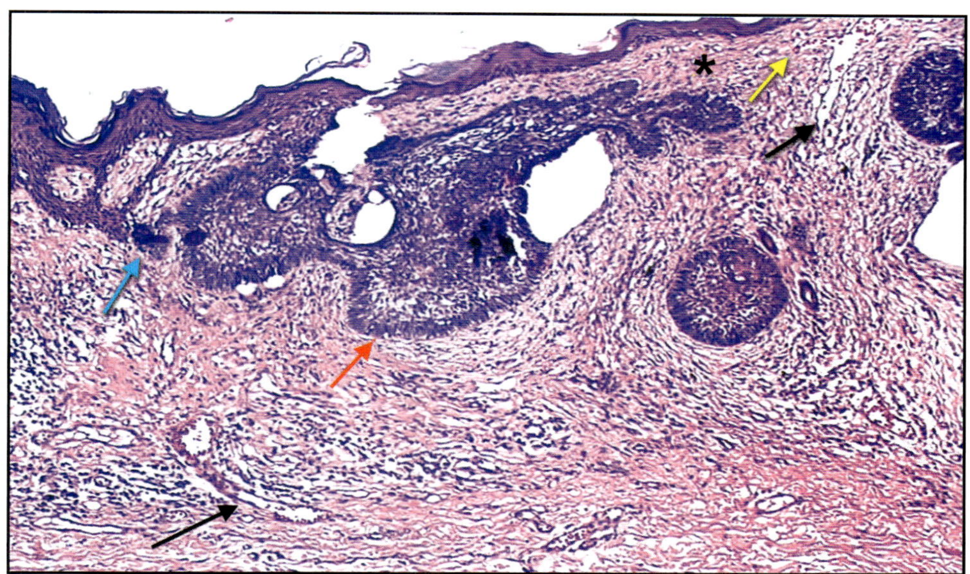

Fig. 16: Dermoscopy-histopathologic correlation: Large vessels (black arrows) correspond to arborizing blood vessels on dermoscopy. Small vessel (yellow arrow) corresponds to superficial fine telangiectatic vessel on dermoscopy. Tumor nests connected to epidermis and characterized by finger-like projections having pigment aggregates (blue arrow) correspond to spoke wheel areas on dermoscopy. Collagen alteration (star) corresponds to white shiny streaks due to birefringence of collagen. Multifocal tumor nests containing tumor aggregates connected to each other by lobular extensions (red arrow) correlate with the dermoscopic maple leaf like areas. Multiple melanophages in the papillary and reticular dermis corresponds dermoscopically to blue gray dots.

NONPIGMENTED BASAL CELL CARCINOMA

KEY DERMOSCOPIC FEATURES

- Arborizing vessels
- Superficial fine telangiectasis
- Multiple small erosions
- Shiny white-red structureless areas
- Tiny white streaks.

DISCUSSION

One of the important dermoscopic hallmarks of BCC, arborizing vessels, are vessels of large caliber, branching irregularly into terminal capillaries of lesser diameters. They are in-focus and bright red due to their superficial location on the surface of the tumor. They represent dilated vessels in the dermis which are supportive vasculature of the carcinoma tissue.

Superficial fine telangiectasias are small, fine, and focused linear vessels which rarely branch. They can be correlated with the vessels in the papillary dermis.

Multiple small erosions may be covered by minute brown-yellow crusts.

Shiny white-red structureless areas appear dermoscopically as translucent to opaque white to red areas. They correspond dermal fibrosis or fibrosis of the tumoral mass.

Tiny white streaks dermoscopically shows orthogonal short and thick crossing lines. They correlate well with the collagenous stroma and dermal fibrosis.

CASE 1 (FIGS. 17 TO 23)

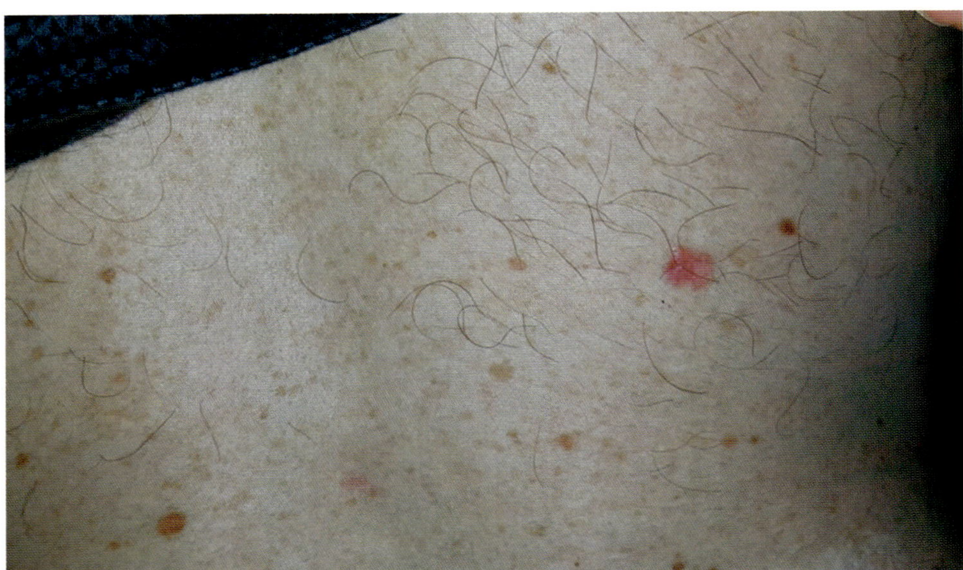

Fig. 17: A small plaque on the right side of the back of a middle-aged male for almost 1 year.

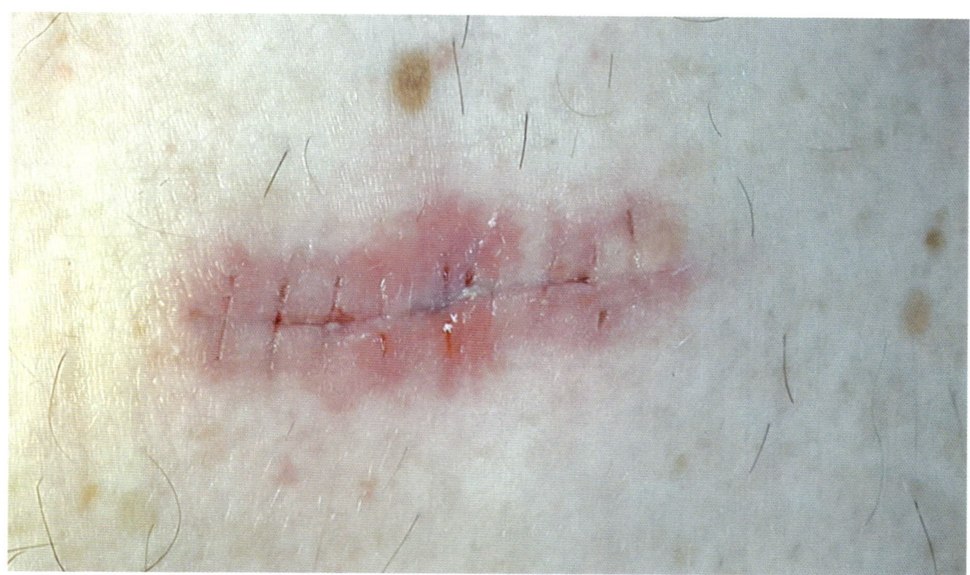

Fig. 18: It was excised and sent for histopathology.

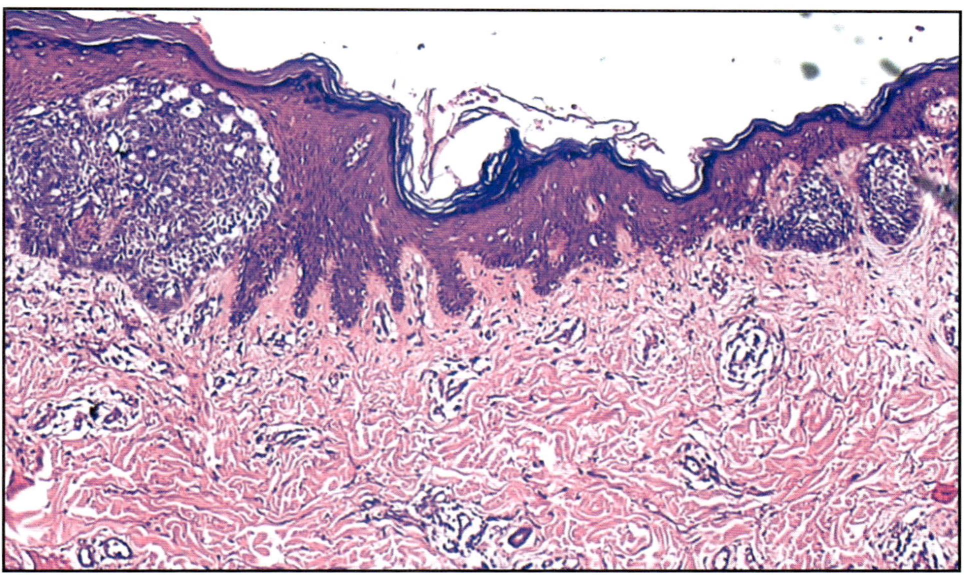

Fig. 19: Biopsy shows an epithelial neoplasm that shows connection with surface epidermis at several places. The tumor islands are made up of small round cells that show peripheral palisading and are restricted to the papillary dermis. The nuclei of these cells are uniformly stained and dark and show no nucleoli. The nuclei are closely crowded but do not show a nucleolus or nuclear pleomorphism. Occasional pyknotic cells are scattered between these cells. The surrounding stroma shows mucin and a moderately dense perivascular lymphoplasmocytic infiltrate with numerous melanophages. The tumor islands are separated from the underlying dermis by a cleft at a few places. Impression: Basal cell carcinoma (superficial spreading).

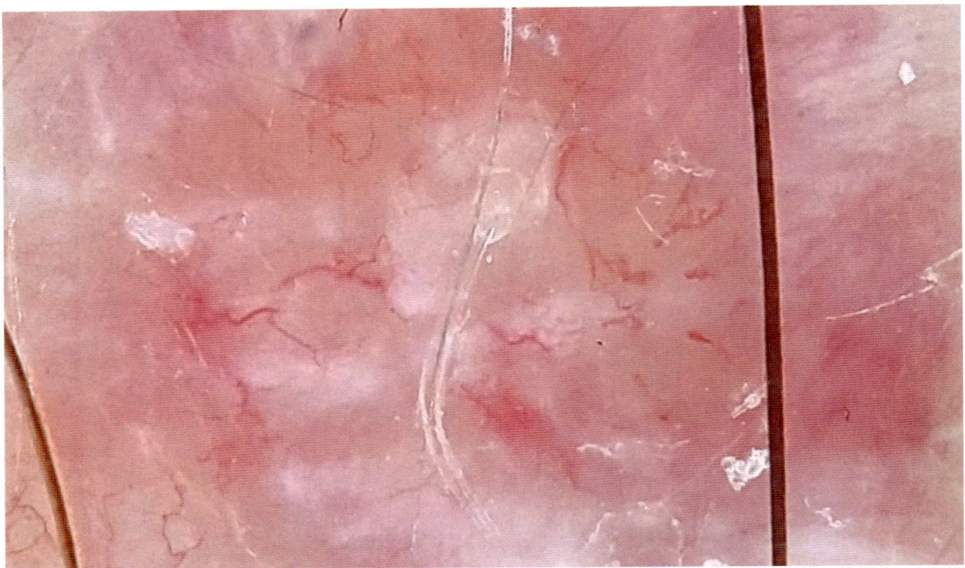

Fig. 20: Dermoscopy reveals arborizing red vessels, superficial fine telangiectatic vessels, and white shiny structures.

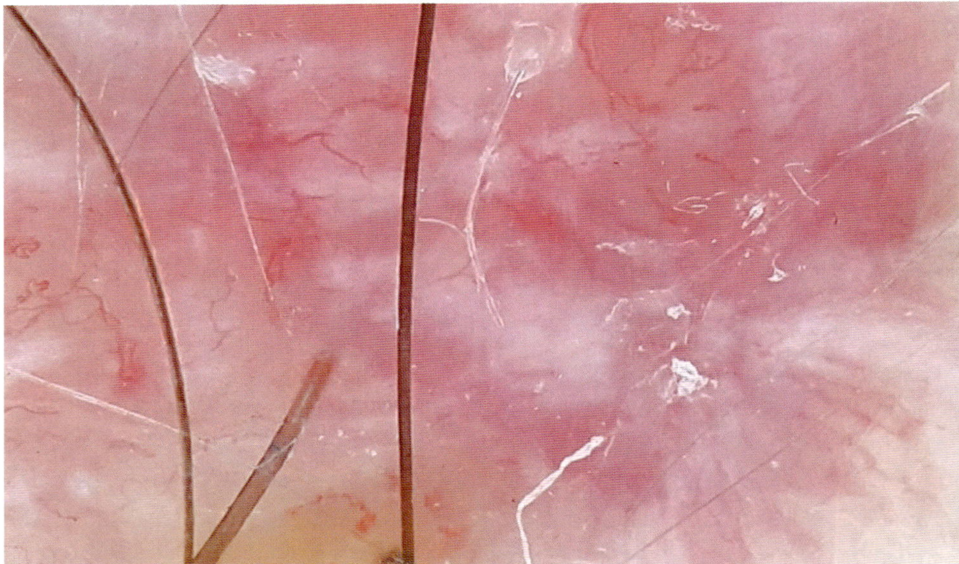

Fig. 21: Dermoscopic detection of arborizing vessels is highly predictive of BCC. SCC and other nonpigmented cutaneous tumors can be distinguished by this criterion. (BCC: Basal cell carcinoma; SCC: Squamous cell carcinoma).

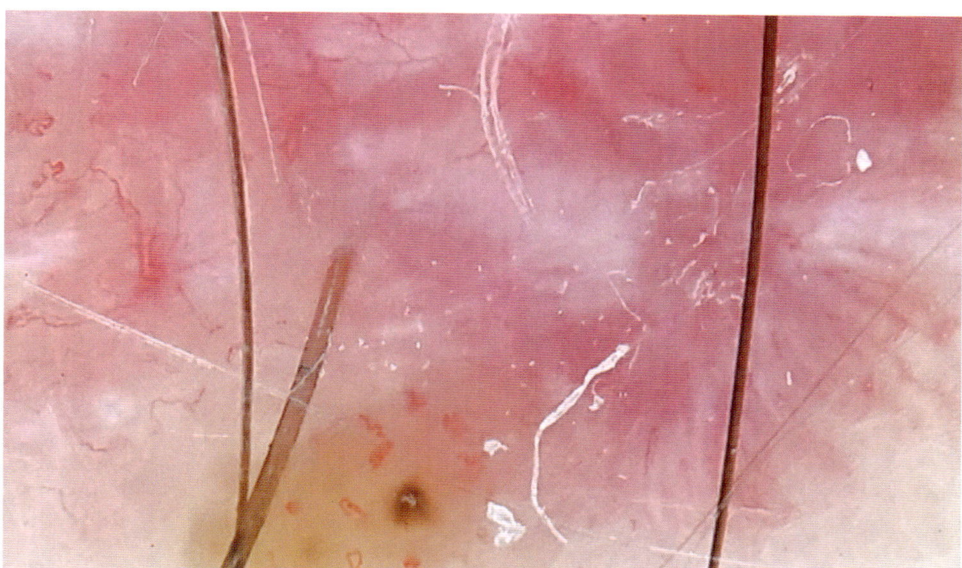

Fig. 22: Besides white shiny structures and superficial fine telangiectasias, a rosette is also seen.

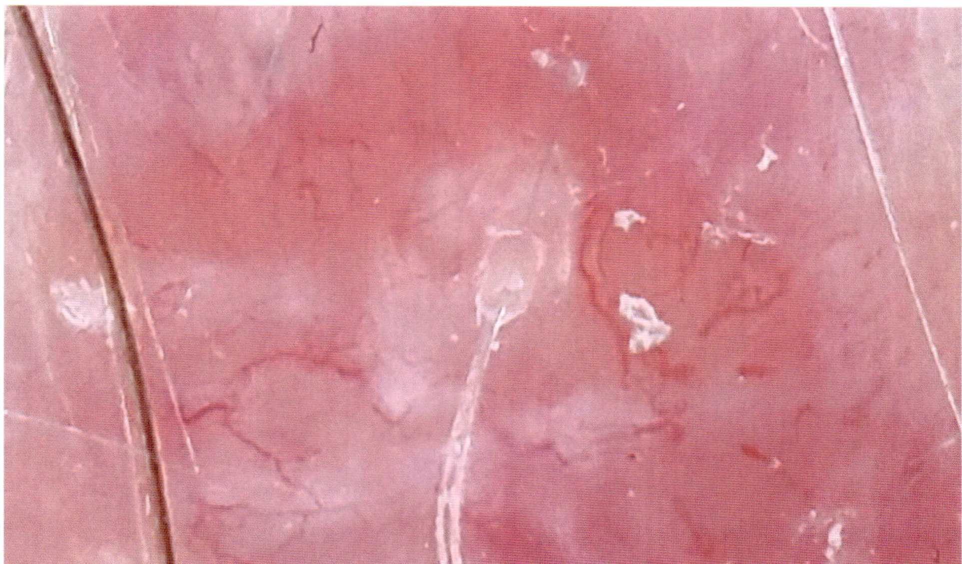

Fig. 23: Arborizing vessels are in-focus due to their superficial location on tumor surface. They represent neovascularization of the tumor.

CASE 2 (FIGS. 24 TO 26)

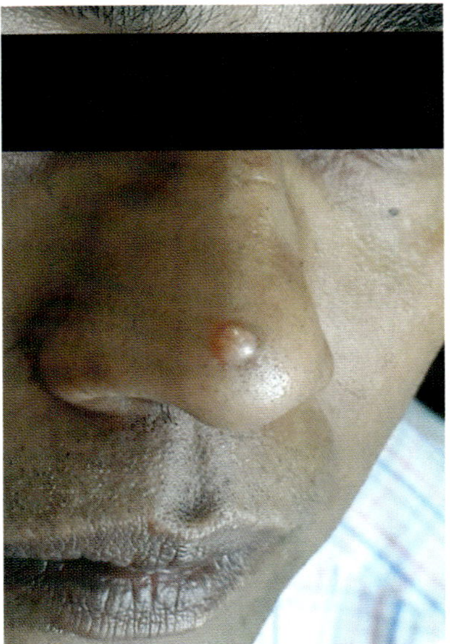

Fig. 24: Asymptomatic skin colored to pinkish nodule on the nose.

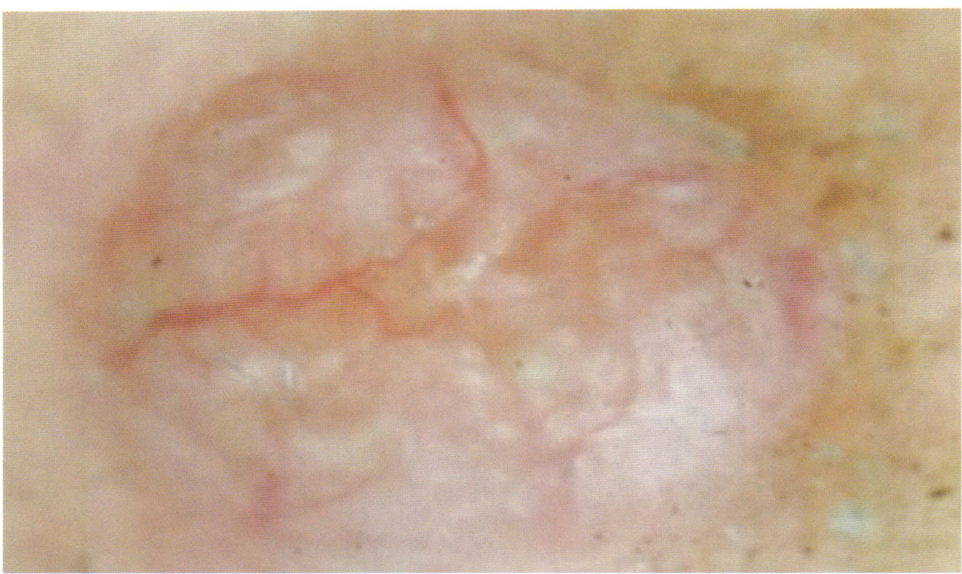

Fig. 25: Dermoscopy reveals bright red, in focus (due to its superficial location) arborizing vessels with a main stem branching into finer terminal capillaries.

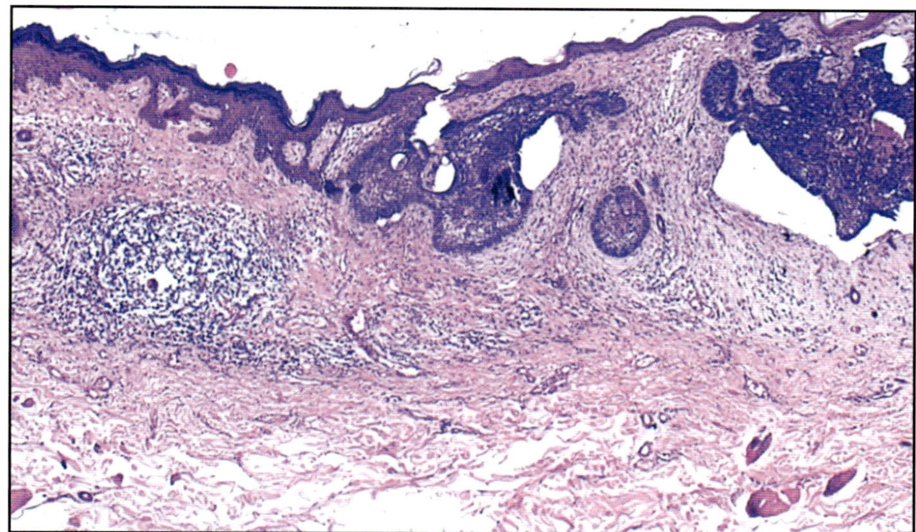

Fig. 26: Histopathology showing tumor islands made up of small round cells that show peripheral palisading.

KEYNOTE

- Dermoscopy enhances the clinical diagnosis of BCC at an early stage when the full blown clinical picture is still nonconspicuous.
- Detection of arborizing vessels is a valuable dermoscopic criteria of BCC, distinguishing it from squamous cell carcinoma (SCC), and other nonpigmented skin tumors.
- Dermoscopic diagnosis of pigmented BCC is usually uncomplicated because it displays maple leaf-like areas, spoke wheel areas, and concentric structures which correspond well to dermoepidermal melanin distribution.
- The author encountered dermoscopically a combination of blue, black, red, yellow, and white color giving a kaleidoscopic appearance that can be correlated well with histopathological findings in pigmented noduloulcerative BCC.
- Dermoscopy seems inadequate to differentiate between BCC and dermoscopic mimickers of BCC, such as adnexal tumors, milia, etc.[3]

REFERENCES

1. Lallas A, Apalla Z, Argenziano G, et al. The dermatoscopic universe of basal cell carcinoma. Dermatol Pract Concept. 2014;4(3): 11-24.
2. Steven Q, Menzis SW. Nonmelanocytic lesion, basal cell carcinoma. In: Ashfaq A (Ed). Atlas of Dermoscopy, 2nd edition. New York: Informa Healthcare; 2012. p. 40.
3. Malakar S, Mukherjee SS. Vascular pattern of milia on dermatoscopy. Our Dermatol Online. 2017;8(4):497-8.

MYCOSIS FUNGOIDES

INTRODUCTION

In mycosis fungoides (MF), the skin is infiltrated by patches or lumps of lymphocytes. It is more common in men than women. Its cause is unknown but in some patients, it is associated with a pre-existing contact allergic dermatitis or infection with a retrovirus (Fig. 27).

Mycosis fungoides has an indolent clinical course and may persist in one stage for a long time before it progresses to next stage.

In patch stage MF, the skin lesions are flat and hypopigmented. Most often there are oval or annular pink dry patches on covered skin. They may spontaneously disappear, remain the same size, or slowly enlarge. The skin may be atrophic, and may or may not itch.

KEY DERMOSCOPIC FEATURES (FIGS. 28 TO 31) [1]

- Orange-yellow patchy areas
- Fine short linear vessels
- Spermatozoa-like vessels
- *Demodex folliculorum* (personal observation).

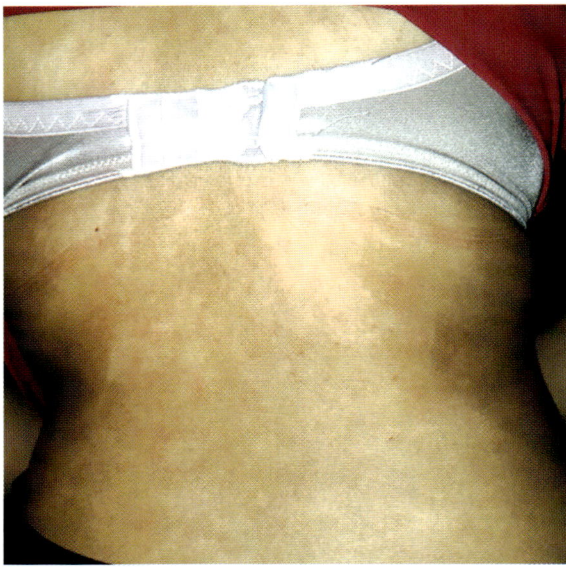

Fig. 27: A-30-year-old female having asymptomatic hypopigmented patches over the back for the last 2 years. Similar lesions were present on abdomen and extremities.

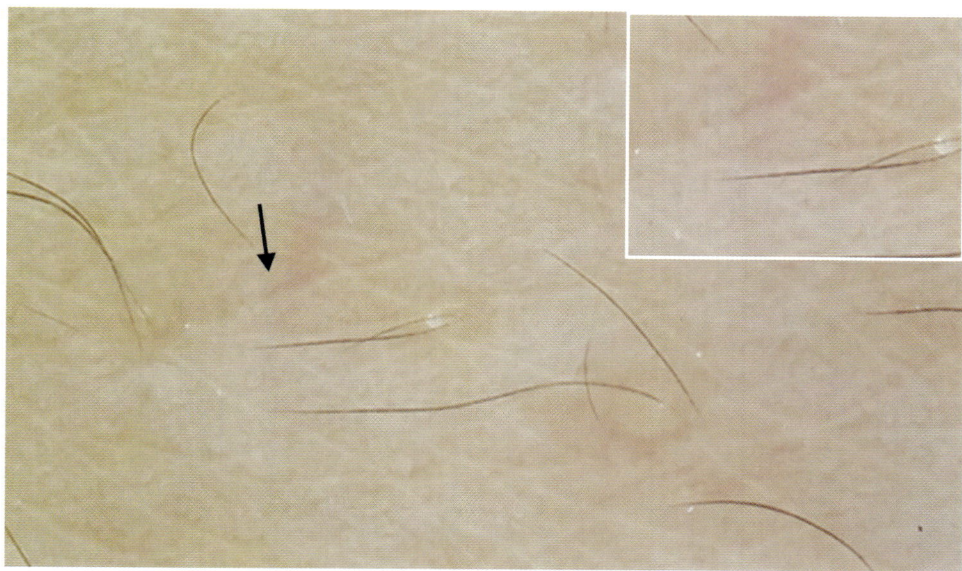

Fig. 28: Orange-yellow patches and fine short linear vessel (arrow).

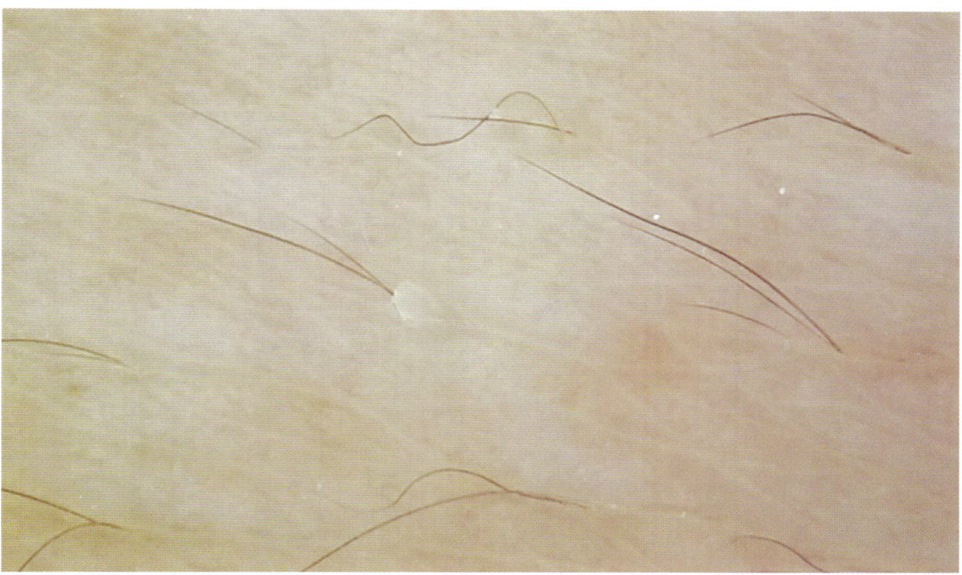

Fig. 29: Orange-yellow patches. Note: *Demodex folliculorum* at the center of the field, probably due to loss of local immunity as a result of the disease.

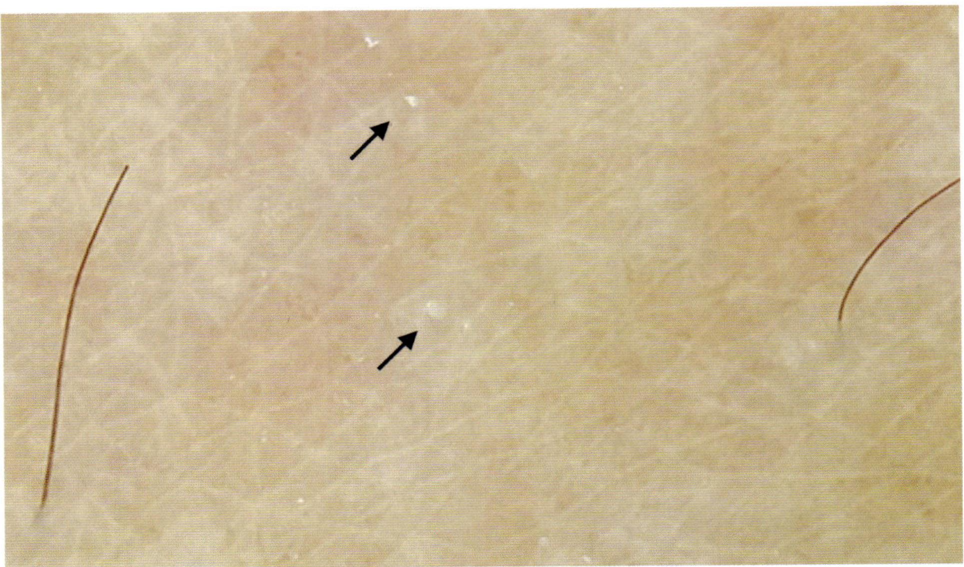

Fig. 30: More *Demodex folliculorum* in this field and faint orange-yellow patches (arrows).

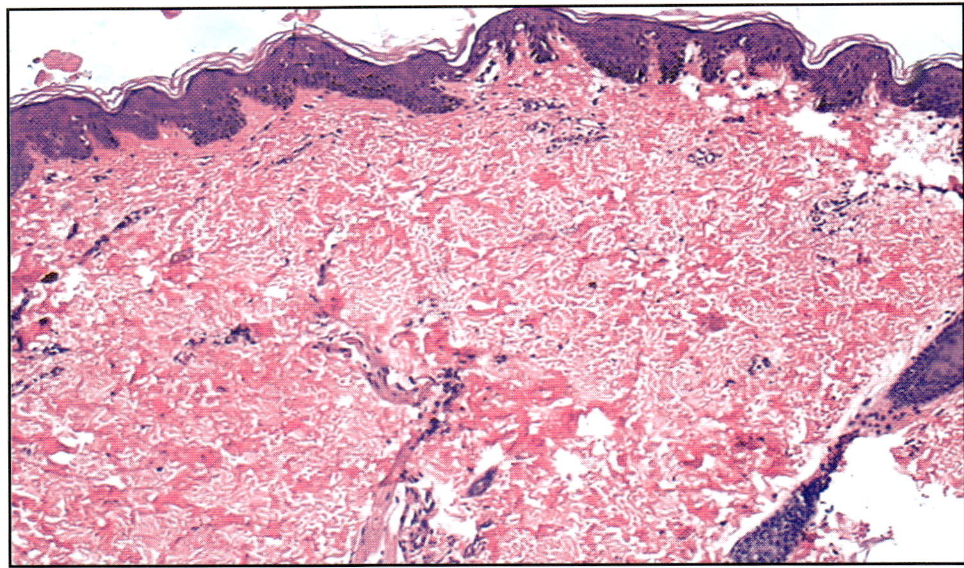

Fig. 31: Biopsy shows sparse superficial perivascular infiltrate of lymphocytes. The epidermis shows slight psoriasiform hyperplasia and infiltration by numerous small and large lymphocytes without much spongiosis. Several lymphocytes are aligned along the basal layer in toy soldier pattern. There is no granuloma nor is there any infiltrate around arrector pilorum muscles or nerves. Diagnosis: Mycosis fungoides (patch stage).

REFERENCE

1. Errichetti E, Stinco G. Dermoscopy in general dermatology: a practical overview. Dermatol Ther (Heidelb). 2016;6(4):471-507.

INVASIVE SQUAMOUS CELL CARCINOMA

INTRODUCTION

Cutaneous SCC present as enlarging scaly or crusted growth (Fig. 32). Typically it arises within pre-existing actinic keratosis or intraepidermal carcinoma. The characteristics of SCC are the followings: (a) Usually located on sun-exposed areas, such as face, lips, and ears; sometimes it may also be seen on the legs, (b) It grows over weeks to months, (c) It may ulcerate, (d) Commonly it is tender or painful, and (e) Size ranges from few mm to several cm in diameter.

KEY DERMOSCOPIC FEATURES[1] (FIGS. 33 TO 35)

- White circles (targetoid hair follicles)
- Central keratin and blood spots
- White structureless area
- Highly polymorphous vascular structures.

DISCUSSION

The dermoscopic criterion of white circles corresponds on histology to acanthosis and hypergranulosis of infundibular epidermis. The white circle is centered around a dilated infundibulum filled with keratin plug. This keratin plug appears as a yellow or orange clod on dermoscopy.

Invasive SCC exhibits highly polymorphous vascular structures; hairpin vessels along with dotted and/or linear irregular vessels are observed commonly. The vessels are seen on a whitish background.

Ulceration and blood crusts appear as reddish-orange to brownish-black blotches on the surface of the tumor.[2,3]

KEYNOTE

Dermoscopically keratin turned out to be a clue to differentiate between keratoacanthoma (KA) and SCC. Keratin located centrally is the single most criterion that separates KA from SCC. In a recent report by Rosendahl et al.,[1] central keratin is more frequently present in both the retrospective (51.2% vs 30.0%) and prospective parts (72.4% vs 40.6%) of their study. This is supported by the findings in histopathology that a central keratin plug is an architectural criterion for the diagnosis of KA.

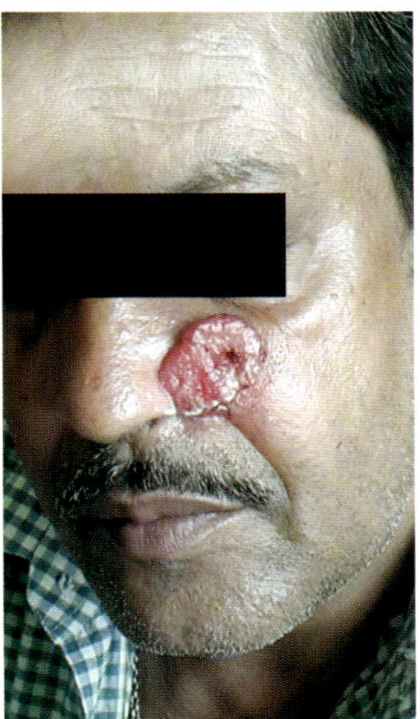

Fig. 32: Squamous cell carcinoma (SCC) is the second most common cause of cutaneous malignancy. SCC is usually found on sun-exposed areas. It may appear as plaques or nodules with variable degrees of scale, crust, or ulceration.

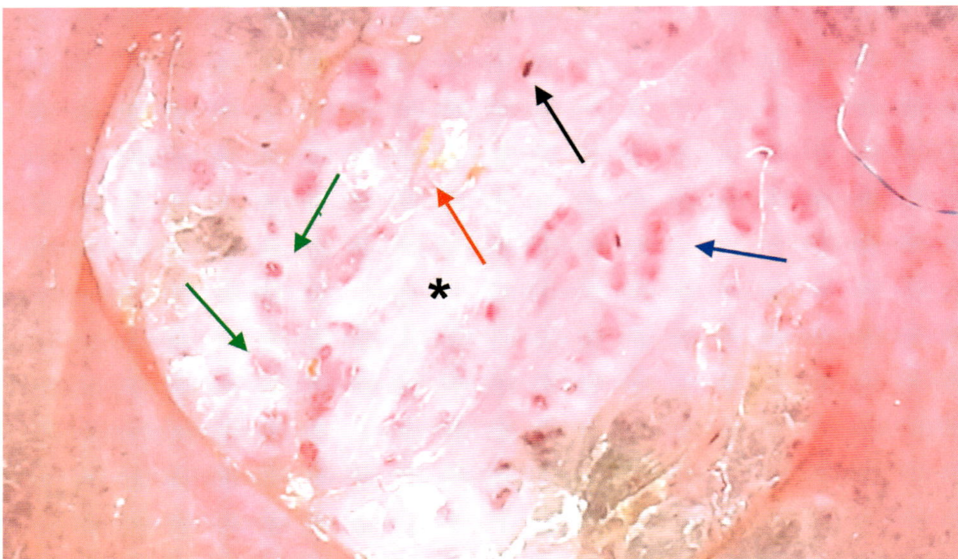

Fig. 33: White circles (green arrows), central keratin (red arrow), blood spots (black arrow), white structureless area (star), and polymorphous vascular structures (blue arrow). White circle is a new criterion and a valuable clue to KA and SCC. Rosendahl et al. suggested that histopathology should be considered in a raised, nonpigmented lesion where white circle is found on dermoscopy. (KA: Keratoacanthoma; SCC: Squamous cell carcinoma).

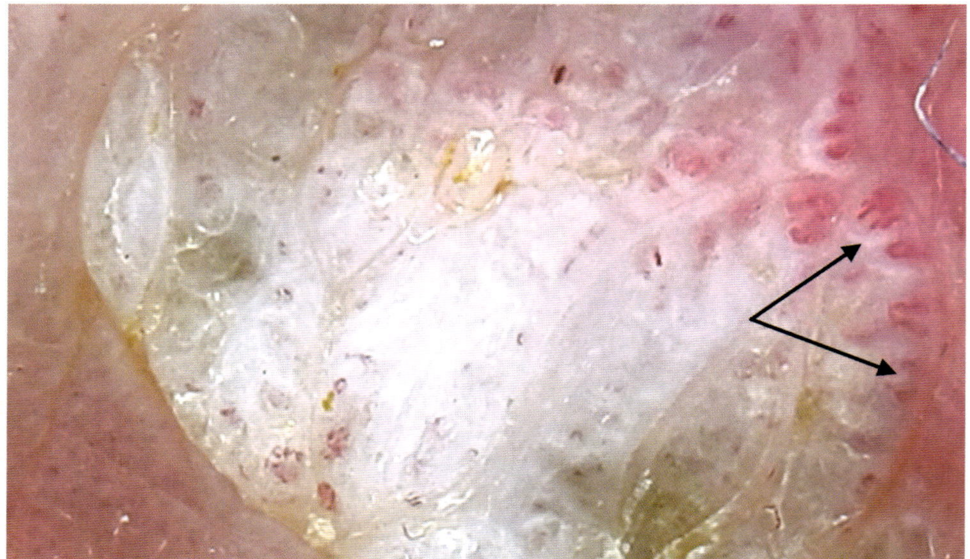

Fig. 34: White structureless areas may also be a valuable clue to SCC and KA, especially in some situations where white circles and keratin are missing. Invasive SCC exhibits highly polymorphous vascular structures; especially hairpin vessels of varying shape and distribution that are usually long (arrow) which may be associated with dotted or linear irregular vessels. The vessels are seen on a whitish background. (KA: Keratoacanthoma; SCC: Squamous cell carcinoma).

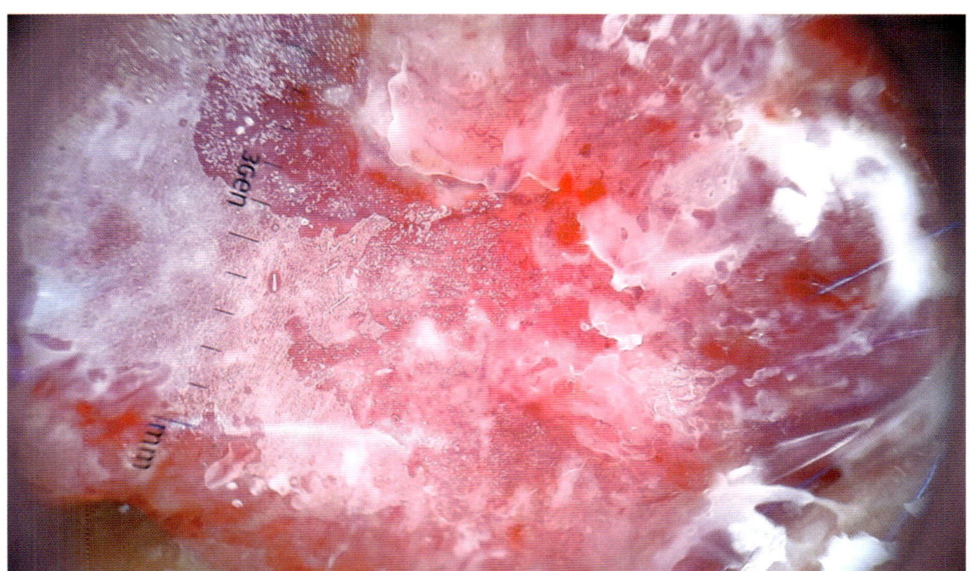

Fig. 35: Structureless homogeneous area with blood spots.

REFERENCES

1. Rosendahl C, Cameron A, Argenziano G, et al. Dermoscopy of squamous cell carcinoma and keratoacanthoma. Arch Dermatol. 2012;14288(12):1386-92.
2. Felder S, Rabinovitz H, Oliviero M, et al. Dermoscopic differentiation of a superficial basal cell carcinoma and squamous cell carcinoma in situ. Dermatol Surg. 2006;32(3):423-5.
3. Pan Y, Chamberlain AJ, Bailey M, et al. Dermatoscopy aids in the diagnosis of the solitary red scaly patch or plaque-features distinguishing superficial basal cell carcinoma, intraepidermal carcinoma, and psoriasis. J Am Acad Dermatol. 2008;59(2):268-74.

CHAPTER 10

Autoimmune Dermatoses

Subrata Malakar

ACUTE CUTANEOUS LUPUS ERYTHEMATOSUS

INTRODUCTION

Cutaneous lupus erythematosus (LE) has been classified as LE specific and LE nonspecific inflammatory conditions and the presentations may overlap. Acute cutaneous lupus erythematosus (ACLE) is a form of LE-specific cutaneous LE and is frequently associated with exposure to sunlight.[1]

Acute cutaneous lupus erythematosus affects at least 50% of patients with systemic lupus erythematosus (SLE). Specific features of acute cutaneous LE may include: (a) Malar eruption, (b) Erythematous papular rash on arms, (c) Photosensitivity, (d) Cheilitis or mouth ulcers, and (e) Blisters or erosions.[1]

KEY DERMOSCOPIC FEATURES (FIGS. 1 TO 7) (PERSONAL OBSERVATION)

- White scales
- Multicomponent vascular patterns
- Red starburst pattern
- Red-pink background.

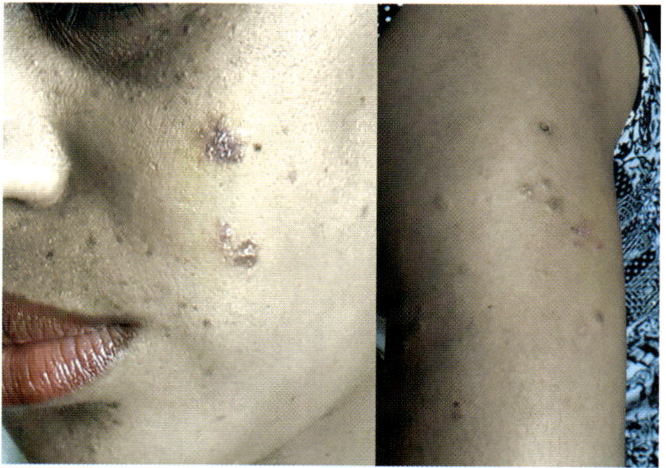

Fig. 1: Erythematous macules and papules becoming confluent in a generalized photo distributed pattern. Note the sparing of nasolabial folds.

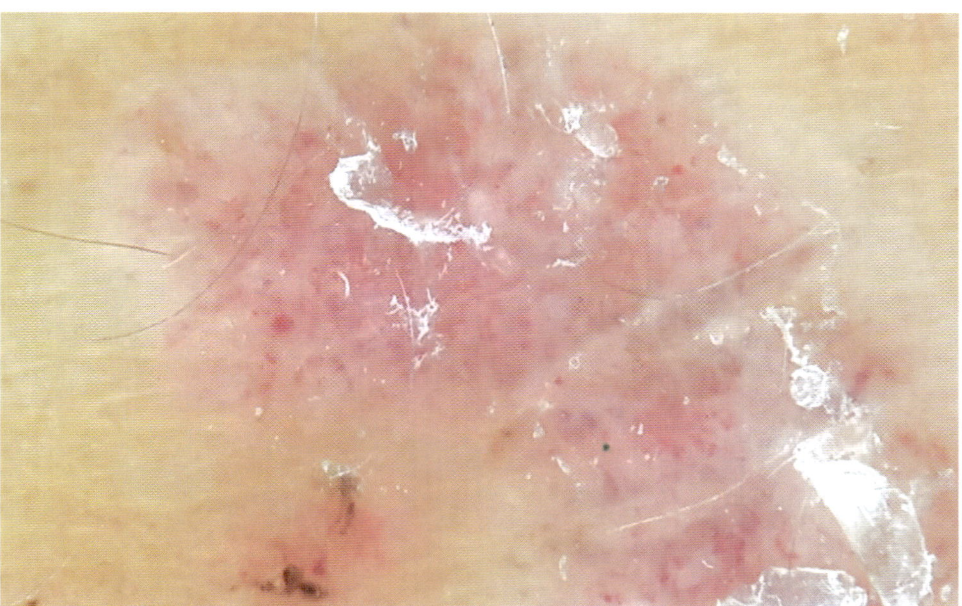

Fig. 2: White scales, multicomponent vascular pattern showing dotted, linear and linear irregular vessels, and red-pink background.

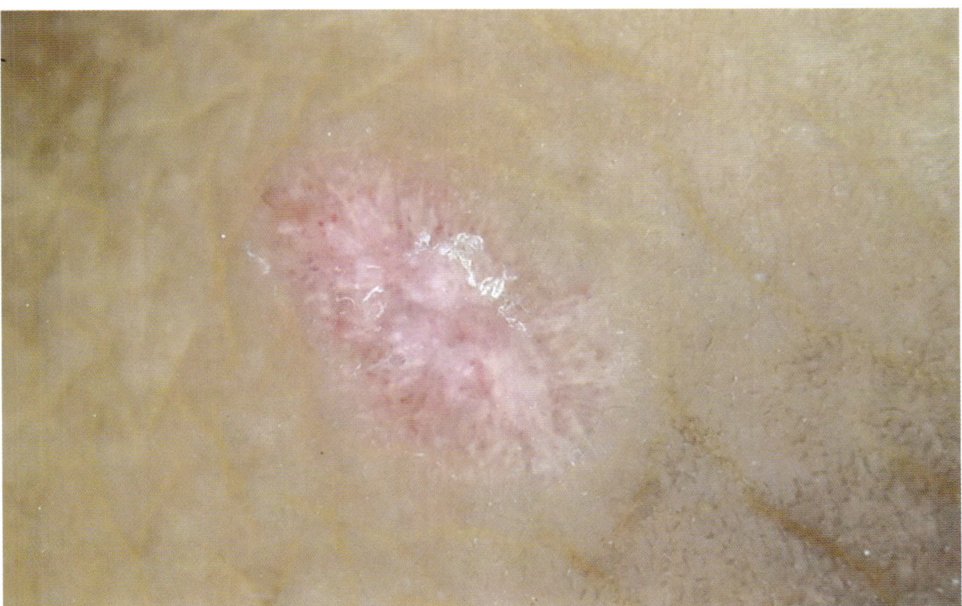

Fig. 3: Red starburst pattern, linear and dotted vessels, and white scales.

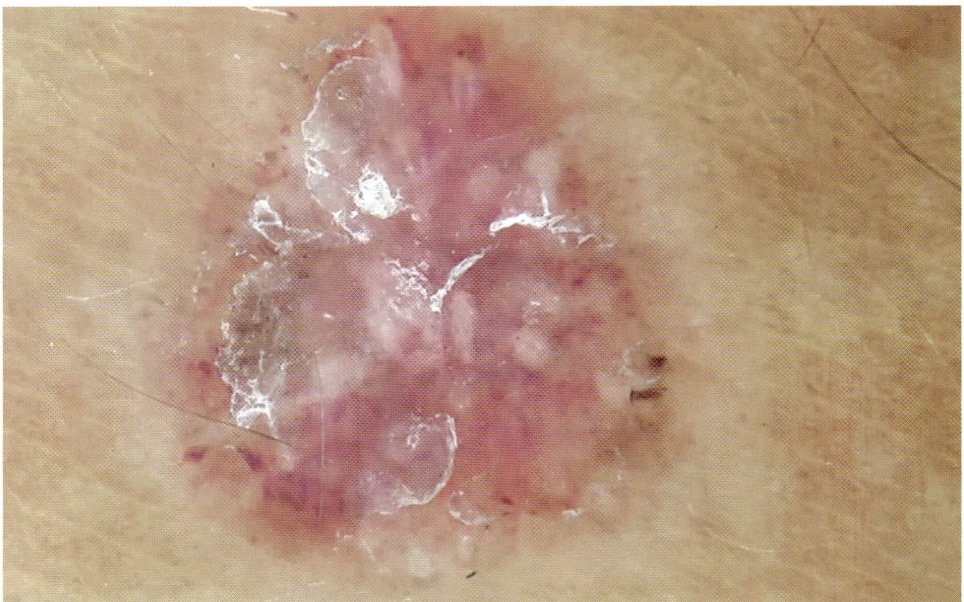

Fig. 4: White shiny structures, multicomponent vascular pattern, white scales, and red-pink background. At the periphery of the lesion, few pigment dots and globules are visible.

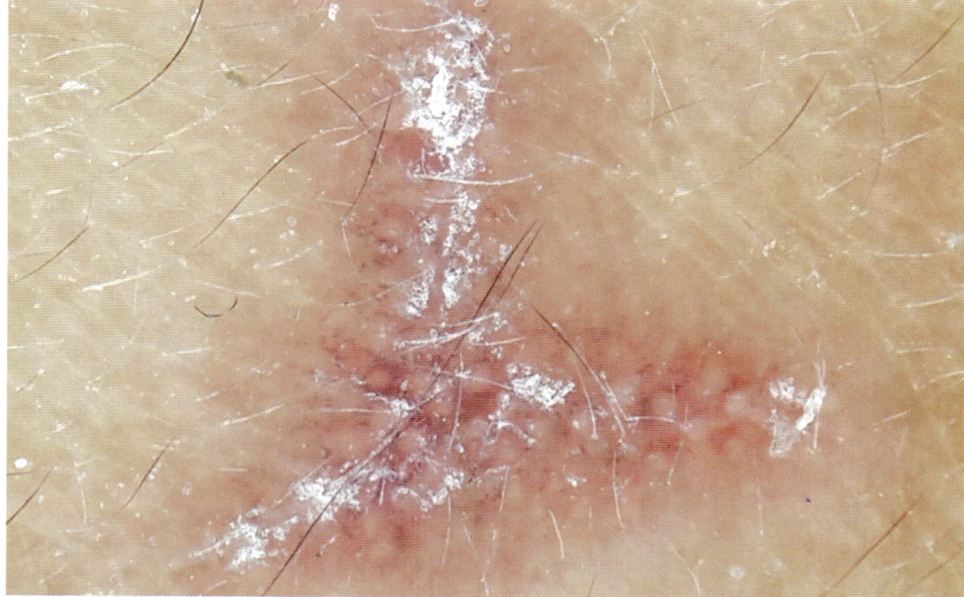

Fig. 5: Erythematous background, pigment dots and globules, and white scales. Some amorphous globular structures are also seen.

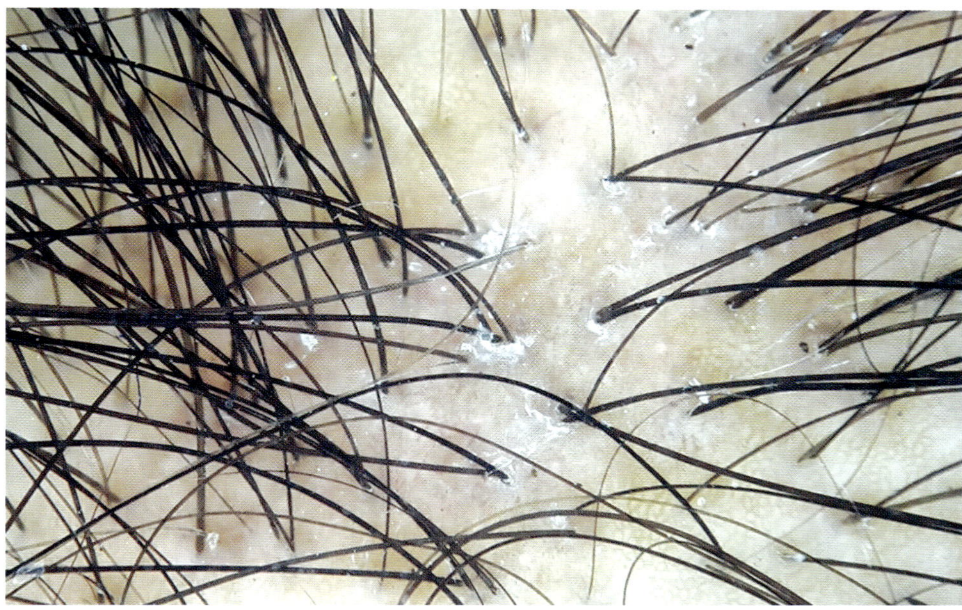

Fig. 6: Scalp is also involved which on dermoscopy reveals erythema, scaling mainly perifollicular, and most importantly speckled pigmentation.

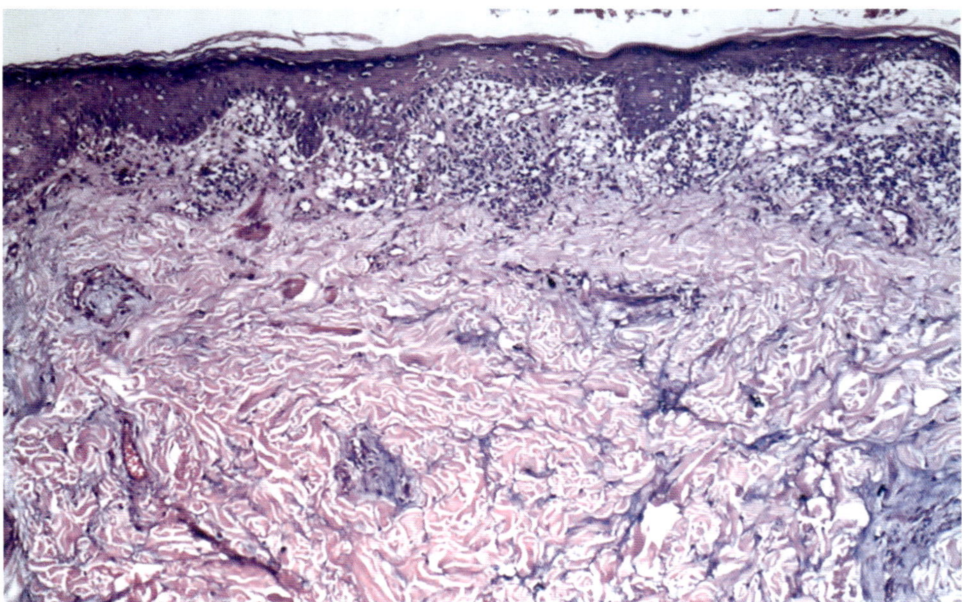

Fig. 7: Biopsy shows sparse superficial and deep perivascular infiltrate of lymphocytes. The papillary dermis is edematous and there is extravasation of red blood cells (RBCs). Basal layer shows vacuolization and interface infiltration by lymphocytes. Reticular dermis shows small amount of mucin. Marked papillary dermal edema with incipient blister formation can also be seen. *Diagnosis:* Acute cutaneous lupus erythematosus.

REFERENCE

1. Kuhn A, Meuth AM, Bein D, et al. Revised Cutaneous Lupus Erythematosus Disease Area and Severity Index (RCLASI): a modified outcome instrument for cutaneous lupus erythematosus. Br J Dermatol. 2010;163(1):83-92.

DERMATOMYOSITIS

INTRODUCTION

Dermatomyositis (DM) primarily affects the skin and the muscle along with other organs. Heliotrope rash and Gottron papules are cutaneous pathognomonic sign of DM. Dermoscopic features of the nails and hair have been described in the literature.

KEY DERMOSCOPIC FEATURES[1] (FIGS. 8 TO 11)

- Enlarged polymorphous interfollicular vessels
- Capillary loss
- Enlarged twisted capillaries
- Bushy capillaries
- Cuticle hemorrhage.

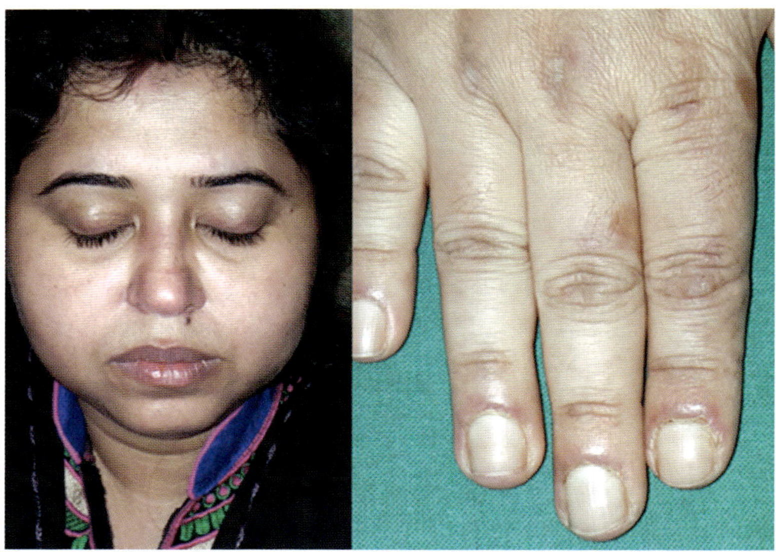

Fig. 8: Facial erythema, especially around the eyes known as heliotrope rash and Gottron papules in a case of dermatomyositis.

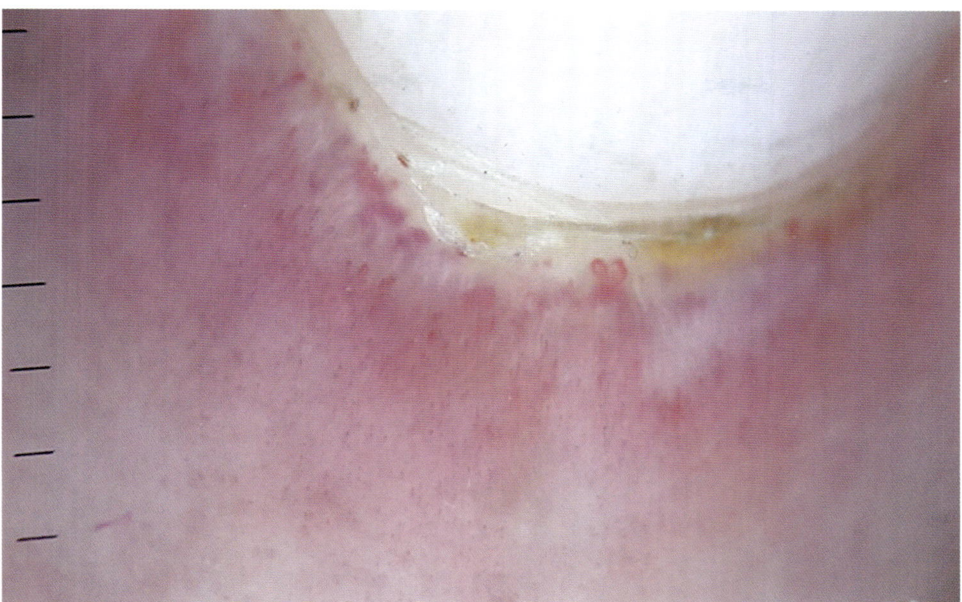

Fig. 9: Dermoscopy reveals both enlarged twisted capillaries and capillary loss. Some bushy capillaries are also seen.

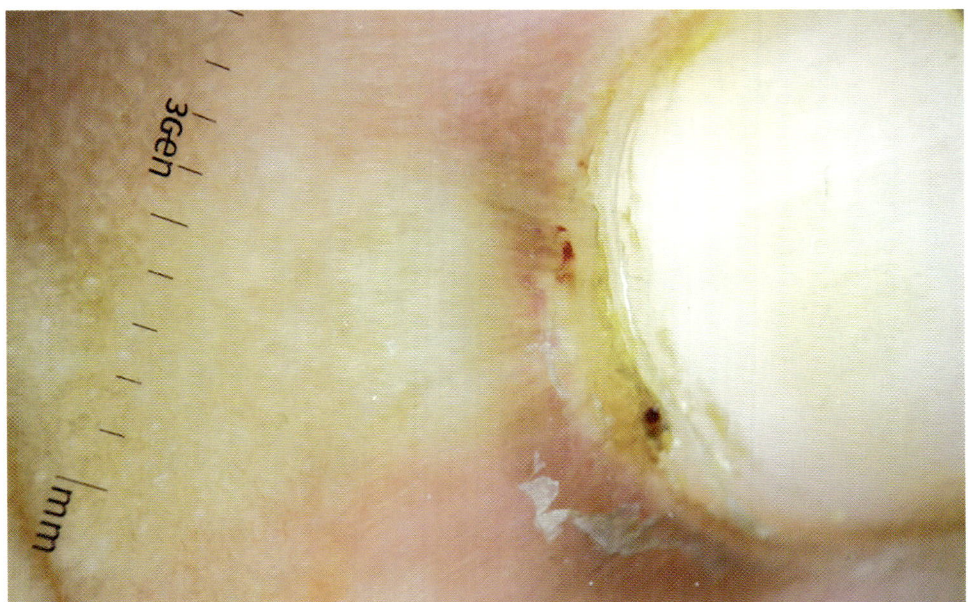

Fig. 10: Capillary loss and cuticle hemorrhage.

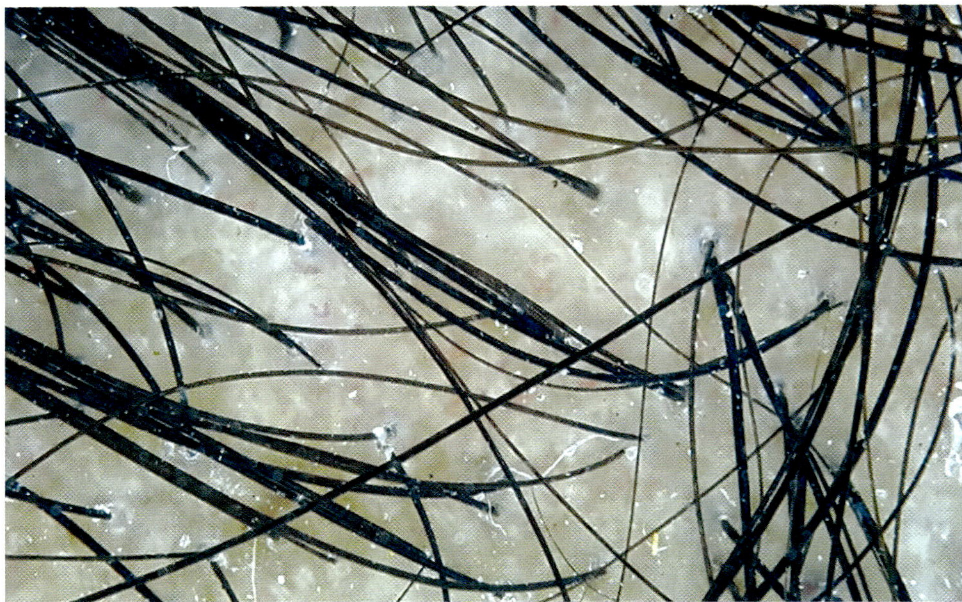

Fig. 11: Dermoscopy of hairs shows enlarged polymorphous interfollicular vessels.

REFERENCE

1. Souvik S, Malakar S. Trichoscopy in autoimmune connective tissue diseases. In: Malakar S (Ed). Trichoscopy: A Text and Atlas. New Delhi: Jaypee Brothers Medical Publishers (P) Ltd; 2017. p. 300.

DISCOID LUPUS ERYTHEMATOSUS

INTRODUCTION

Discoid lupus erythematosus (DLE) is the most common variant of cutaneous LE and may occur independently or as a manifestation of SLE. DLE most commonly occurs over scalp and is characterized by circumscribed inflammatory papules which develop into atrophic scars (Fig. 12). Dermoscopy can differentiate the scarring alopecias of scalp such as scalp DLE, lichen planopilaris, frontal fibrosing alopecia, etc.[1,2]

Sometimes differentiating DLE from inflammatory, infectious, and neoplastic cutaneous conditions are challenging and biopsies may be required to come to a diagnostic conclusion.

The following data describes dermoscopic features of DLE on other locations except scalp.

KEY DERMOSCOPIC FEATURES (FIGS. 13 TO 29)

Dermoscopic features of DLE depend upon its stage of progression.

Early Lesions

- Perifollicular whitish halo
- Follicular plugging
- White scales.

Long-standing Lesions

- Telangiectatic vessels
- Pigmentation structures
- White structureless areas.

Unclassified

- Follicular red dots.

PERSONAL OBSERVATIONS (FIGS. 17 TO 22)

- Palisade pigmentation (may be due to peripheral pigmentary incontinence in the lesion confirmed by biopsy).
- Red starburst pattern (corresponds to epidermal hyperplasia and hyperkeratosis).
- White shiny structures.
- Rosettes.

Unclassified

- Follicular red dots.

DISCUSSION

Scalp DLE has been extensively studied to differentiate it from other causes of scarring alopecias such as lichen planopilaris, frontal fibrosing alopecia, pseudopelade of Brocq, etc.[1,3] Until recently, before the study of Lallas et al.,[4] limited data was available concerning dermoscopic features of DLE over other parts of body barring the scalp.

Peripilar whitish halo is present most commonly and can be correlated histologically to perifollicular fibrosis. Scarring alopecia in DLE starts from the hair follicle, which destroys the perifollicular elastic sheath. As the disease progresses, the scarring spreads gradually to involve the dermis of interfollicular areas. Thus, the end-stage DLE demonstrate diffuse fibrosis histologically that reflects whitish structureless area dermoscopically.[5,6] Al-Refu K et al. in an experiment using C8/144B monoclonal antibody, demonstrated the absence of stem cells at hair follicle bulge of DLE lesions. Thus, they provided evidence that in DLE pilosebaceous unit is the primary target of the inflammatory process.[7]

White scales represent hyperkeratosis.

Dermoscopy highlights the follicular plugs[8] and can well be correlated with follicular hyperkeratosis in histology. Follicular hyperkeratosis is a valid clinicohistopathologic criterion of DLE, but in case of diffuse hyperkeratosis that covers the whole surface of the lesion, the follicular plugs may be missed by naked eye examination. Follicular plugs may be detected by dermoscopy in such situations (Figs. 22 to 25).

Dermoscopic features of long-standing lesions are telangiectatic vessels, pigmentation structures, and white structureless areas, often observed in combination.[4] Diffuse dermal fibrosis, pigmentary changes, and telangiectasias correspond to late histopathological features of DLE.[9] Pigmentary changes represent presence of numerous melanophages in the late stage of DLE (Figs. 26 to 28).

Follicular red dots are important feature of scalp DLE,[1,2] although in nonscalp DLE, its frequency is less.[4] Lallas explained its lower frequency in nonscalp DLE due to anatomical site characteristic or differences in disease duration. Histologically follicular red dots have been correlated with perifollicular extravasation of erythrocytes.

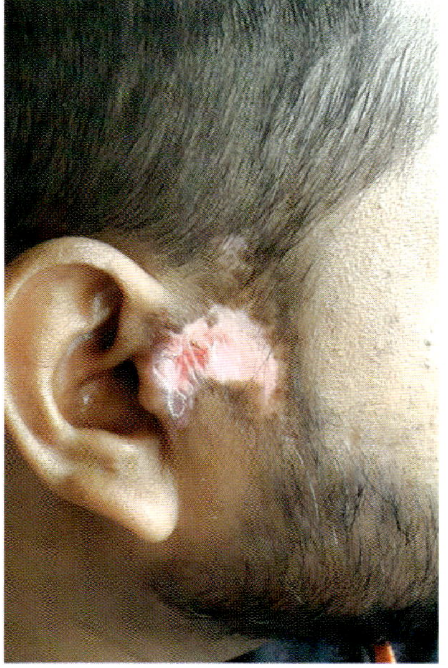

Fig. 12: Discoid lupus erythematosus.

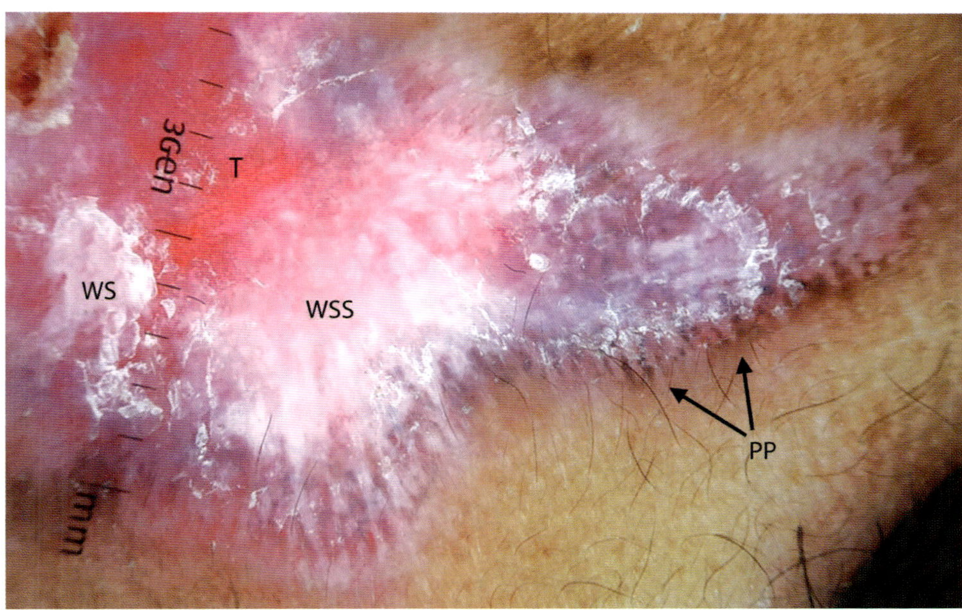

Fig. 13: Dermoscopy reveals the following features: Telangiectasia (T), white shiny structures (WSS), white scales (WS), and palisade pigmentation (PP). Except the white scales, all other features are regarded as a late feature of DLE dermoscopically. White scales correspond to hyperkeratosis.[4] Telangiectatic vessels correlate to histopathologic telangiectasias.[4] Pigmentation structures represent pigmentary incontinence histopathologically;[4] the incontinence may not involve the entire dermis but is present focally or segmentally to produce the characteristic palisade pigmentation. Altered collagen produce dermoscopic white shiny structures.[10]

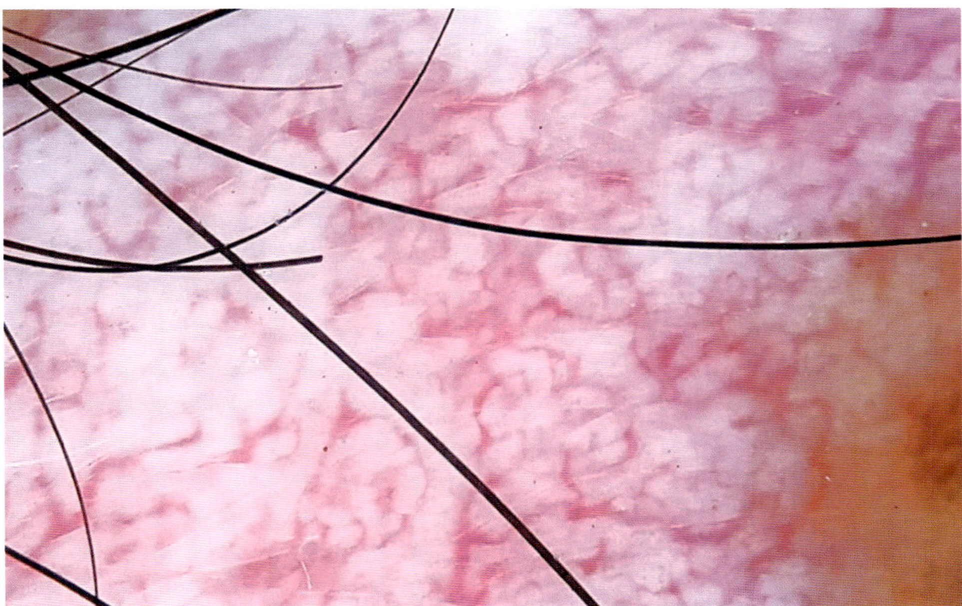

Fig. 14: Advanced lesion of discoid lupus erythematosus (DLE) dermoscopically shows white structureless areas corresponding histopathologically to diffuse fibrosis. The process of fibrosis begins perifollicularly, producing perifollicular white halo; the fibrosis spreads further to other follicles and intervening areas.

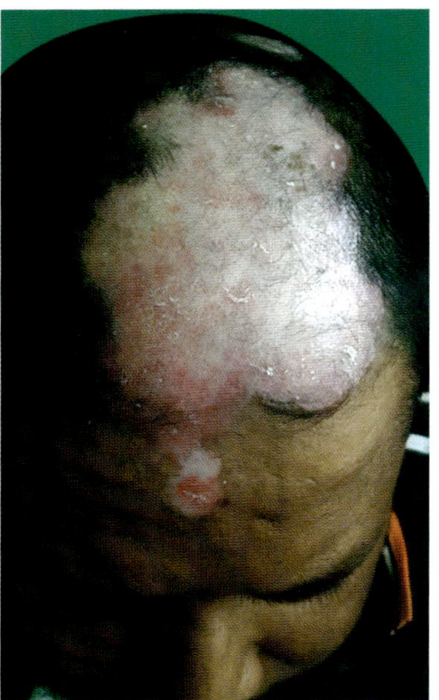

Fig. 15: A case of late discoid lupus erythematosus.

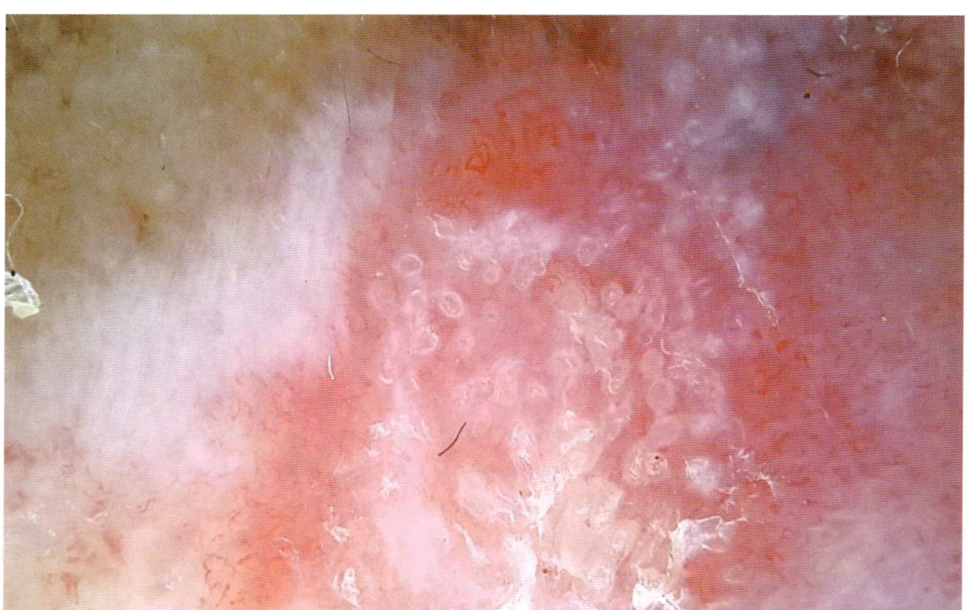

Fig. 16: Dermoscopy reveals follicular plugging, white structureless area, telangiectasia, and other vascular patterns such as linear irregular, comma, and hairpin vessels. Rosettes are also seen. Follicular plugging/hyperkeratosis is a typical clinical, histopathological, and also a dermoscopical criterion of discoid lupus erythematosus (DLE). This feature differentiates DLE from actinic keratosis and Bowen's disease.

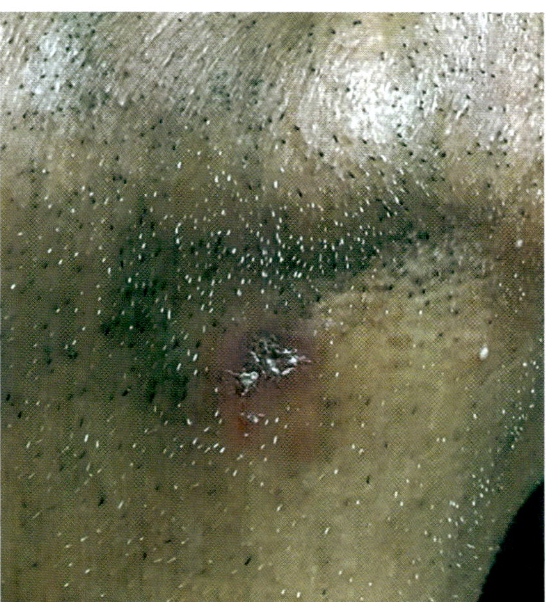

Fig. 17: A case of long-standing discoid lupus erythematosus (DLE).

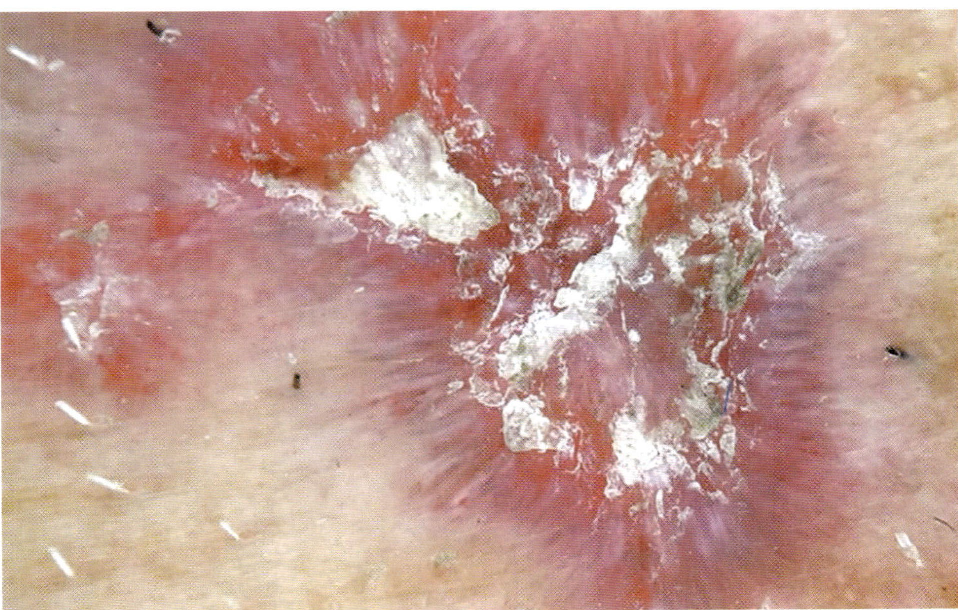

Fig. 18: Dermoscopy reveals a new pattern, the "red starburst pattern". Telangiectasia is usually a late feature of DLE. The combination of telangiectasias, epidermal hyperplasia, and diffuse dermal fibrosis may be the cause of this red starburst pattern. Thick white scales and follicular plugging are also evident in this dermoscopic field.

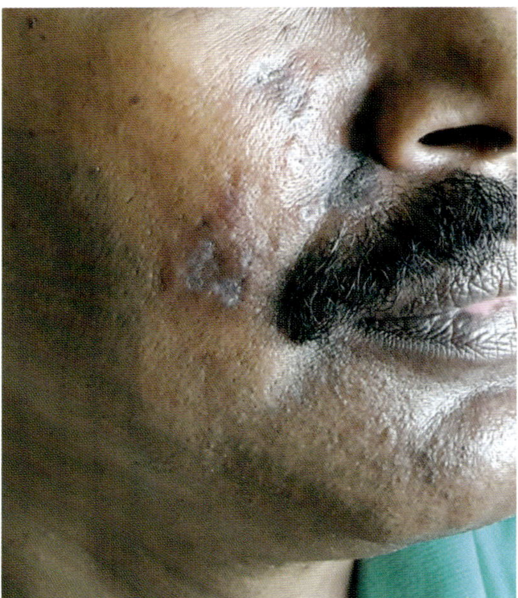

Fig. 19: Plaques of discoid lupus erythematosus (DLE) on sun exposed areas since 5 months.

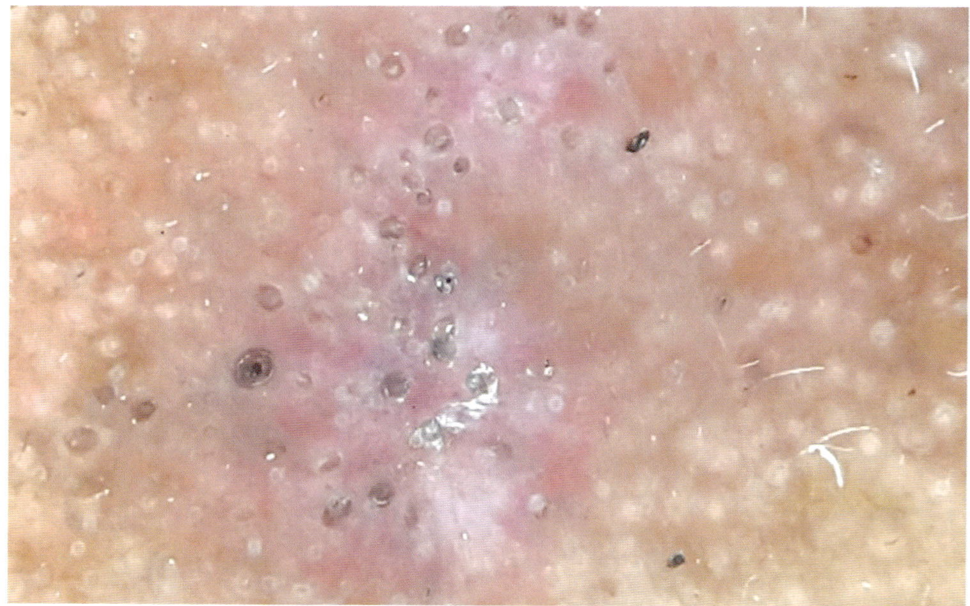

Fig. 20: Sometimes accentuation of follicular plugs is overlooked clinically. Dermoscopy highlights this hallmark feature of discoid lupus erythematosus (DLE). Rosettes, white shiny structures, and erythema are also visible.

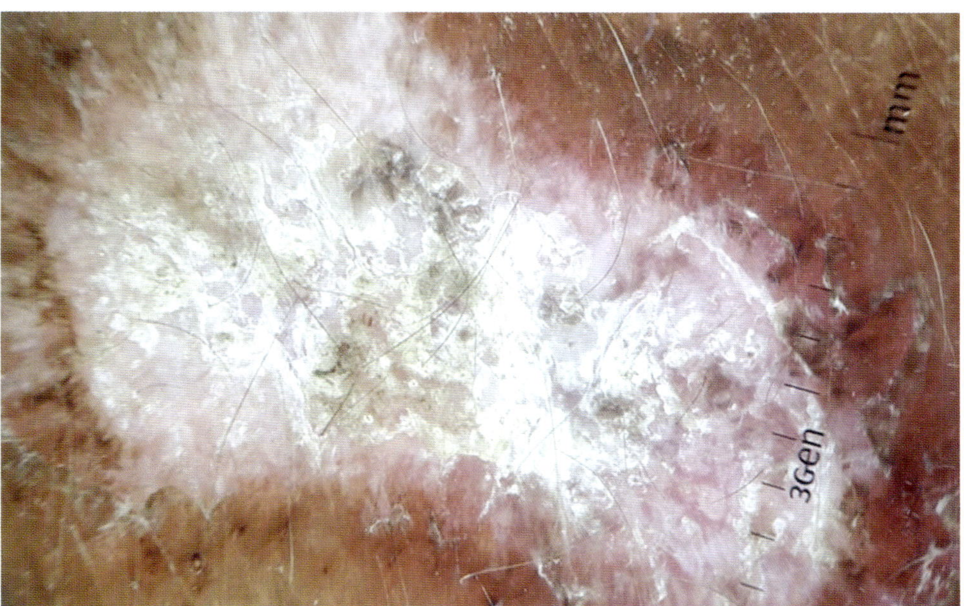

Fig. 21: Falisade pigmentation, white shiny structures[10,11] and thick white scales.

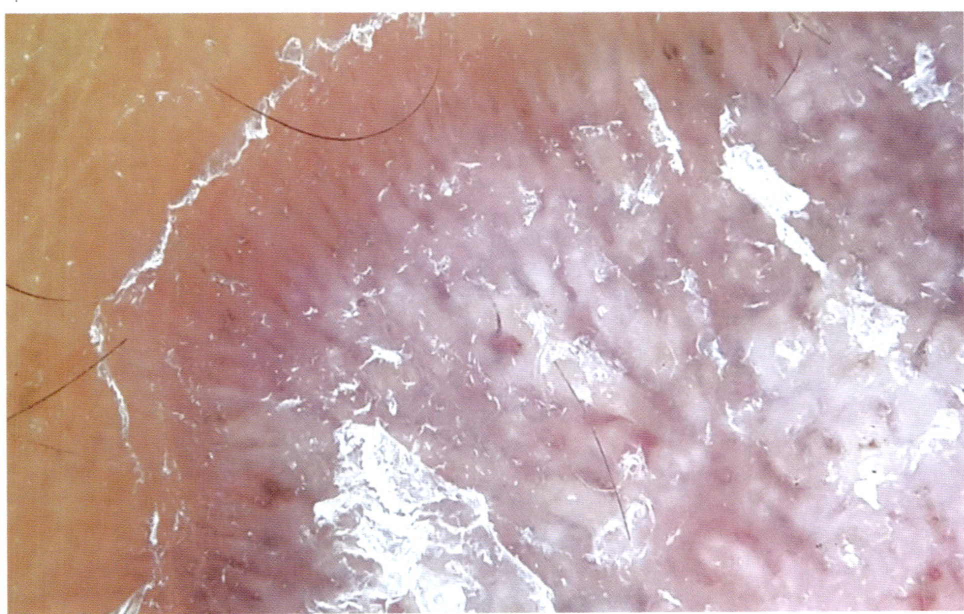

Fig. 22: Red starburst pattern with follicular plugging and white scales in this dermoscopic field.

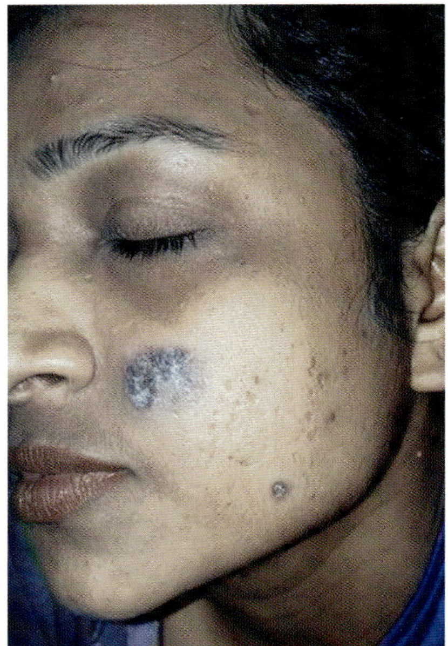

Fig. 23: Discoid lupus erythematosus (DLE) in a young female since 6 months.

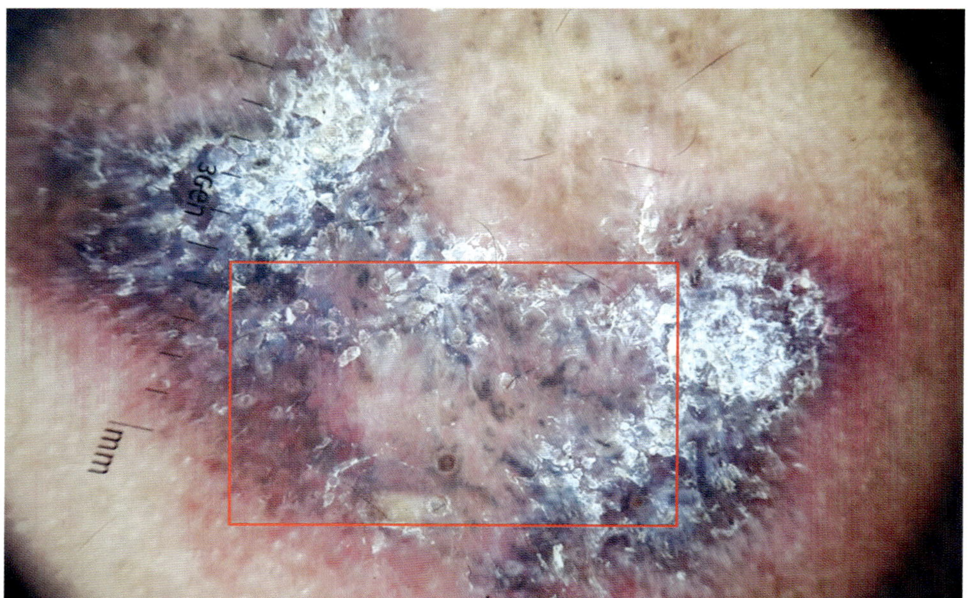

Fig. 24: Follicular plugging/hyperkeratosis may at times be overlooked, especially when hyperkeratosis is prominent and covers most of the lesional plaque. The area enclosed by red rectangle has been reobserved on magnification in the next picture.

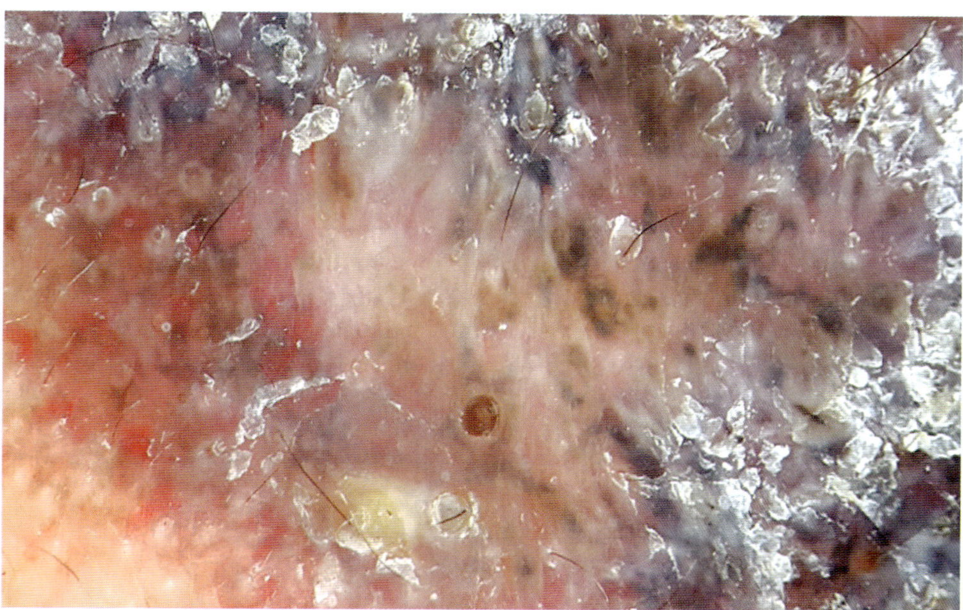

Fig. 25: Prominent follicular pluggings are evident. Note: Some pigmentation structures, which show pigment dots, globules, and clods. At the periphery, linear vessels are visible.

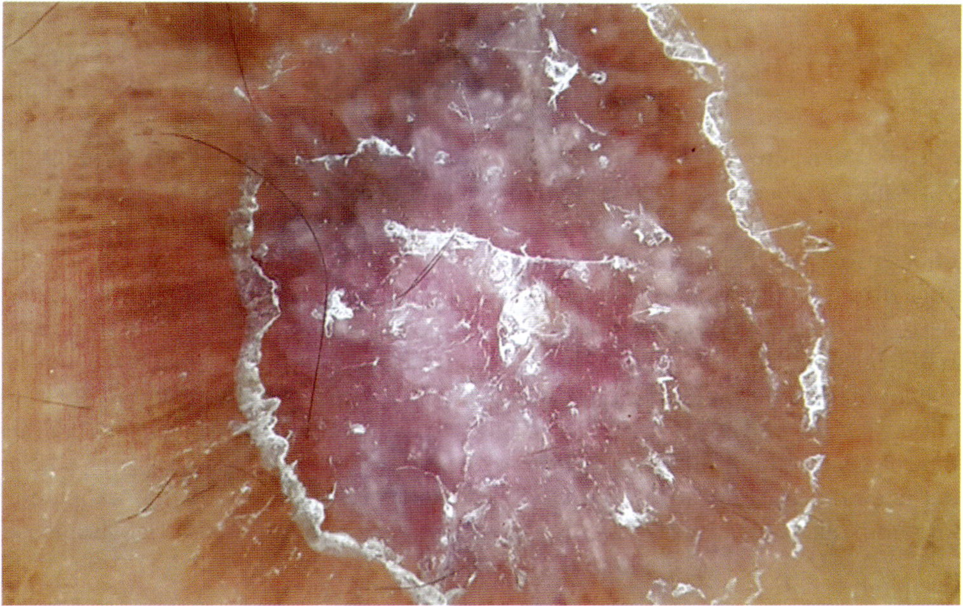

Fig. 26: White starburst pattern, white shiny structures, and palisade pigmentation.

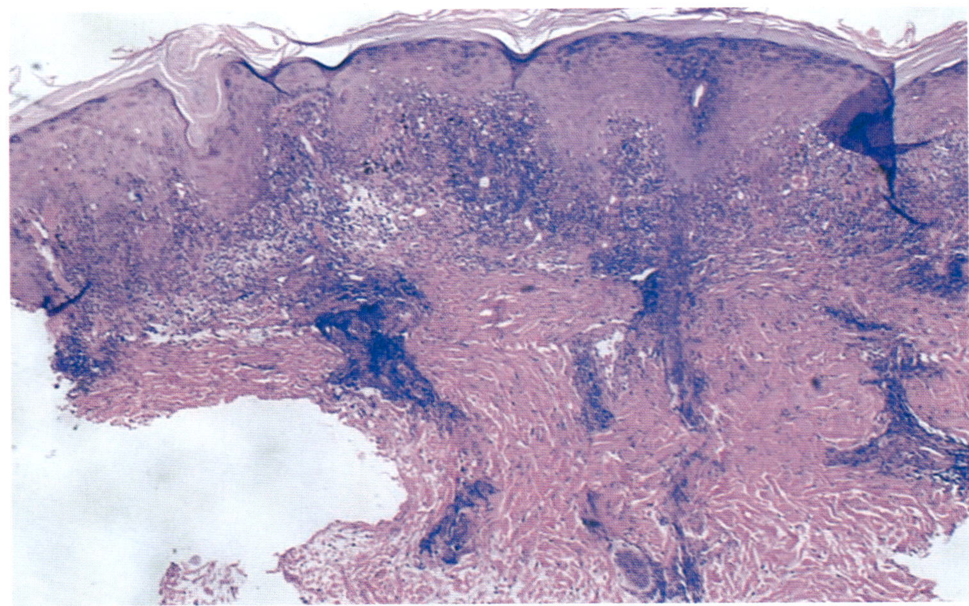

Fig. 27: Histopathology of the above case on 10 X.

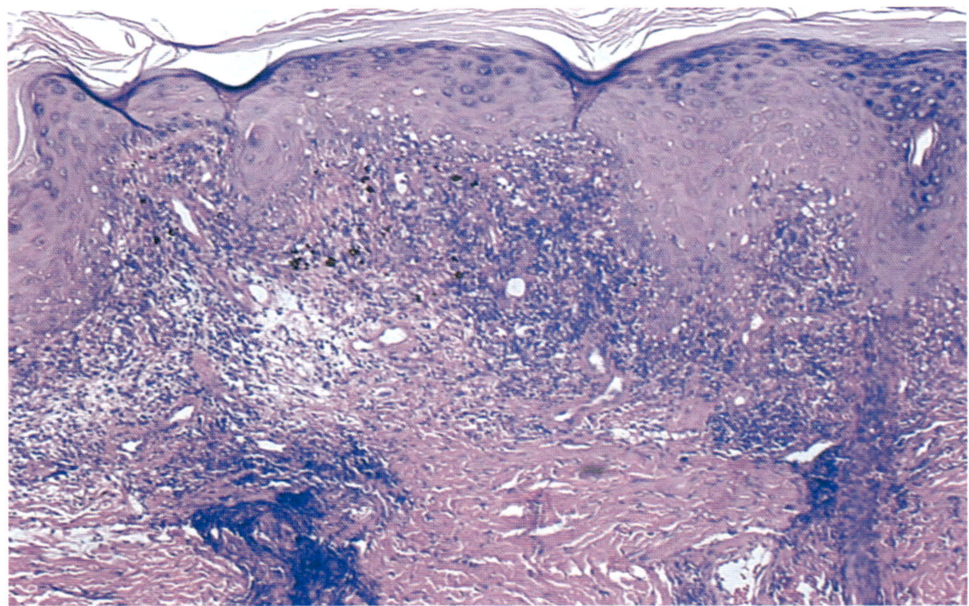

Fig. 28: Biopsy shows moderately dense superficial and midperivascular infiltrate of lymphocytes with focal interface vacuolar change. The infiltrate is more dense in the papillary dermis where it has a lichenoid appearance. The papillary dermis is edematous and shows scattered colloid bodies. The dermoepidermal junction is smudged and shows occasional necrotic keratinocytes. Scant mucin is present within the reticular dermis.

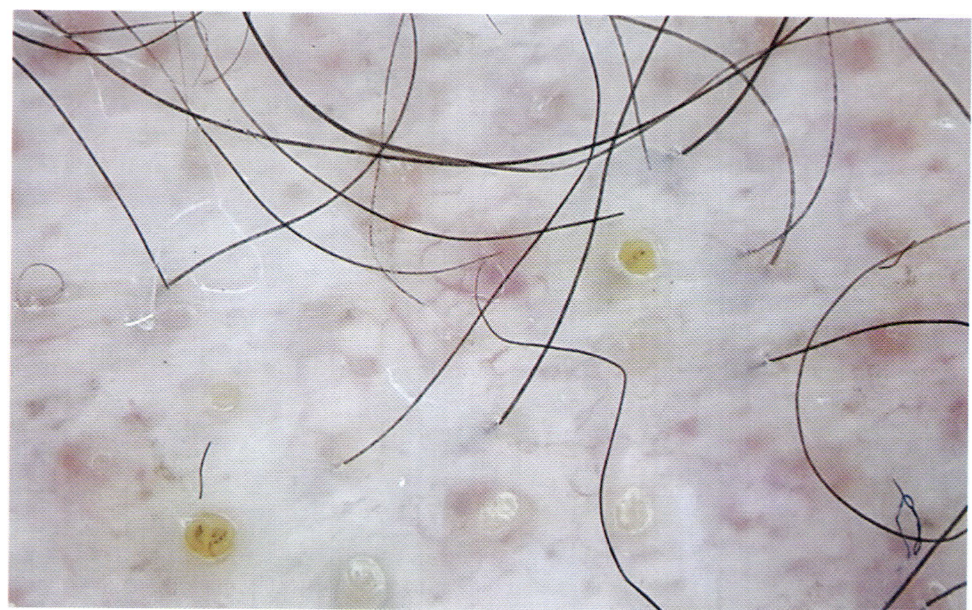

Fig. 29: Dermoscopy of long-standing discoid lupus erythematosus (DLE) showing prominent telangiectatic vessels and white scar like structures. Note the prominent follicular plugging with a yellow hue due to inspissated sebum.

REFERENCES

1. Tosti A, Torres F, Misciali C, et al. Follicular red dots: a novel dermoscopic pattern observed in scalp discoid lupus erythematosus. Arch Dermatol. 2009;145:1406-9.
2. Malakar S. Trichoscopy: A Text and Atlas. New Delhi: Jaypee Brothers Medical Publishers (P) Ltd; 2017.
3. Ross EK, Vincenzi C, Tosti A. Videodermoscopy in the evaluation of hair and scalp disorders. J Am Acad Dermatol. 2006;55:799-806.
4. Lallas A, Apalla Z, Lefaki I, et al. Dermoscopy of discoid lupus erythematosus. Br J Dermatol. 2013;168(2):284-8.
5. Elston DM, McCollough ML, Warschaw KE, et al. Elastic tissue in scars and alopecia. J Cutan Pathol. 2000;27:147-52.
6. Fabbri P, Amato L, Chiarini C, et al. Scarring alopecia in discoid lupus erythematosus: a clinical, histopathologic and immunopathologic study. Lupus. 2004;13:455-62.
7. Al-Refu K, Edward S, Ingham E, et al. Expression of hair follicle stem cells detected by cytokeratin 15 stain: implications for pathogenesis of the scarring process in cutaneous lupus erythematosus. Br J Dermatol. 2009;160:1188-96.
8. Lopez-Tintos BO, Garcia-Hidalgo L, Orozco-Topete R. Dermoscopy in active discoid lupus. Arch Dermatol. 2009;145:358.
9. McKee P, Calonje E, Granter S. Idiopathic connective tissue disorders. In: McKee P (Ed). Pathology of the Skin with Clinical Correlations, 3rd edition. Amsterdam: Elsevier Mosby; 2005. pp. 775-803.
10. Marghoob AA, Cowell L, Kopf AW, et al. Observation of chrysalis structures with polarized dermoscopy. Arch Dermatol. 2009;145:168.
11. Liebman TN, Rabinovitz HS, Balagula Y, et al. White shiny structures in melanoma and BCC. Arch Dermatol. 2012;148(1):146.

LICHEN SCLEROSUS (EXTRAGENITAL)

INTRODUCTION

Lichen sclerosus (LS) is a chronic inflammatory dermatosis of unknown etiology that may involve genital and extragenital areas. In females LS has bimodal onset in prepubertal and postmenopausal age group.[1] The most common presentation in vulvar LS is itching whereas urinary or sexual dysfunction in a case of penile LS.

Lichen sclerosus is characterized by sharply defined, tiny, ivory white, slightly raised, and flat topped papules a few millimeters in diameter that progresses in size and ultimately coalesces into plaques of various sizes (Fig. 30). The diagnosis is usually clinical, but occasionally might be a dilemma in its early stage.[2]

Dermoscopy, a noninvasive tool instantly unveils the subsurface structures as well as highlights the skin surface parameters.

KEY DERMOSCOPIC FEATURES (FIGS. 31 TO 42)

- Comedo-like openings
- White structureless areas
- Chrysalis structures
- Linear branching vessels
- Nonbranching vessels such as dotted, comma like, and hairpin.

DISCUSSION

"Comedo-like openings" appear early in the course of the disease and is the dermoscopic hallmark of extragenital LS; histopathologically it closely corresponds to follicular plugging.[3,4]

White structureless areas represent the predominant dermoscopic feature of LS and indicate epidermal atrophy and fibrosis of the upper dermis (Fig. 43).[4] Chrysalis structure was reported in extragenital LS of a 22-year-old male.[5] In the author's opinion this feature is more common than is reported.

Linear and dotted vessels are commonly observed additional features in the genital and extragenital lesions.[5] Comma vessels and hairpin vessels have been reported in a small number of lesions.[5,6]

KEYNOTE

If there is no genital involvement, the differentiation of LS from other atrophic plaques, especially in the early stage of the disease may be a difficult task. At this point dermoscopy aids in revealing comedo-like openings, that represent an extremely valuable finding; accordingly invasive investigation can be avoided.

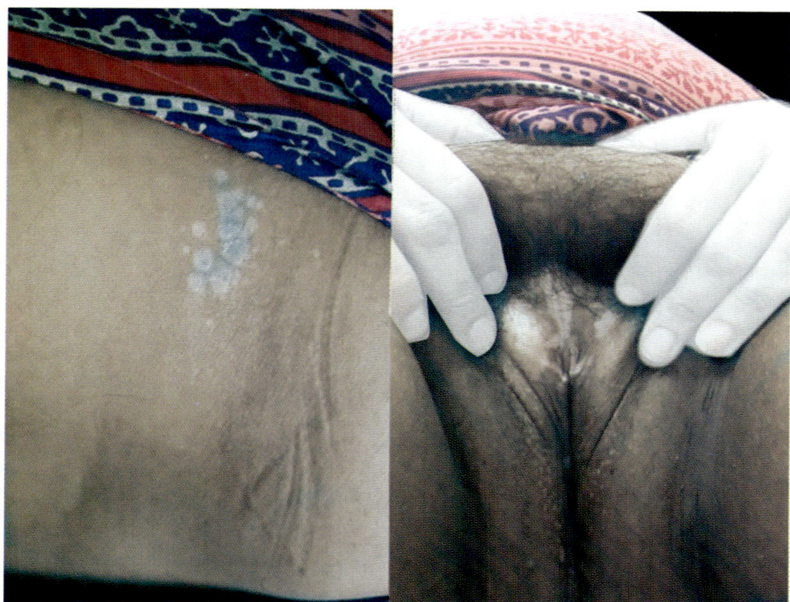

Fig. 30: A lady of 42 years presented with asymptomatic white lesions on middle of her back, gradually increasing in number since the last 8 months. The patient also complained about dyspareunia and vulva itching. On examination, the lesion on trunk revealed multiple ivory white papules and plaques. Examination of the genital area showed the involvement of both the labia majora and minora.

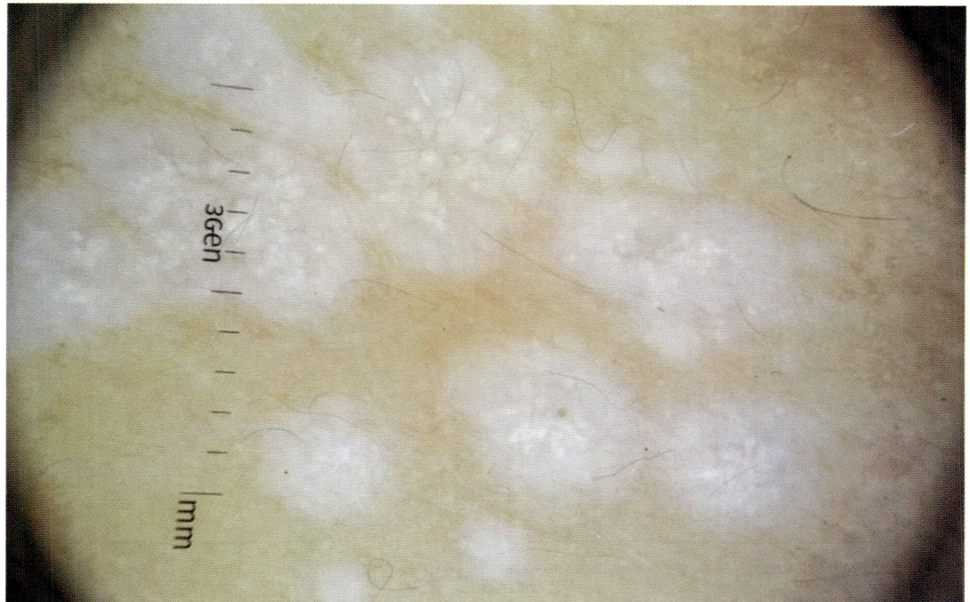

Fig. 31: Comedo-like opening (CLO), white structureless areas (WSAs), and white shiny structures (WSSs).

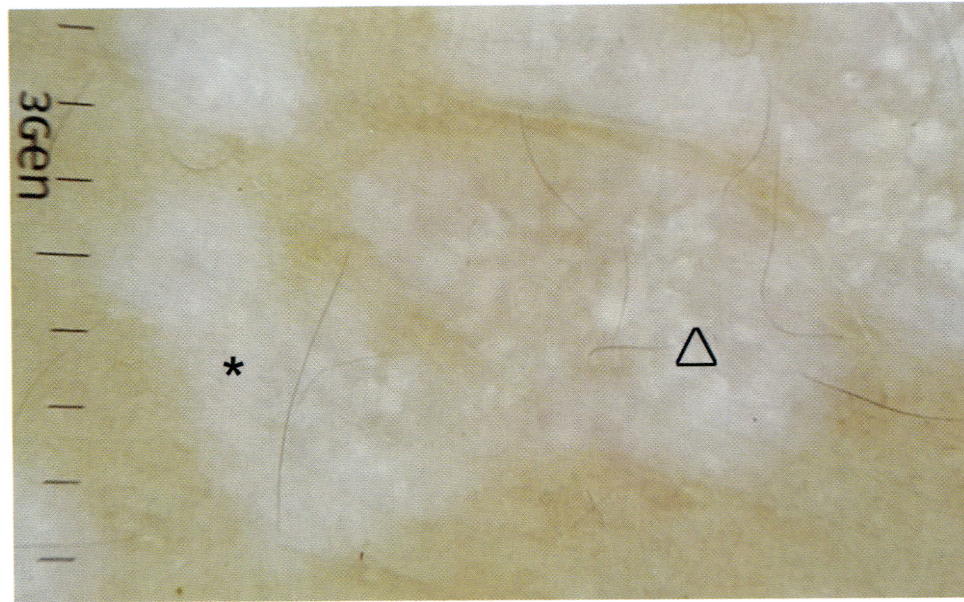

Fig. 32: WSA - star, WSS - triangle. (WSA: White structureless area; WSS: White shiny structure)

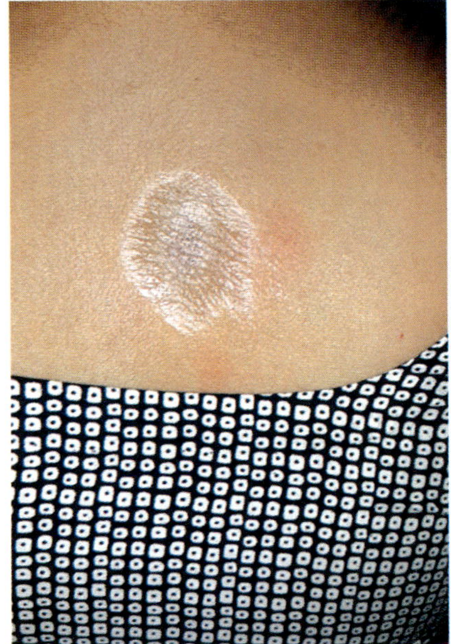

Fig. 33: A 45-year-old lady presented with 1 year history of an asymptomatic ivory white plaque on the upper back; few tiny satellite whitish papules are seen on the lower right side of the plaque.

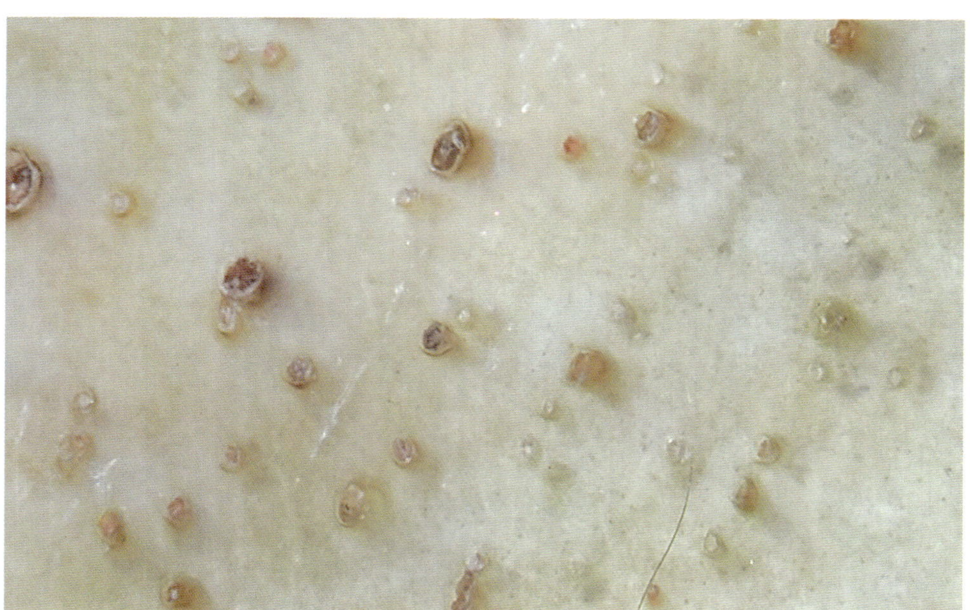

Fig. 34: Comedo-like openings (CLOs) and white structureless area (WSA).

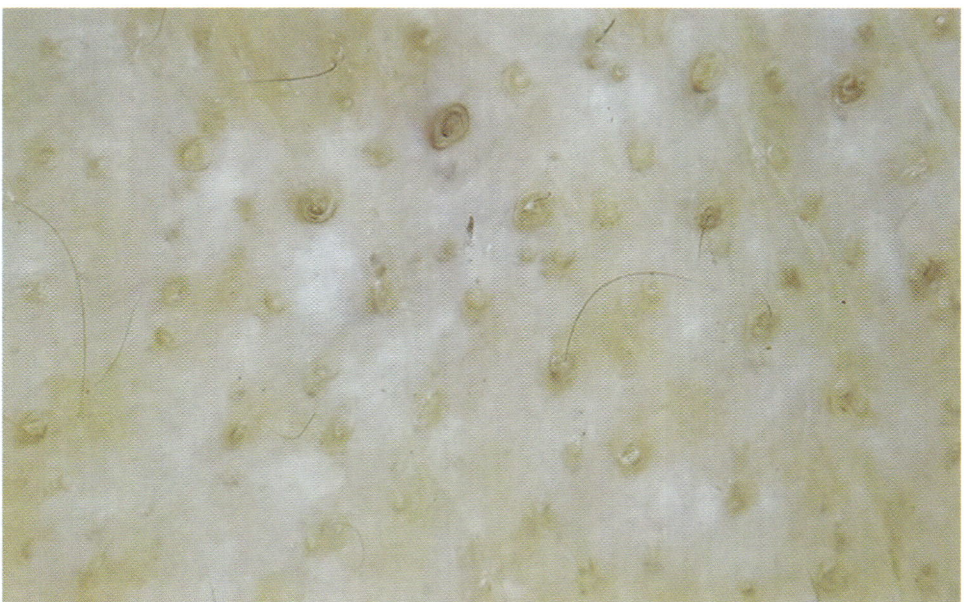

Fig. 35: CLO, WSS. (CLO: Comedo-like opening; WSS: White shiny structure)

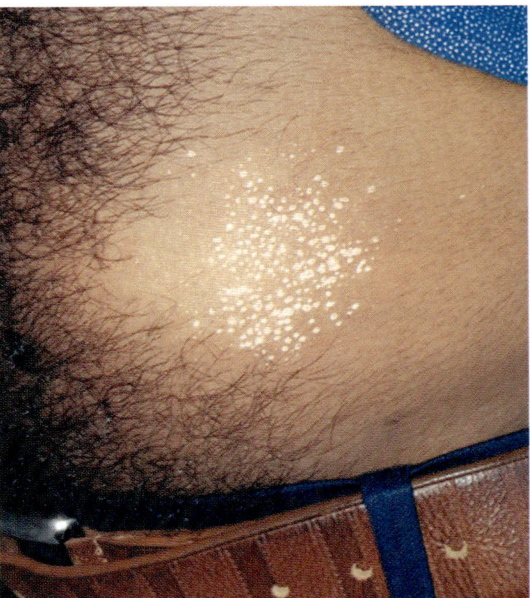

Fig. 36: A 35-year-old male presented with multiple hypopigmented whitish atrophic macules over abdomen for last 5 months.

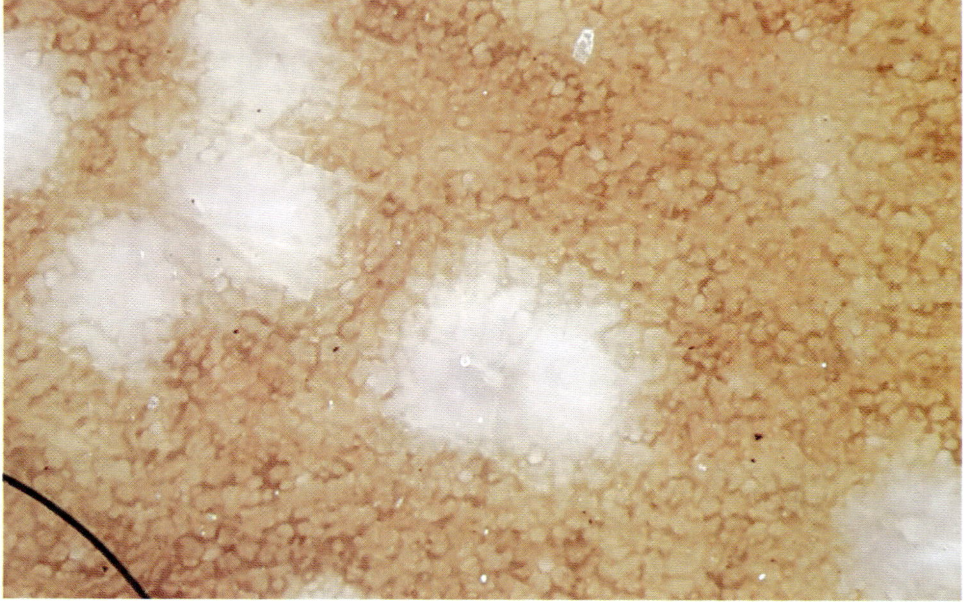

Fig. 37: WSA, CLO. (CLO: Comedo-like opening; WSA: White structureless area)

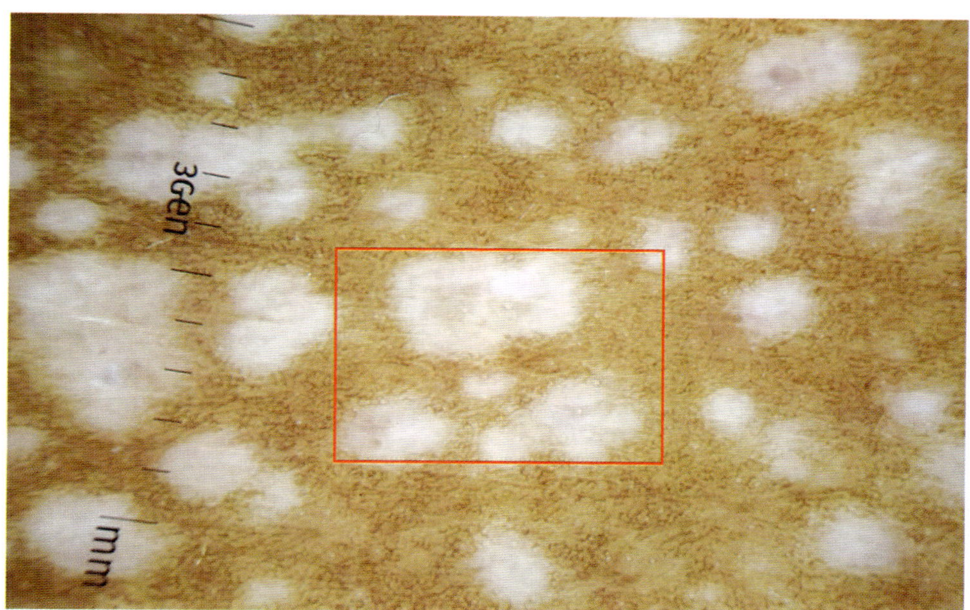

Fig. 38: WSA, CLO. The area in rectangle has been magnified to show the prominent CLO in the next picture. (CLO: Comedo-like opening; WSA: White structureless area)

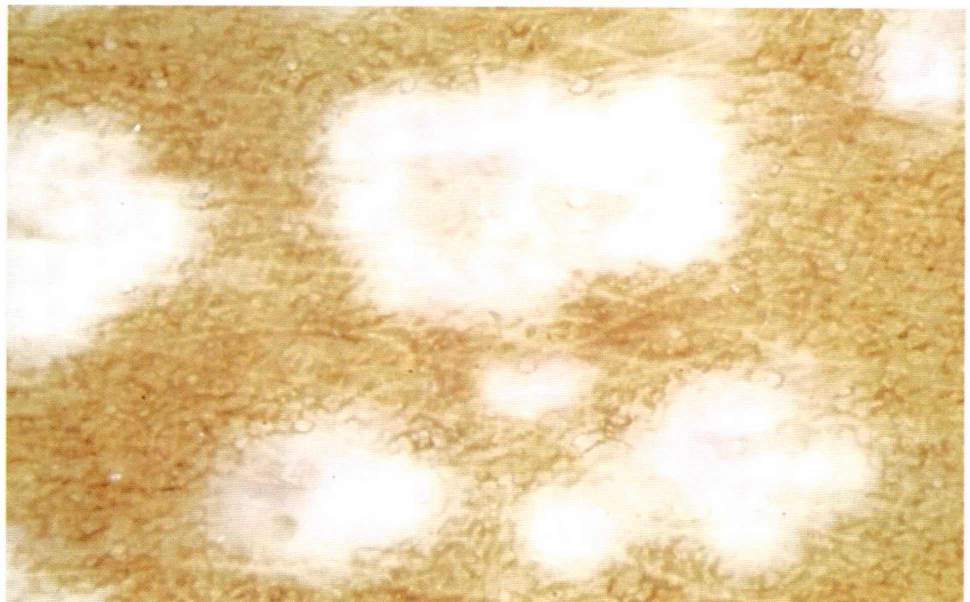

Fig. 39: CLO, WSA. (CLO: Comedo-like opening; WSA: White structureless area)

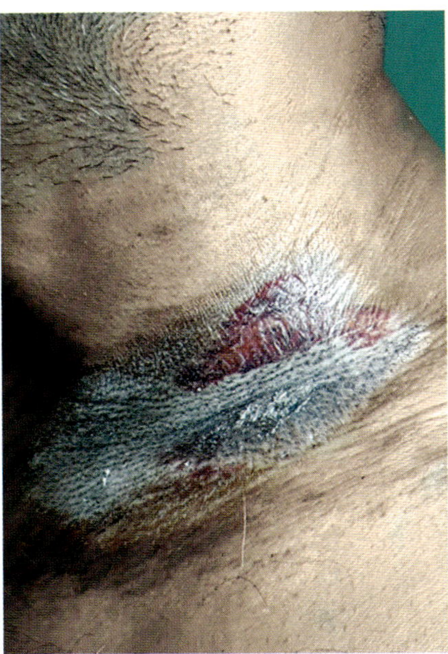

Fig. 40: Extragenital lichen sclerosus (LS) may have an atypical presentation such as development of vesiculobullous lesions that involve predominantly trunk and neck. Presentation with hemorrhagic blisters is less frequent.

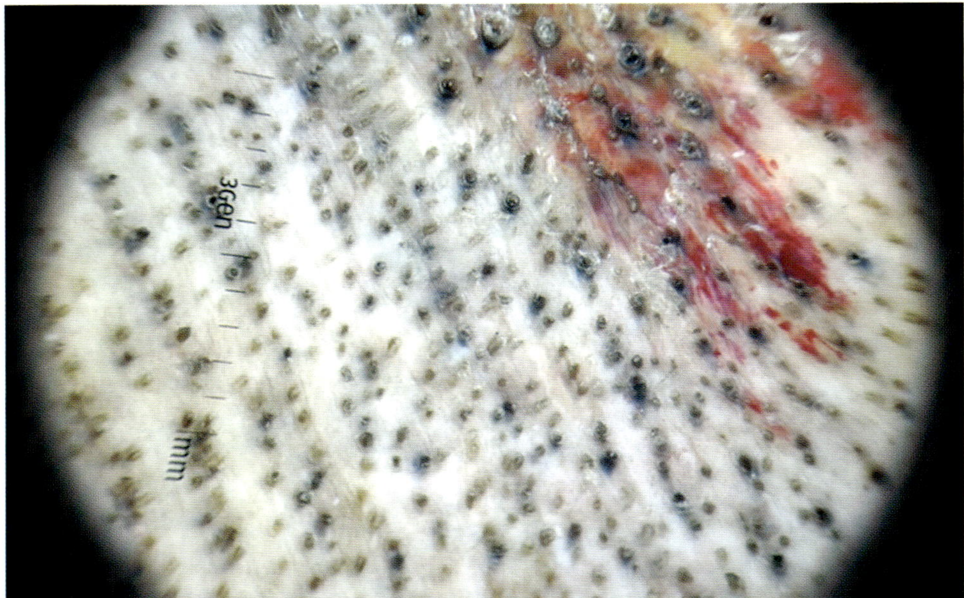

Fig. 41: CLO, WSA, and hemorrhagic area dermoscopically reveals lacunae and orange-yellow areas. (CLO: Comedo-like opening; WSA: White structureless area)

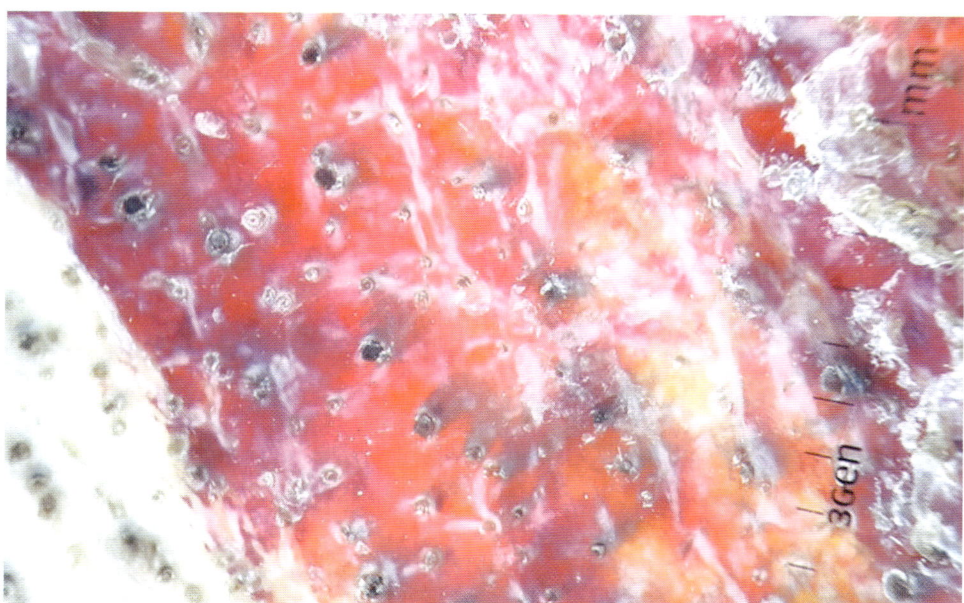

Fig. 42: Orange-yellow areas, white shiny structures, follicular pluggings, and white structureless area (WSA).

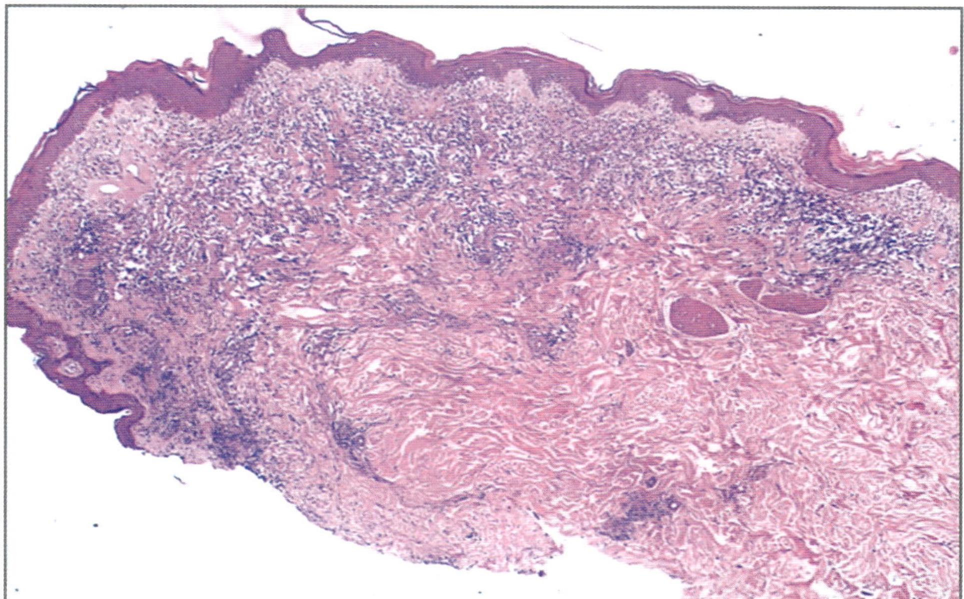

Fig. 43: Scanner view—Biopsy shows lichenoid interface vacuolar dermatitis with epidermal atrophy. The epidermis is compact flat with compact orthokeratosis and follicular plugging. There is dense lichenoid lymphocytic infiltrate with subepidermal hyalinization and subepidermal split at single foci.

REFERENCES

1. Goodfield MJ, Jones SK, Veale DJ. The connective tissue diseases. In: Burns T, Breathnach S, Cox N, Griffiths C (Eds). Rook's Textbook of Dermatology, 8th edition. West Sussex: Wiley-Blackwell; 2010. pp. 112-8.
2. Carlson JA, Lamb P, Malfetano J, et al. Clinicopathologic comparison of vulvar and extragenital lichen sclerosus: Histologic variants, evolving lesions, and etiology of 141 cases. Mod Pathol. 1998;11:844-54.
3. Larre Borges A, Tiodorovic-Zivkovic D, Lallas A, et al. Clinical, dermoscopic and histopathologic features of genital and extragenital lichen sclerosus. J Eur Acad Dermatol Venereol. 2013;27:1433-9.
4. Garrido-Rıos AA, Alvarez-Garrido H, Sanz-Munoz C, et al. Dermoscopy of extragenital lichen sclerosus. Arch Dermatol. 2009;145:1468.
5. Ankad BS, Beergouder SL. Dermoscopic patterns in lichen sclerosus: A report of three cases. Indian Dermatol Online J. 2015;6:237-40.
6. Shim WH, Jwa SW, Song M, et al. Diagnostic usefulness of dermatoscopy in differentiating lichen sclerous et atrophicus from morphea. JAAD. 2012;66:690-1.

MORPHEA

INTRODUCTION

It is an autoimmune disorder characterized clinically by localized plaques of cutaneous sclerosis.[1] Superficial plaque type morphea begins as skin-colored, erythematous patches which evolve into firm, hyperpigmented, or ivory-colored plaques with or without a surrounding lilac inflammatory zone; in darker skin the lilac zone is difficult to appreciate (Fig. 44).

The ivory plaques may resemble LS. Dermoscopy is very helpful in differentiating the two conditions.

KEY DERMOSCOPIC FEATURES (FIGS. 45 TO 54)

Superficial Morphea

- White fibrotic beam
- Linear branching vessels
- White shiny structures (personal observation).

Deep Morphea (Personal Observation)

- Fibrotic beams
- Pigment patterns include pigmentation around hair follicles, spoke and wheel pattern, and dots and globules
- Linear vessels
- Few white shiny structures.

DISCUSSION

The hallmark of dermoscopic features of morphea consists of white fibrotic beams, which are frequently crossed by linear branching vessels. The fibrotic beams indicate dermal sclerosis on histopathology.[2] In some lesions, white shiny structures are also observed (Figs. 55 and 56).

KEYNOTE

Sometimes differentiation of morphea and LS, especially in extragenital sites, is a diagnostic dilemma. Before performing histopathology, dermoscopy may solve the problem. Because both the conditions show characteristic dermoscopic findings, to differentiate between them, morphea is characterized by fibrotic beams and crossing linear vessels while LS reveals comedo-like openings and white patches.

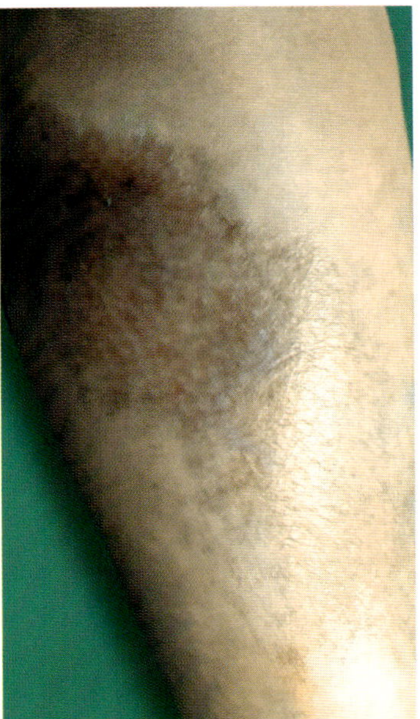

Fig. 44: The patient presented with an asymptomatic hyperpigmented plaque on her elbow since past 6.5 months. Onset was insidious.

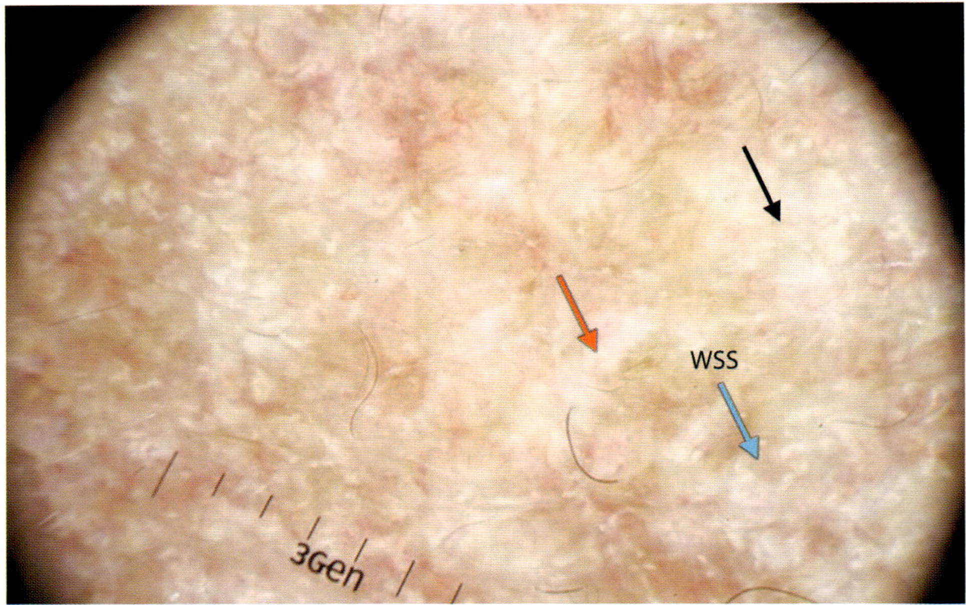

Fig. 45: Dermoscopy reveals fibrotic beams (red arrow). Linear vessels are also seen in the upper and extreme right side of the field. Some of the vessels are seen crossing the fibrotic beams (black arrow). White shiny structures (WSS) are also present.

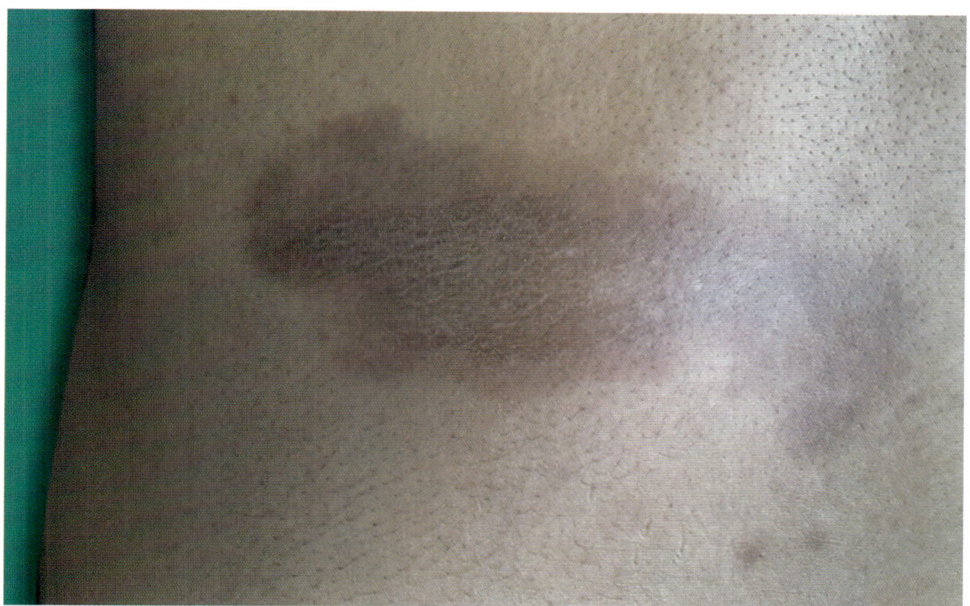

Fig. 46: A case of circumscribed superficial morphea.

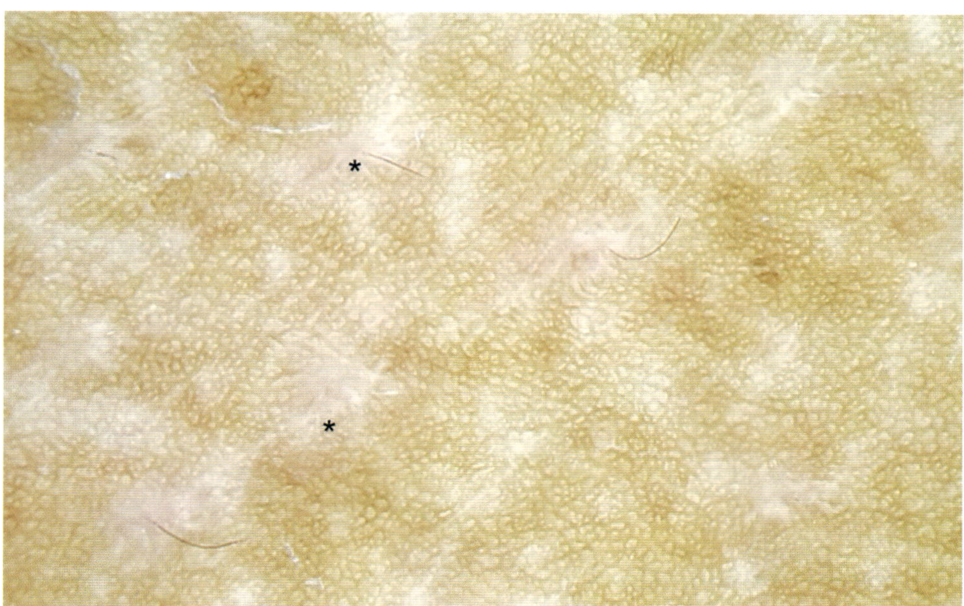

Fig. 47: Fibrotic beams are only visible dermoscopically here (stars). Note: The honeycomb appearance of the melanocytic network.

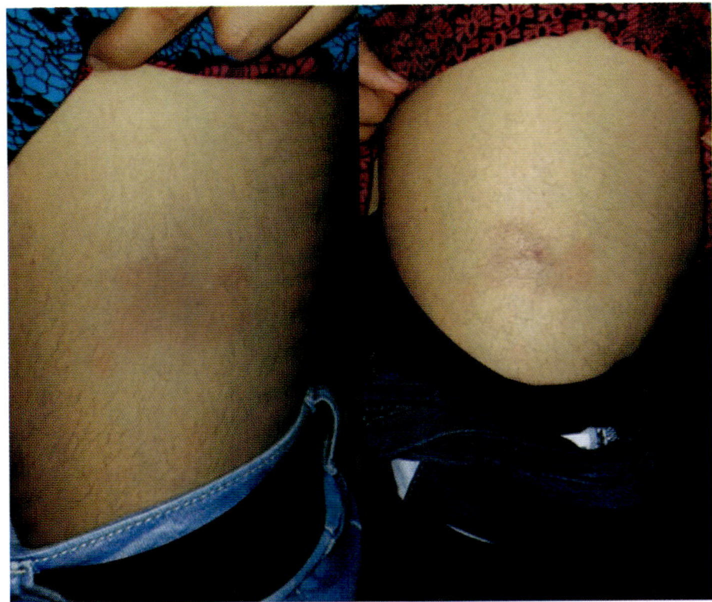

Fig. 48: A young female presented with an asymptomatic erythematous patch over the left thigh since 4 months.

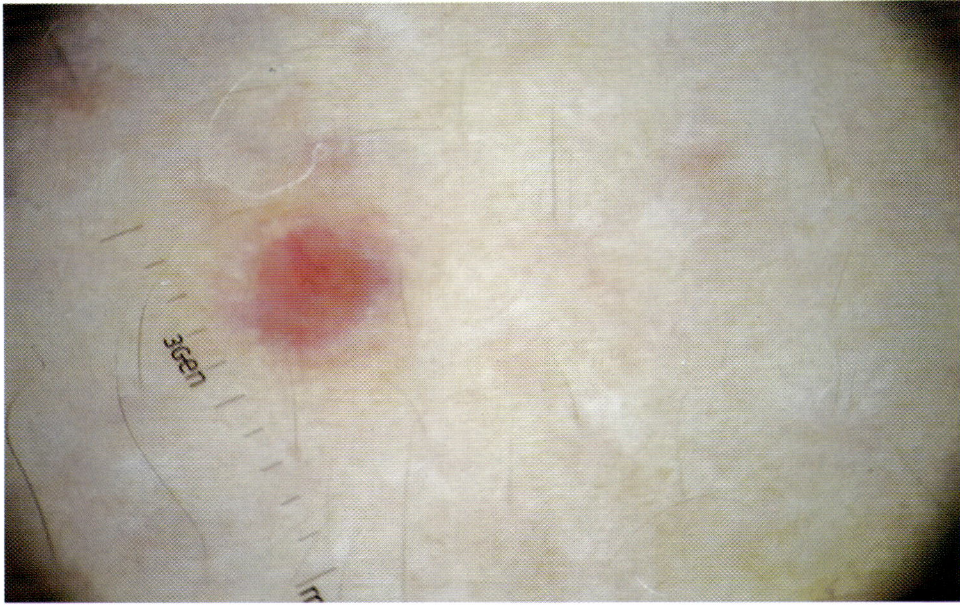

Fig. 49: Fibrotic beams.

Fig. 50: Fibrotic beams (star) and some faint linear vessels.

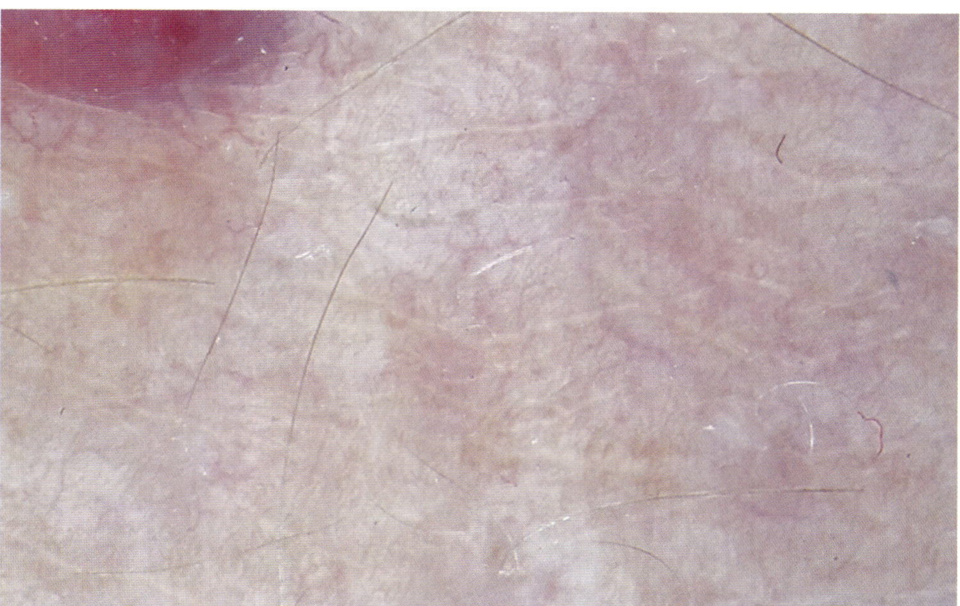

Fig. 51: Linear vessels and fibrotic beams. Note: The intense erythema at the extreme upper left corner (site of biopsy).

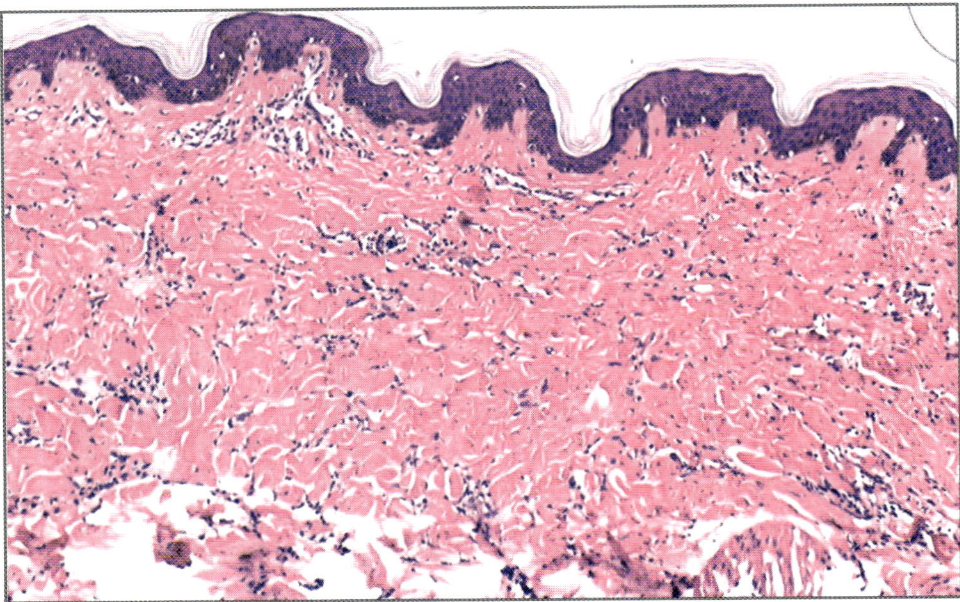

Fig. 52: The biopsy shows sparse superficial and deep perivascular and interstitial lymphocytic infiltrate with occasional plasma cells. There is marked thickening of collagen bundles in reticular and papillary dermis. The thickened bundles are closely packed so as to give hyalinized appearance.

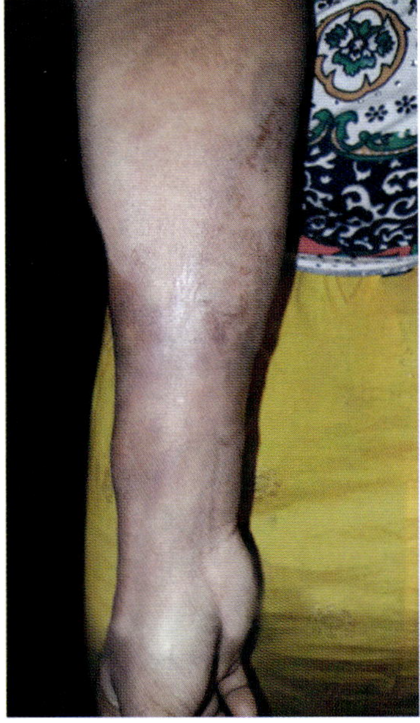

Fig. 53: Panniculitic morphea. Deep variant of morphea primarily involves the deep layers of skin such as fascia and muscle and is characterized by bound down sclerotic plaque. The epidermis may be indurated or atrophic, or may remain uninvolved. The lesions are typically hyperpigmented.

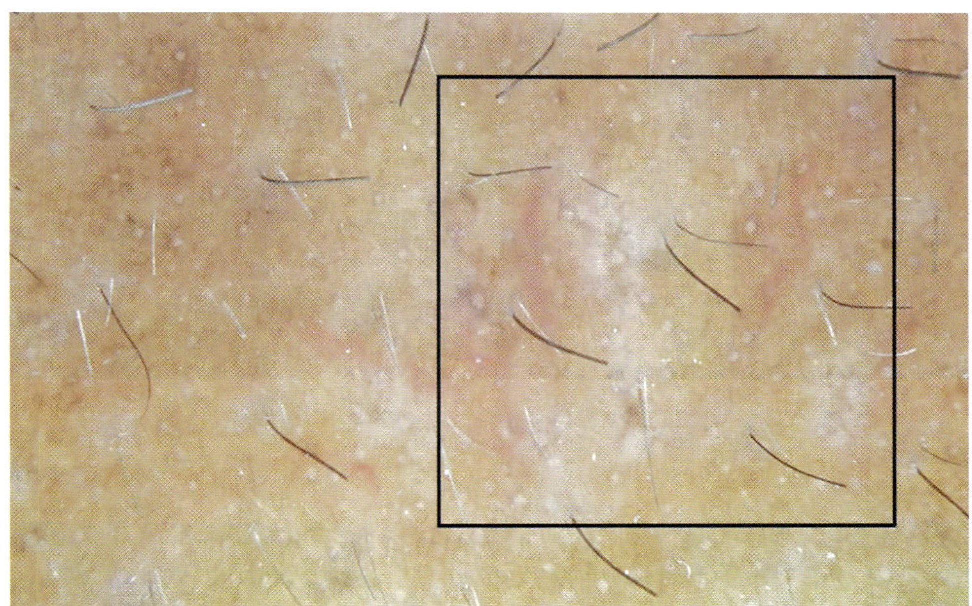

Fig. 54: Fibrotic beams, white shiny structures (WSS). Pigment structures include pigmentation around sweat glands/follicles, spoke and wheel pattern, and dots and globules, vascular pattern reveals linear vessels. Rosettes are also visible. The area in black square has been magnified in the next figure to show the features more significantly.

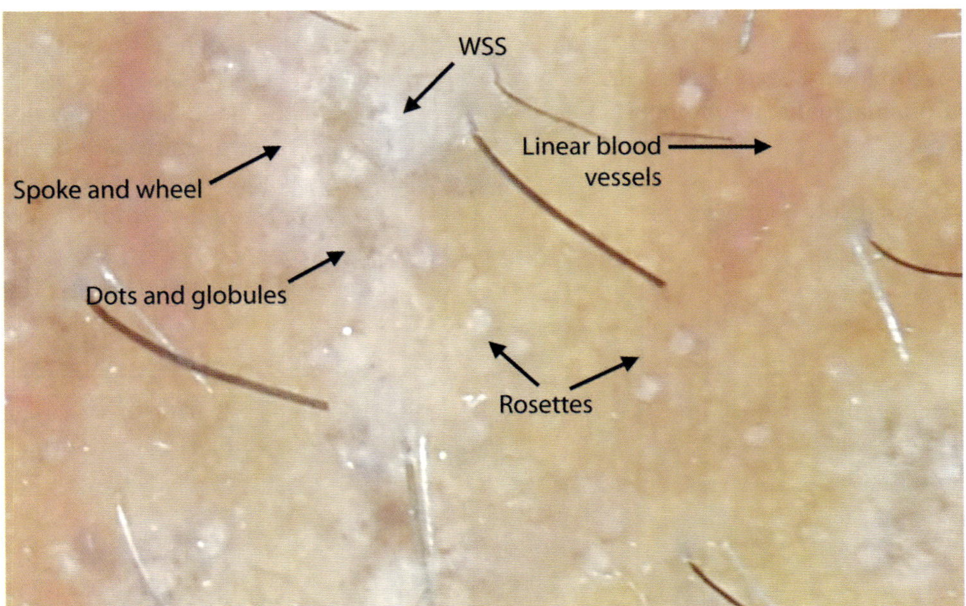

Fig. 55: Another dermoscopic field of the same patient (WSS: White shiny structures).

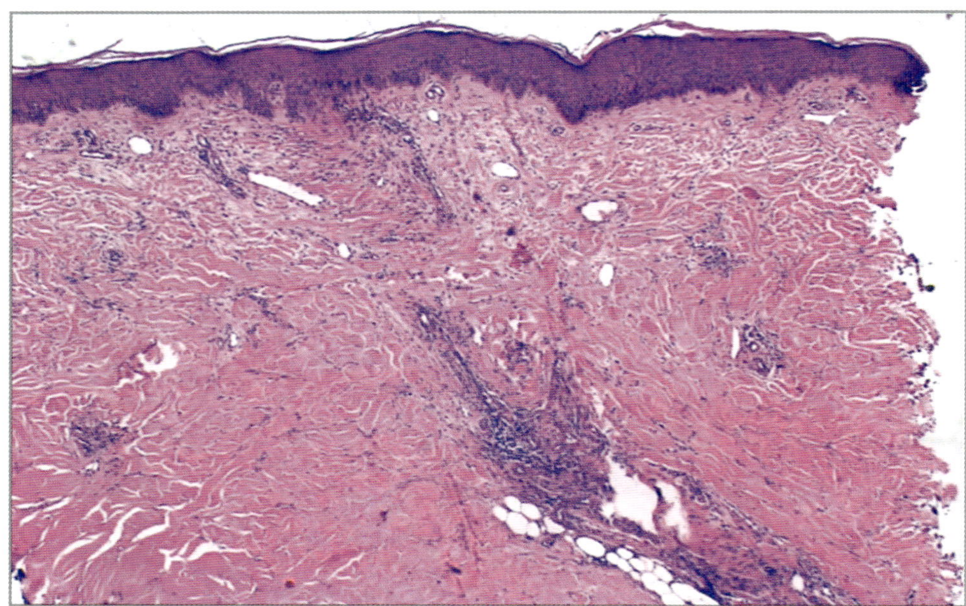

Fig. 56: Biopsy shows sparse superficial and deep perivascular and periappendageal lymphohistiocytic infiltrate with occasional plasma cells. There is marked thickening of collagen bundles in reticular and papillary dermis. The thickened bundles are closely packed so as to give hyalinized appearance. The upper reticular dermis shows telangiectasia and eccrine units appear to be present in the thickened midreticular dermis. The subcutaneous fat shows marked septal thickening with hyalinization of collagen and moderately dense lymphoplasmocytic infiltrate.

REFERENCES

1. Pope E, Laxer RM. Diagnosis and management of morphea and lichen sclerosus and atrophicus in children. Pediatr Clin North Am. 2014;61(2):309-19.
2. Shim WH, Jwa SW, Song M, et al. Diagnostic usefulness of dermatoscopy in differentiating lichen sclerous et atrophicus from morphea. JAAD. 2012;66:690-1.

SYSTEMIC LUPUS ERYTHEMATOSUS

INTRODUCTION

Cutaneous manifestations of systemic lupus erythematosus (SLE) include malar rash, photosensitivity, and discoid lupus. Discoid lesions can develop in 25% of patients with SLE. It was reported that patients with discoid lesions rarely progressed to SLE.

Hair loss is a typical complaint in patients with SLE. Presentations may be acute telogen effluvium (TE), patchy nonscarring alopecia, or patchy scarring alopecia (discoid LE).

KEY DERMOSCOPIC FEATURES[1]

- Dermoscopic features due to discoid lesions (described in *discoid lupus erythematosus* section).
- Dilated telangiectatic vessels.
- *Scalp:* Enlarged branching vessels, red dots, keratotic plugs, speckled pigmentation, and upright regrowing hairs.
- *Nail:* Dilated tortuous vessels, cuticle hemorrhage.

CASE 1 (FIGS. 57 AND 58)

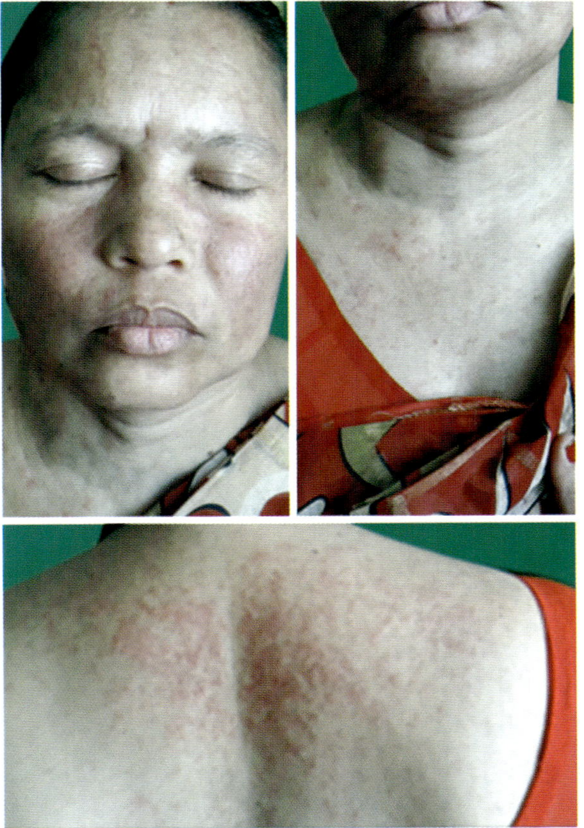

Fig. 57: A patient of systemic lupus erythematosus (SLE) with malar rash and photosensitive rash.

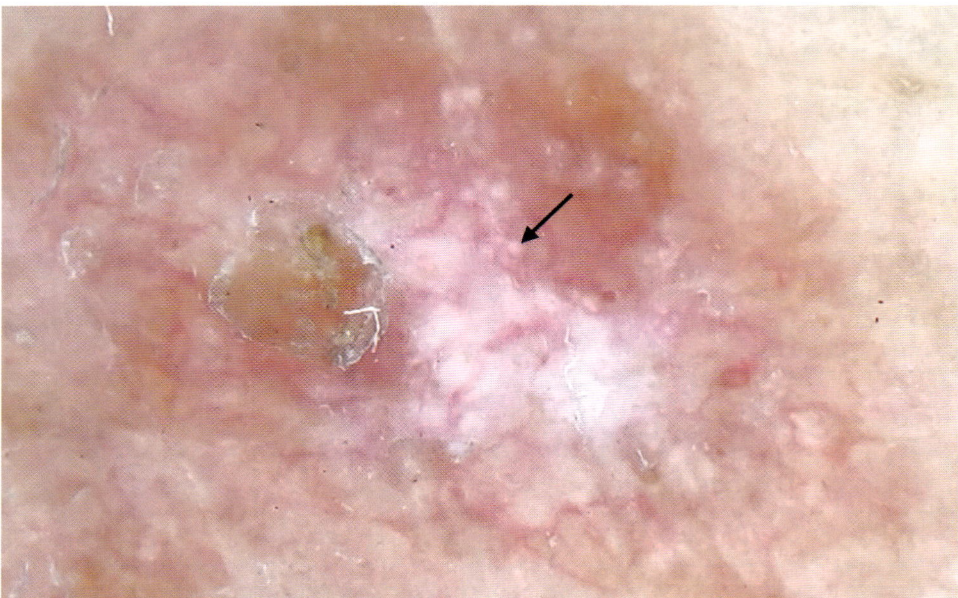

Fig. 58: Dermoscopy of rash on chest show follicular plugging, enlarged branching vessels, whitish area, and rosette-like structures (arrow).

CASE 2 (FIGS. 59 TO 64)

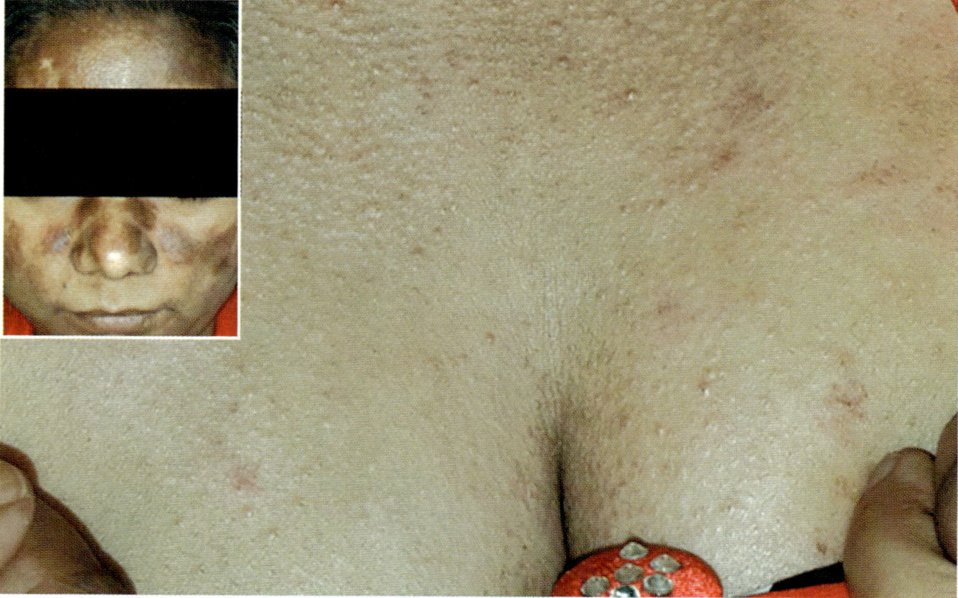

Fig. 59: A patient of systemic lupus erythematosus (SLE) showing butterfly rash and scaly erythematous rash on chest.

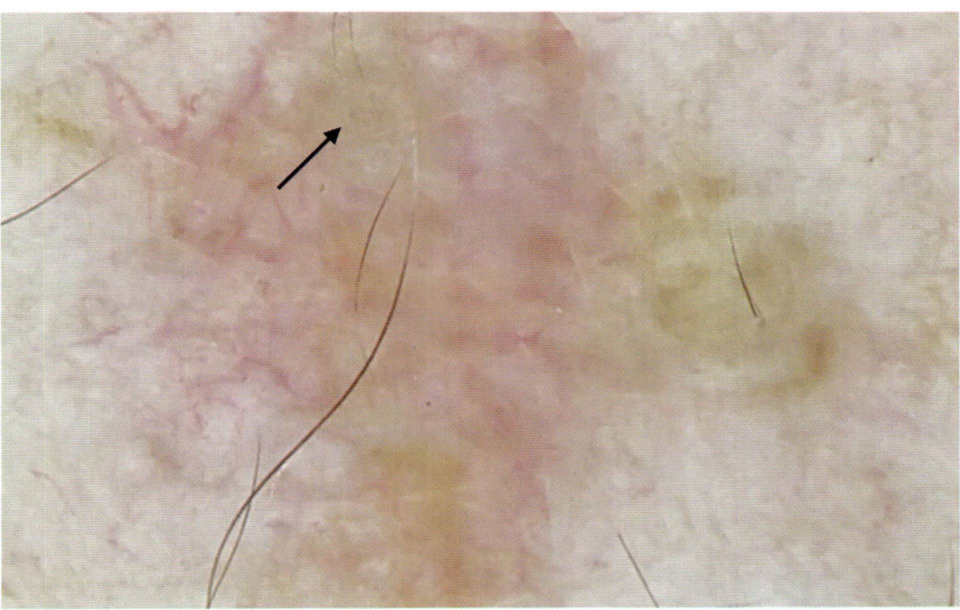

Fig. 60: Dermoscopy of the lesions over chest reveals dilated enlarged vessels, follicular plugging (arrow), and some pigmentation structures, which correspond to the interface dermatitis and pigment incontinence on histopathology.

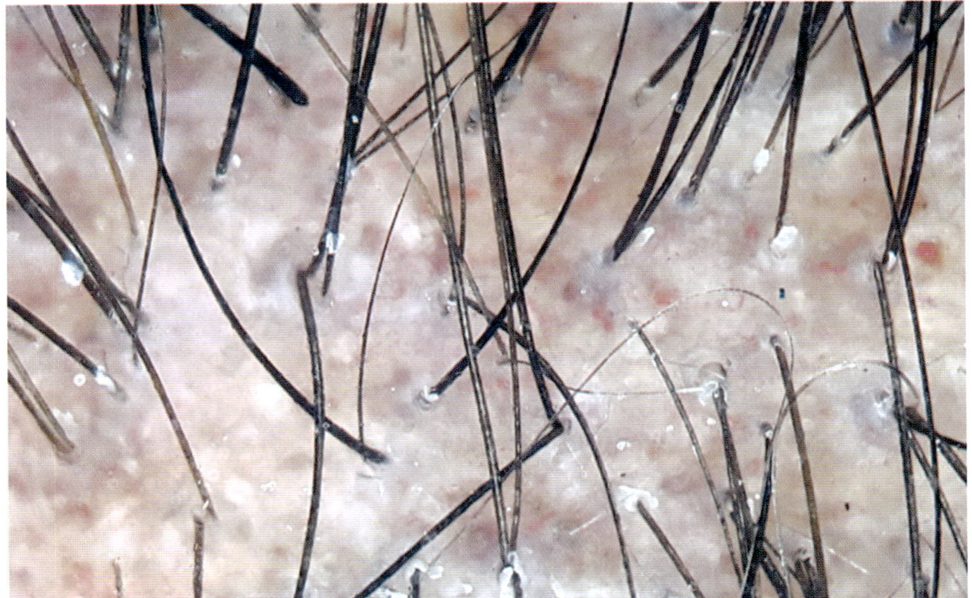

Fig. 61: Dermoscopy of scalp shows dilated vessels, red dots, and follicular plugs associated with grayish speckled pigmentation.

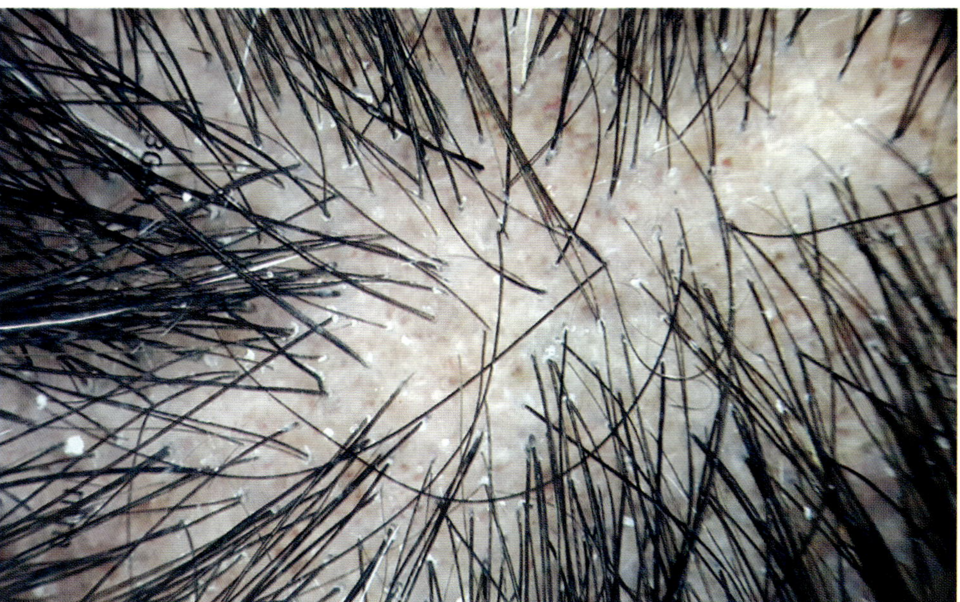

Fig. 62: On scalp grayish speckled pigmentation is seen interfollicularly along with some vascular structures.

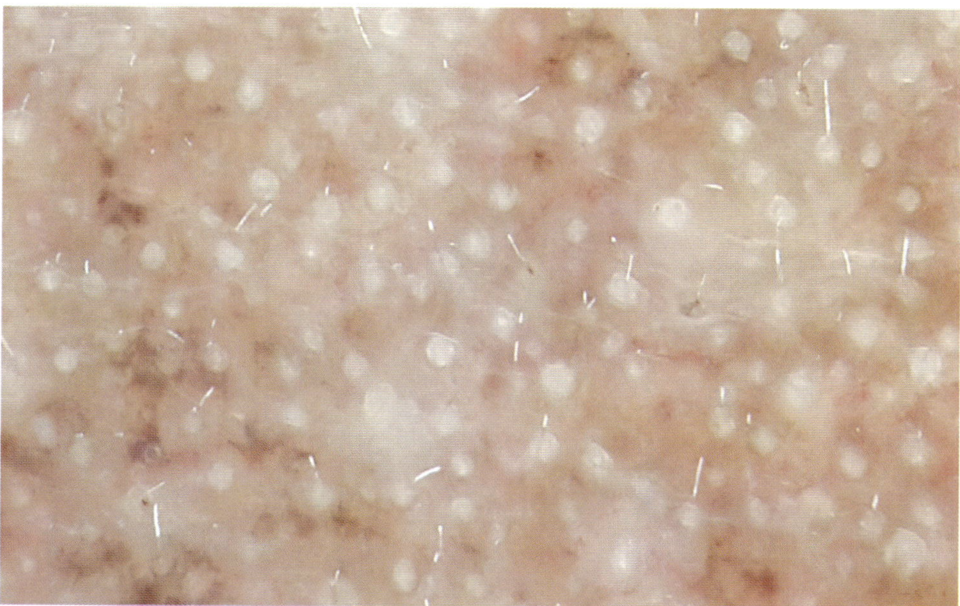

Fig. 63: Dermoscopy of facial rash showing numerous rosettes, which are nonspecific features of many conditions. Note: Background erythema.

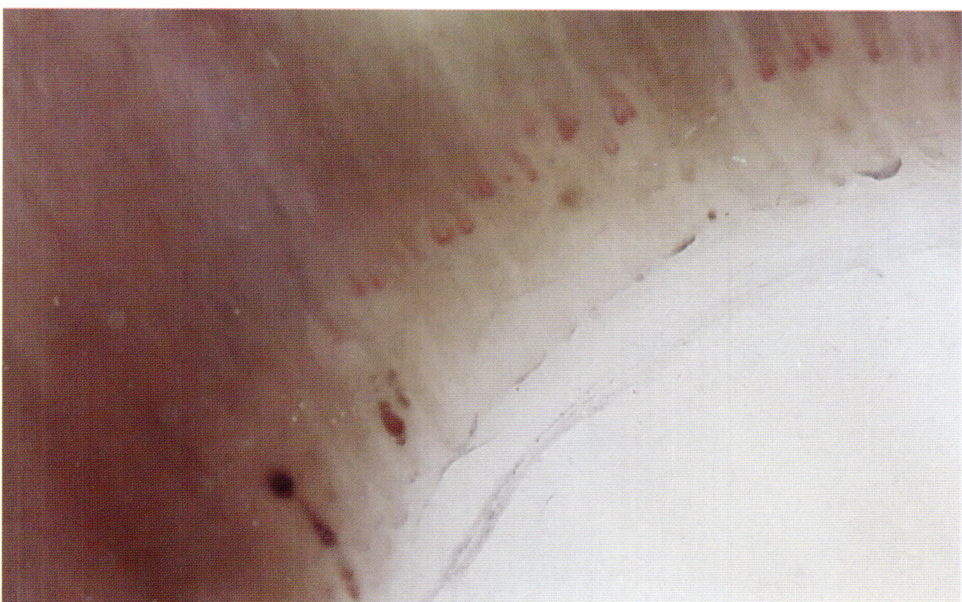

Fig. 64: Dilated tortuous capillaries and cuticular hemorrhage are seen on dermoscopy of the nails.

CASE 3 (FIGS. 65 TO 68)

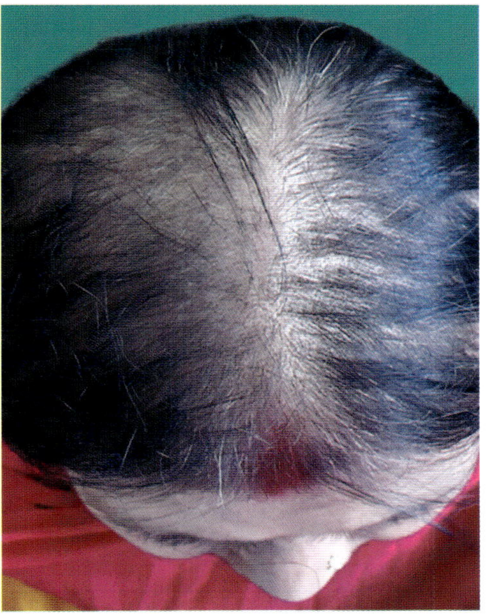

Fig. 65: Pretreatment clinical picture of a patient of systemic lupus erythematosus (SLE) showing diffuse nonscarring alopecia over scalp.

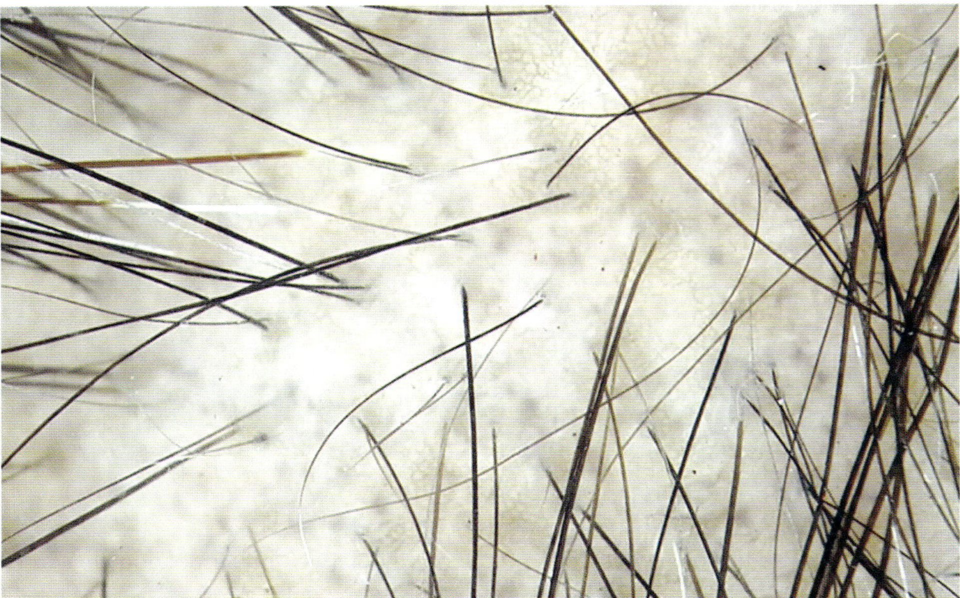

Fig. 66: Trichoscopic image of the previous patient showing predominance of single hair-bearing follicles, reduced hair follicle density. Also note upright regrowing hairs which indicates telogen effluvium.

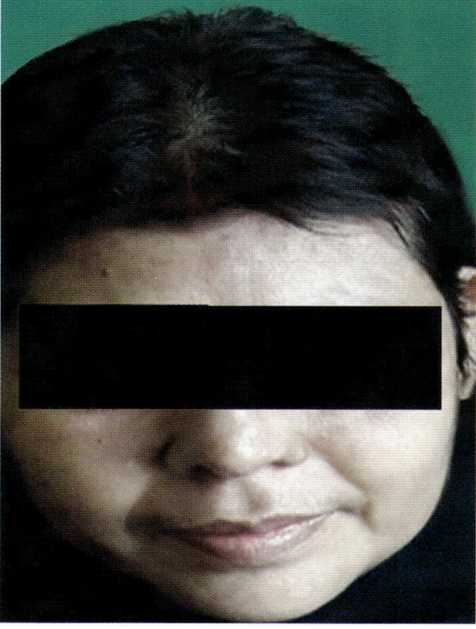

Fig. 67: After 4 months of treatment, the same patient showing remarkable improvement in the diffuse alopecia.

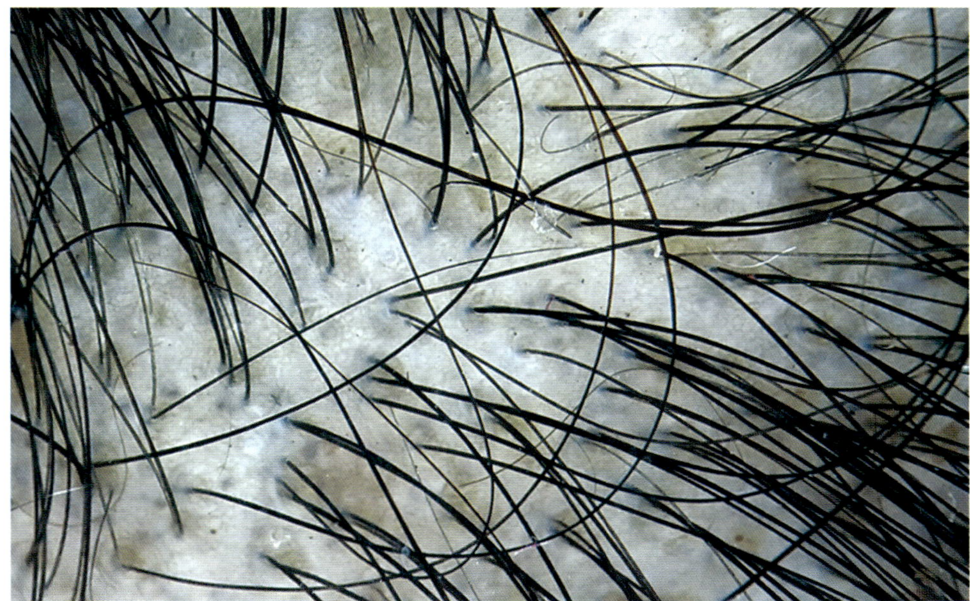

Fig. 68: Trichoscopic image of the same patient (posttreatment) showing increased hair density. Please note the increased number of two and three unit hair follicles as well as remarkable reduction of blue-gray dots.

REFERENCE

1. Souvik S, Malakar S. Trichoscopy in autoimmune connective tissue diseases. In: Malakar S (Ed). Trichoscopy: A Text and Atlas. New Delhi: Jaypee Brothers Medical Publishers (P) Ltd; 2017. p. 300.

CHAPTER 11

Granulomatous Dermatoses

Subrata Malakar, Jayasree Puravoor

INTRODUCTION

The dermoscopic marker of granulomatous skin diseases (GSDs) is the orange-yellow patches of round or oval shape. In darker skin, the orange-yellow patches may be masked by different shades of brown color, or the patches may have brown-yellow shades instead of orange yellow (personal observation). This dermoscopic pattern is highly indicative of dermal granulomas such as sarcoidosis, lupus vulgaris, cutaneous leishmaniasis, and granulomatous rosacea.

Granulomatous skin diseases have additional features like linear or branching vessels, however, in granuloma annulare vascular features are less evident or absent.

Dermoscopy may give a guide to the diagnosis of GSDs but histological assessment is needed to reach a definitive diagnosis of the different GSDs.

CUTANEOUS LEISHMANIASIS

INTRODUCTION

Cutaneous leishmaniasis (CL) is caused by different species of *Leishmania*, which are transmitted by sandflies. The lesion appears usually over the face and limbs and presents as a slow growing, erythematous papule, or nodule, which ultimately forms a central crust and ulcer. CL usually appears on uncovered areas such as face and limbs.

The diagnosis is confirmed by the demonstration of amastigotes in the infected lesion or by the growth of promastigotes in culture medium.[1-3] Dermoscopy can refine the clinical diagnosis of CL.

KEY DERMOSCOPIC FEATURES[4]

- Generalized erythema
- Hyperkeratosis
- Central erosion/ulceration
- Yellow tears
- White starburst-like pattern
- Vascular structures like comma vessels, linear irregular vessels, dotted vessels, hairpin vessels, and polymorphous vessels.

DISCUSSION

Erythema is the most frequent dermoscopic feature seen in CL. Generalized erythema and vascular structures present in all the lesions and correspond histologically to the dilated and telangiectatic vessels. Erosions, ulcerations, and hyperkeratosis are present in more than one-third of the cases toward the late phase of the disease. In more than 50% of cases of CL, "yellow tears" may be seen which corresponds to the follicular plugging; tumoral lesion of CL compresses the hair follicle laterally by its growth. "White starburst-like" pattern is attributed to the hyperkeratosis and parakeratosis around the lesion. Among the vascular lesions, the most frequent pattern reported is comma vessels. Linear irregular, dotted, polymorphous/atypical, arborizing, corkscrew, and glomerular vascular patterns have also been described in the lesions of CL. At least one vascular feature is present in every lesion.

Lambrich et al.[4] have described two main dermoscopic patterns during different stages of the lesion. CL begins with a papular lesion, which shows yellow tears and vascular structures. In more advanced CL, that consists of tumoral lesion with central ulceration/crust, there is hyperkeratosis with starburst pattern, erosion/ulceration and vascular structures at the periphery. Occasionally a combination of these two patterns is seen.

REFERENCES

1. Garcia-Almagro D. Leishmaniasis cutanea. Actas Dermosifiliogr. 2005;96:1-24.
2. Herwaldt BL. Leishmaniasis. Lancet. 1999;354:1191-9.
3. Vega-Lopez F. Diagnosis of cutaneous leishmaniasis. Curr Opin Infect Dis. 2003;16:97-101.
4. Lambrich A, Zaballos P, Terrasa F, et al. Dermoscopy of cutaneous leishmaniasis. Br J Dermatol. 2009;160(4):756-61.

CUTANEOUS SARCOIDOSIS

INTRODUCTION

Sarcoidosis is a multisystem granulomatous disease characterized histologically by the presence of noncaseating epithelioid granulomas. Cutaneous sarcoidosis occurs in up to one-third of patients with systemic sarcoidosis. Because sarcoidosis can exhibit different morphologies, it is known as the great imitator in dermatology. Specific presentations include papules, plaques, scar sarcoidosis, lupus pernio, etc. (Figs. 1 and 2).

Correct diagnosis of sarcoidosis may be a challenge.

KEY DERMOSCOPIC FEATURES (FIGS. 3 TO 7)

- Orange-yellow areas
- Linear vessels
- Central scar-like areas
- Rosettes.

KEYNOTE

The dermoscopic detection of orange-yellow areas is suggestive of granulomatous skin disease that includes sarcoidosis, cutaneous tuberculosis, leishmaniasis, and granulomatous rosacea. However, a biopsy is a must to differentiate between them.

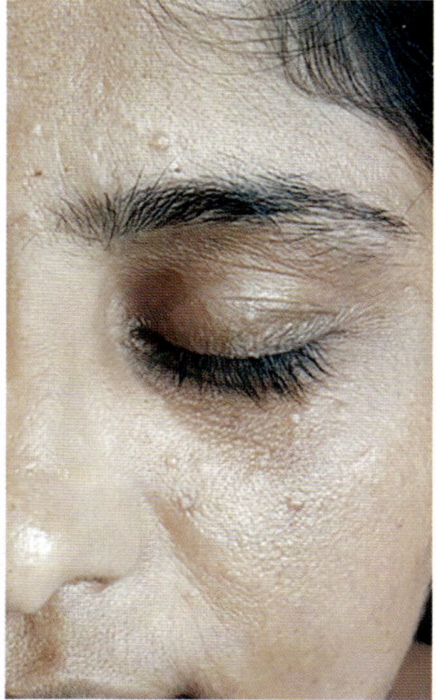

Fig. 1: A 32-year-old lady presented with asymptomatic skin lesions over the face since 7 months which was not earlier treated.

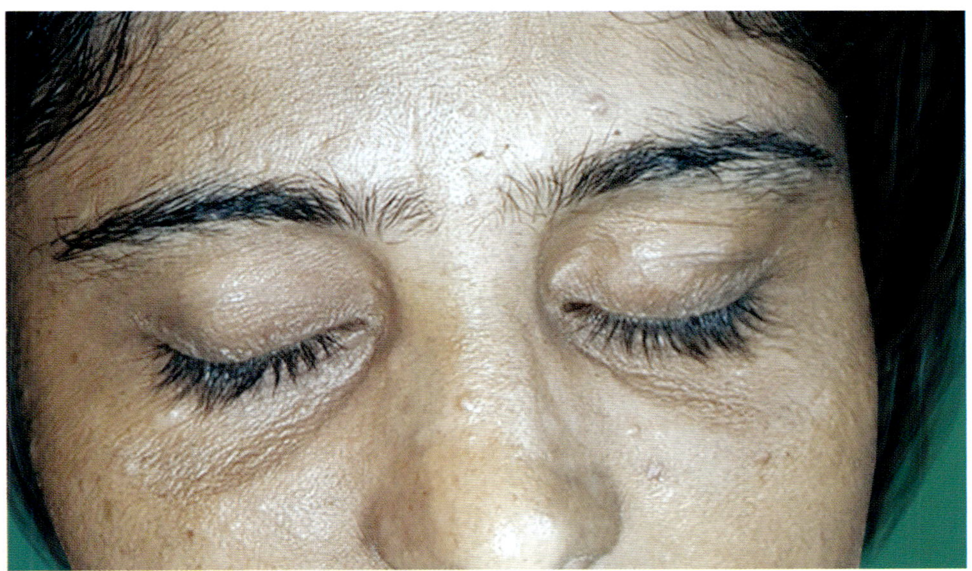

Fig. 2: Cutaneous examination showing multiple skin-colored papular lesions distributed over the upper half of the face.

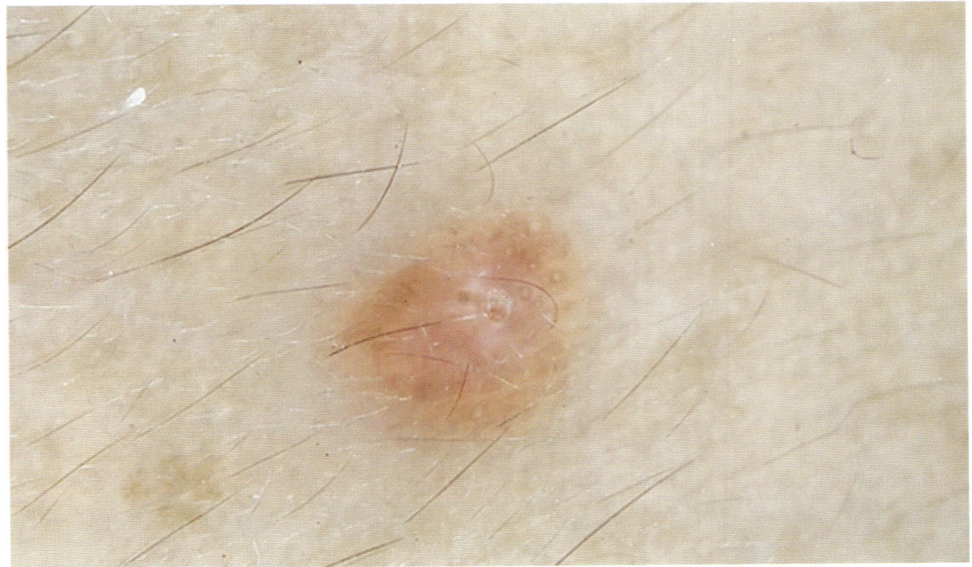

Fig. 3: Dermoscopy reveals orange-yellow background and central whitish scar-like area.

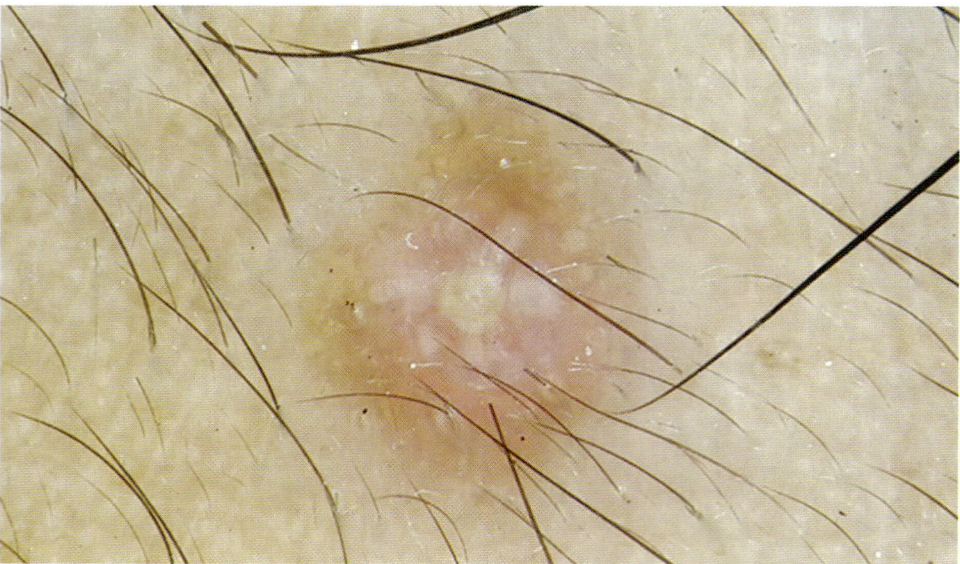

Fig. 4: Central scar-like area.

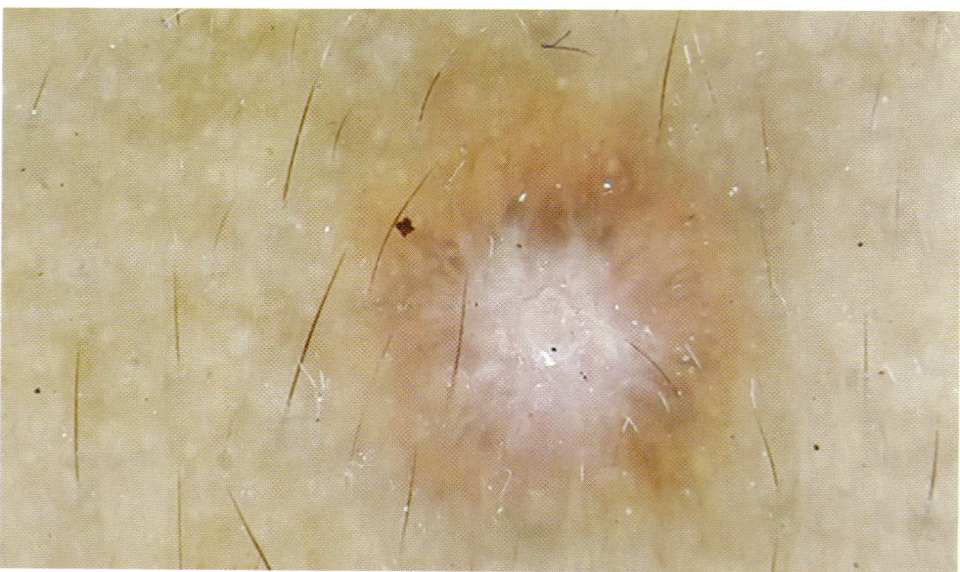

Fig. 5: Central scar-like area and linear vessels. Background color is orange-yellow.

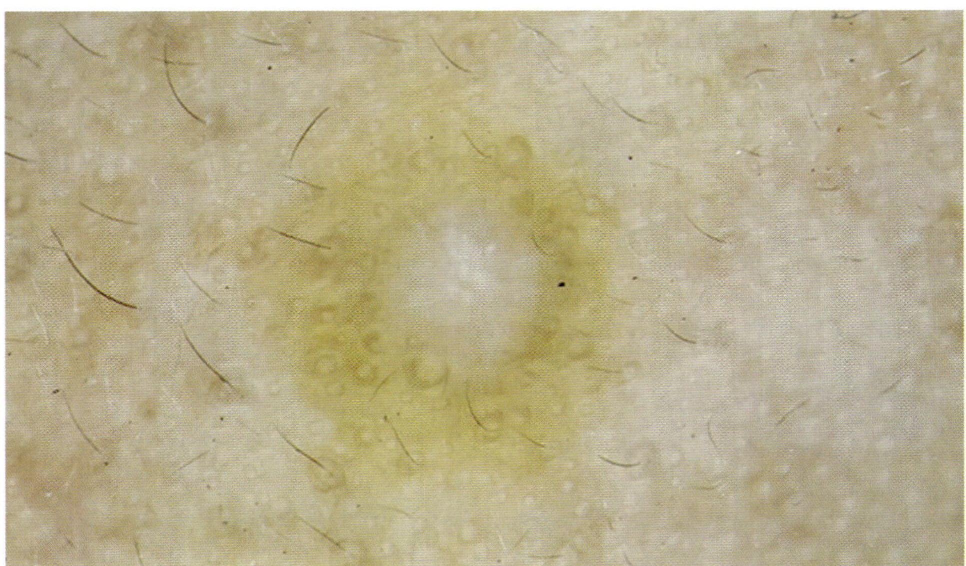

Fig. 6: Dermoscopy of a papule of sarcoid shows a classical rosette.

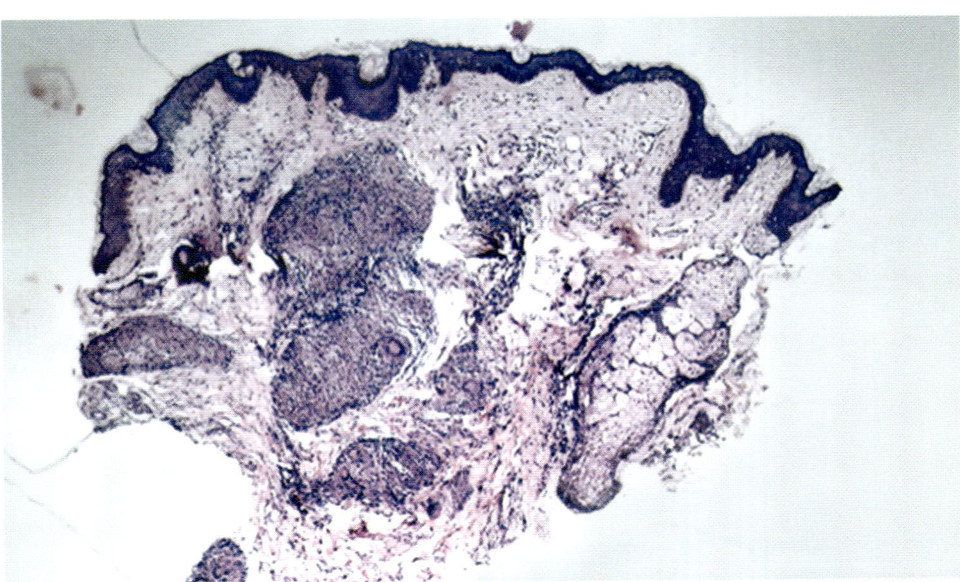

Fig. 7: Biopsy shows nodular tuberculoid granulomatous inflammation throughout the upper dermis. Granuloma consists of lymphocytes, histiocytes, epithelioid cells, and occasional Langhans and foreign body giant cells. Overlying epidermis shows focal thinning. There are no organisms seen. A nerve in deep dermis is spared by the granuloma. Impression: Consistent with sarcoidosis.

GRANULOMA ANNULARE[1-3]

INTRODUCTION

Granuloma annulare (GA) usually presents clinically as an annular plaque without scales, the border of which consists of numerous small papules (Figs. 8 to 11). Several clinical variants of GA have been recognized such as localized, generalized, subcutaneous, perforating and arcuate dermal erythema. Type IV cell-mediated immunity, immune complex vasculitis, and abnormality of tissue monocytes are proposed mechanism of pathogenesis.

KEY DERMOSCOPIC FEATURES (FIGS. 12 TO 16)

- Peripheral structureless orange-reddish borders
- Unfocused vessel.

DISCUSSION

Dermoscopy of GA is characterized by peripheral yellow-orange rim surrounding the structureless center. It usually lacks vessels but when present, they include unfocused vessels with variable appearance such as dotted, branching, and linear-irregular vascular patterns on a reddish-pink background. Yellow-orange at the periphery corresponds to the "palisading granuloma" on histology.

KEYNOTE

Evaluation using dermoscopy often help to narrow the clinical differentials. This is true for necrobiosis lipoidica (NL) and GA when investigating using dermoscopy; arborizing vessels are present in NL whereas in GA vessels are scant to absent.[4]

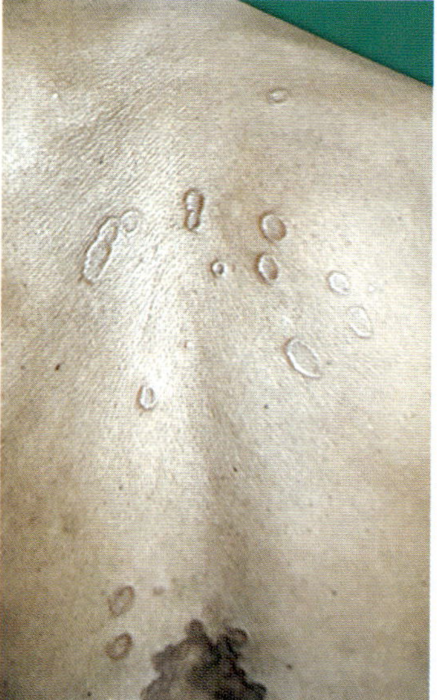

Fig. 8: A middle-aged man presented with erythematous annular lesions with mild pruritus of 9 months duration.

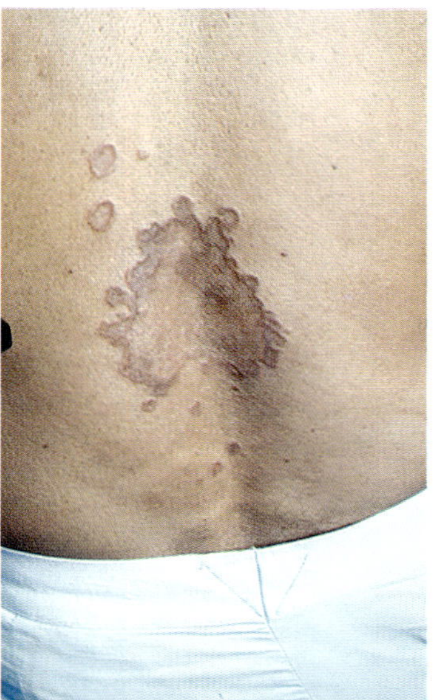

Fig. 9: Closer examination reveals annular dull erythematous plaques with central clearing and raised margins devoid of scales.

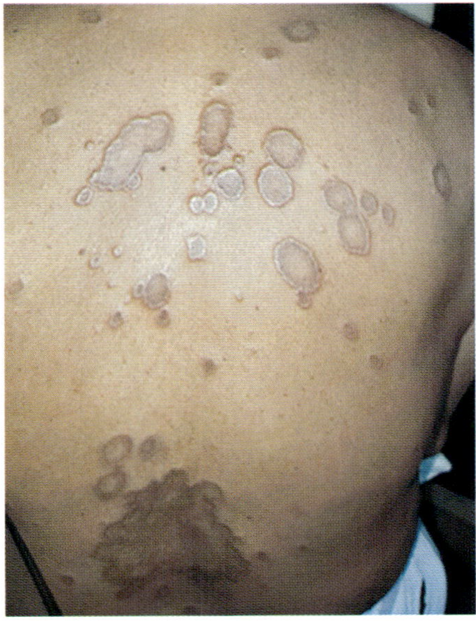

Fig. 10: A geriatric patient presented with asymptomatic patches over the back since 5 months that were relatively asymptomatic.

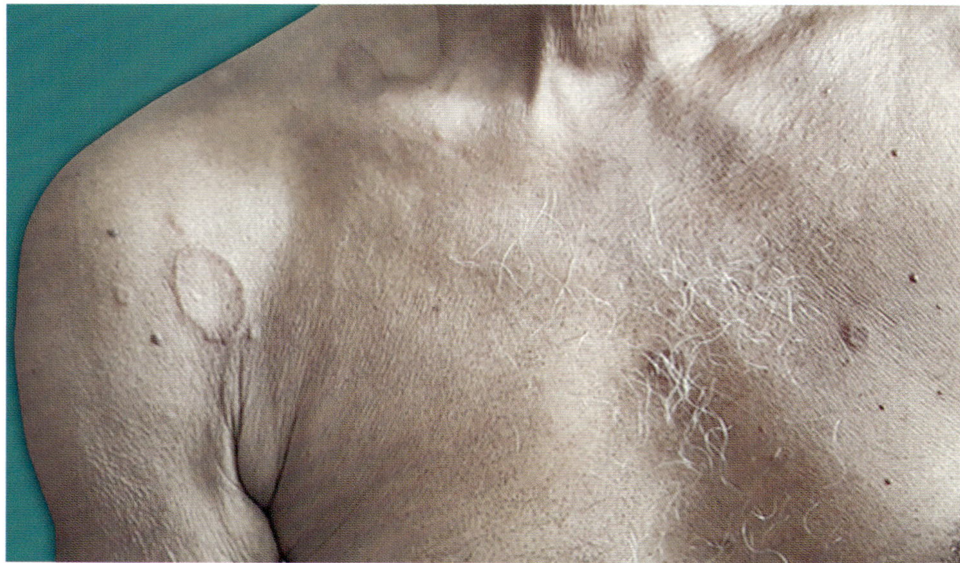

Fig. 11: The same patient showing annular lesions with central clearing and raised margin suggestive of granuloma annulare.

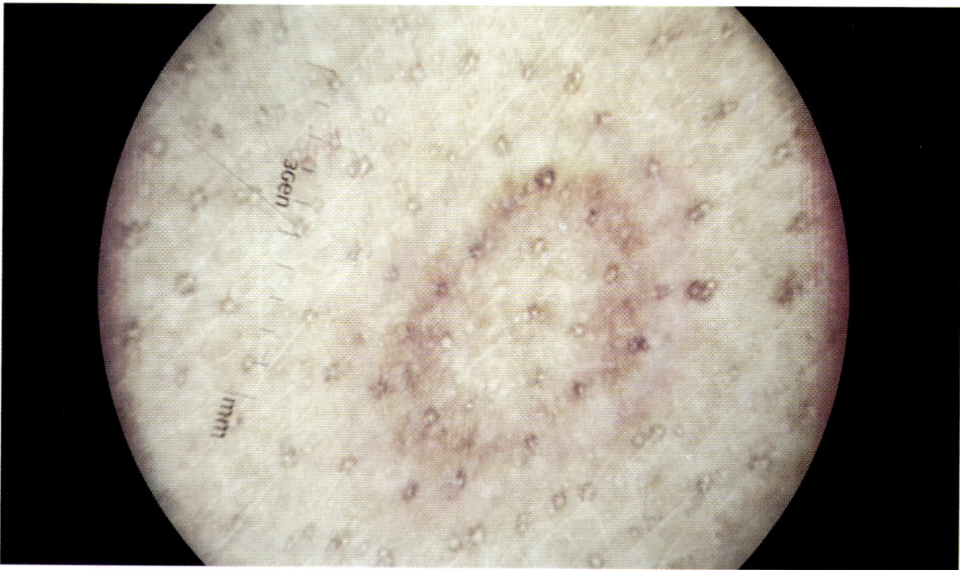

Fig. 12: Dermoscopic overview shows annular lesion with central structureless area surrounded by yellow-orange zone with erythema.

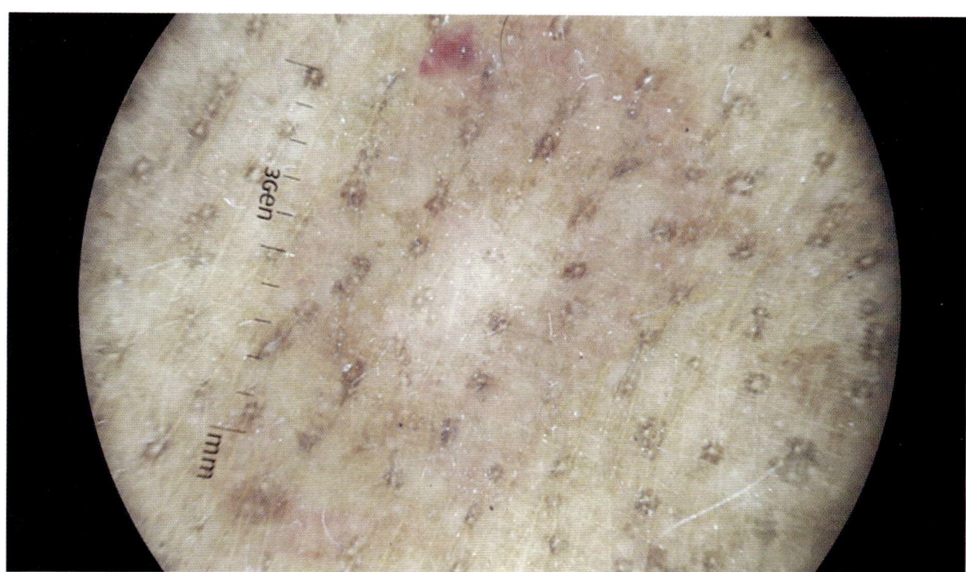

Fig. 13: Yellow-orange background with erythema.

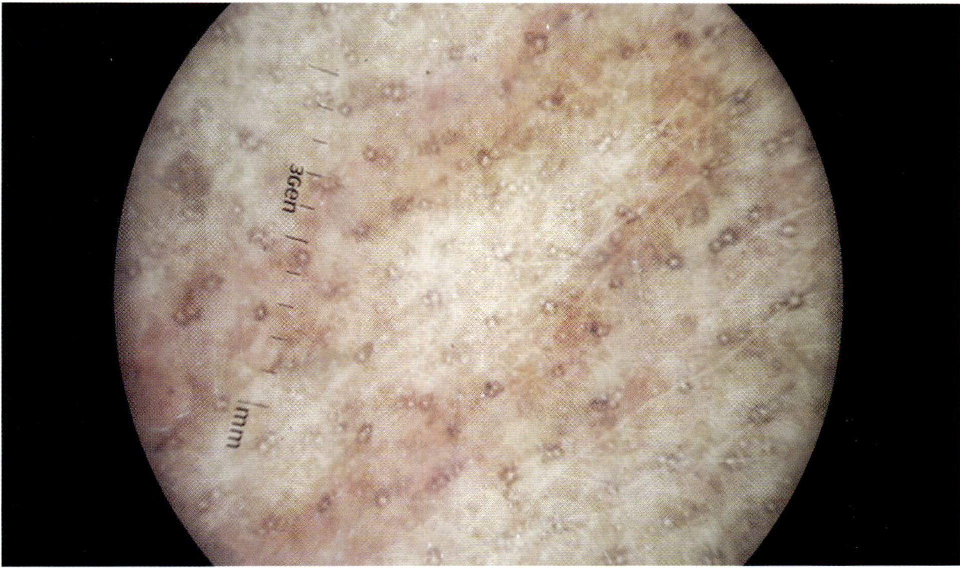

Fig. 14: Structureless center is surrounded by yellow-orange periphery.

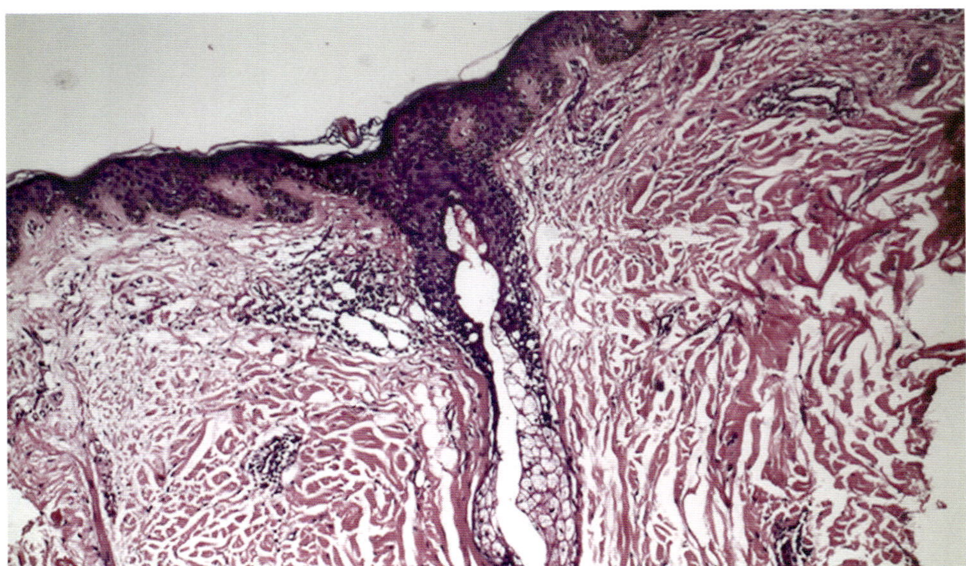

Fig. 15: Biopsy shows a sparse superficial and deep perivascular lymphocytic infiltrate with numerous histiocytes seen scattered in the interstitium of reticular dermis. Between the histiocytes is seen abundant mucin. Overlying epidermis is unaffected. Impression: Granuloma annulare—interstitial variety.

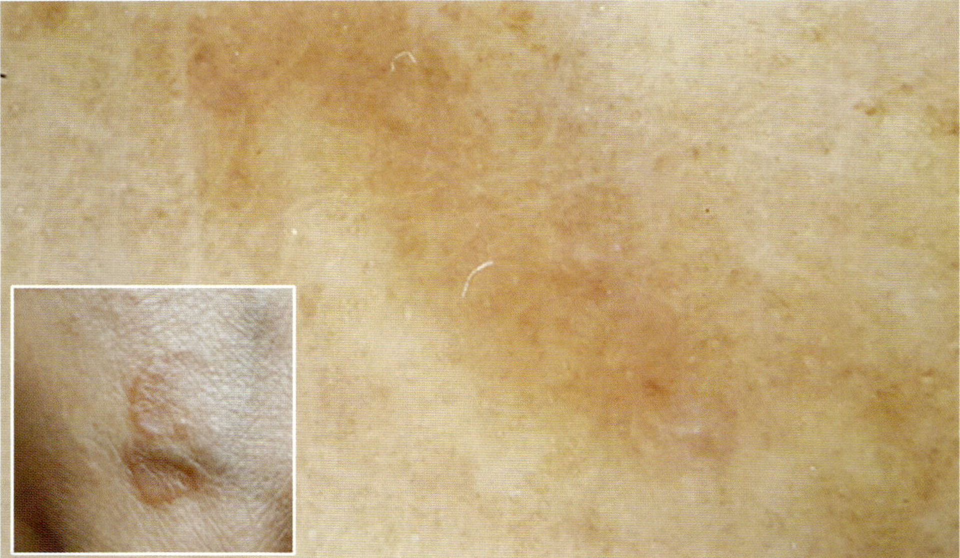

Fig. 16: Some unfocused vessels are seen on a yellow-orange background.

REFERENCES

1. Errichetti E, Lallas A, Apalla Z, et al. Dermoscopy of granuloma annulare: a clinical and histological correlation study. Dermatology. 2017;233(1):74-9.
2. Pellicano R, Caldarola G, Filabozzi P, et al. Dermoscopy of necrobiosis lipoidica and granuloma annulare. Dermatology. 2013;226(4):319-23.
3. Navarrete-Dechent C, Puerto CD, Bajaj S, et al. Dermoscopy of elastosis perforans serpiginosa: a useful tool to distinguish it from granuloma annulare. J Am Acad Dermatol. 2015;73(1):e7-9.
4. Lallas A, Zaballos P, Zalaudek I, et al. Dermoscopic patterns of granuloma annulare and necrobiosis lipoidica. Clin Exp Dermatol. 2013;38:425-7.

LUPUS VULGARIS

INTRODUCTION

It is the most frequent form of cutaneous tuberculosis, which occurs in patients previously sensitized to *Mycobacterium tuberculosis.*[1] It consists of a solitary reddish-brown papule that evolves to form a plaque with serpiginous borders. Lupus vulgaris (LV) progresses by central healing and peripheral extension resulting in central scarring and atrophy. Regardless of this classical presentation, the correct diagnosis is challenging as the list of differentials are long and poses a diagnostic dilemma to the treating physician.

KEY DERMOSCOPIC FEATURES (FIGS. 17 TO 21)

- Fine focused telangiectasias
- Yellow to golden-colored background
- Milia-like cysts
- Whitish reticular streaks.

DISCUSSION

The hallmark of granulomatous skin diseases is the presence of structureless orange-yellow areas. Dermoscopy and diascopy of orange-yellow patches of cutaneous sarcoidosis and LV may reveal individual yellowish nodules (*grains of sand*), or yellow-brown discoloration (*apple-jelly* sign). Although not predictable of a particular granulomatous disease, orange-yellow areas are highly suggestive of underlying dermal granulomas seen in LV, cutaneous sarcoidosis, granulomatous rosacea, and CL.

Lupus vulgaris is commonly associated with focused linear or branching vessels.

Other additional findings include milia-like cysts, whitish reticular streaks, erythema, and white or yellow scales.

KEYNOTE

Although the dermoscopic features of LV are not highly specific, truly speaking the combination of fine-focused telangiectasias, yellow-golden background, milia-like cysts, and whitish reticular streaks, is typical of LV.

The most characteristic dermoscopic finding in LV is the golden-yellow colored background, which represent the so-called "apple-jelly" sign under diascopy.

CASE 1 (FIGS. 17 TO 21)

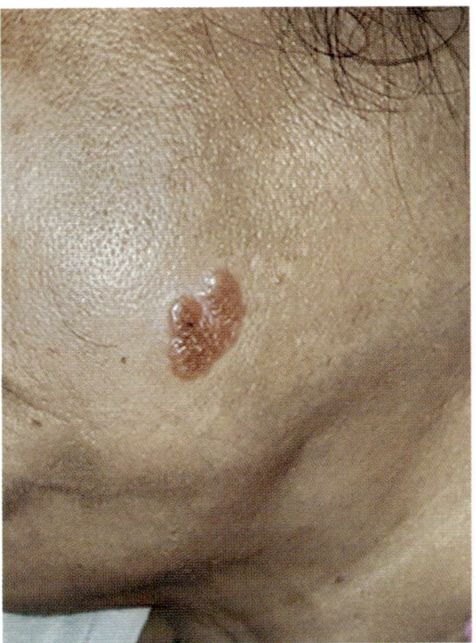

Fig. 17: Solitary enlarging erythematous infiltrated plaque on the left cheek of a middle-age female. Note: The central scarring.

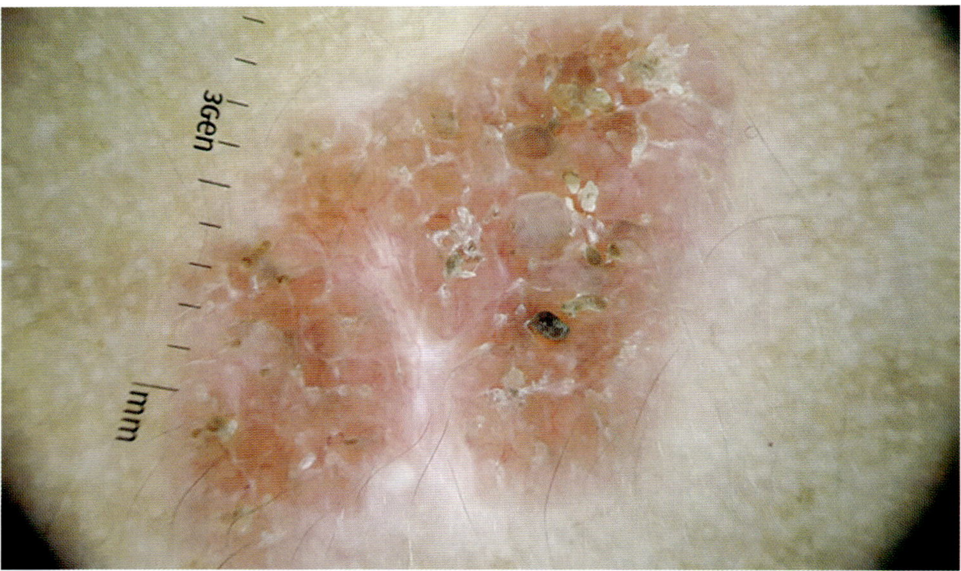

Fig. 18: Yellow-golden colored background, whitish reticular streaks.

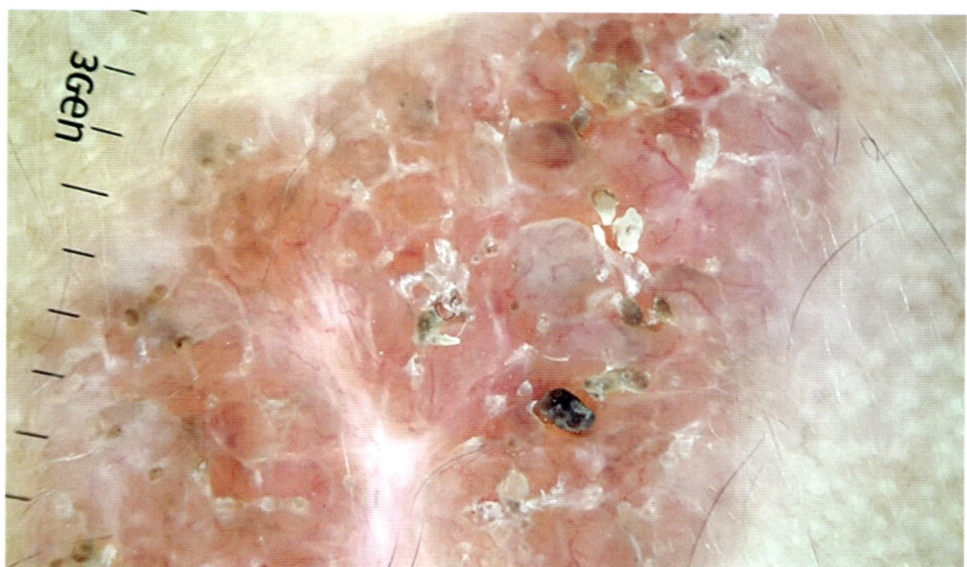

Fig. 19: Yellow-golden colored background, whitish reticular streaks, and fine-focused telangiectasias.

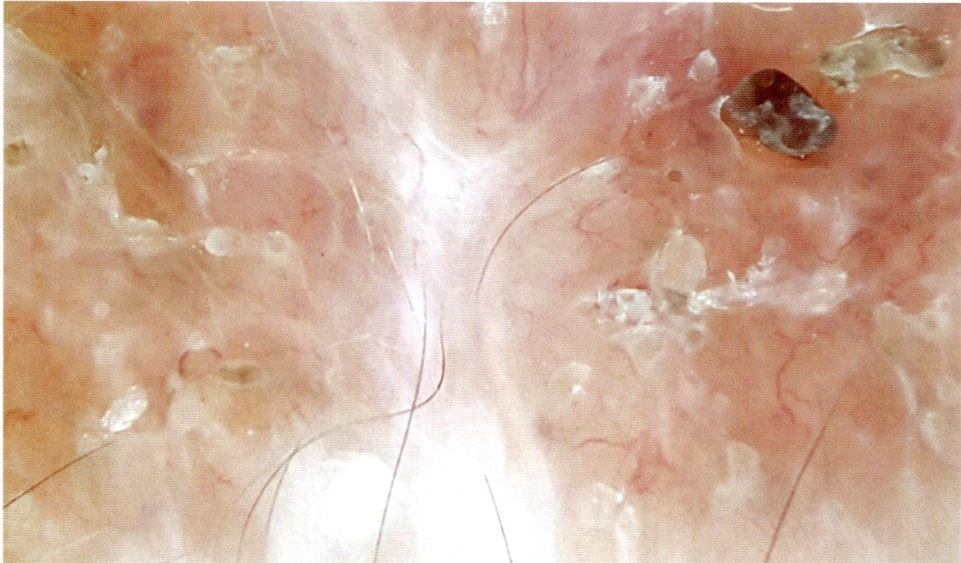

Fig. 20: White shiny structures and fine-focused telangiectasia. Note: The *Demodex* parasites due to loss of local immunity.

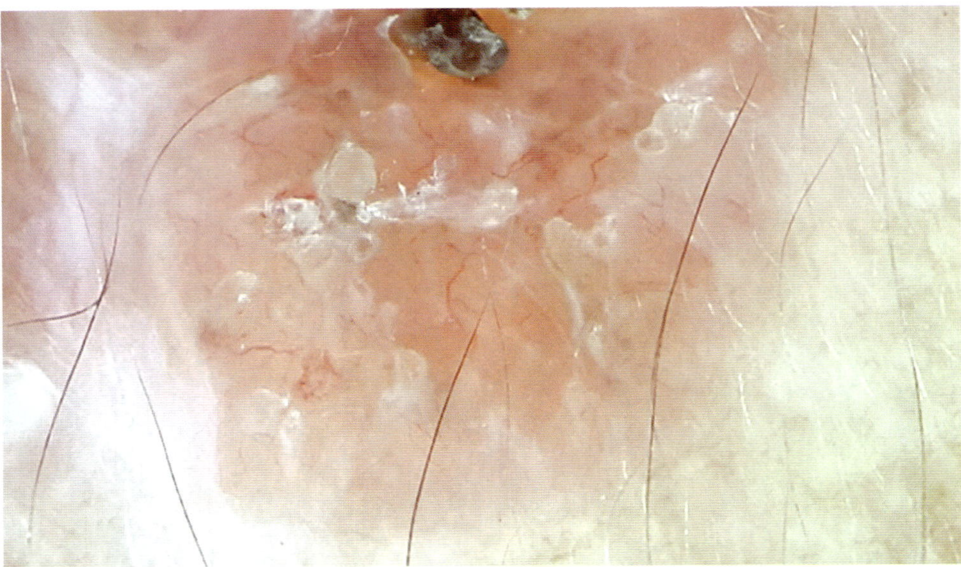

Fig. 21: Fine-focused telangiectasia on a yellow-gold background. Few *Demodex folliculorum* are also seen in this field.

CASE 2 (FIGS. 22 TO 25)

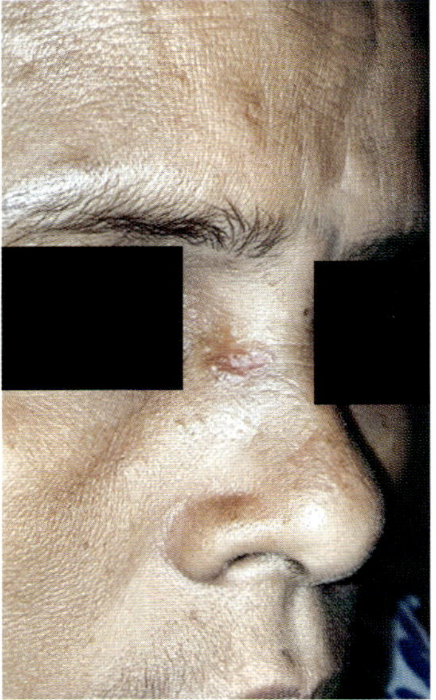

Fig. 22: A small erythematous plaque on the nasal bridge for 5 months duration.

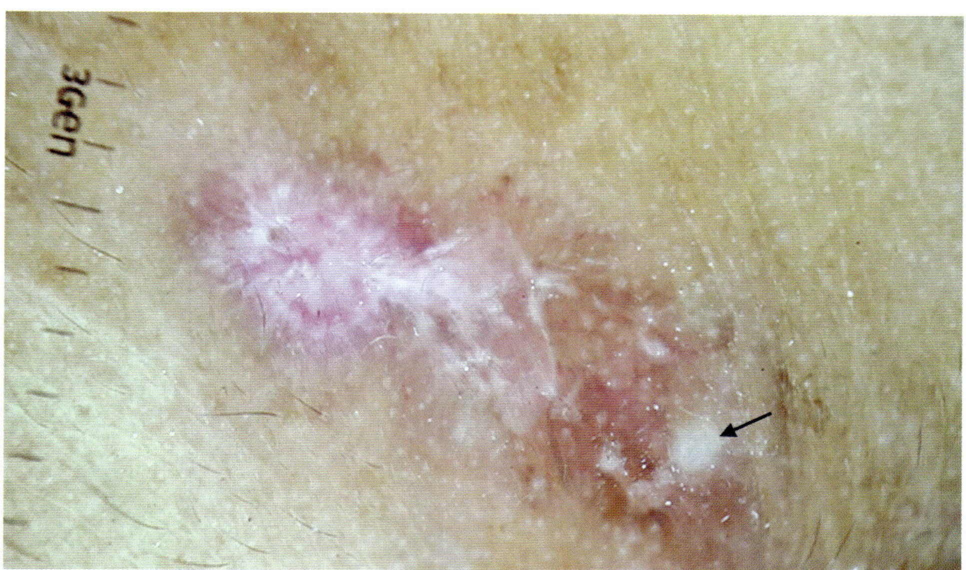

Fig. 23: Background color is brown-yellow rather than golden-yellow in this dark complexioned patient. Homogeneous erythema with linear vessels and white reticular streaks. Note: One milia-like cyst (arrow).

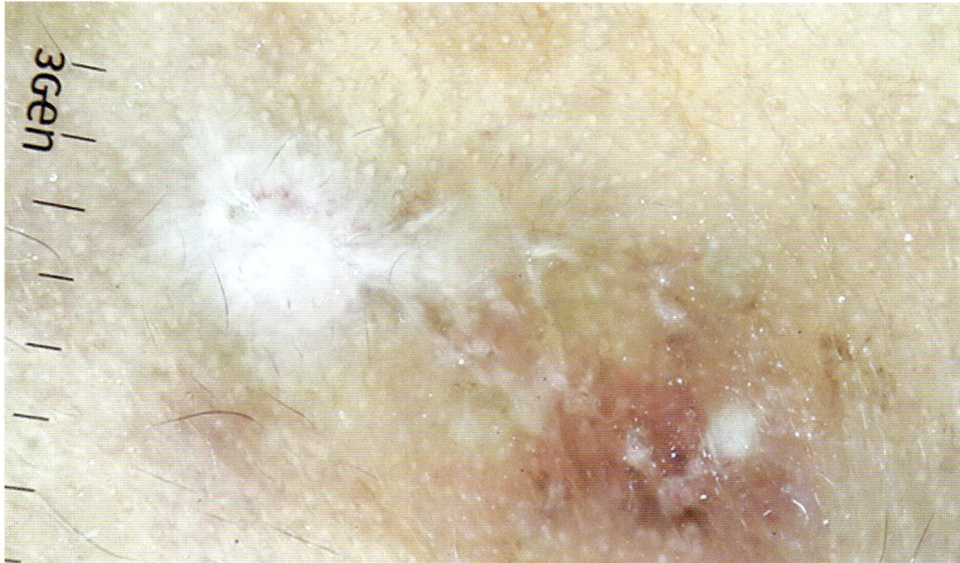

Fig. 24: Fine-focused telangiectasia, white reticular streaks, and milia on a yellow-brown background.

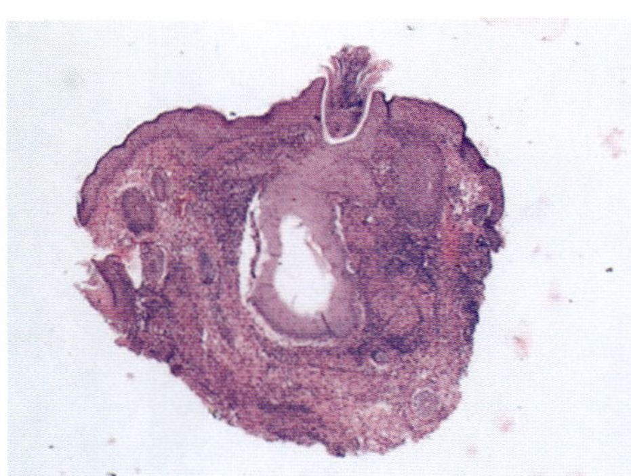
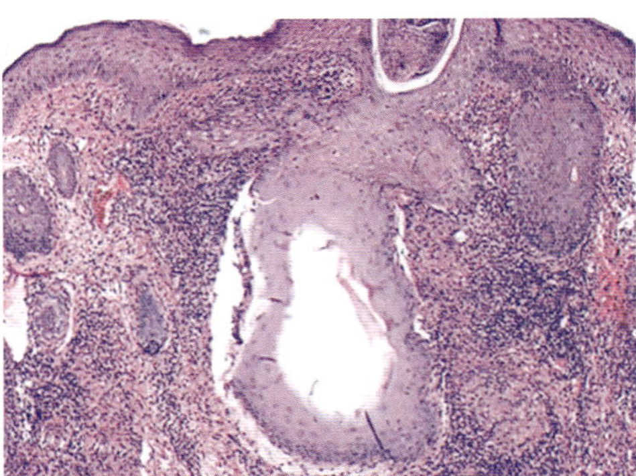

Fig. 25: Biopsy shows patchy nodular tuberculoid granulomatous infiltrate made up of lymphocytes, plasma cells, histiocytes, and epithelioid cells with occasional Langhans giant cells. Overlying epidermis shows moderate spongiotic psoriasiform change. Underlying dermis shows fibroplasia. Impression: Lupus vulgaris.

REFERENCE

1. Wozniacka A, Schwartz RA, Sysa-Jedrzejowska A, et al. Lupus vulgaris: report of two cases. Int J Dermatol. 2005;44:299-301.

NECROBIOSIS LIPOIDICA

INTRODUCTION

Necrobiosis lipoidica (NL) is a disorder of collagen degeneration with a granulomatous response. Most cases of NL present with shiny red-brown patches that gradually enlarge and progress to yellow, atrophic plaques; pretibial region is most commonly affected (Fig. 26). Histopathology is characterized by parallel layers of palisading granuloma and degenerated collagen.[1] Often it is associated with diabetes mellitus.[2] The diagnosis is usually based on clinical presentation and histopathologic findings. However, atypical presentations can be associated with diagnostic challenge.[2,3]

KEY DERMOSCOPIC FEATURES (FIGS. 27 TO 29)[4,5]

- Orange-yellow areas
- Dermoscopic findings of vessels vary according to the duration of the disease: (a) Comma-shaped vessels in the early lesions, (b) Fine network of vessels in the full form lesions, and (c) In the advanced stage of NL, irregular pattern of arborizing vessels.
- Whitish structures on a pink background.
- Pigmented reticulum and brown background in advanced lesions.

DISCUSSION

In the early lesions of NL, dermoscopy shows comma vessels, while more developed lesions reveal a fine network of vessels; irregular pattern of arborizing vessels are seen in advanced stage of the disease. These findings correspond to the papillary vessels in the initial stage, and later, as the atrophy progresses the deeper plexus becomes more visible.[4]

The whitish structures correlate histologically to the degenerated collagen and the orange-yellow patches to the dermal granuloma. Advanced stage lesions such as pigmented reticulum and brown background are due to the postinflammatory melanocyte stimulation (Fig. 28).[4]

KEYNOTE

Dermoscopy is a very useful investigatory tool for the diagnosis of early stage NL and NL in the atypical site. Moreover, it is often difficult to differentiate plaque form of cutaneous sarcoidosis and NL; both have almost similar findings dermoscopically. Regardless of the similar dermoscopic features, more close observation could reveal the longer and more branching telangiectatic vessels in the lesion of NL caused by atrophic changes; the atrophic changes are not seen in cutaneous sarcoidosis.

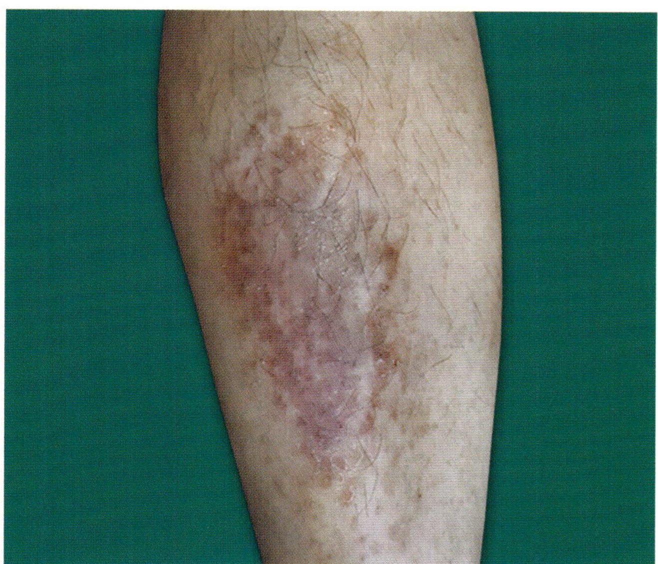

Fig. 26: Slightly raised shiny red-brown patch on the skin of a patient with uncontrolled diabetes mellitus.

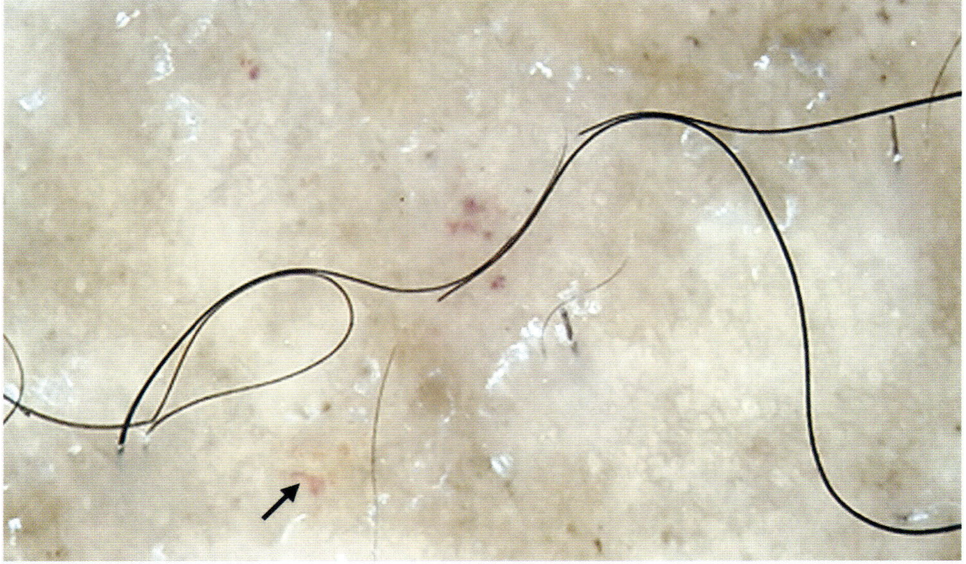

Fig. 27: Dermoscopy shows comma vessels (arrow) on an orange-yellow background.

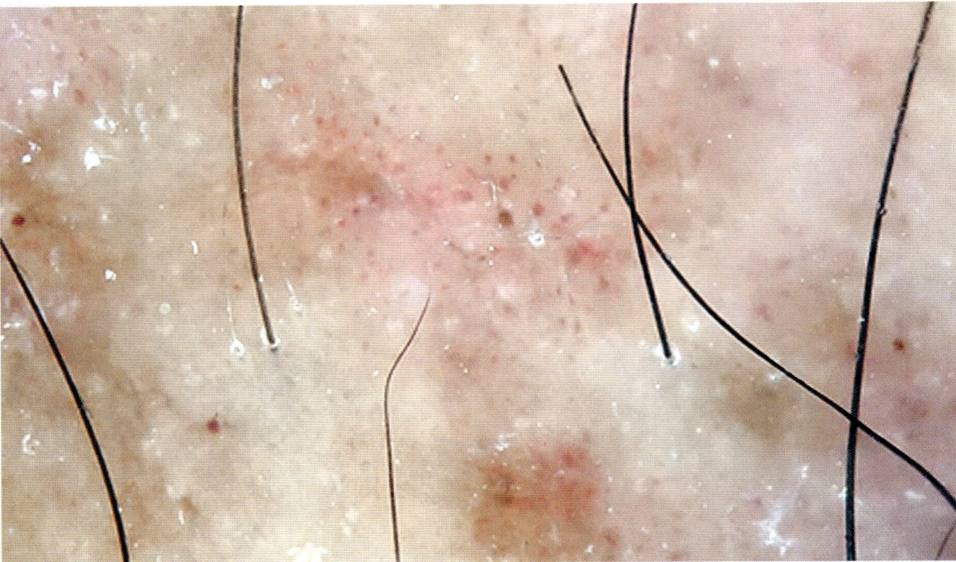

Fig. 28: Dotted vessels over a pinkish-yellow background.

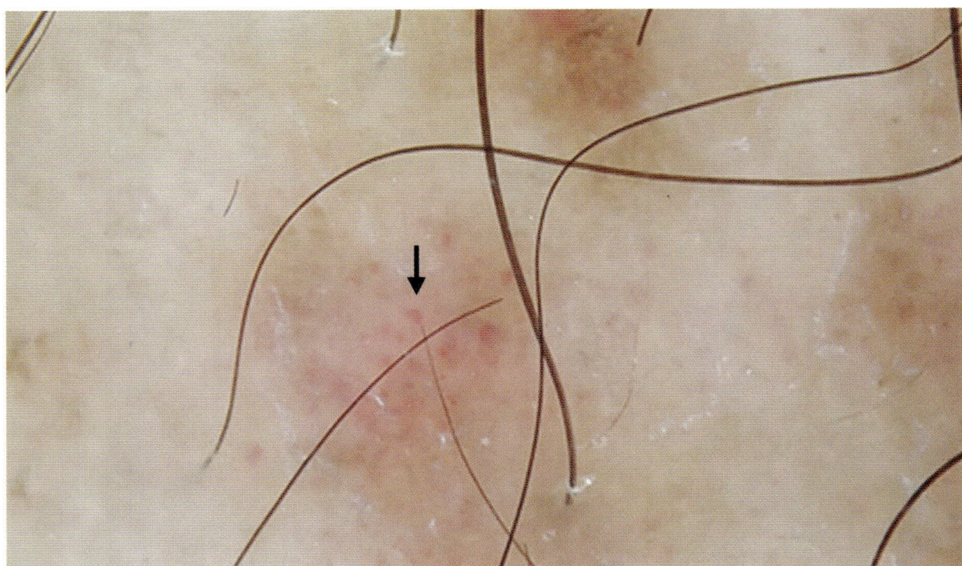

Fig. 29: Comma vessels (arrow).

REFERENCES

1. Lynch JM, Barrett TL. Collagenolytic (necrobiotic) granulomas: part II—the red granulomas. J Cutan Pathol. 2004;31:409-18.
2. Roche-Gamon E, Garcia-Melgares ML, Vilata-Corell JJ. Necrobiosis lipoidica. Piel. 2006;2:180-7.
3. Peyrí J, Moreno A, Marcoval J. Necrobiosis lipoidica. Semin Cutan Med Surg. 2007;26:87-9.
4. Conde-Montero E. Dermatoscopia de la necrobiosis lipoídica. Actas Dermosifiliogr. 2013;104:534-7.
5. Errichetti E, Stinco G. Dermoscopy in general dermatology: a practical overview. Dermatol Ther. 2016;6:471-507.

CHAPTER 12

Pigmentary Disorders

Balachandra S Ankad, Balakrishna Nikam, Niti Khunger

12A. DERMOSCOPY OF HYPOPIGMENTARY DISORDERS

Balachandra S Ankad, Balakrishna Nikam

INTRODUCTION

Dermoscopy of hypopigmentary disorders is a diagnostic challenge to the clinician many a times due to close resemblance to each other. There may be reduction or complete absence of melanin leading to either hypo or depigmentation. Since melanin is the primary factor that gives rise to various dermoscopic patterns, the reduction or absence of this pigment gives relatively subtle dermoscopic patterns. Although many hypopigmented lesions are benign and easy to diagnose, some lesions require histopathological confirmation of diagnosis. Dermoscopy, being a noninvasive diagnostic tool, demonstrates characteristic patterns of hypopigmented lesions.

IDIOPATHIC GUTTATE HYPOMELANOSIS

INTRODUCTION

Idiopathic guttate hypomelanosis (IGH) is characterized by 3–5 mm porcelain white macules on the extremities of older individuals (Fig. 1). IGH is commonly seen on sun-exposed areas.[1] Close differential diagnoses include guttate vitiligo, lichen sclerosus et atrophicus (LSEA). Hyperkeratosis, atrophic epidermis, reduced number of melanocytes, and decreased melanin content are noted in histopathology. Similar features are seen in guttate vitiligo making it difficult to differentiate both conditions.[1]

Dermoscopy demonstrates characteristic patterns in IGH. Four different patterns have been described.[2,3]

KEY DERMOSCOPIC FEATURES

- Ameboid pattern
- Feathery pattern
- Petaloid pattern
- Nebuloid pattern.
- Occasionally, perifollicular and perilesional pigmentation and linear vessels are noted.

DISCUSSION

Ameboid pattern is the most common with diffuse structureless white areas in the center, which extend peripherally in the normal skin as pseudopods appearing as ameba. Hence, it is denoted as ameboid pattern (Fig. 2).

When borders extend in a feather-like manner it is described as feathery pattern (Fig. 3).

Petaloid pattern is characterized by well-defined borders resembling petals of a flower (Fig. 4).

Nebuloid pattern is least distinctive of all with ill-defined borders. It closely resembles guttate vitiligo (Fig. 5).

It is interesting to note that recent lesions generally show nebuloid and older IGH demonstrate ameboid, feathery, or petaloid pattern.

Authors have described two aspects of dermoscopic patterns in IGH.[4] One is cloudy sky-like pattern with multiple small irregular or polycyclic macules, with both well- and ill-defined edges, surrounded by patchy hyperpigmented network and another is cloudy pattern in which well or ill-defined roundish homogeneous whitish areas surrounded by patchy hyperpigmented network are noted. This difference is probably attributable to the color of the skin and duration of lesions.

Guttate vitiligo reveals dense and glowing diffuse white areas with well to ill-defined borders with perifollicular pigmentation.[5] The histological findings associated with IGH are hyperkeratosis, an atrophic epidermis, and flattened rete ridges and decreased melanin content, and reduced numbers of melanocytes.[1] These features are well correlated with dermoscopic patterns.

Personal observation of one of the authors (BSA) shows perifollicular and perilesional pigmentation suggesting presence of melanin in the lesional skin (Fig. 6). Linear and branching vessels are also visible in IGH but with a magnification higher than 20X (Fig. 7). Nevertheless affirmation of this preliminary observation is recommended by studies on a larger scale.

KEYNOTE

Idiopathic guttate hypomelanosis demonstrates characteristic dermoscopic patterns, which delineate it from other similar depigmented lesions. This is of utmost importance because it alleviates the apprehension associated with hypopigmented lesions among patients, especially in Indian subcontinent.

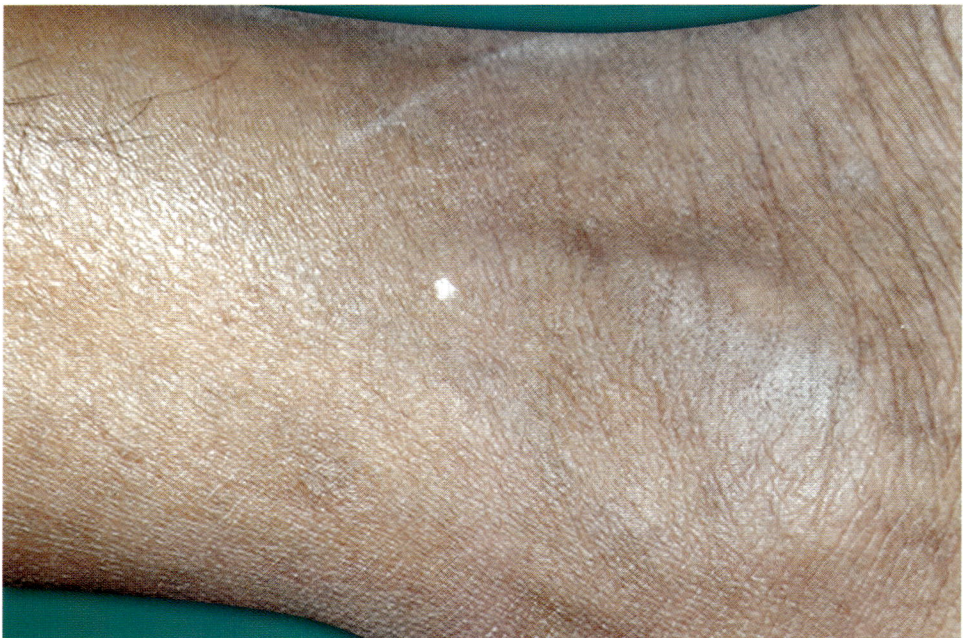

Fig. 1: Porcelain white macule on the ankle.

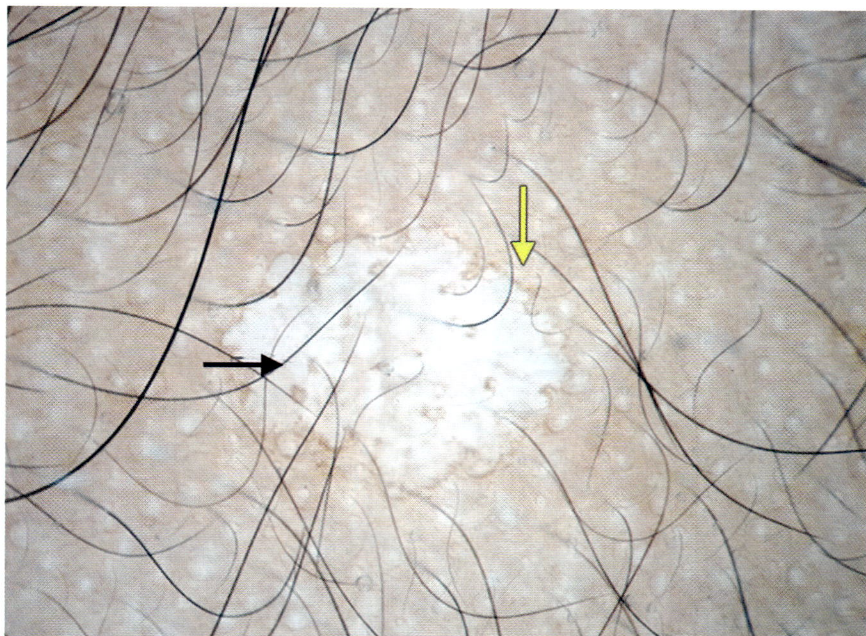

Fig. 2: Ameboid pattern showing pseudopods. Note: The perifollicular (black arrow) and perilesional pigmentation (yellow arrow).

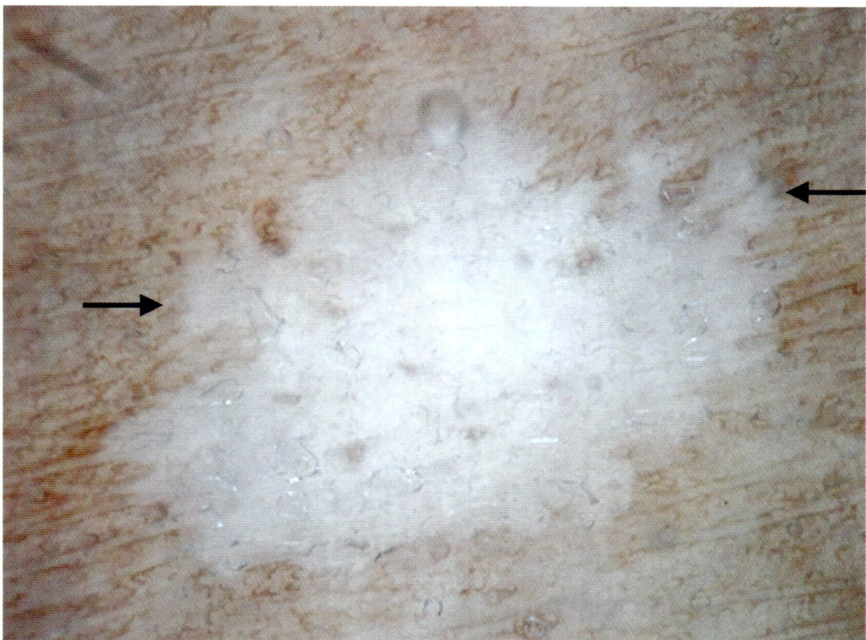

Fig. 3: Feather-like projections (arrows) at periphery with pigmented globules in feathery pattern.

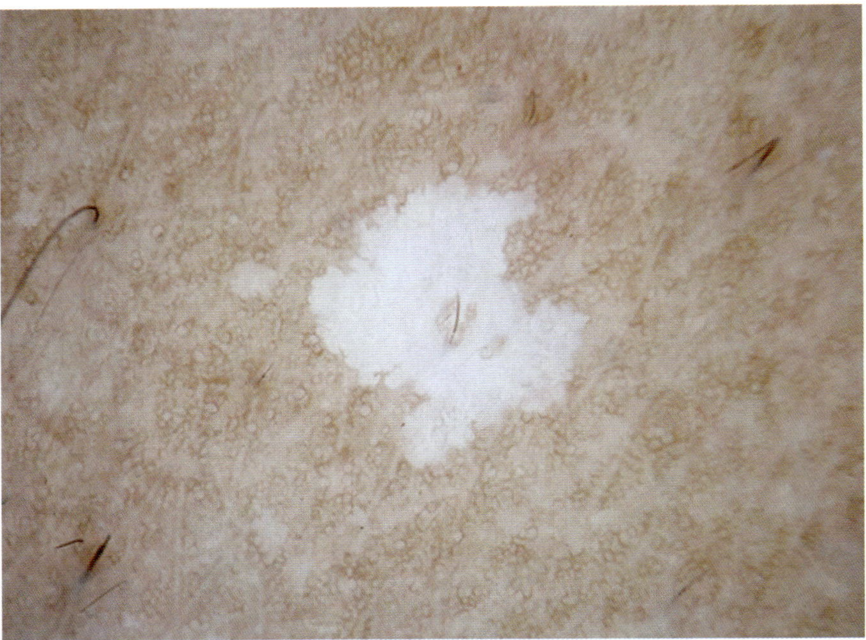

Fig. 4: Petaloid pattern with extensions resembling petals with perifollicular pigmentation.

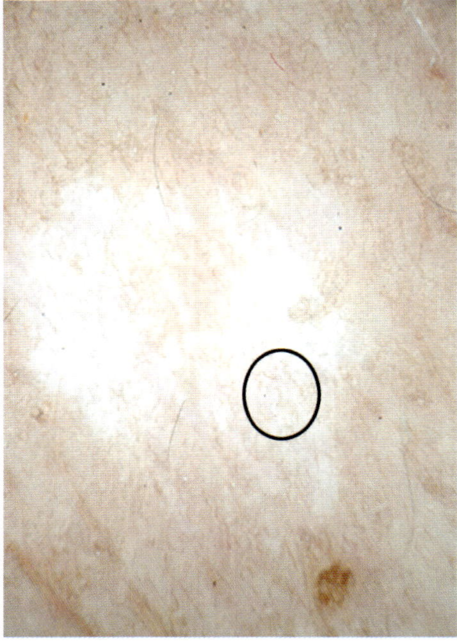

Fig. 5: Indistinct borders with subtle pigmentation in whitish areas are seen in nebuloid pattern. Note: The broken pigment network (black circle).

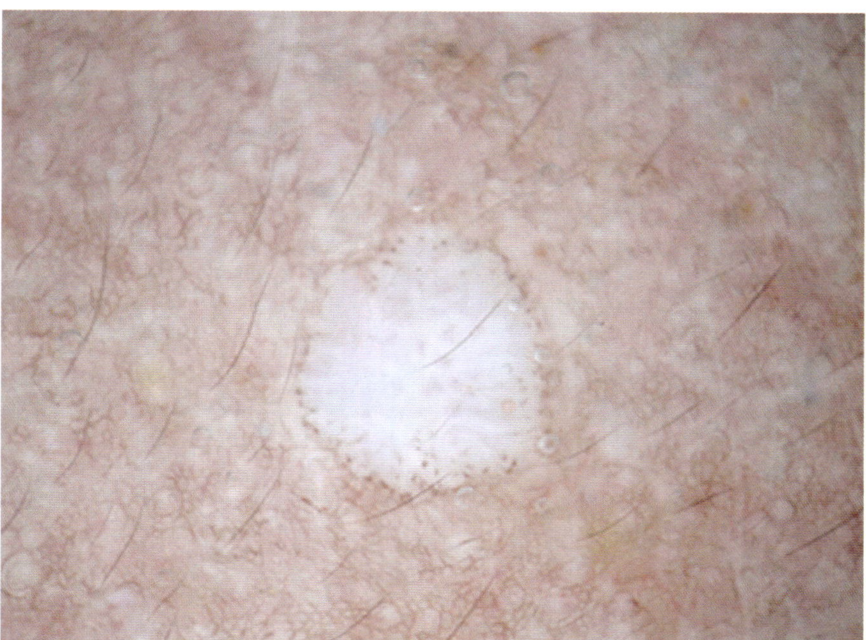

Fig. 6: Prominent perilesional pigment is well appreciated in this image.

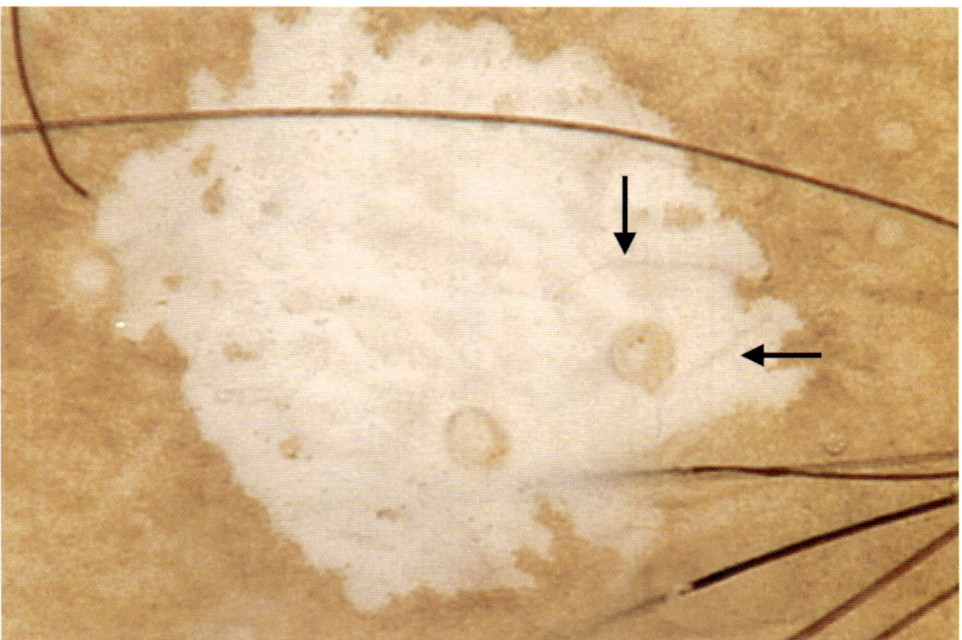

Fig. 7: Linear and branching vessels (arrows) are noted with higher magnification (20X).

REFERENCES

1. Kim SK, Kim EH, Kang HY, et al. Comprehensive understanding of idiopathic guttate hypomelanosis: clinical and histopathological correlation. Int J Dermatol. 2010;49:162-6.
2. Ankad BS, Beergouder SL. Dermoscopic evaluation of idiopathic guttate hypomelanosis: a preliminary observation. Indian Dermatol Online J. 2015;6:164-7.
3. Bambroo M, Pande S, Khopkar U. Dermoscopy in the differentiation of idiopathic guttate hypomelanosis (IGH) and guttate vitiligo. In: Khopkar S (Ed). Dermoscopy and Trichoscopy in Diseases of the Brown Skin: Atlas and Short Text, 1st edition. New Delhi: Jaypee Brothers Medical Publishers (P) Ltd; 2012. pp. 97-103.
4. Errichetti E, Stinco G. Dermoscopy of idiopathic guttate hypomelanosis. J Dermatol. 2015;42:1118-9.
5. Errichetti E, Stinco G. Dermoscopy in general dermatology: a practical overview. Dermatol Ther (Heidelb). 2016;6(4):471-507.

LICHEN SCLEROSUS ET ATROPHICUS

INTRODUCTION

Lichen sclerosus et atrophicus is a chronic inflammatory condition characterized by milky white macules or patches affecting anogenital areas (Fig. 8). Extragenital lesions are less common (Fig. 9). Clinical differentiation from guttate vitiligo and IGH is challenging owing to similar clinical features. Histopathologic studies would help in the diagnosis. However, dermoscopy is a rapid and noninvasive technique, which demonstrates characteristic patterns in LSEA.

KEY DERMOSCOPIC FEATURES

Early Lesions

- White structureless areas and follicular plugs (comedo-like openings).[1,2]

Late Lesions

- White structureless areas with chrysalis strands.[1,2]
- Other less common patterns include delicate branching telangiectasia of variable diameter, black or gray dots, and pigment-like structures.[3]
- Anogenital lesions show similar patterns but with more prominent vascular patterns on a diffuse whitish background.[4]

DISCUSSION

Dermoscopy provides specific patterns in LSEA, which correlate well with histopathology changes. Histopathology of established early lesions of LSEA demonstrates hyperkeratosis, follicular plugging, thinning of epidermis, and vacuolar changes in basal layer. Late lesions show more sclerotic changes with eosinophilia.[5]

In early lesions, white structureless areas and comedo-like openings (Fig. 10) suggest hyperkeratosis, homogenization of collagen, and follicular plugging, respectively.[2] Whereas comedo-like openings are absent in late lesions owing to the fibrosis of lesions with destruction of follicles in the dermis. Whitish areas become prominent in chronic lesions showing characteristic chrysalis strands in polarized mode (Fig. 11). Brown or gray dots represent either epidermal or dermal melanin, respectively. Dilated capillaries are seen as delicate linear or branching telangiectasia. Hairpin and comma vessels are also described in LSEA.[2,3]

Similar patterns are seen in anogenital lesions. Authors noted sparse vessels without a specific arrangement. Dotted vessels were observed in the early stage of the disease (Fig. 12). Whitish to pinkish-white structureless areas on white background was a distinctive and constant dermoscopic feature (Fig. 13). Peppered arrangement of gray-blue dots corresponding to dermal melanophages was also frequently seen.[4]

KEYNOTE

Lichen sclerosus et atrophicus gives characteristic dermoscopic patterns, which are beneficial in clinical diagnosis and prompt treatment. Patterns vary depending on the duration and location of lesions as well.

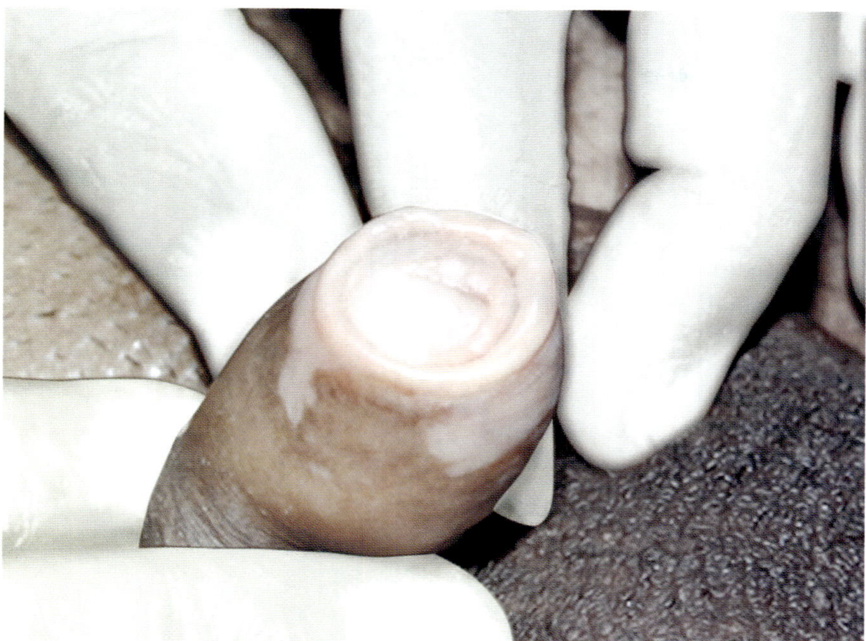

Fig. 8: Depigmented patches on the prepuce in genital lichen sclerosus et atrophicus.

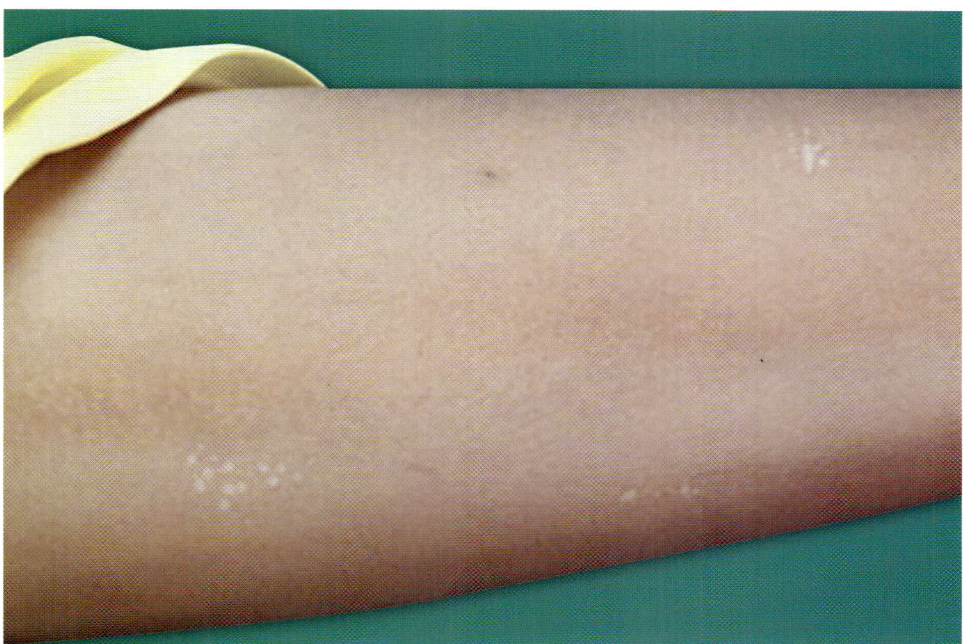

Fig. 9: Multiple milky white macules on the leg in a girl.

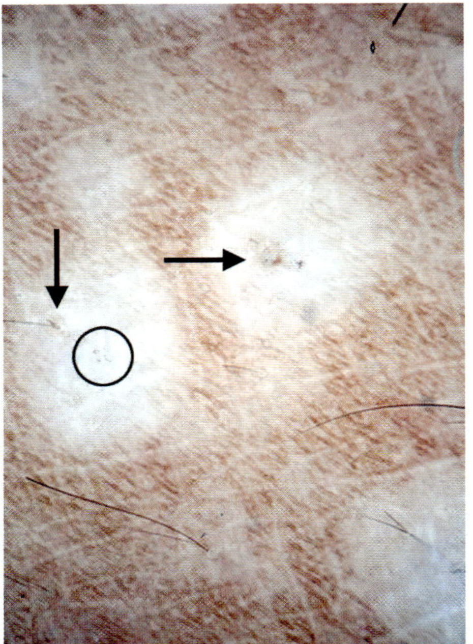

Fig. 10: Dermoscopy of early lesions shows white structureless areas, comedo-like openings (arrows), and gray dots in peppered arrangement (circle).

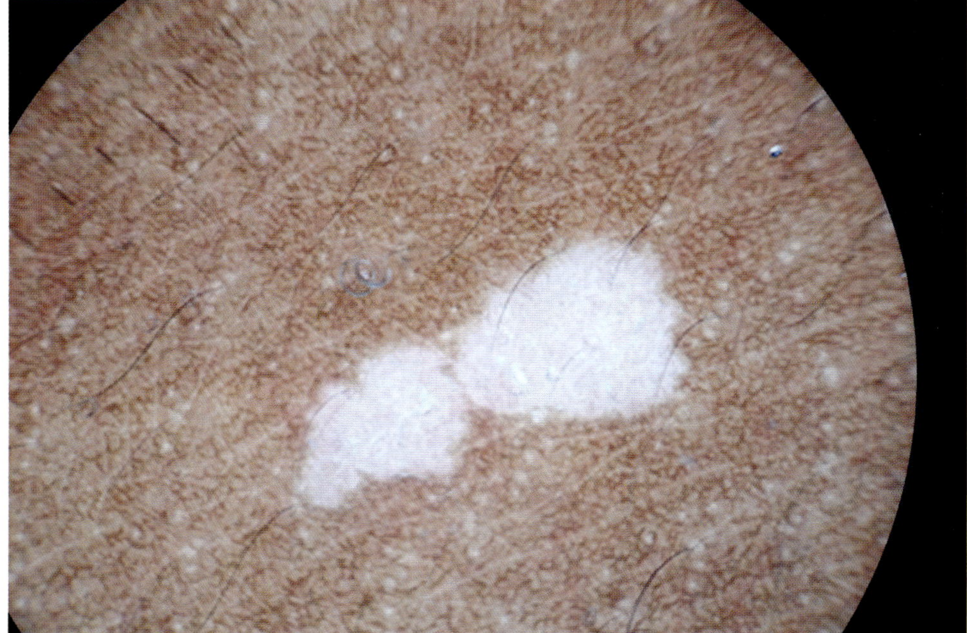

Fig. 11: Dermoscopy of late lesions reveals white structureless areas.

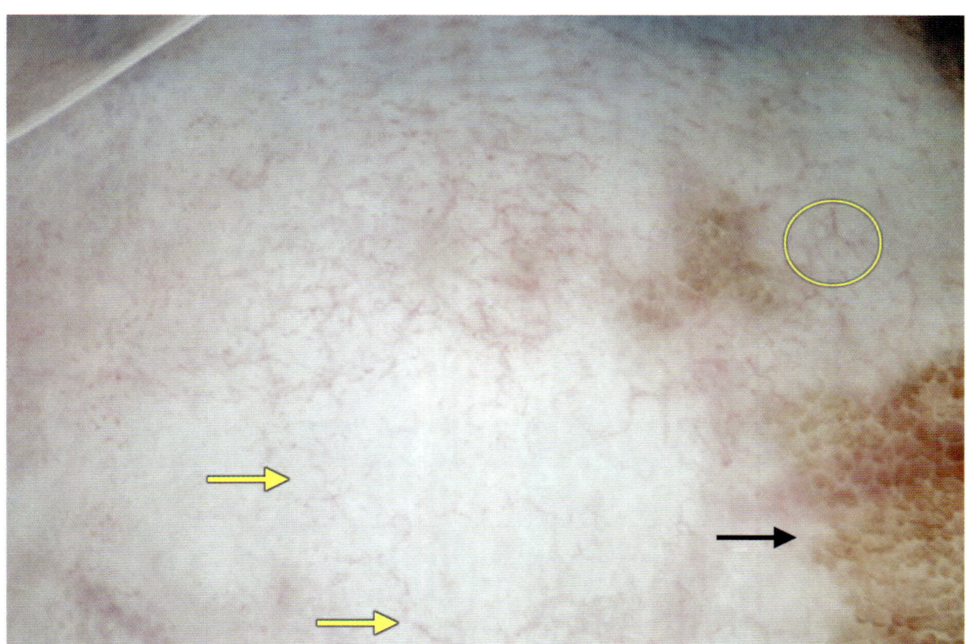

Fig. 12: Dermoscopy of genital lesions shows whitish-pink background with numerous branching (yellow circle) and linear vessels (yellow arrows). Pigment network is also seen (black arrow).

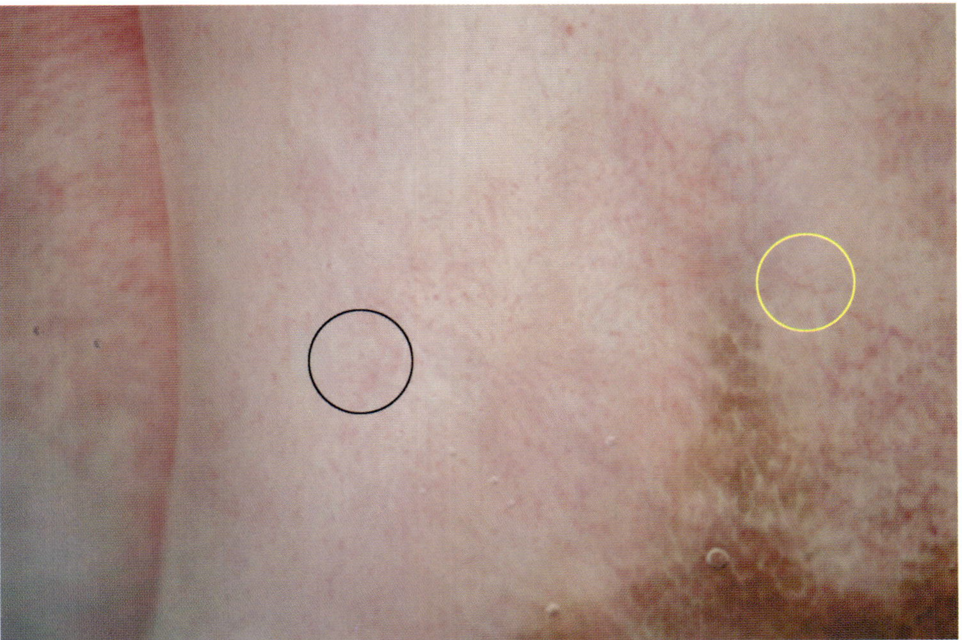

Fig. 13: Dermoscopy of genital lichen sclerosus et atrophicus shows predominantly dotted vessels (black circle) with branching vessels (yellow circle). Note: Whitish-pink background.

REFERENCES

1. Garrido-Ríos AA, Alvarez-Garrido H, Sanz-Muñoz C, et al. Dermoscopy of extragenital lichen sclerosus. Arch Dermatol. 2009;145:1468.
2. Ankad BS, Beergouder SL. Dermoscopic patterns in lichen sclerosus: a report of three cases. Indian Dermatol Online J. 2015;6:237-40.
3. Tiodorovic-Zivkovic D, Argenziano G, Popovic D, et al. Clinical and dermoscopic findings of a patient with co-existing lichen planus, lichen sclerosus, and morphea. Eur J Dermatol. 2012;22:143-4.
4. Borghi A, Corazza M, Minghetti S, et al. Dermoscopic features of vulvar lichen sclerosus in the setting of a prospective cohort of patients: new observations. Dermatology. 2016;232:71-7.
5. Weedon D. Disorders of collagen. In: Weedon D (Ed). Skin Pathology, 2nd edition. Edinburgh: Churchill Livingstone; 2002. pp. 345-80.

NEVUS DEPIGMENTOSUS

INTRODUCTION

Nevus depigmentosus (ND) is a common nevoid depigmentary condition characterized by white patches appearing on the skin at birth or in later stages of life.[1]

Clinically ND is characterized by well-defined depigmented patches with serrated borders (Figs. 14 and 15). Vitiligo, ash leaf macules, and nevus anemicus resemble ND clinically. Dermoscopy can be utilized in this scenario to differentiate these conditions.

KEY DERMOSCOPIC FEATURES[2,3]

- Faint pigment network throughout the lesion
- Perifollicular pigmentation
- Pseudopods at periphery representing serrated borders.

DISCUSSION

Peripheral extensions of white areas appear as pseudopods (Fig. 16). Here, presence of faint or subtle pigmentation in lesion indicates that melanin is definitely present in the epidermis. This feature of ND gives affirmation to fact that melanosomes are not transferred to the keratinocytes in ND even though numbers of melanocytes are normal. Histopathology of ND reveals perivascular lymphohistiocytic infiltrate with normal epidermis. Number of melanocytes is normal whereas amount of melanin is reduced.[4]

Perifollicular pigment is also a prominent feature of ND. Hairs in the lesional skin retain their pigment (Fig. 17).

Vitiligo reveals white structureless areas, though, white areas are dense and glowing. Notably pseudopods are not observed in vitiligo. Instead, perilesional and reverse pigmentation is frequently seen in vitiligo.[15] Dermoscopic evaluation of the borders may reveal trichrome/quadrichrome or pentachrome pattern.

KEYNOTE

Nevus depigmentosus is characterized by depigmented patches which do not change in color or texture throughout life. It has to be differentiated from other treatable depigmentary disease like vitiligo. Dermoscopy by providing useful pattern aides in the diagnosis of ND and also curtails psychological impact of depigmented skin lesions.

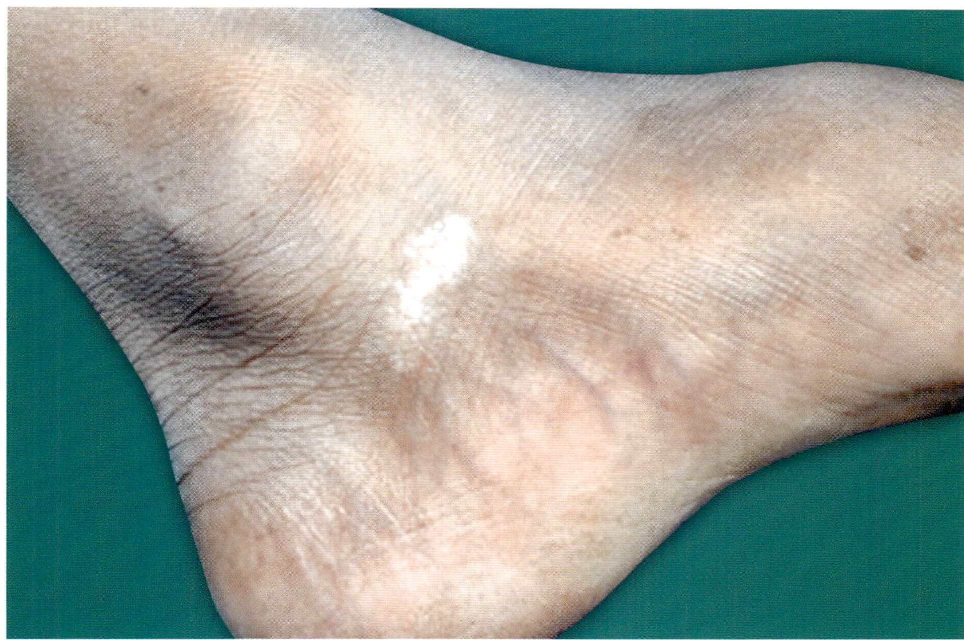

Fig. 14: Well-defined white patch of nevus depigmentosus with serrated borders on the ankle.

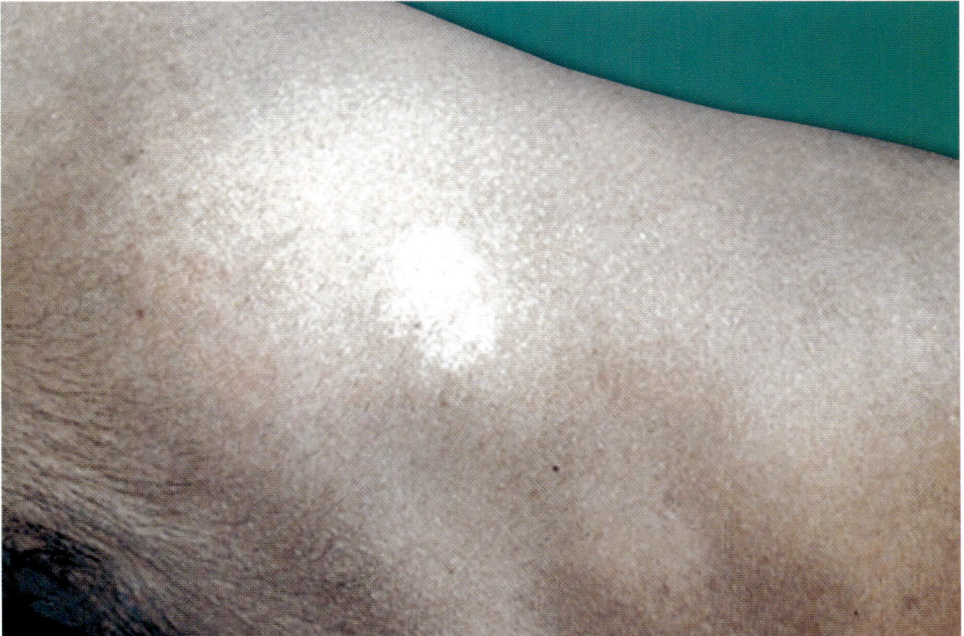

Fig. 15: Clinical image of nevus depigmentosus on the trunk.

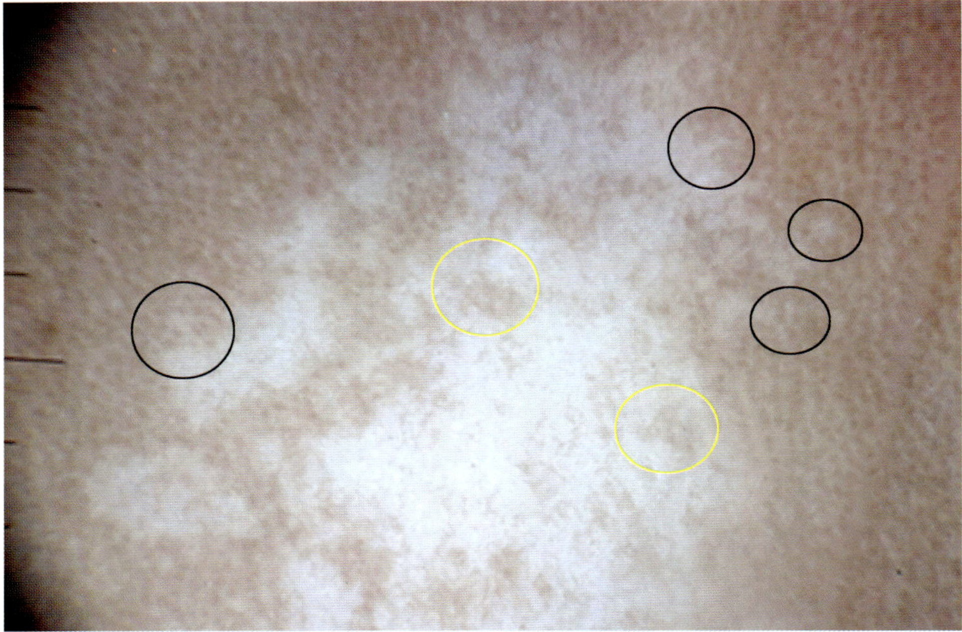

Fig. 16: Dermoscopy shows white structureless areas with subtle pigment network (yellow circles) in white areas. Note: The pseudopods at the periphery (black circles).

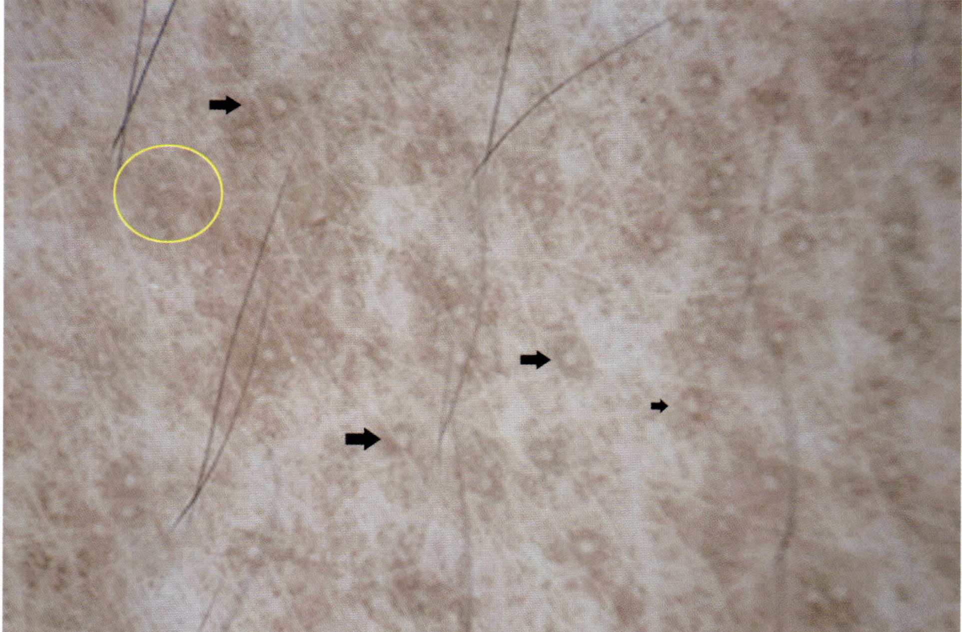

Fig. 17: Dermoscopy reveals white areas, faint pigment network (yellow circle), and normal black colored hairs. White dots (eccrine openings) show peripheral pigmentation (black arrows).

REFERENCES

1. Deb S, Sarkar R, Samanta AB. A brief review of nevus depigmentosus. Pigment Int. 2014;1:56-8.
2. Oiso N, Kawada A. The diagnostic usefulness of dermoscopy for nevus depigmentosus. Eur J Dermatol. 2011;21(4):639-40.
3. Sarma N, Ankad BS. Dermoscopy in nevoid disorders. In: Chattarjee M, Neema S, Malakar S (Eds). Dermoscopy in Darker Skin, 1st edition. New Delhi: Jaypee Brothers Medical (P) Ltd; 2017. pp. 127-33.
4. Lee HS, Chun YS, Hann SK. Nevus depigmentosus: clinical and histopathologic characteristics in 67 patients. J Am Acad Dermatol. 1999;40:21-6.
5. Thatte SS, Khopkar US. The utility of dermoscopy in the diagnosis of evolving lesions of vitiligo. Indian J Dermatol Venereol Leprol. 2014;80:505-8.

VITILIGO

INTRODUCTION

Vitiligo is an acquired spontaneous depigmentation of skin due to progressive destruction of melanocytes. It is characterized by off-white depigmented macules and patches (Fig. 18). Early lesions of vitiligo are difficult to distinguish from other hypopigmented or depigmented lesions.[1] Few reports suggest that dermoscopy can be useful diagnostic aide to affirm the diagnosis of vitiligo.[2]

KEY DERMOSCOPIC FEATURES[3]

- Reduced pigment network
- Absent pigment network
- Perifollicular and perilesional pigmentation
- Reverse pigment network.

DISCUSSION

Dermoscopy in vitiligo gives characteristic and useful patterns. Reduced (Fig. 19) and absent (Fig. 20) pigment network is observed and is expected due to reduced number of melanocytes in the lesions. Vitiliginous lesions show complete loss of melanin from the epidermis and absence of melanocytes. Advancing borders show large melanosomes with increased number of melanocytes. This explains both absent and perilesional pigment network under dermoscopy.[4]

Perifollicular (Fig. 21) and perilesional (Fig. 22) pigment network suggest that lesions are stable or repigmenting. It is known fact that repigmentation starts from the follicular or perilesional melanocytes after therapy in vitiligo. This is visualized under dermoscopy.[3] Evolving lesions of vitiligo demonstrate an entity called as "reverse pigment network" which is a well known feature of melanoma and melanocytic nevus. It describes reversal of normal reticular pigment network. White lines divide hyperpigmentary areas in net-like fashion (Fig. 23). This is exactly opposite to the normal network, hence the name reverse pigment network. This is noted in evolving lesions of vitiligo and can thereby obviate the need for the biopsy in doubtful lesions of vitiligo.[3]

KEYNOTE

Dermoscopic examination of vitiligo lesions shows few particular yet characteristic patterns. These patterns are useful in affirmation of diagnosis of vitiligo when lesions are indiscernible to naked eyes. Dermoscopy probably scores over routine histopathology in vitiligo, in diagnosis as well as treatment monitoring.

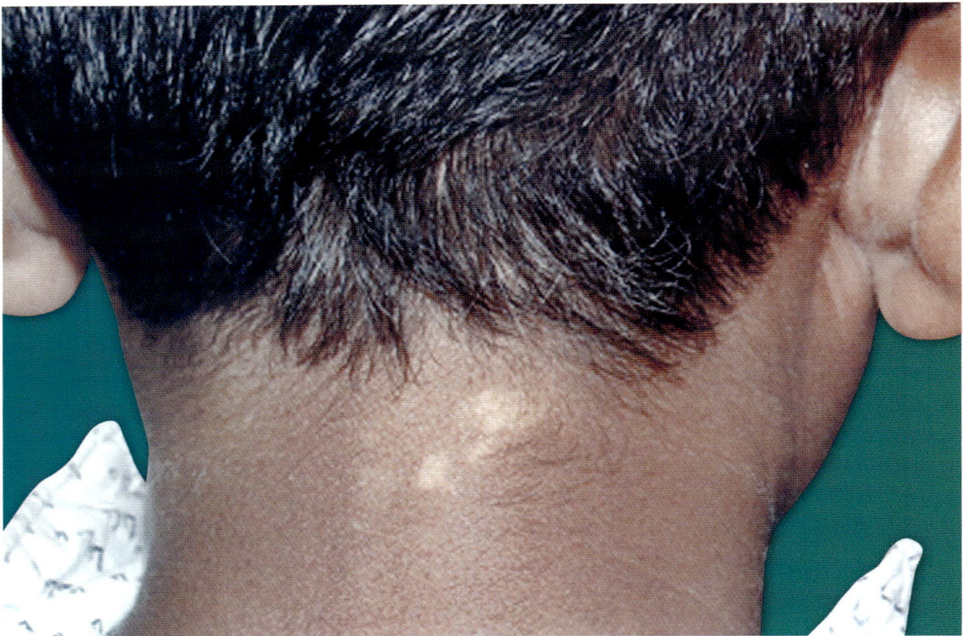

Fig. 18: Well-demarcated depigmented patch on the neck.

Fig. 19: Dermoscopy of vitiligo showing reduced pigment network (arrows) as compared to normal skin.

Fig. 20: Tota absence of pigmentary network in vitiligo patch.

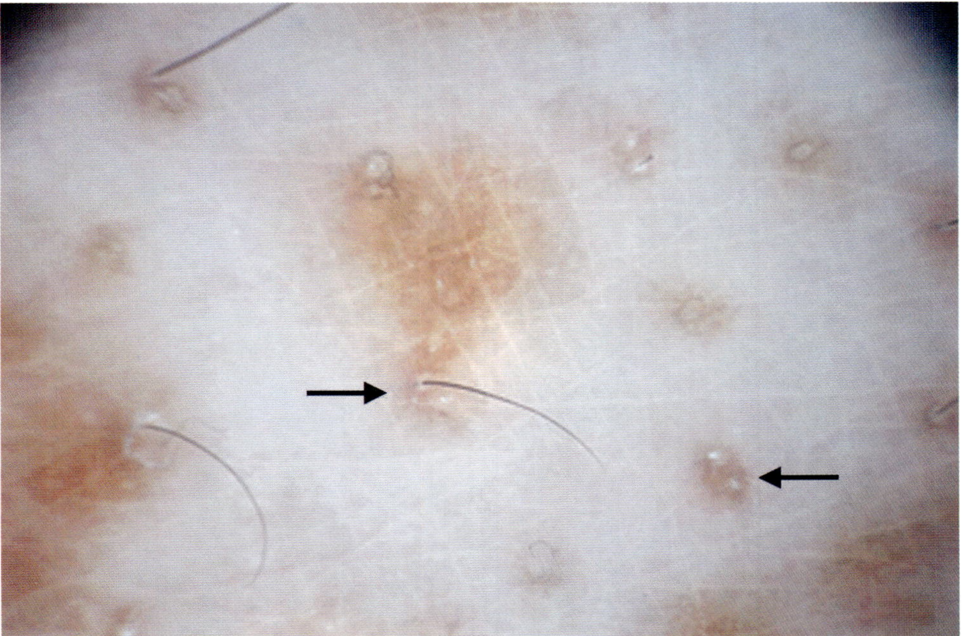

Fig. 21: Perifollicular pigmentation (arrows) is well appreciated.

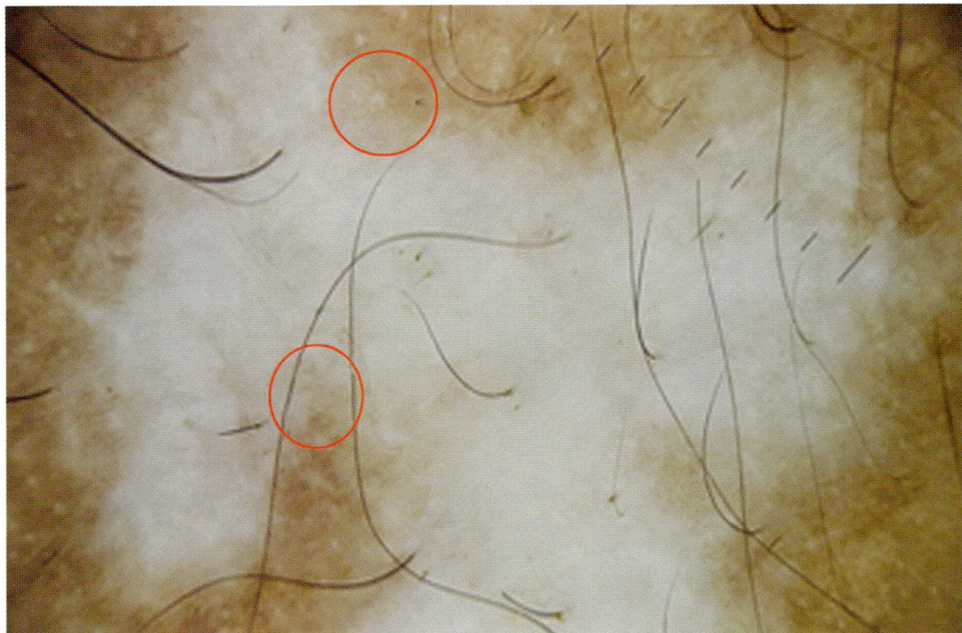

Fig. 22: Perilesional pigment network (red circles) is demonstrated in this image.

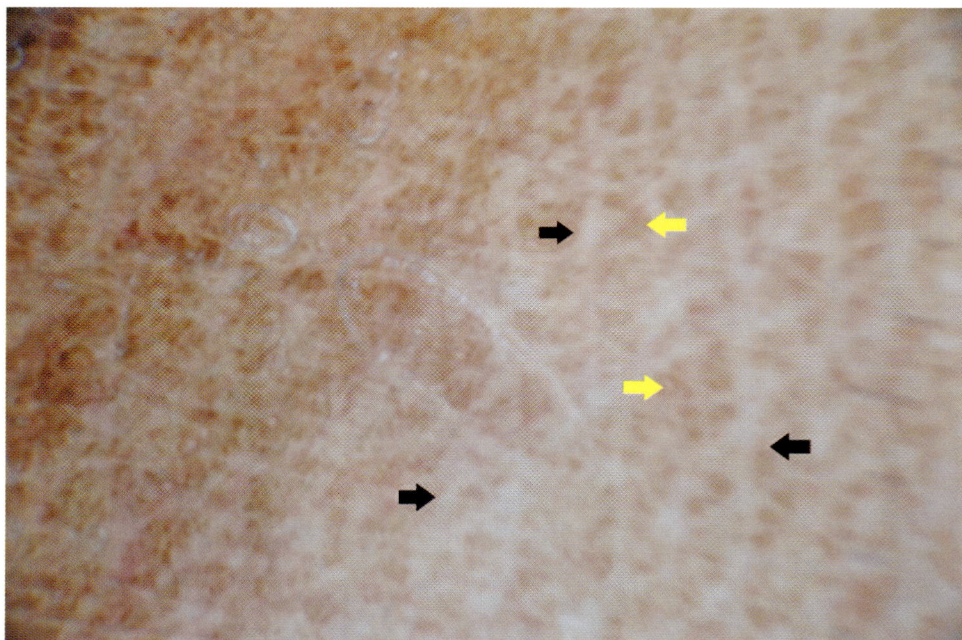

Fig. 23: Reverse pigment network with white lines (black arrows) dividing brown areas (yellow arrows); reverse of normal pigment network.

REFERENCES

1. Chuh AA, Zawar V. Demonstration of residual perifollicular pigmentation in localized vitiligo—a reverse and novel application of digital epiluminescence dermoscopy. Comput Med Imaging Graph. 2004;28:213-7.
2. Errichetti E, Stinco G. Dermoscopy in general dermatology: a practical overview. Dermatol Ther (Heidelb). 2016;6(4):471-507.
3. Thatte SS, Khopkar US. The utility of dermoscopy in the diagnosis of evolving lesions of vitiligo. Indian J Dermatol Venereol Leprol. 2014;80:505-8.
4. Nordlund JJ, Lerner AB. Vitiligo: It is important. Arch Dermatol. 1982;118:5-8.

PITYRIASIS VERSICOLOR

INTRODUCTION

Pityriasis versicolor (PV) manifests as maculosquamous lesions characterized by macules or patches with latent scaling. Many clinical variants are described but hypopigmented (Figs. 24 and 25) is most common presentation followed by hyperpigmented variant. Hypopigmented lesions of PV closely mimic vitiligo, LSEA, pityriasis alba, and progressive macular hypomelanosis.[1]

KEY DERMOSCOPIC FEATURES (FIG. 26)[1,2]

- Diffuse white areas
- Surface scaling which is prominent in skin lines and becomes double edged upon stretching the lesional skin
- Faint and distorted pigmentary network.

DISCUSSION

Pityriasis versicolor provides useful morphological information under dermoscopy for the clinical diagnosis as well as to differentiate it from other hypopigmented lesions. In the literature, dermoscopic patterns of PV are very few. It shows fairly distinct white areas with fine scaling. Scaling is localized to skin lines or furrows (Fig. 27).

Histopathology of PV shows slight or moderate hyperkeratosis and acanthosis. Dermis harbors mild superficial inflammatory infiltrate.[3]

However, white areas with fine scaling are common findings in PV in brown skin. One distinguishing feature is that scales are seen over entire lesion. They become double edged upon stretching the lesional skin (Fig. 28). This is visible under noncontact polarized light (personal observation).

Close differential diagnosis is pityriasis alba which also presents with depigmented patches with fine scaling, especially, when PV appears on the cheek. Dermoscopy of pityriasis alba shows white areas with scaling which are different from that of PV.

KEYNOTE

Pityriasis versicolor demonstrates characteristic dermoscopic patterns which help in distinguishing from other hypopigmented lesions.

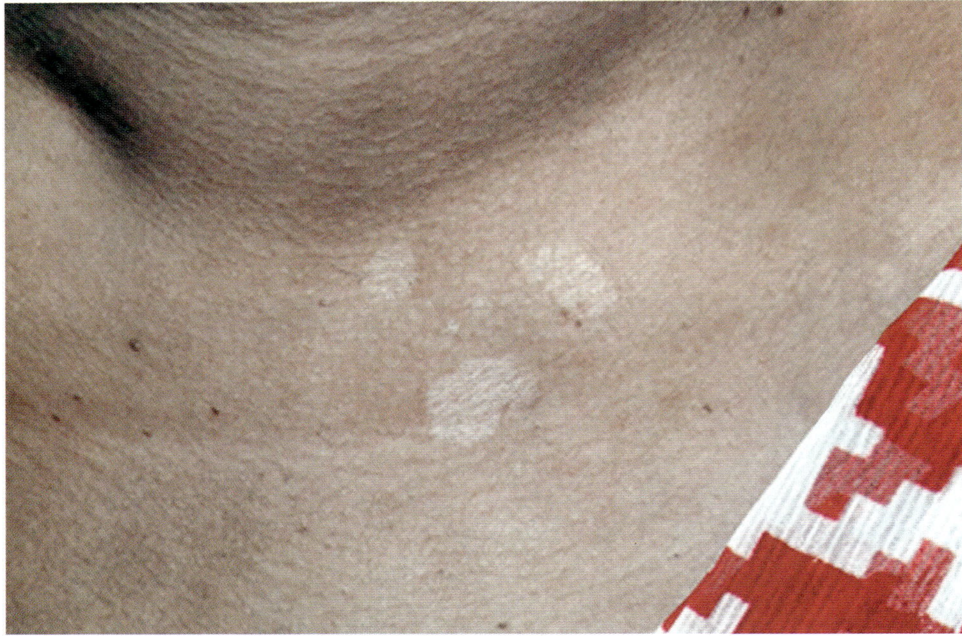

Fig. 24: Well-defined patches with fine scale of pityriasis on the upper chest.

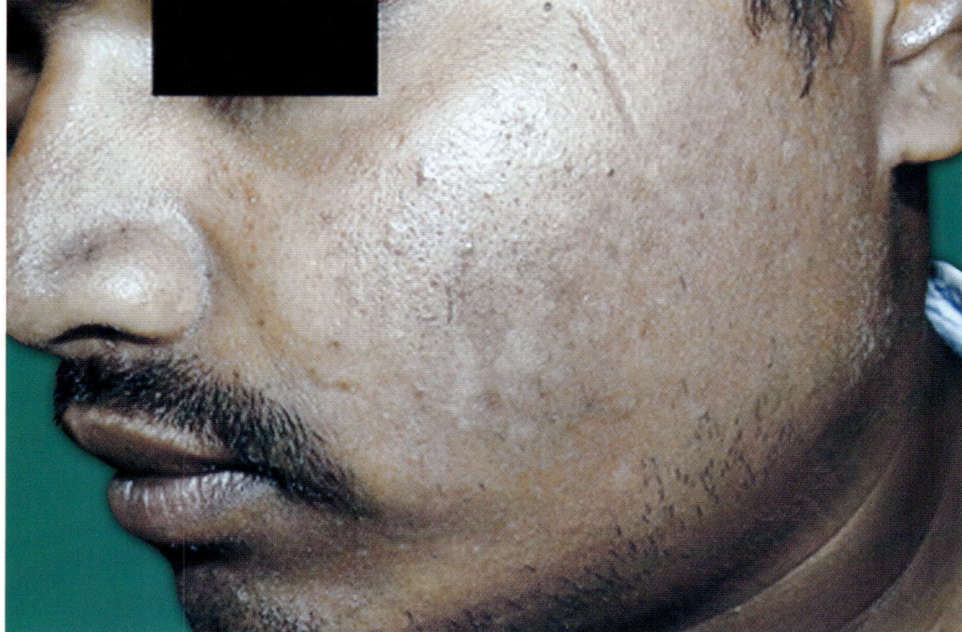

Fig. 25: Well-defined macules coalescing into patches on the face.

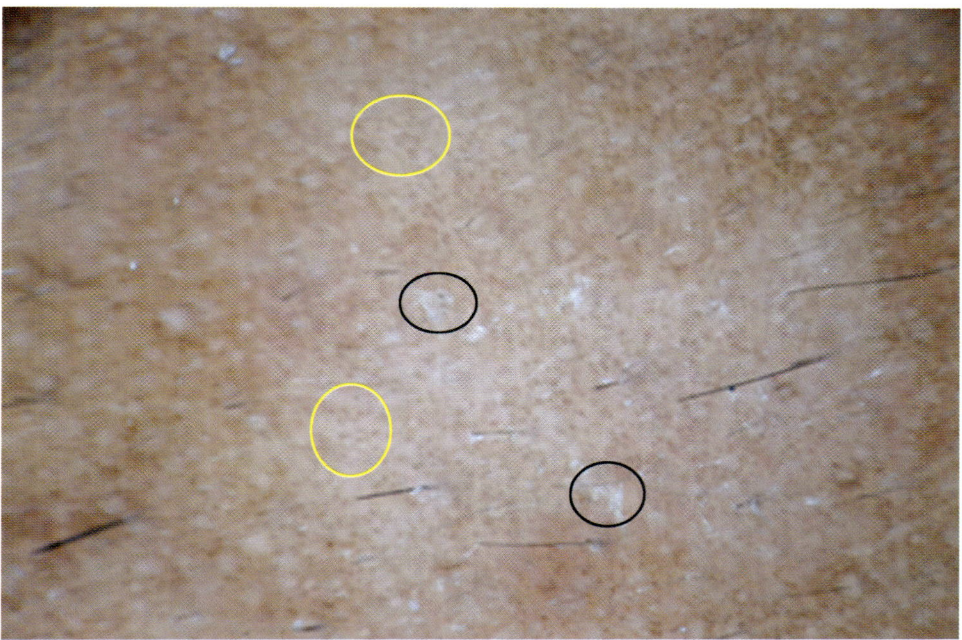

Fig. 26: Dermoscopy shows diffuse white areas, scanty scale (black circles), and brown dots (yellow circles).

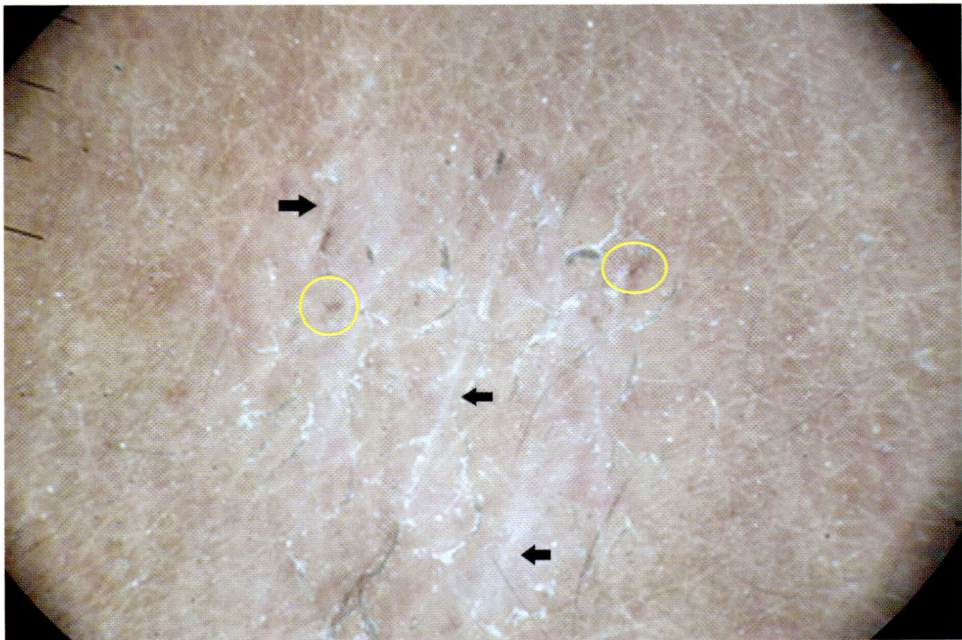

Fig. 27: Dermoscopy shows white areas with scaling on the surface. Note: Brown globules (yellow circles) and prominence of skin lines (black arrows).

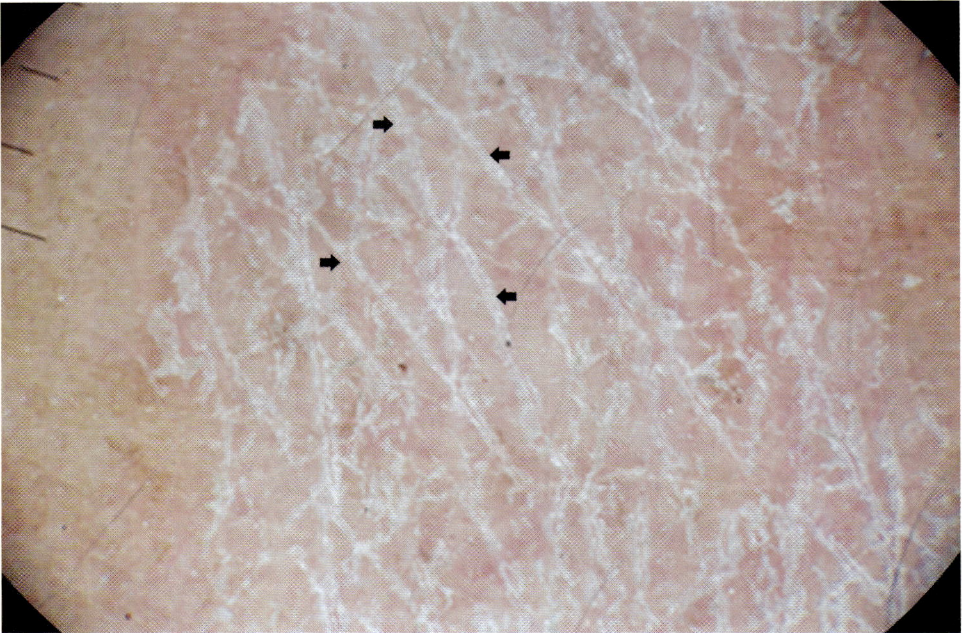

Fig. 28: Dermoscopy of same lesion of Figure 27; upon stretching the skin, scales become double edged (arrows).

REFERENCES

1. Errichetti E, Stinco G. Dermoscopy in general dermatology: a practical overview. Dermatol Ther (Heidelb). 2016;6(4):471-507.
2. Zhou H, Tang XH, De Han J, et al. Dermoscopy as an ancillary tool for the diagnosis of pityriasis versicolor. J Am Acad Dermatol. 2015;73:e205-6.
3. Weedon D. Mycoses and algal infections. In: Weedon D (Ed). Skin Pathology, 2nd edition. Edinburgh: Churchill Livingstone; 2002. pp. 659-90.

PITYRIASIS ALBA

INTRODUCTION

Pityriasis alba consists of variably hypopigmented patches on the face, neck, or shoulders (Fig. 29). It is common in darker individuals. It is considered as postinflammatory hypopigmentation following eczema.[1]

Histopathology shows mild hyperkeratosis, focal parakeratosis, and focal spongiosis with prominent exocytosis of lymphocytes.[2] However, there are no reports on dermoscopic patterns in pityriasis alba.

KEY DERMOSCOPIC FEATURES (PERSONAL OBSERVATION)

- Ill-demarcated whitish areas
- Mild scaling especially in the center of lesion
- Faint pigment network
- Normal hair color.

DISCUSSION

Pityriasis versicolor and pityriasis alba look similar when PV affects cheek. It is difficult to distinguish both. Dermoscopy can be helpful in this situation (Figs. 30 and 31). Dermoscopy of PV also shows white areas, however, scaling is characteristically double edged in the skin furrows.

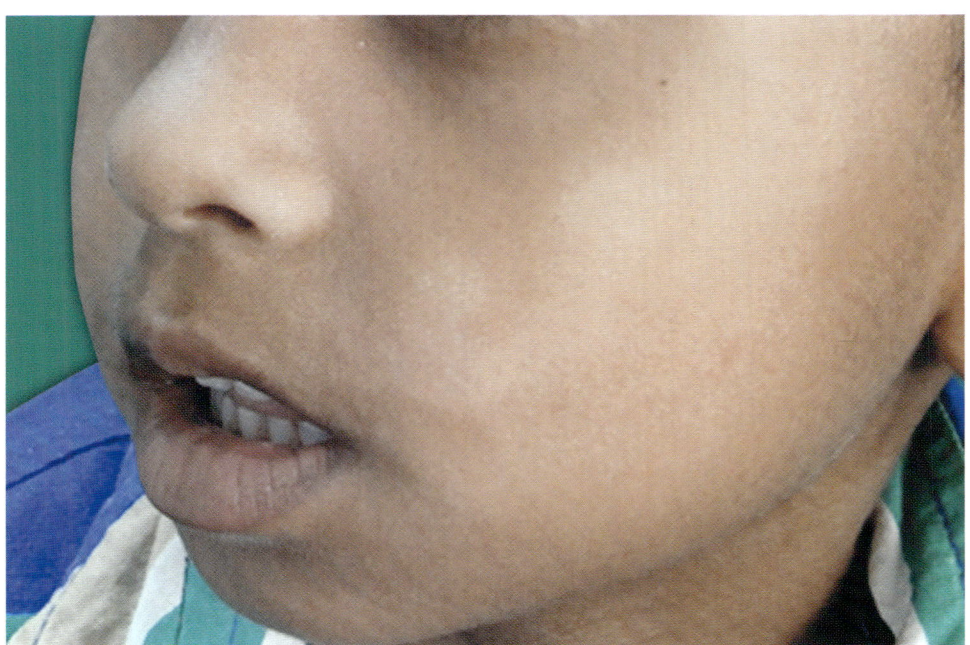

Fig. 29: Dep-gmented patch on the cheek with mild scaling in a child.

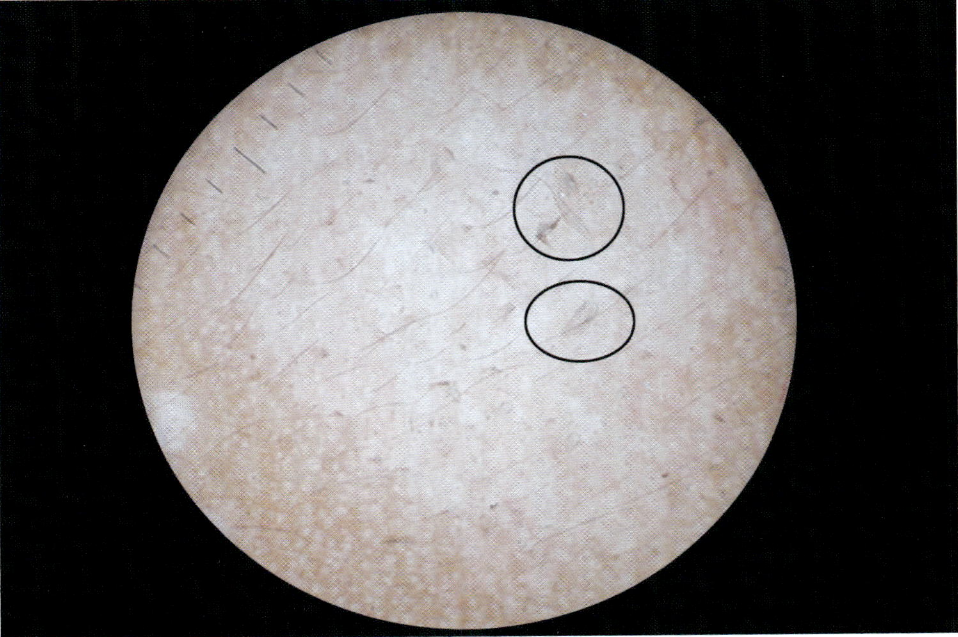

Fig. 30: Dermcscopy demonstrates diffuse white areas with fine scaling (black circles). Note: Faint pigmentary network.

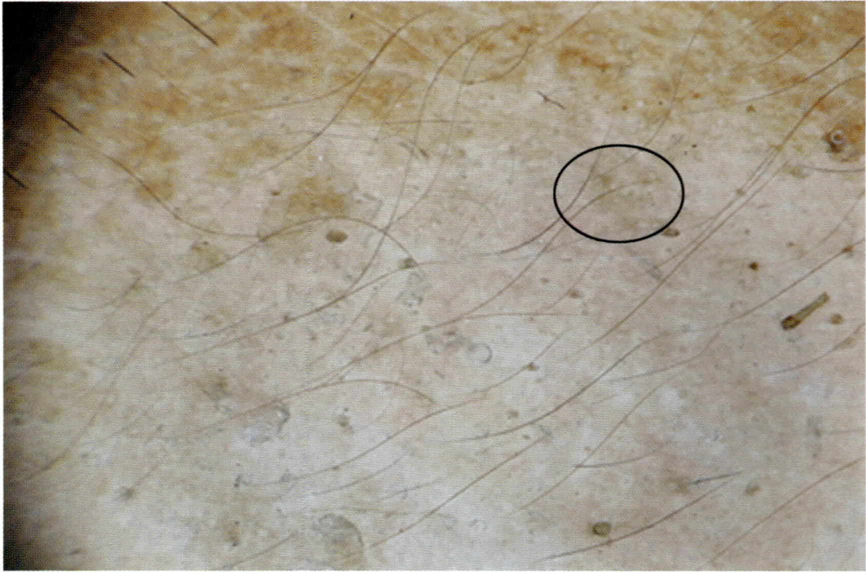

Fig. 31: Dermoscopy reveals white areas with faint pigmentation (black circles).

REFERENCES

1. Hanifin JM. Clinical and basic aspects of atopic dermatitis. Semin Dermatol. 1983;2:5-19.
2. Weedon D. Disorders of pigmentation. In: Weedon D (Ed). Skin Pathology, 2nd edition. Edinburgh: Churchill Livingstone; 2002. pp. 321-41.

ASH LEAF MACULE

INTRODUCTION

Ash leaf macules (ALMs) are characterized by depigmented macules, which are lanceolate in shape (Fig. 32). Less than 6 ALM is considered as normal even though ALM is specific for tuberous sclerosus. It appears even before the other clinical signs of tuberous sclerosus are evident. Sometimes it can be mistaken for vitiligo or ND. Hence, its diagnosis becomes an important aspect in clinical practice. Dermoscopy shows characteristic patterns in ALM.[1]

KEY DERMOSCOPIC FEATURES (FIG. 33)[1]

- White areas
- Zones of total loss of pigment network
- Zones of faint pigment network.

DISCUSSION

The diagnosis of ALM is a warning sign for internal disease like tuberous sclerosus. In children with such lesions, diagnostic tests including skin biopsy may not be practical. Thus, knowledge of dermoscopic pattern in ALM would help in its early diagnosis and prompt treatment. It also alleviates the apprehension associated with hypopigmented lesions like vitiligo.

KEYNOTE

Dermoscopy is a useful aide in the diagnosis of ALM.

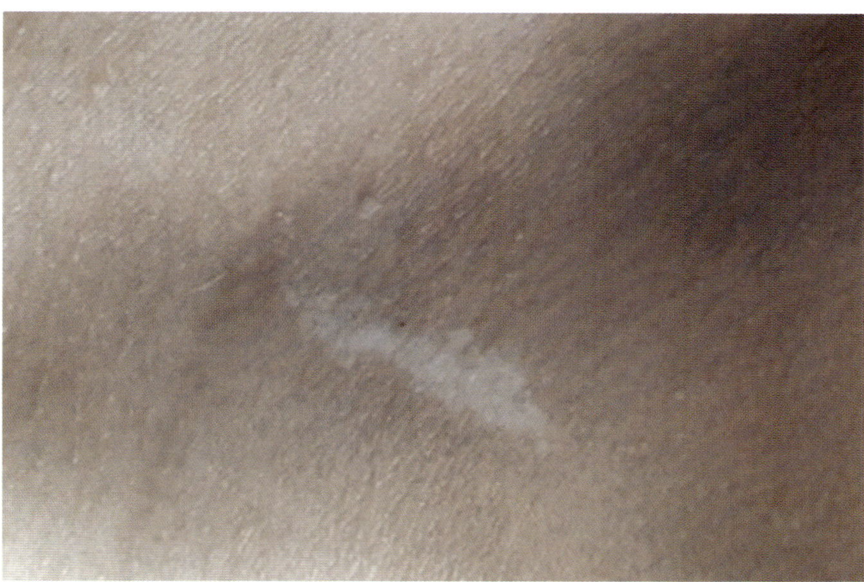

Fig. 32: Depigmented macule on the anterior neck.
Courtesy: Dr Subrata Malakar, Director, Rita Skin Foundation, Kolkata, West Bengal

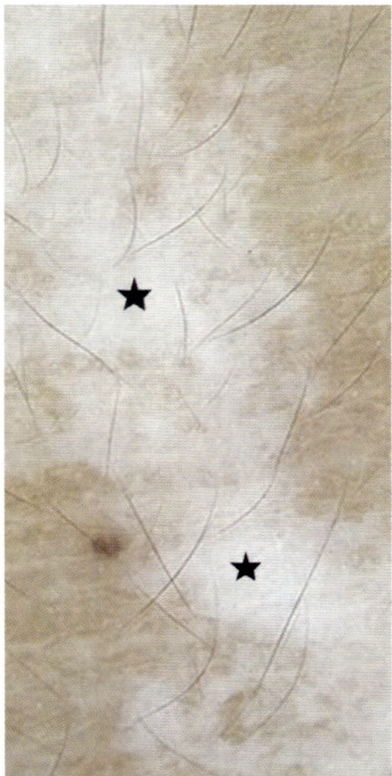

Fig. 33: Dermoscopy of ash leaf macule shows white areas with zones of total loss of pigment network (stars) among the areas of faint pigment network.
Courtesy: Dr Subrata Malakar, Director, Rita Skin Foundation, Kolkata, West Bengal

REFERENCE

1. Malakar SS, Mukharjee S. Differentiation of nevus depigmentosus, ash leaf macule and nevus anemicus. In: Chattarjee M, Neema S, Malakar S (Eds). Dermoscopy in Darker Skin, 1st edition. New Delhi: Jaypee Brothers Medical Publishers (P) Ltd; 2017. pp. 39-41.

LEPROSY

INTRODUCTION

Leprosy is characterized by hypopigmented patches with impairment or total loss of sensation (Fig. 34). Peripheral nerves are thickened and tender. In atypical presentations, it can mimic early vitiligo and other hypopigmentary conditions. Dermoscopy provides useful information by demonstrating characteristic patterns in granulomatous conditions. As a granulomatous disease, leprosy shows characteristic patterns under dermoscopy. Dermoscopy of borderline tuberculoid (BT) leprosy is reported in the literature.[1]

KEY DERMOSCOPIC FEATURES (BORDERLINE TUBERCULOID LEPROSY) (FIG. 35)

- White areas, prominent on skin furrows
- Reduced pigment network, prominent in perifollicular areas
- Decreased hairs
- Decreased white dots (eccrine opening).

Above-mentioned patterns are seen in hypopigmented and noninfiltrated lesions of BT leprosy affecting nonfacial skin. Infiltrated lesions and facial lesions show different dermoscopic patterns.

DISCUSSION

Generally, hypopigmented lesions are anesthetic and diagnosis is not difficult in typical clinical features. White areas and reduced pigment network suggests decreased number of melanocytes. Decreased hairs and white dots indicate destruction of hair follicles and eccrine glands by the granuloma. Infiltrated and facial lesions show yellow areas and telangiectasia. These patterns are identical to dermoscopic patterns of lupus vulgaris and sarcoidosis (granulomatous conditions).

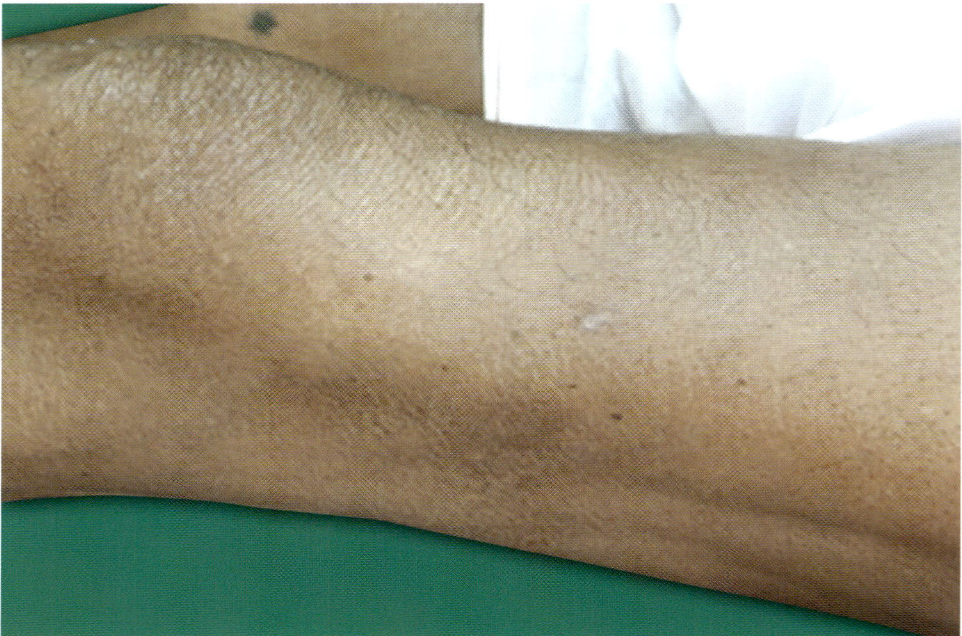

Fig. 34: Clinical image of borderline tuberculoid leprosy showing ill-defined patch on the thigh.

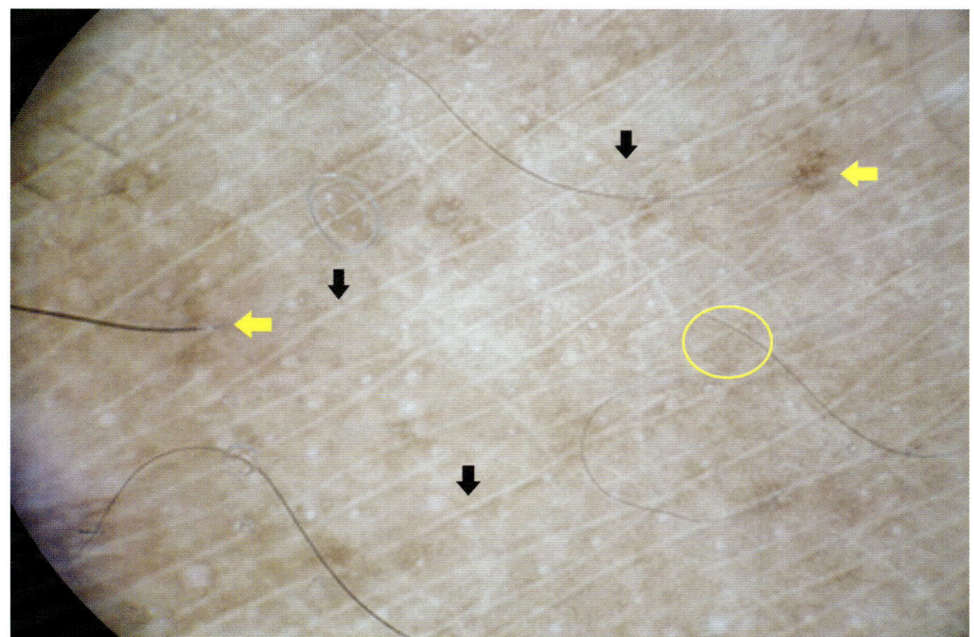

Fig. 35: Dermoscopy of Figure 34 shows diffuse white areas, prominence of skin furrows (black arrows). Reduced numbers of white dots and hair are noted. Pigment is faint (yellow circle) and is prominent in perifollicular areas (yellow arrows).

KEYNOTE

Dermoscopic patterns vary in different type of lesions in BT leprosy. Thus, dermoscopy plays an additional role in the diagnosis of BT leprosy.

REFERENCE

1. Ankad BS, Sakhare PS. Dermoscopy of borderline tuberculoid leprosy. Int J Dermatol. 2017. [Epub ahead of print].

12B. DERMOSCOPY IN HYPERPIGMENTATION

Niti Khunger

INTRODUCTION

Dermoscopy is a specialized noninvasive technique that allows a rapid and magnified in vivo observation of the skin with the visualization of morphologic features that are invisible to the naked eye. The term dermatoscopy was first introduced by the German dermatologist Johann Saphier in 1920 to describe the examination of the skin using an instrument resembling a binocular microscope with a built-in light source. This surface microscopy was further described as dermoscopy by Goldman in the United States in the 1950s, who was the first dermatologist to evaluate pigmented skin lesions with a dermascope.[1] Today dermoscopy has become an essential tool to evaluate pigmented skin lesions, both melanocytic and nonmelanocytic. It has been shown that dermoscopy increases diagnostic accuracy by 5–30% over clinical examination alone.[2]

Though it was traditionally introduced for evaluation of suspicious nevi and early diagnosis of cutaneous malignancies such as malignant melanoma and basal cell carcinoma, its role has expanded vastly to include other pigmentary abnormalities such as melasma, ochronosis, lichen planus, vitiligo, etc. The advantage of dermoscopy is that it opens up a new dimension of clinical morphology, is more accurate than clinical examination, and it can reduce the need for biopsy or help to select the correct site of biopsy. Digital dermoscopy allows easy storage and retrieval and opens the door for monitoring, teledermoscopy, and automated diagnosis. This chapter will give the dermoscopic approach to common pigmentary disorders.

BASIC PRINCIPLES IN PIGMENTATION

The colors seen on dermoscopy depend on depth of the melanin and other structures. There are eight basic colors in dermoscopy. Black, dark brown, light brown, gray, and blue are seen in melanocytic lesions, depending of the depth of the lesions.[3] The others are red, yellow, and white. The melanin in the stratum corneum appears black, darker brown in the upper epidermis, lighter brown in the dermoepidermal junction, and grayish blue in the dermis due to the Tyndall effect. Free melanin or melanophages appear grayish. This is an advantage in distinguishing if the lesion is epidermal, dermal, or mixed. Lack of melanin, calcium deposits, or fibrosis appears white. Keratin in the stratum corneum and lipid collections appears yellow. Vascularity can be picked up early as red hues and telangiectasia can be easily observed.

PATTERN ANALYSIS

Dermoscopy of pigmented lesions follows the two-step approach. The first is to decide if the lesion is melanocytic or nonmelanocytic. Seborrheic keratosis, basal cell carcinoma, and vascular lesions are examples of nonmelanocytic lesions. If the lesion is melanocytic or unknown, the next step is whether it is benign or malignant. This is based on the pattern analysis. The pattern analysis includes a description of the global pattern and the local pattern.

CRITERIA FOR MELANOCYTIC LESIONS

There are basic five criteria for melanocytic lesions: (1) A pigment network, (2) Aggregated globules, (3) Branched streaks, (4) A homogeneous pigmentation, or (5) A parallel pattern.[3] If one of these criteria is observed on dermoscopy, the lesion is likely to be melanocytic; and, if not, the lesion will be nonmelanocytic.

Pigment Network and Pseudonetwork

A reticulated pigment network shows a grid-like or honeycomb pattern composed of pigmented lines that correspond to the rete ridge pattern of the epidermis with melanin in the keratinocyte and melanocyte and hypopigmented holes correspond to the tips of the dermal papillae. The pigment network may be typical as observed in benign lesions, seen as lines of uniform thickness and color, a regular patterned network with fading in the periphery. An atypical network as seen in malignancy is seen as lines of varying thickness and color, darker broader lines, heterogeneous holes, and abrupt transition to the periphery. A pseudonetwork is usually seen in pigmented lesions on the face, where the rete ridge pattern is attenuated, the adnexal openings of the hair follicles, and sweat gland appear as holes of the pseudonetwork.

Dots and Globules

Dots are small, roundish colored structures less than 0.1 mm in diameter. The color depends on the depth of the pigment and appears as black dots representing pigment in the stratum corneum. Brown dots represent small melanocytic nests at the tips of the rete ridges, at the dermal-epidermal junction, or in the epidermis. Blue-gray dots represent free melanin in the dermis or in macrophages. Blood vessels appear as red dots.

Globules are symmetrical, round to oval structures larger than 0.1 mm. Brown, black, and blue globules correspond to nests of pigmented melanocytes at the dermal-epidermal junction or in the dermis. Red globules represent blood vessels.

DERMOSCOPY OF NORMAL FACIAL SKIN IN DARKER SKINS

Dermoscopy of normal facial skin shows a background of diffuse pigmentation interspersed with openings of sweat glands and hair follicles, exhibiting a pseudonetwork pattern. Melanin is the main chromophore and vessels appear red (Fig. 1).

The dermoscopic patterns of some common pigmented lesions are discussed in the chapter, particularly in relation to darker skin types.

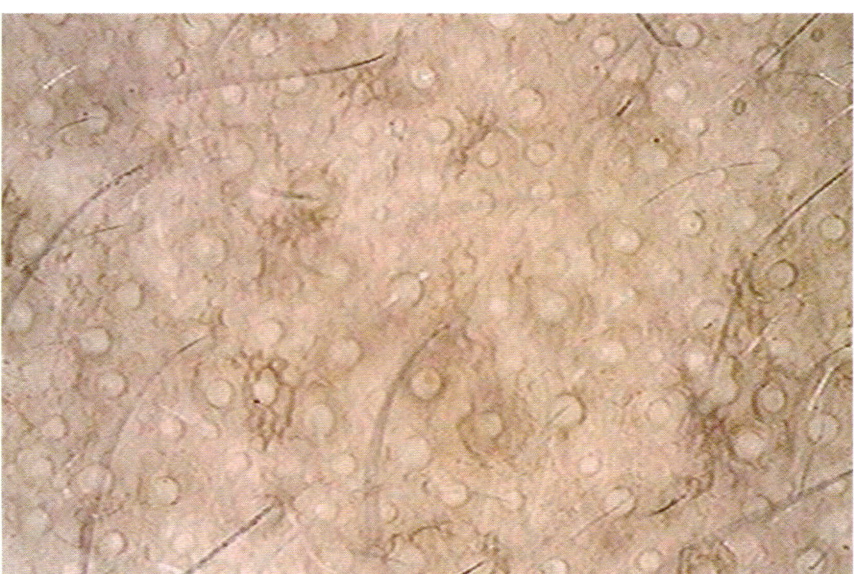

Fig. 1: Dermoscopy of normal facial skin showing a background of diffuse pigmentation, interspersed with holes of sweat glands, forming a pseudonetwork pattern, and vessels appearing red.

REFERENCES

1. Braun RP, Rabinovitz HS, Oliviero M, et al. Dermoscopy of pigmented skin lesions. J Am Acad Dermatol. 2005;52:109-21.
2. Kittler H, Pehamberger H, Wolff K, et al. Diagnostic accuracy of dermoscopy. Lancet Oncol. 2002;3(3):159-65.
3. Tanaka M. Dermoscopy basics and melanocytic lesions. Hong Kong J Dermatol Venereol. 2013;21:124-9.

MELASMA

INTRODUCTION

Melasma is a common, acquired pigmentary skin disease predominantly involving sun-exposed areas like cheeks, forehead, upper lip, and occasionally the extensor aspect of the forearms (Fig. 2A).

It is clinically characterized by brownish to grayish black, symmetrical hyperpigmented macules with irregular borders, and histopathologically by increased melanin in the epidermis, increase in melanosomes in the melanocytes and keratinocytes in epidermal melasma. There is increased vascularity and solar elastosis in the dermis. In addition, there are melanophages in the dermis, with increased free melanin in mixed epidermal and dermal melasma (Fig. 2B).

Dermoscopy in melasma plays an important role as it can help in judging the depth of melasma, whether epidermal, dermal, or mixed, and can also assist to rule out exogenous ochronosis that can be a complication of melasma treatment.

KEY DERMOSCOPIC FEATURES

The key dermoscopic features of melasma include a diffuse brown reticular pigmentation with sparing of follicles and sweat gland openings producing an exaggerated pseudonetwork pattern. The borders are concave which is referred to as "jelly sign" (Fig. 2C).[1] Varied dermoscopic patterns have been described in melasma such as reticuloglobular, perifollicular brown-black globules, arcuate, annular, honeycomb or granular pigmented pattern, or unpatterned patchy brown-black pigment.[2] Tamler et al.[3] classified melasma based on dermoscopy and correlated it with Wood's lamp examination. Brownish pigment with a regular pigment network was epidermal, blotchy bluish-gray pigment was dermal, and a mixed pattern was seen in mixed melasma. In another study of 100 patients of melasma, the reticuloglobular pattern was most common, seen in 83% of patients, granular pigment in 28%, and unpatterned patchy brown-black pigment was seen in 17% patients. Perifollicular brown-black globules were seen in 60% of patients, but also in 62% of controls were not specific for melasma. A higher percentage of patients showed telangiectasia as compared to controls. This may be a result of increased vascularity of melasma or more commonly due to topical steroid abuse, which is rampant in melasma (Table 1).

DISCUSSION

Though it is easy to diagnose melasma on clinical grounds, dermoscopy in melasma has therapeutic and prognostic significance. A dermal or mixed pattern on dermoscopy implies that treatment will be prolonged and melasma will be more difficult to treat. The chances of recurrence of mixed melasma are higher due to sparing of deeper melanocytes following treatment. Dermoscopy not only differentiates the type of melasma but also helps to differentiate between melasma and ochronosis. Due to a striking similarity of ochronosis with melasma, clinicians require a high index of suspicion in order to make an early diagnosis. This is important to prevent worsening of pigmentation due to overuse of hydroquinone.

KEYNOTE

Dermoscopy helps to differentiate epidermal from mixed melasma, which has therapeutic and prognostic significance. It is also valuable to rule out exogenous ochronosis that can be a complication of melasma treatment.

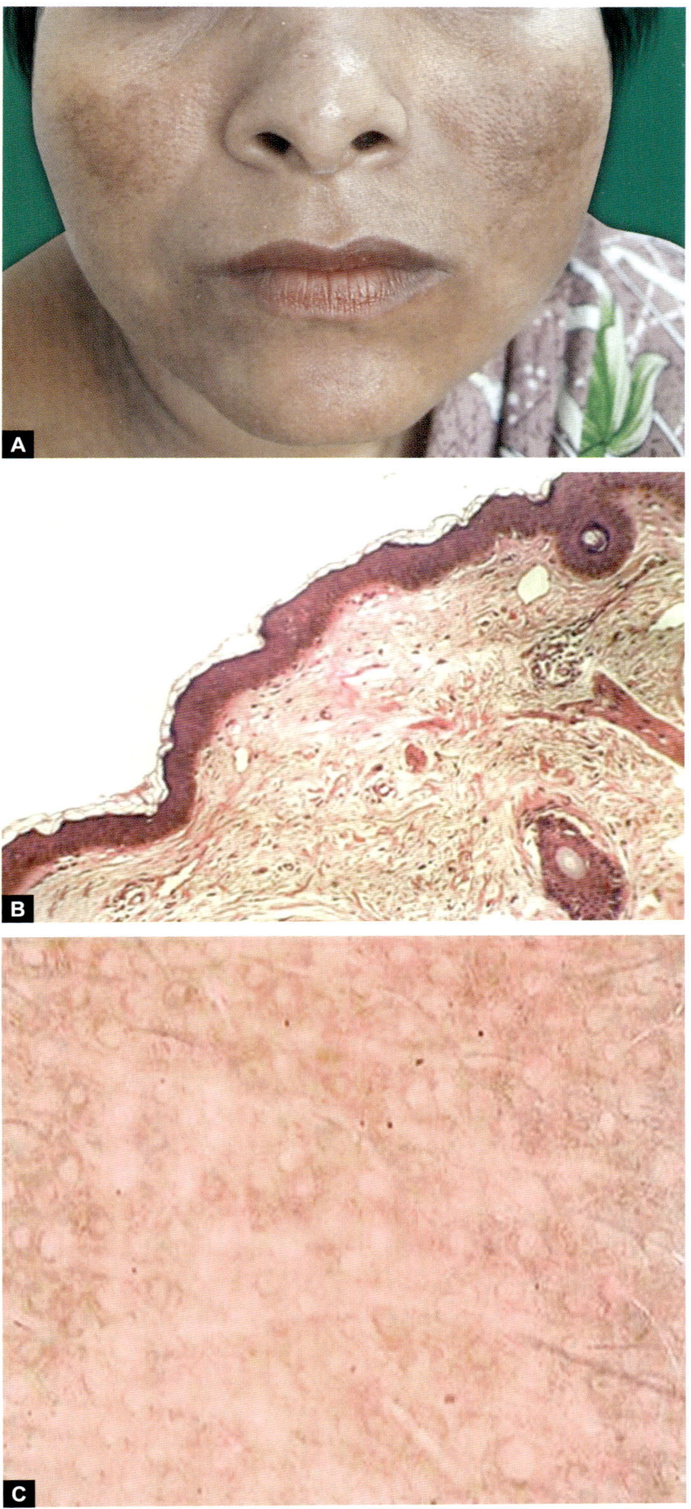

Figs. 2A to C: (A) Brownish, symmetrical hyperpigmented macules with irregular borders in a case of melasma; (B) Increased melanin in the epidermis. There is increased vascularity and solar elastosis along with melanophages and increased free melanin in the dermis on histopathology in melasma; and (C) Dermoscopy of melasma showing pseudonetwork pattern, brownish to bluish-gray pigment globules and dots, and prominent vessels.

Table 1: Dermoscopic pattern of various histopathological types of melasma.

Types of melasma	*Pattern*	*Color*	*Vascularity*
Epidermal	• Regular pigment network • Homogeneous brown pigmentation • Reticuloglobular • Perifollicular pattern	Brown	May be present
Dermal	• Irregular mixed network	Bluish gray	May be present
Mixed	• Diffuse • Unpatterned with mixture of both patterns • Bluish-gray arcuate, annular, and star-shaped morphologies with sparing of follicles	Brown and bluish gray	May be present
Ochronosis	• Dark brown globules • Elongated and curvilinear worm-like structures • Blue-gray amorphous areas that may obliterate follicular openings.	Dark brown globules with blue-gray amorphous areas	May be present

REFERENCES

1. Khopkar US. Dermoscopy and Trichoscopy in Diseases of the Brown Skin—Atlas and Short Text. New Delhi: Jaypee Brothers Medical Publishers (P) Ltd; 2014. pp. 50-62.
2. Neema S, Chatterjee M. Dermoscopic characteristics of melasma in Indians: a cross-sectional study. Int J Dermoscopy. 2017;1(1):6-10.
3. Tamler C, Fonseca RM, Pereira FB, et al. Classification of melasma by dermoscopy: comparative study with Wood's lamp. Surg Cosmet Dermatol. 2009;1(3):115-9.

EXOGENOUS OCHRONOSIS

INTRODUCTION

Ochronosis is an accumulation of brown-yellow or ochre-colored pigment in connective tissue. It can be exogenous or endogenous in origin. Exogenous ochronosis manifests as asymptomatic hyperchromia of the skin, usually on the sun-exposed areas of the face, particularly bony prominences, back, and the extensor surfaces of the extremities (Fig. 3A).

It is often associated with prolonged application of various topical agents, such as hydroquinone, phenol, resorcinol, mercurials, and picric acid, as well as with quinine injections and oral antimalarial agents. Dogliotti described three clinical stages of exogenous ochronosis:[1]

- *Stage 1:* Erythema and hyperpigmentation
- *Stage 2:* Hyperpigmentation, pigmented colloid milium (caviar-like lesions), and atrophy
- *Stage 3:* Papulonodular lesions.

In the early first stage, it can be clinically indistinguishable from melasma. In such cases, dermoscopy might help to differentiate it from melasma.

KEY DERMOSCOPIC FEATURES

- Dermoscopy shows irregular, brownish to grayish, globular, annular, and arciform structures along with brown-gray amorphous areas at times obliterating the follicular structures rather than just surrounding them.[2] Multiple thick globular structures may be seen overlying the melasma patch. The structures are curvilinear with a "worm-like" pattern that corresponds to the banana-shaped yellowish brown ochre bodies seen on histopathology (Figs. 3B and C).
- Confetti-like depigmentation can be seen as white dots and telangiectasia as red dots and red linear lesions.

DISCUSSION

Exogenous ochronosis is probably more common than diagnosed. Sometimes it is difficult to differentiate exogenous ochronosis from melasma especially in its early stages. In such cases, dermoscopy can act as a handy noninvasive tool in differentiating the two.[3] Melasma is characterized by normal pseudoreticular pigment network along with dark brown globules and granules sparing the follicles and sweat gland openings whereas in exogenous ochronosis amorphous and globular structures obliterate hair follicle openings along with confetti-like depigmentation. As histopathology is the gold standard to diagnose ochronosis, dermoscopy can assist in selection of the proper site of biopsy. Early diagnosis will necessitate immediate discontinuation of hydroquinone rather than increasing it in attempt to clear the hyperpigmentation.

KEYNOTE

Dermoscopy can be employed as a rapid screening test for exogenous ochronosis. The clinical presence of coarse texture of the skin, fine telangiectasias, and hyperchromia with speckling or reticulation along with confetti-like depigmentation should alert the clinician to resort to a dermoscopic examination, particularly in patients who are reluctant to get a facial biopsy.

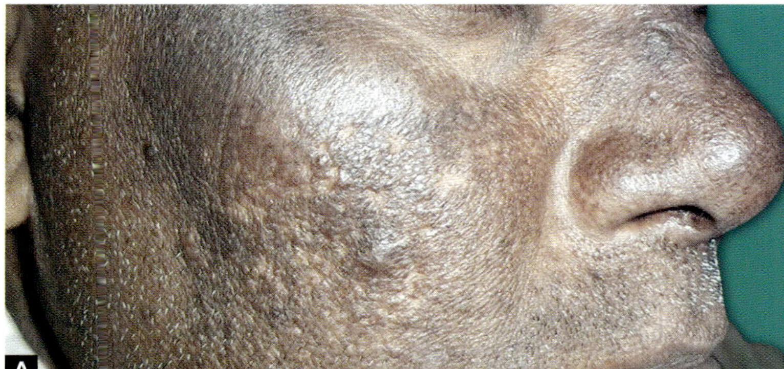

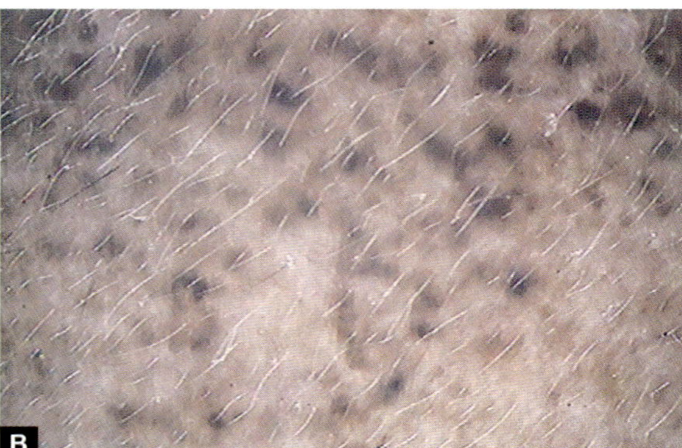

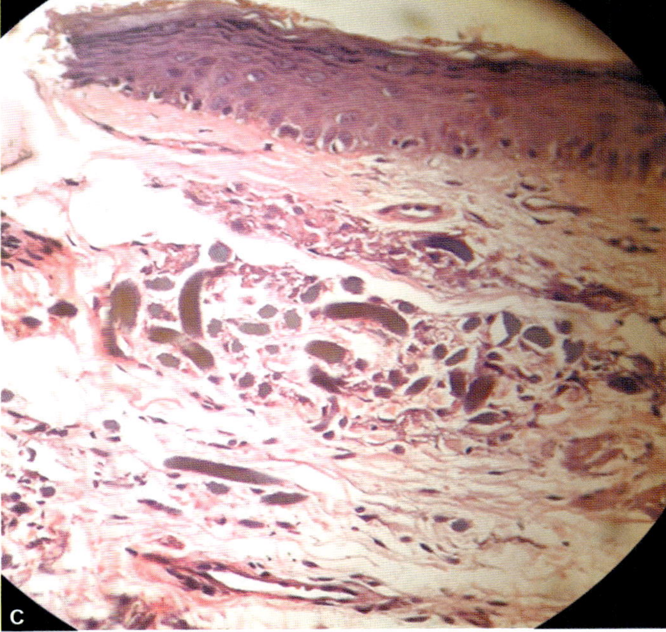

Figs. 3A to C: (A) Asymptomatic hyperchromia of the skin, usually on the sun-exposed areas of the face, particularly bony prominences in exogenous ochronosis; (B) Irregular, brownish to grayish, globular, annular, and arciform structures along with brown-gray amorphous areas at times obliterating the follicular structures on dermoscopy in exogenous ochronosis; and (C) Banana-shaped yellowish-brown ochre bodies in the dermis on histopathology of exogenous ochronosis.

REFERENCES

1. Tamler C, Fonseca RM, Pereira FB, et al. Classification of melasma by dermoscopy: comparative study with Wood's lamp. Surg Cosmet Dermatol. 2009;1(3):115-9.
2. Charlín R, Barcaui CB, Kac BK, et al. Hydroquinone-induced exogenous ochronosis: a report of four cases and usefulness of dermoscopy. Int J Dermatol. 2008;47(1):19-23.
3. Khunger N, Kandhari R. Dermoscopic criteria for differentiating exogenous ochronosis from melasma. Indian J Dermatol Venereol Leprol. 2013;79(6):819-21.

PIGMENTARY DEMARCATION LINES

INTRODUCTION

Pigmentary demarcation lines (PDLs) are physiological, abrupt transition zones from deeper pigmented skin to lighter pigmented skin (Fig. 4A).[1]

The pathogenesis of PDLs is unclear, although some believe that the axial-neural theory is at play as these lines coincide with cutaneous nerve distribution, whereas others believe that they are due to pigmentary mosaicism. They are classified into eight types A–H, depending on their location. The facial PDLs (FPDLs) F, G, and H are more important as they occur on the cosmetic areas of the face.[2] They are often misdiagnosed with melasma as they share certain clinical similarities such as the presence of facial hyperpigmented macules and predominant occurrence in women, yet they are discrete entities and can be differentiated clinically. They may even be coexistent. It is important to differentiate from melasma as the etiology, treatment, and prognosis varies widely. Though the diagnosis is mainly clinical, dermoscopic examination can be a useful entity.

KEY DERMOSCOPIC FEATURES

- Dermoscopic pictures of FPDL have not been elaborated sufficiently. Dermoscopy of FPDL does not show a specific pattern. There is exaggeration of the normal pseudonetwork pattern at the global level and a blotchy, globular, or granular pigmentation at the local level or combinations of these (Fig. 4B).
- In a personal study of 20 patients of FPDL, four patterns of pigmentation were observed. The most common pattern observed was a blotchy pattern seen in 8/20 patients (40%), followed by a blotchy and granular pattern in seven patients (35%), a granular pattern in four patients (20%), and a blotchy and globular pattern in a single patient.

DISCUSSION

Facial pigmentary demarcation lines are a distinct entity with specific patterns of pigmentation. Though they share certain common features with melasma, they can be differentiated clinically by their brownish, patterned pigmentation with well-defined borders. Dermoscopically there are subtle differences in the patterns, but have not been adequately studied. In a personal study, it was observed that under the dermoscope, melasma appears to involve the entire face, whereas dermoscopic changes in FPDL are confined to the lesional skin.

KEYNOTE

Dermoscopy of PDLs shows a pattern of exaggerated pseudonetwork of the skin along with blotchy, globular, or granular pattern of pigmentation that is confined to the lesion with well-defined borders.

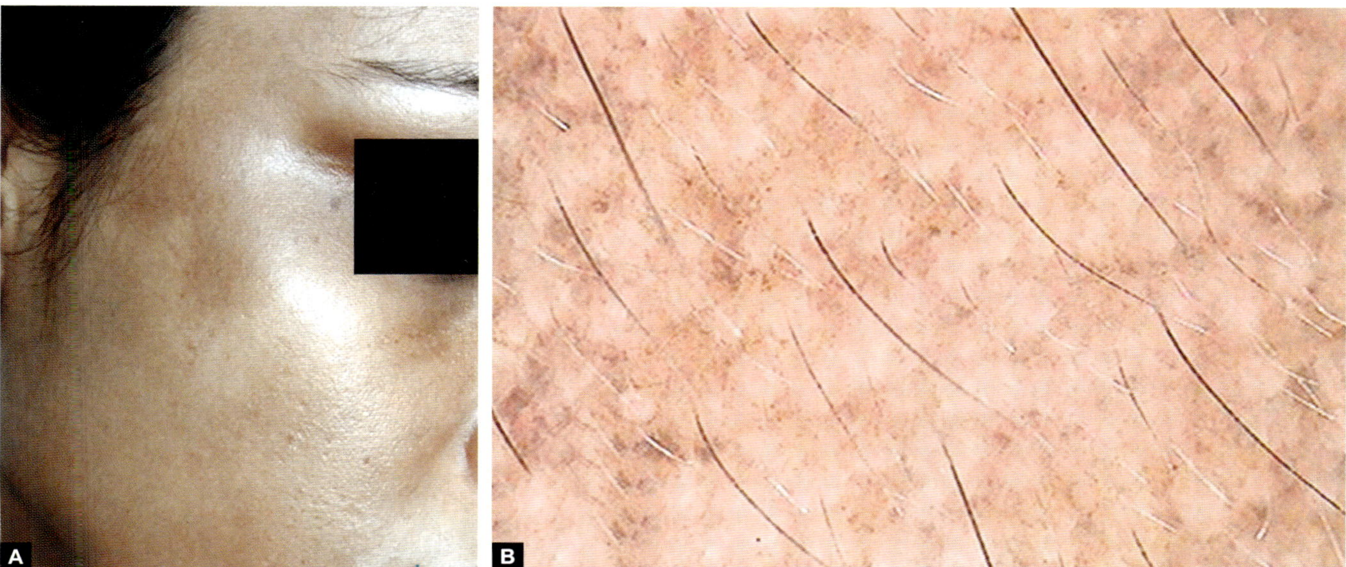

Figs. 4A and B: (A) Pigmentary demarcation line in a young female; and (B) Dermoscopy of facial pigmentary demarcation line (FPDL) showing pseudonetwork of the skin along with blotchy and globular pattern of pigmentation which is confined to the lesion with well-defined borders.

REFERENCES

1. Malakar S, Dhar S. Pigmentary demarcation lines over the face. Dermatology. 2000;200(1):85-6.
2. Somani VK, Razvi F, Sita VN. Pigmentary demarcation lines over the face. Indian J Dermatol Venereol Leprol. 2004;70:336-41.

PIGMENTED COSMETIC DERMATITIS (RIEHL'S MELANOSIS)

INTRODUCTION

Pigmented contact dermatitis (Riehl's melanosis) is a type of melanosis characterized by diffuse or reticulated brown, slate gray, or bluish brown pigmentation observed on the face and neck (Fig. 5A).

It is low-grade contact dermatitis, often due to antigens present in cosmetics, textiles, airborne antigens, and fragrances. Occasionally it may be due to occupational allergens like coal tar, asphalt, mineral oil, and chromates. The site of involvement depends on the contact allergen.[1] Pigmented contact dermatitis due to cosmetics begins on forehead, temples, and zygomatic region and then spreads to involve rest of the face, followed by the neck, chest, hands, and forearms, while those due to textiles involve the anterior aspect of thighs and axillae, with sparing of the vault. It is more common in women, particularly with darker skin types. The patch test may be positive in some patients.

KEY DERMOSCOPIC FEATURES

- Pseudonetwork pattern with gray dots, granules, and telangiectatic vessels are the most common features.
- These correspond to pigmentary incontinence. Perifollicular whitish halo and keratotic plugs may be seen in few patients. In addition, flour-like white scales may be seen, suggestive of preceding low-grade inflammation (Fig. 5B).[2]

DISCUSSION

Pigmented cosmetic dermatitis is a common facial pigmentary disorder. Dermoscopy may help to differentiate it from lichen planus pigmentosus (LPP), which it can clinically resemble.

KEYNOTE

The clinical presentation of bluish gray pigment, predominant on the lateral part of the face, with features of a pseudonetwork pattern, follicular sparing, whitish halo in the perifollicular region, and pigmented gray dots and globules should raise the suspicion of pigmented cosmetic dermatitis.

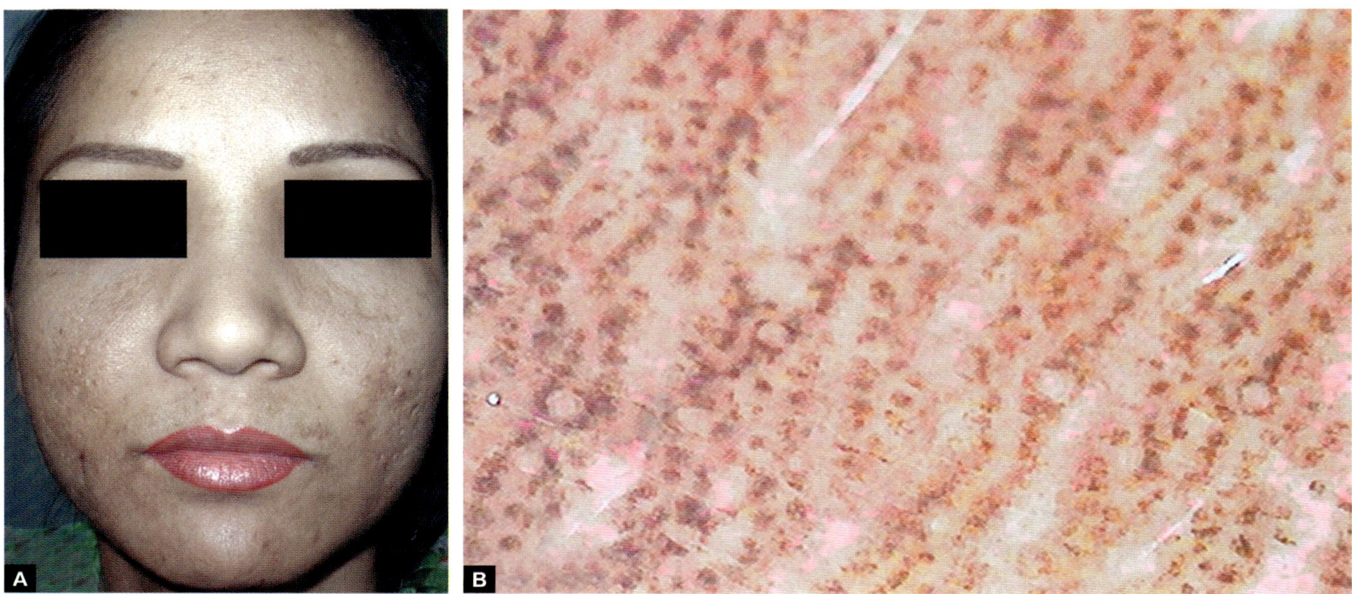

Figs. 5A and B: (A) Pigmented cosmetic dermatitis in a female with diffuse to reticulated brown pigmentation on the face; (B) Pseudonetwork pattern, follicular sparing, whitish halo in the perifollicular region, and pigmented gray dots and globules in Riehl's melanosis.

REFERENCES

1. Shenoi SD, Rao R. Pigmented contact dermatitis. Indian J Dermatol Venereol Leprol. 2007;73:285-7.
1. Wang L, Xu AE. Four views of Riehl's melanosis: clinical appearance, dermoscopy, confocal microscopy and histopathology. J Eur Acad Dermatol Venereol. 2014;28:1199-206.

LICHEN PLANUS PIGMENTOSUS

INTRODUCTION

Lichen planus pigmentosus is a macular variant of lichen planus, which presents as diffuse ill-defined violaceus to grayish-black macules predominantly on the sun-exposed areas that gradually extend to the trunk and limbs (Fig. 6A).

Lichen planus pigmentosus inversus is a variant of LPP, where brownish, bluish gray to black pigmentation is observed in the flexural areas.

KEY DERMOSCOPIC FEATURES

- In LPP three patterns have been described:[1] (1) Diffuse pattern is characterized by brownish diffuse structureless areas, (2) Dotted pattern which is characterized by brownish to bluish gray dots that correspond to dermal melanophages, and (3) Mixed pattern, which is a combination of diffuse and dotted pigmentation. A reticular variant of LPP has also been described (Fig. 6B).[2]

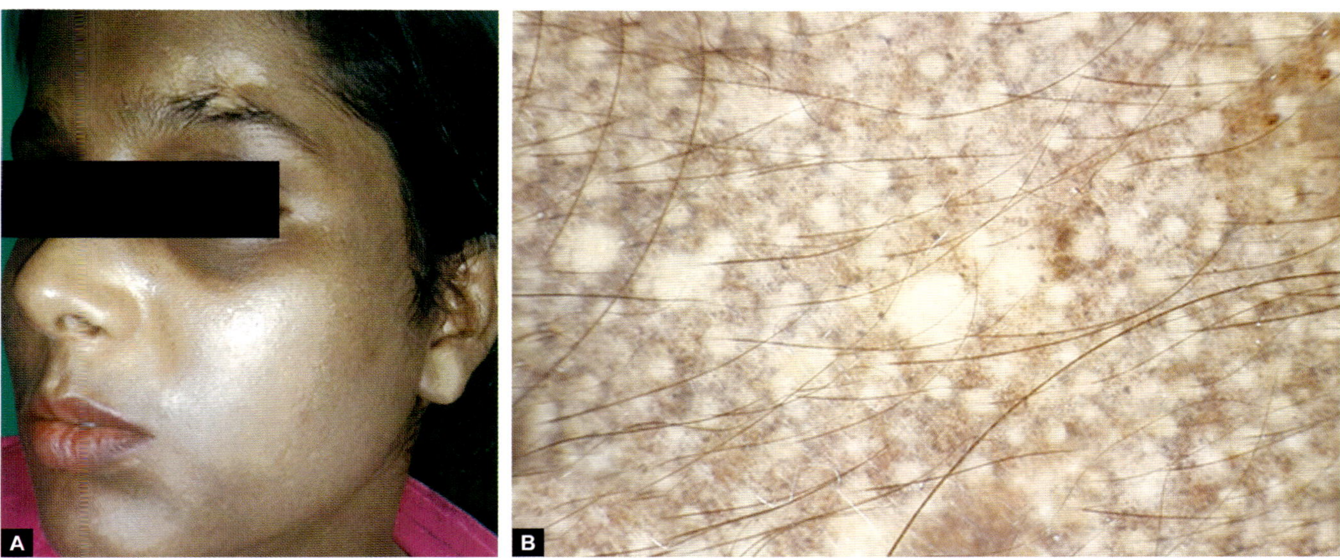

Figs. 6A and B: (A) Lichen planus pigmentosus in a female; (B) Brownish dots and globules in a sheet-like pattern with perifollicular accentuation in a case of lichen planus pigmentosus.
(*Courtesy:* Dr Subrata Malakar).

REFERENCES

1. Vázquez-López F, Maldonado-Seral C, López-Escobar M, et al. Dermoscopy of pigmented lichen planus lesions. Clin Exp Dermatol. 2003;28(5):554-5.
2. Vishwanath T, Agrawak S, Shukla D, et al. Utility of dermoscopy in diagnosing reticular variant of lichen planus pigmentosus. Int J Dermoscop. 2017;1:32-4.

ASHY DERMATOSIS

INTRODUCTION

Ashy dermatosis (AD) is an acquired pigmentary dermatosis, more common in women, characterized by mildly pruritic bluish-gray color macules, of variable shapes and size, and frequently involving the trunk and the arms. AD is more common in adults and is often preceded by reddish raised itchy lesions.

KEY DERMOSCOPIC FEATURE

Grayish-blue dots over a bluish background are dermoscopic features of AD. In contrast, LPP shows as brownish background with brownish to bluish-gray dots that are larger than those of AD.[1]

DISCUSSION

Dermoscopy can help in the differential diagnosis of AD from LPP, which it closely resembles. Dermoscopy in LP may show Wickhams striae, which will be absent in AD. Pigmented globules in LPP are more brownish and larger than those of AD, where they are more bluish gray and smaller as they are deeper melanophages.[1]

KEYNOTE

Dermoscopy is a useful tool for diagnosis as well as therapeutic tool to assess treatment response.

REFERENCE

1. Khopkar US. Dermoscopy and Trichoscopy in Diseases of the Brown Skin Atlas and Short Text, 1st edition. New Delhi: Jaypee Brothers Medical Publishers (P) Ltd; 2012. pp. 60-1.

NEVUS OF OTA

INTRODUCTION

Nevus of Ota is a dermal melanocytic hamartoma that presents typically as bluish to slate-gray hyperpigmentation distributed unilaterally on areas supplied by the ophthalmic and maxillary division of trigeminal nerve (forehead, temple, nose, eyelid, ear, and occasionally scalp). Few patients have ocular lesions such as pigmentation of sclera, cornea, iris, and retina. It can rarely involve the hard palate and rarely be bilateral (Fig. 7A).

It usually presents in childhood or at adolescence. Histopathological findings include melanocytes dispersed in a ribbon-like pattern in between collagen fibers and around the neurovascular bundles of mid and upper dermis. Most patients seek treatment due to cosmetic concerns. Q-switched neodymium-doped yttrium aluminum garnet (Nd:YAG) laser has revolutionized the treatment of nevus of Ota and has become the mainstay of therapy.

KEY DERMOSCOPIC FEATURES

- Bluish-gray reticular pigmentation with some white areas and areas of dark brown color are the key dermoscopic features.[1]
- The pigmented network appears distorted and the pigmented lines are thick and broad.
- Hypopigmented areas surrounded by pigmented background are seen (Fig. 7B).

DISCUSSION

Dermoscopy can be a noninvasive diagnostic tool to differentiate nevus of Ota from other similar looking lesions over face such as melasma or ochronosis. Dermoscopy can also be used as method to evaluate response to laser therapy (Fig. 7C).

KEYNOTE

Dermoscopy can be sensitive noninvasive tool to diagnose nevus of Ota and assess response to therapy.

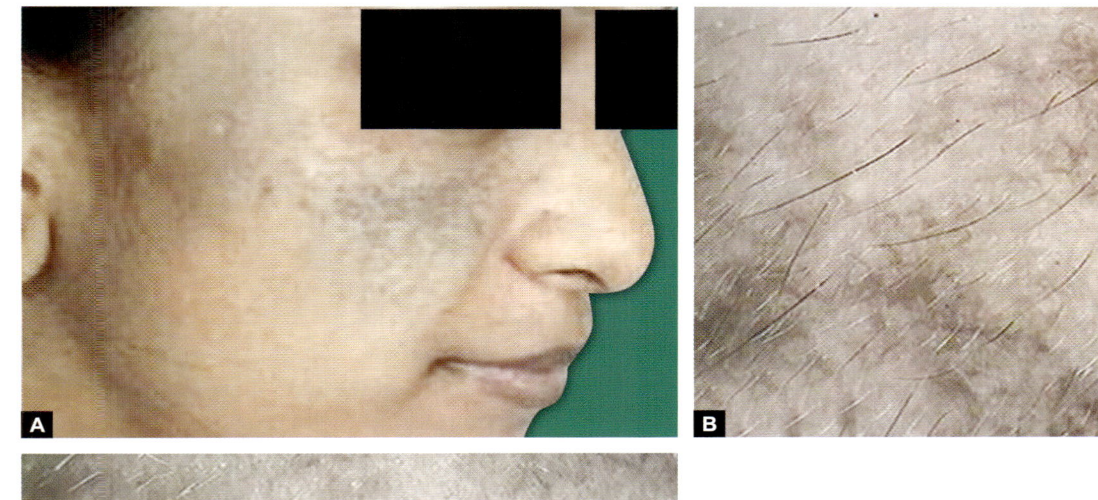

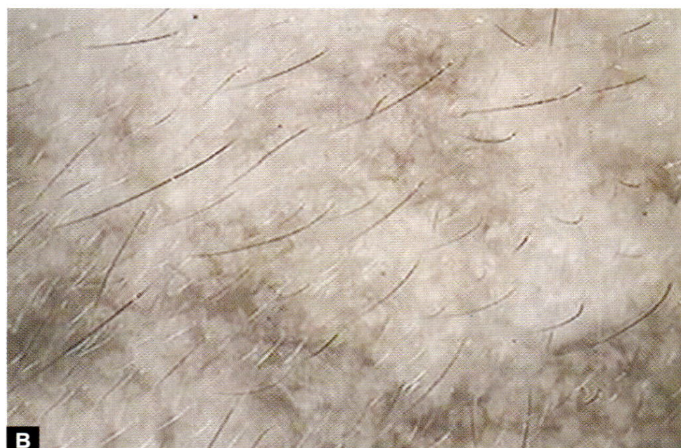

Figs. 7A to C: (A) Nevus of Ota in a young female; (B) Dermoscopic features of nevus of Ota showing bluish-gray reticular pigmentation, with white and brown areas; and (C) Reduction in pigmentation in Nevus of Ota on dermoscopy following treatment with Q-switched neodymium-doped yttrium aluminum garnet (Nd:YAG) laser at 1,064 nm.

REFERENCE

1. Khopkar US. Dermoscopy and Trichoscopy in Diseases of the Brown Skin Atlas and Short Text, 1st edition. New Delhi: Jaypee Brothers Medical Publishers (P) Ltd; 2012. pp. 60-1.

BECKER'S NEVUS

INTRODUCTION

Becker nevus (also called Becker melanosis/Becker pigmentary hamartoma/pigmented hairy epidermal nevus) is not a true nevus because it lacks nevus cells, but is a hamartoma. It was first described by Samuel William Becker in 1949, who reported two males with the characteristic pigmented lesion. It is more common in males, appears around puberty, and is characterized by a circumscribed, brownish to bluish-gray macule with irregular geographical borders, on the shoulder or clavicular region. However, it may present on other areas of the body, may be seen in females, and rarely may be congenital or multiple (Fig. 8A).

It is commonly associated with hypertrichosis and acneiform eruptions. It may rarely be associated with ipsilateral breast hypoplasia, polythelia (supernumerary nipples), and skeletal abnormalities as part of Becker nevus syndrome.

KEY DERMOSCOPIC FEATURES

The key dermoscopic features include a well-defined pigment network, focal hypopigmentation, furrow hypopigmentation, perifollicular hypopigmentation, focal thickening of network lines, and presence of vessels and hair follicles (Fig. 8B).[1]

DISCUSSION

Sometimes it may be difficult to differentiate between large congenital melanocytic nevi (CMN) and Becker's nevus (BN). Besides histopathology dermoscopy will help to differentiate the two conditions. Ingordo et al.[1] in their analysis of 127 male patients with CMN and 64 patients with BN found that focal thickening of network lines, pigment globules on a background of homogeneous diffuse pigmentation, along with blotches, and hyperpigmented areas were more frequently observed in CMN than in BN, whereas a well-defined pigment network, focal, skin furrow, and perifollicular hypopigmentation along with hair follicles and vessels were more common in BN. They concluded that dermoscopy may provide some clues to differentiate the two conditions.

KEYNOTE

Dermoscopy may be useful in differentiating between CMN and BN.

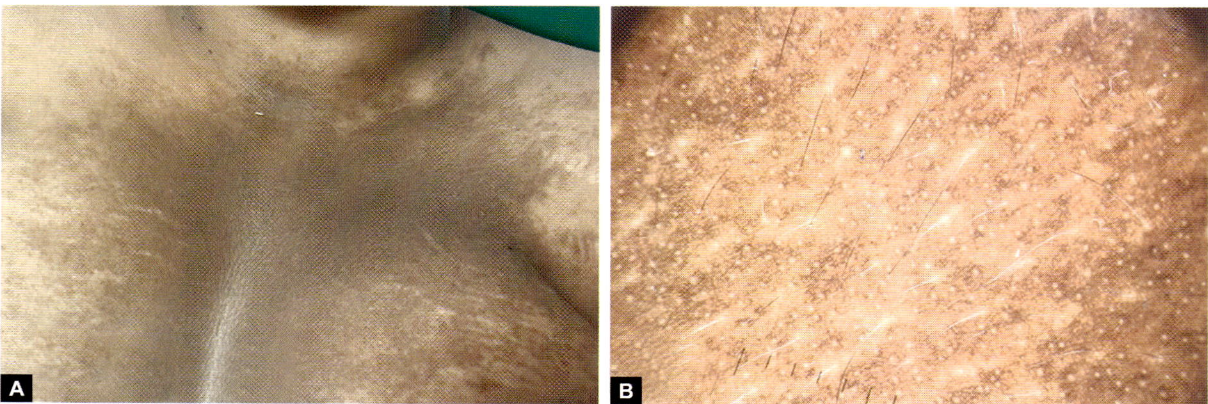

Figs. 8A and B: (A) Becker's nevus in a female; (B) Dermoscopic features of Becker's nevus showing a well-defined pigment network with focal hypopigmentation.
(*Courtesy:* Dr Purva Mehta).

REFERENCE

1. Ingordo V, Iannazzone SS, Cusano F, et al. Dermoscopic features of congenital melanocytic nevus and becker nevus in an adult male population: an analysis with a 10-fold magnification. Dermatology. 2006;212(4):354-60.

CHAPTER 13

Disorders of Keratinization

Subrata Malakar, Priya Diwaker, Surit Malakar

DARIER'S DISEASE (KERATOSIS FOLLICULARIS)

INTRODUCTION

Also known as Darier–White disease, it is characterized clinically by persistent greasy scaly papules mainly in the seborrheic areas (Figs. 1 to 4). It may have some atypical presentations including linear pattern, flat freckle-like lesion, blistered papules, etc. The clinical use of dermoscopy, in addition to being a possible diagnostic tool, highlights the recognition of subtle but important features of Darier's disease (DD).

KEY DERMOSCOPIC FEATURES[1,2] (FIGS. 5 TO 12)

- Polygonal star-like or round oval-shaped yellow-brown areas of various sizes surrounded by a thin white halo (pseudocomedones).
- Dotted/linear/irregular vessels.
- Whitish scaling over a reddish-yellow background.

DISCUSSION

Dermoscopy of DD displays centrally located polygonal star-like or round oval-shaped yellow-brown areas of various sizes surrounded by a thin white halo that overlies a pinkish homogeneous area; whitish scales and dotted or linear vessels may or may not be present. The central polygonal star-shaped area corresponds histopathologically to compact hyperkeratosis and the whitish halo to acanthosis (Fig. 5).[3]

The pinkish background along with the presence of vessels of different patterns indicates dermal inflammation.[1,3]

Recently, Errichetti et al. described a case of type 1 segmental DD with the same dermoscopic pattern as described for classical DD. They pointed out the usefulness of such noninvasive procedure in recognition of this variant of DD. Even though the diagnostic confirmation of such a dermatosis depends on histopathology, dermoscopy may be used as an auxiliary tool to rule out the other inflammatory papular conditions presenting in a Blaschko linear fashion, e.g. lichen planus, psoriasis, and lichen striatus.[2]

KEYNOTE

Polygonal brownish areas seen on dermoscopy of Darier's correspond to hyperparakeratosis histopathologically. This feature is highly helpful to rule out other dermatosis with similar presentations.

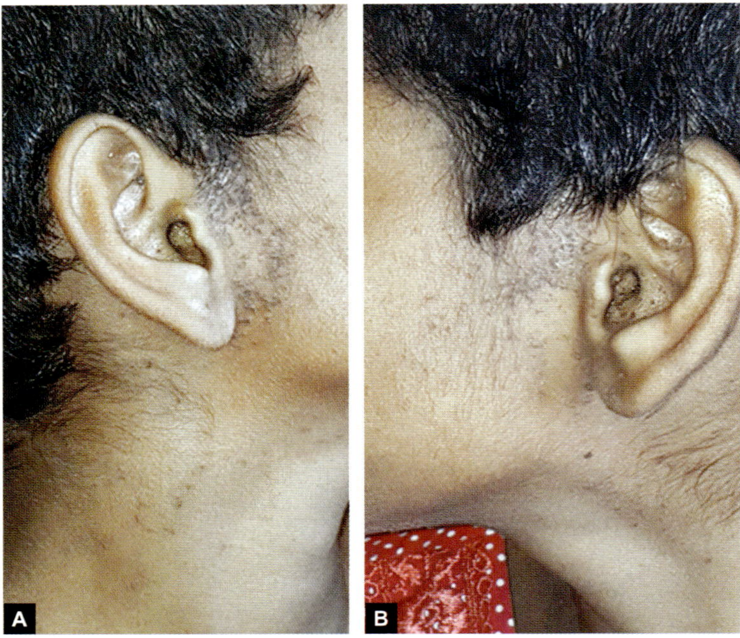

Figs. 1A and B: A 13-year-old girl presented with 3 years history of these greasy brown papules over seborrheic areas.

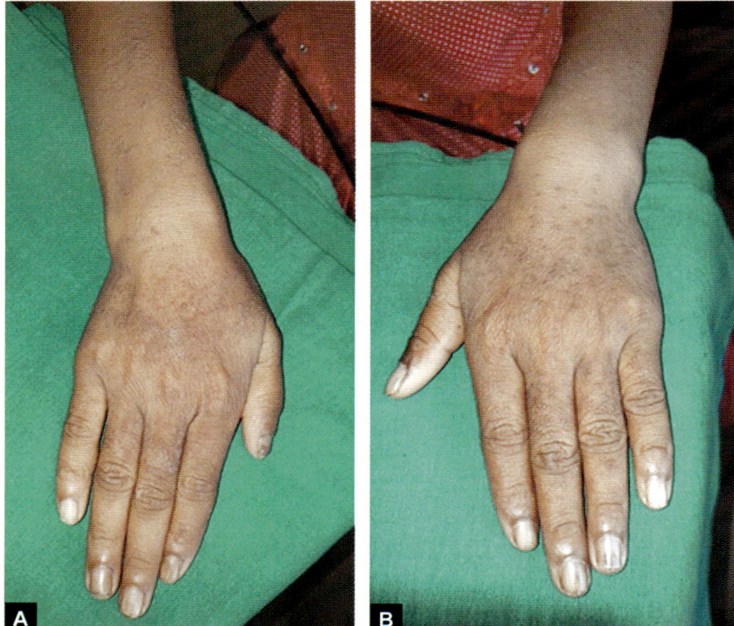

Figs. 2A and B: Clinical evaluation reveals the presence of multiple hyperkeratotic papules on the dorsum of both the hands which should be distinguished from acrokeratosis verruciformis of Hopf.

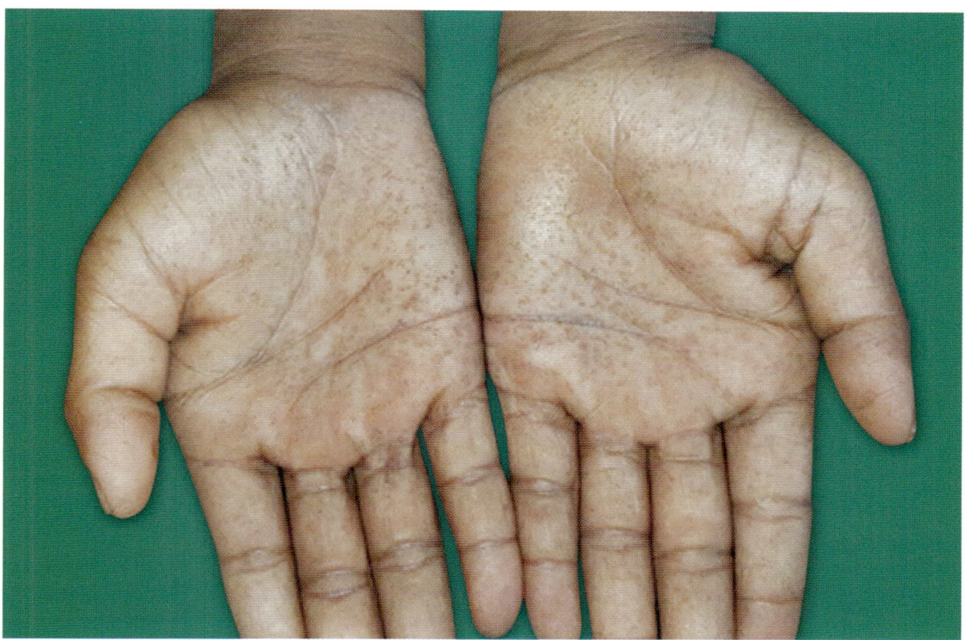

Fig. 3: On close inspection, lesions on the palms include pits and punctate keratosis.

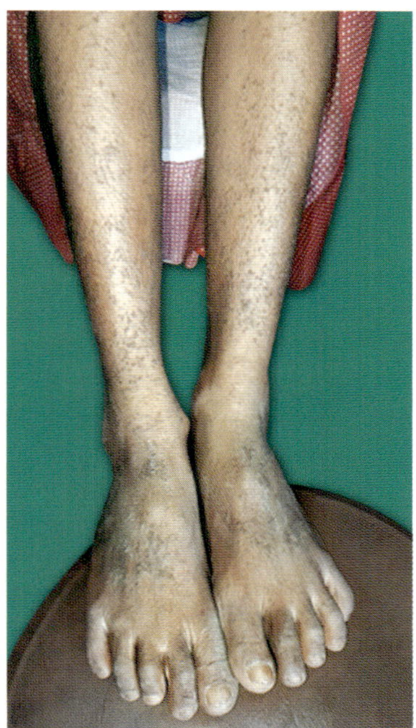

Fig. 4: Similar warty papules seen over both the legs.

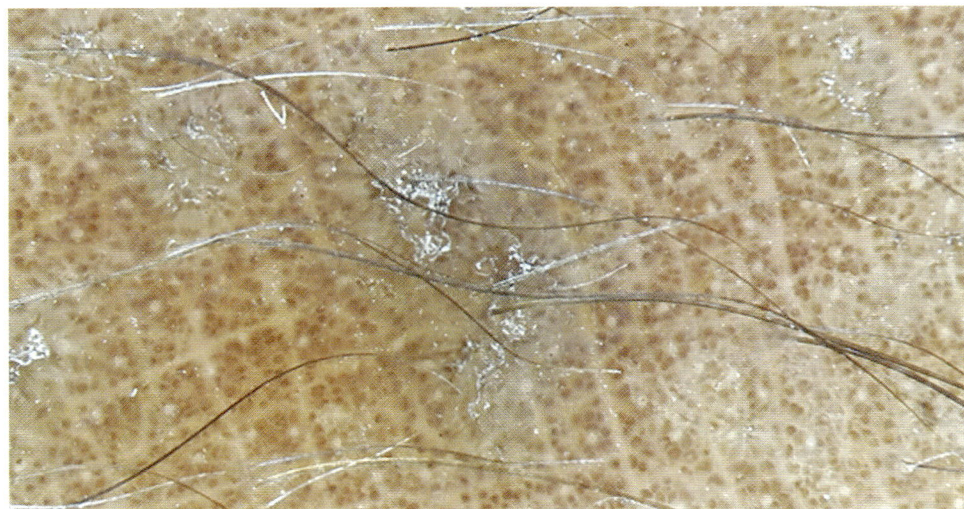

Fig. 5: Dermoscopy revealed polygonal brown areas surrounded by a thin whitish halo (pseudocomedones).

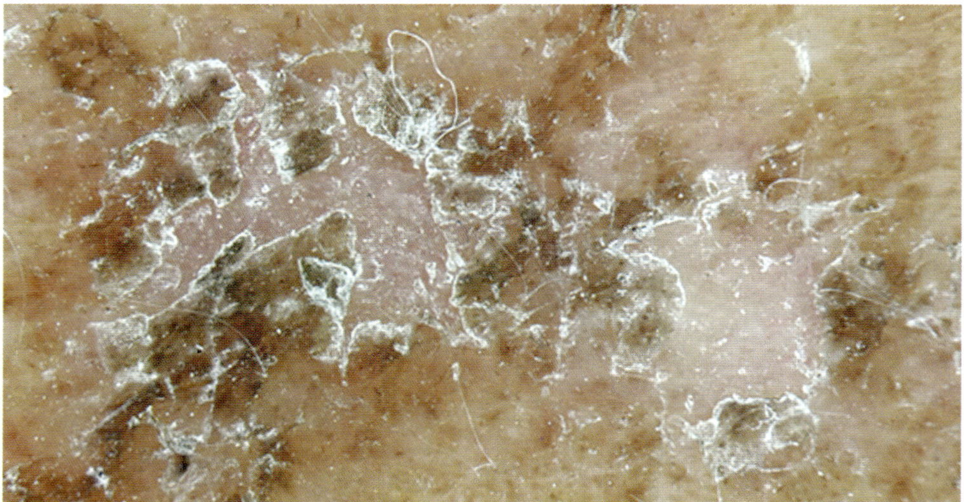

Fig. 6: Whitish scales are seen over yellowish-red background.

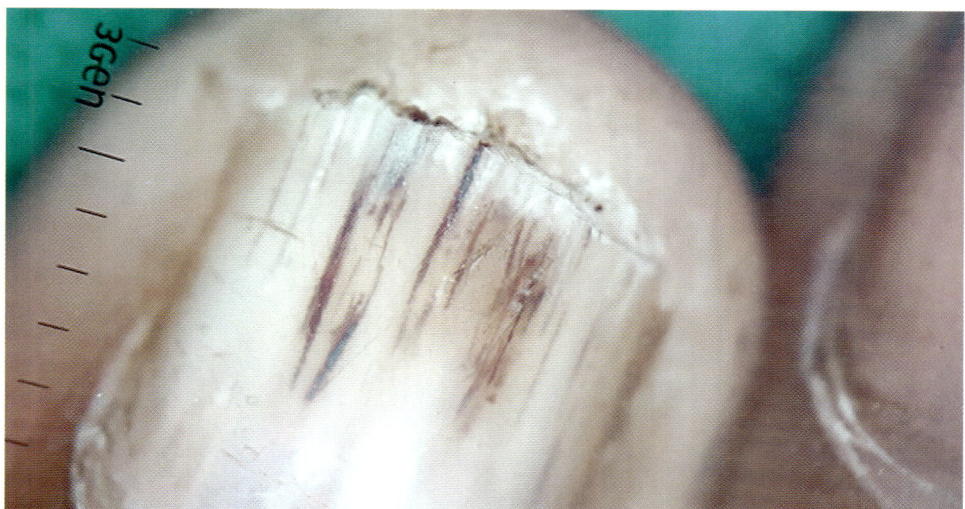

Fig. 7: Dermoscopy of nail highlights the clinical features like longitudinal ridges, red and white lines, and V-shaped nicks.

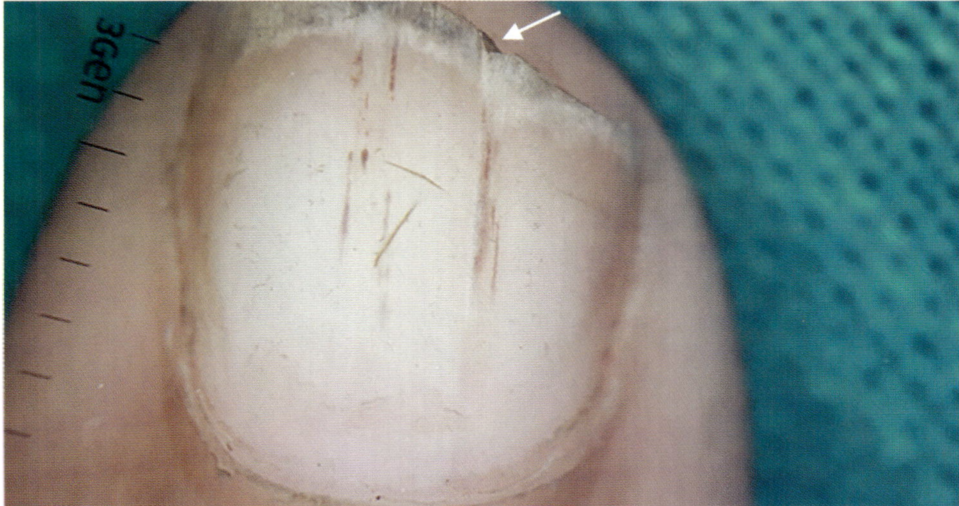

Fig. 8: Dermoscopically, a V-shaped nick (arrow) at the free margin of the nail becomes obvious. It is the most pathognomonic nail finding of Darier's.

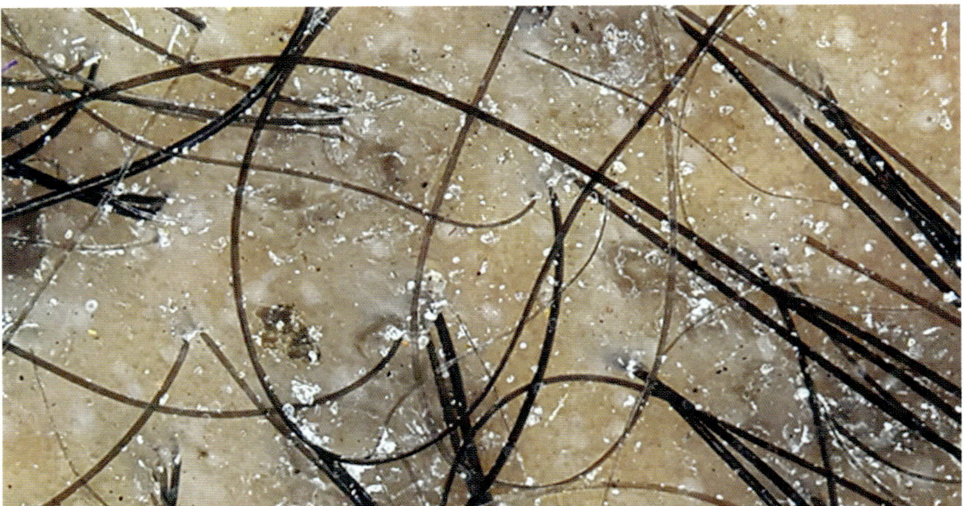

Fig. 9: Dermoscopy of scalp shows the dirty appearance along with few scattered pseudocomedones.

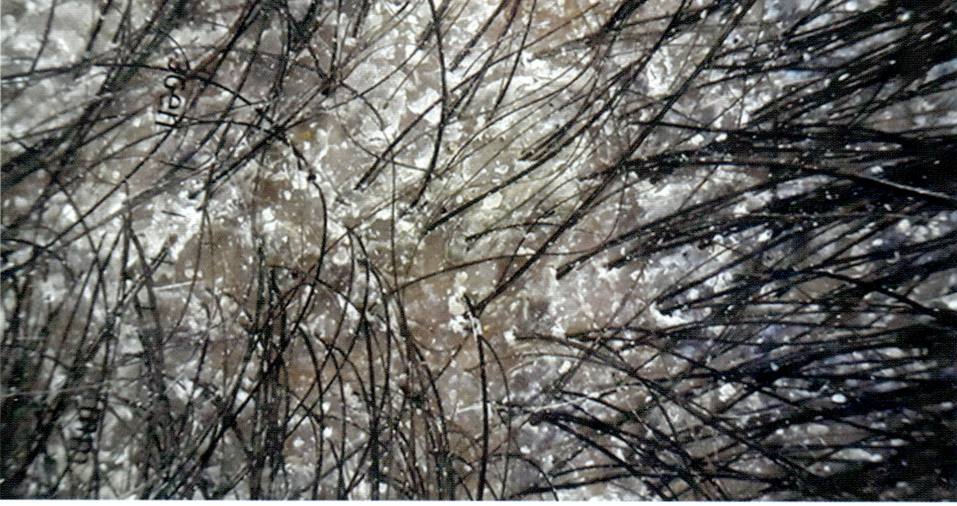

Fig. 10: Scalp is studded with greasy scales.

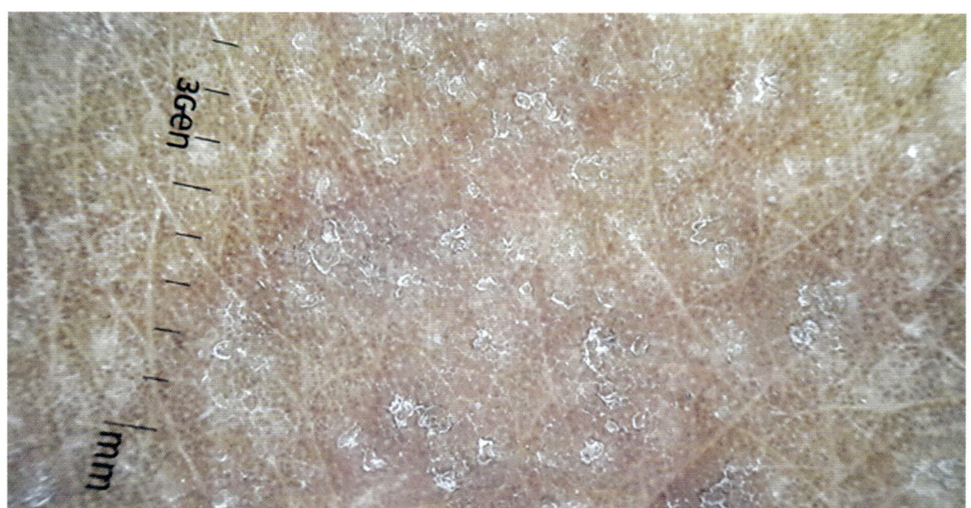

Fig. 11: Dermoscopy of dorsum of hand showing plenty of pseudocomedones with whitish halos.

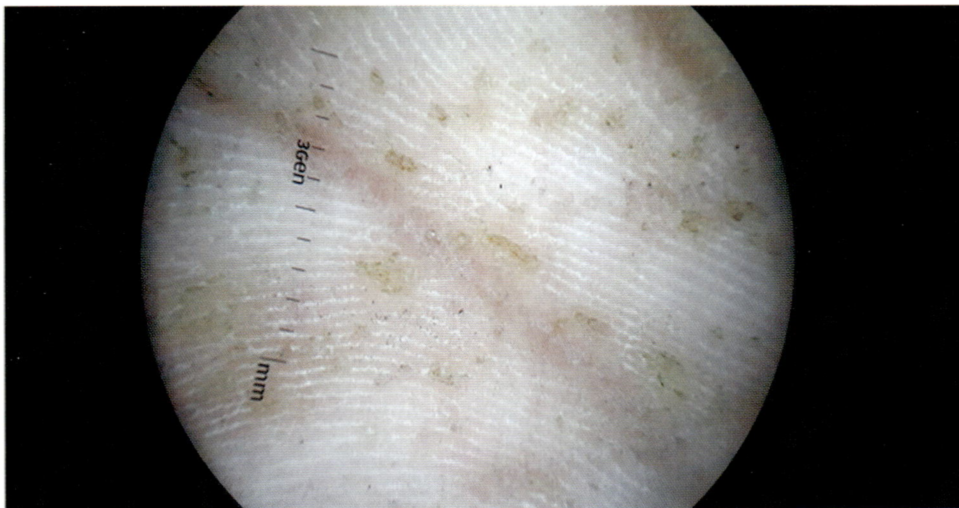

Fig. 12: Dermoscopy of palm enhances the pits and punctate keratosis.

REFERENCES

1. Lacarrubba F, Verzì AE, Errichetti E, et al. Darier disease: dermoscopy, confocal microscopy, and histologic correlations. J Am Acad Dermatol. 2015;73:e97-9.
2. Errichetti E, Maoine V, Pegolo E, et al. Dermoscopy: a useful auxillary tool in the diagnosis of type 1 segmental Darier's disease. Dermatol Pract Concept. 2016;6(2):10.
3. Errichetti E, Stinco G, Lacarrubba F, et al. Dermoscopy of Darier's disease. J Eur Acad Dermatol Venereol. 2016;30(8):1392-4.

GROVER'S DISEASE (TRANSIENT ACANTHOLYTIC DERMATOSIS)

INTRODUCTION

The patient usually presents with recurrent papulovesicular itchy rash on the trunk, which is exacerbated by heat and sweating.

The histopathology of the disease is characterized by acantholysis with or without dyskeratosis; spongiotic dermatitis may also be present.

KEY DERMOSCOPIC FEATURES[1,2]

Early Stage (Erythematous Papule)

- Pinkish-white background
- Central glomerular vessels
- Linear and hairpin vessels at the periphery.

Late Stage (Erythematous Papule with Central Keratotic Plug)

- Central, yellowish-brown, and star-like pattern
- A white radiating halo
- Linear and hairpin vessels at the periphery.

DISCUSSION

Grover's disease essentially evolves from a nonspecific early stage to a specific late stage characteristic appearance, as is reflected by the spectrum of dermoscopic-histopathologic changes of initial and late lesions.[3]

In the early stage, pink-white background, and vessel patterns correspond to mild superficial perivascular inflammatory infiltrates.

In the late stage, central, yellowish-brown, and star-like pattern corresponds to a central keratotic plug. The white radiating halo correlates to suprabasal acantholysis with acanthosis and dyskeratosis. The linear and hairpin vessels at the periphery corresponds to prominent capillary vessels vertically arranged in the elongated rete ridges.[3]

REFERENCES

1. Giacolel J, Zalaudek I, Argenziano G. Dermatoscopy of Grover's disease and solitary acantholytic dyskeratome shows a brown, star-like pattern. Australas J Dermatol. 2012;53:315-6.
2. Specchio F, Argenziano G, Tiodorovic-Zivkovic D, et al. Dermoscopic clues to diagnose acantholytic dyskeratosis. Dermatol Pract Concept. 2015;5:11.
3. de Abreu L, Cordeiro NG, Buçard AM, et al. Dermoscopy of Grover disease. J Am Acad Dermatol. 2017;76(2 Suppl 1):S60-3.

HAILEY–HAILEY DISEASE (FAMILIAL BENIGN PEMPHIGUS)

INTRODUCTION

It is a chronic autosomal dominant disorder with incomplete penetrance. In 75% of these patients, there is a positive family history of similar complaints. Multiple relapses and remissions characterize this disease (Figs. 13 and 14). Decreased number of desmosomes is the proposed etiopathogenesis of this condition giving rise to the classical dilapidated brick wall appearance on histology (Fig. 15).

The clinical recognition might be generally easy, but in some cases with unusual presentation, dermoscopy can help.[1]

KEY DERMOSCOPIC FEATURES[2] (FIGS. 16 TO 24)

- Combination of pink and white areas resembling a cloud
- Irregular whitish areas separated by pink furrows (iceberg pattern)
- Small erosions and ulcerations.

DISCUSSION

Dermoscopic pattern of Hailey–Hailey disease is combination of pink and white areas.

In some areas of the disease, it reveals irregular combination of pink and white color resembling clouds. Some other places show irregular white areas separated by pink furrows, which is reminiscent of iceberg.

The white areas probably represent acanthosis and dyskeratosis histologically whereas pink areas correspond to the exposed basal layer and dermis due to acantholysis of the whole epidermis.

KEYNOTE

The characteristic combination of pink and white areas is a useful clue to Hailey–Hailey disease when differential diagnosis of intertriginous rashes is a dilemma.

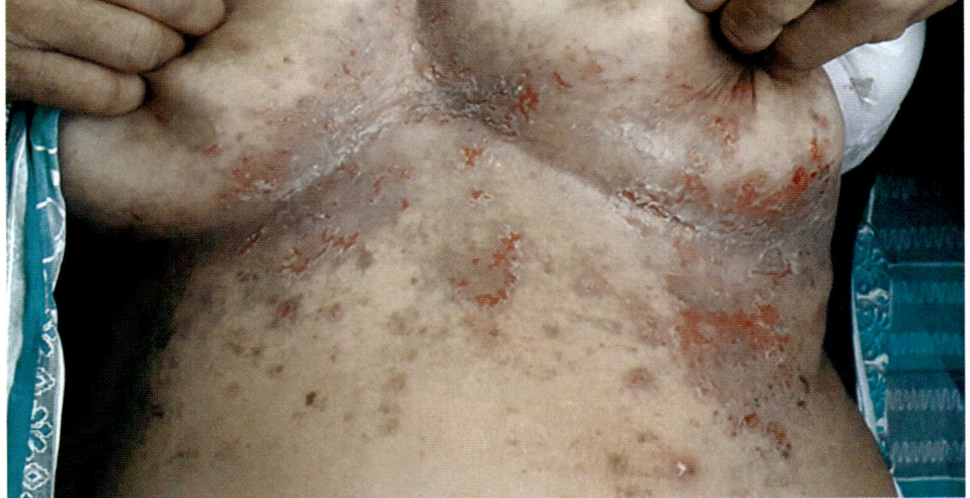

Fig. 13: A middle-aged lady presented with weeping lesions over the body folds, having seasonal recurrence since 7 years.

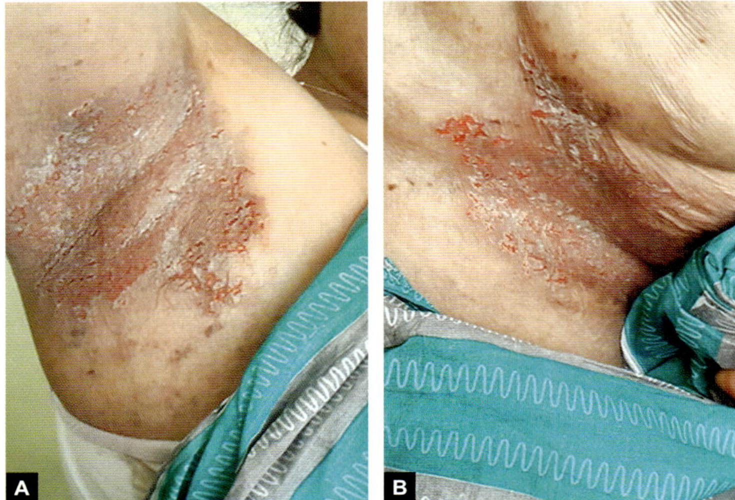

Figs. 14A and B: Other intertriginous areas show erythematous plaques with linear erosions, cracks, and whitish areas.

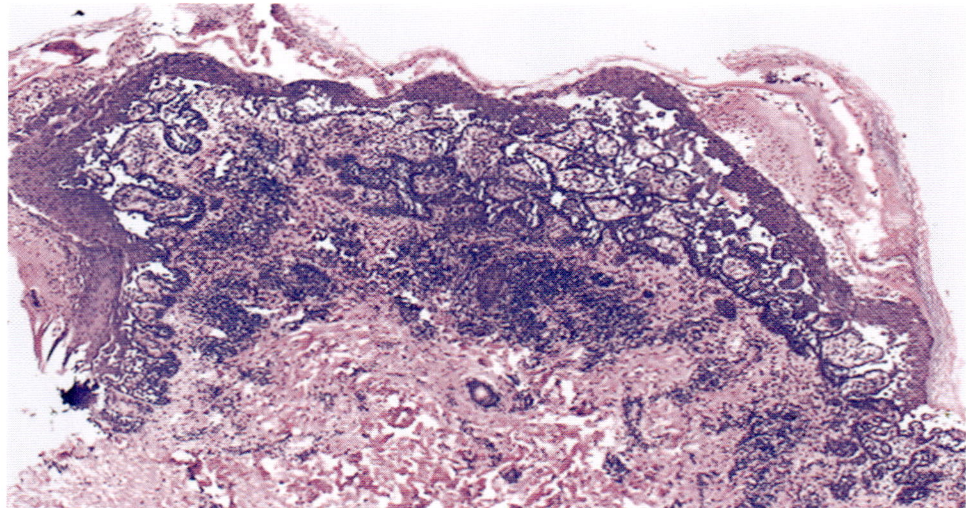

Fig. 15: Histopathology shows suprabasal acantholysis, dyskeratosis, and the classic description of dilapidated brick wall appearances.

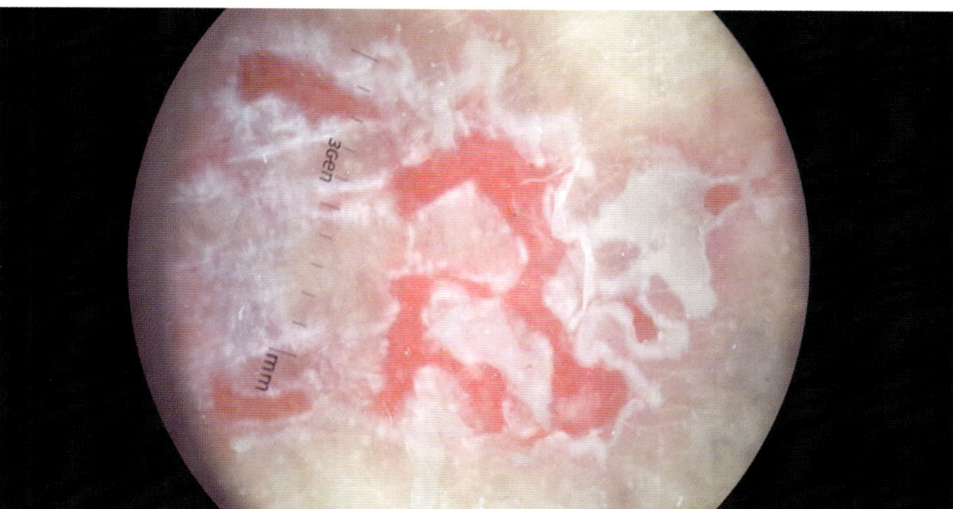

Fig. 16: Dermoscopy shows pink and white areas which resembles a cloud.

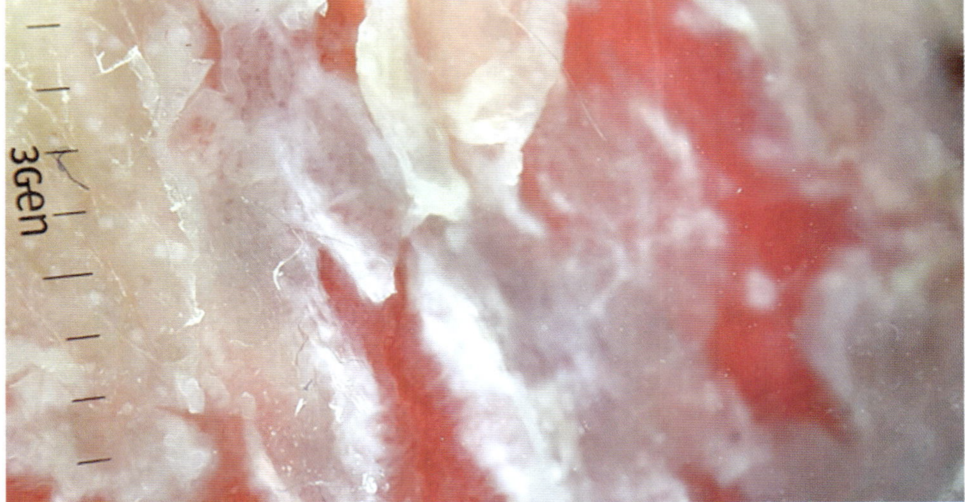

Fig. 17: Irregular white areas separated by pink furrows forming a pattern called iceberg pattern.

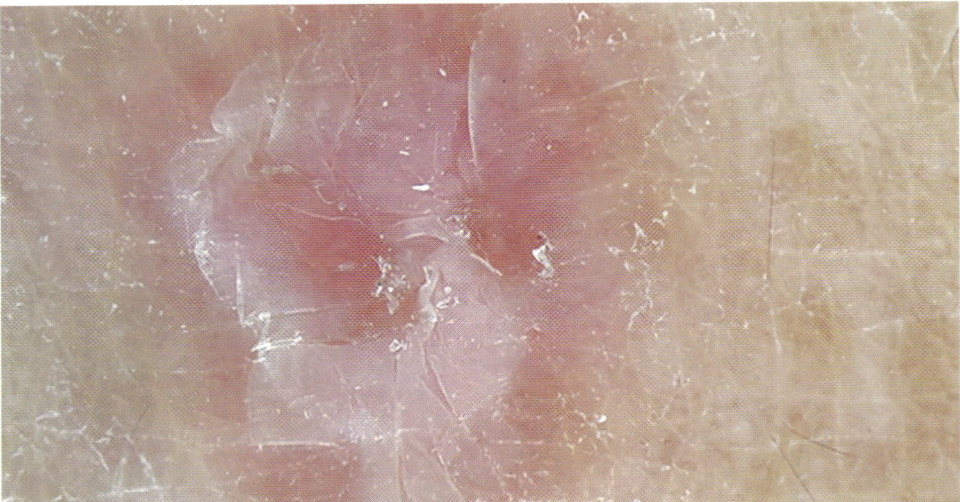

Fig. 18: A small intact vesicle with central depression looks like the petals of a flower.

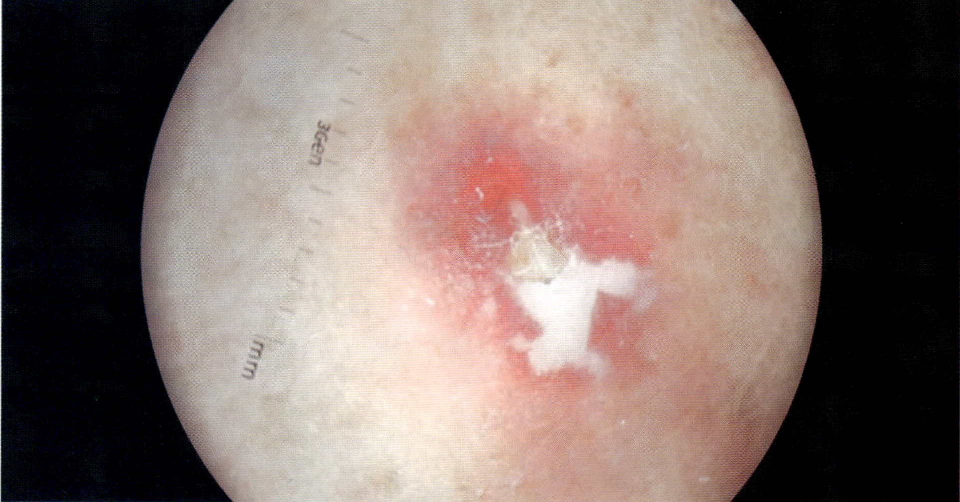

Fig. 19: Dermoscopy shows active stage of the disease with erosion and pus.

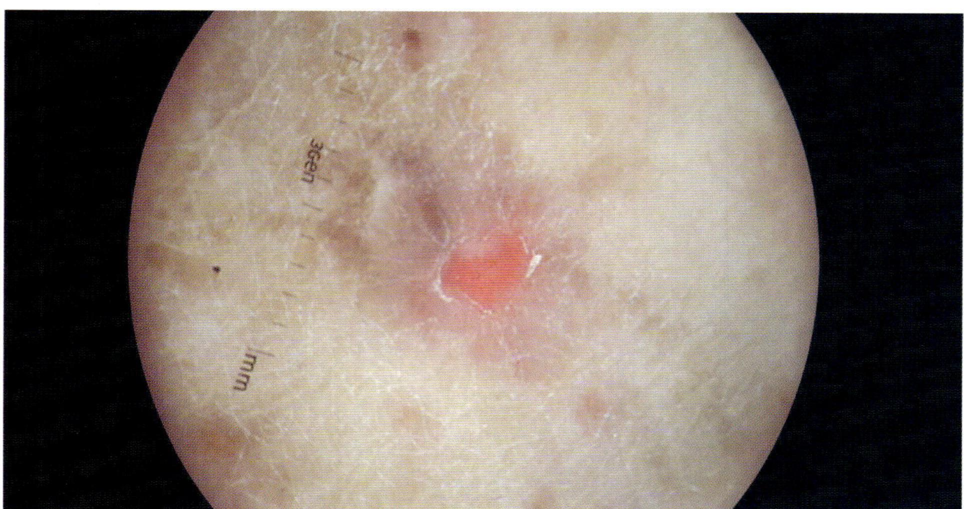

Fig. 20: A vesicle, postrupture, and deroofing shows a small erosion.

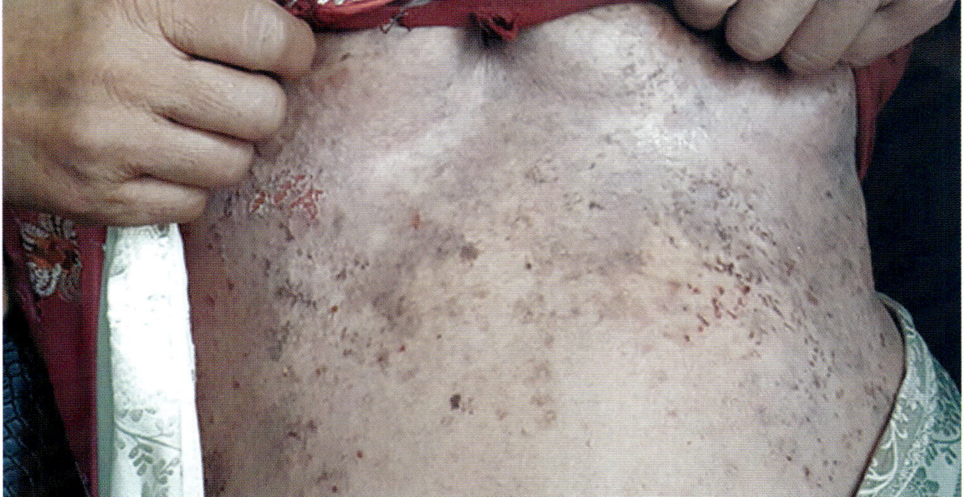

Fig. 21: Same patient after 3 weeks of treatment with oral retinoid.

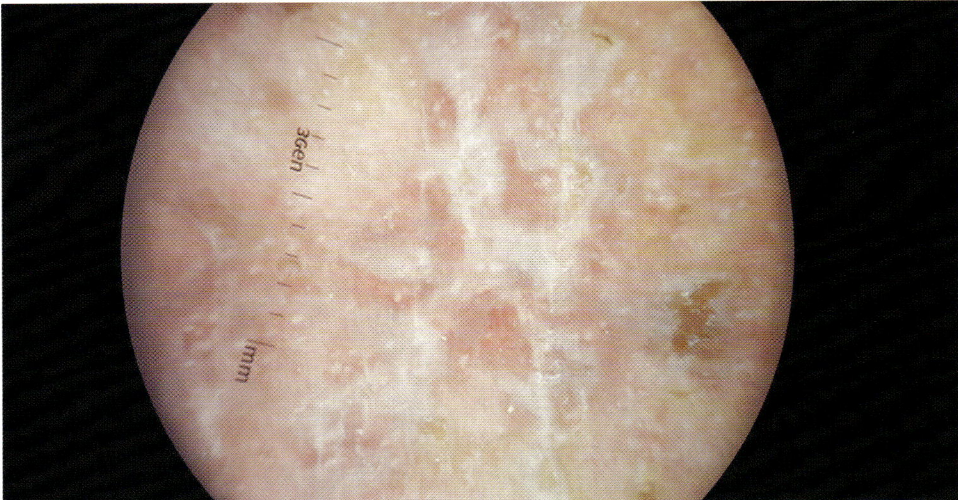

Fig. 22: The earlier pink and white areas resolved post-treatment and thereafter shows reticular yellow-white pattern on dermoscopy.

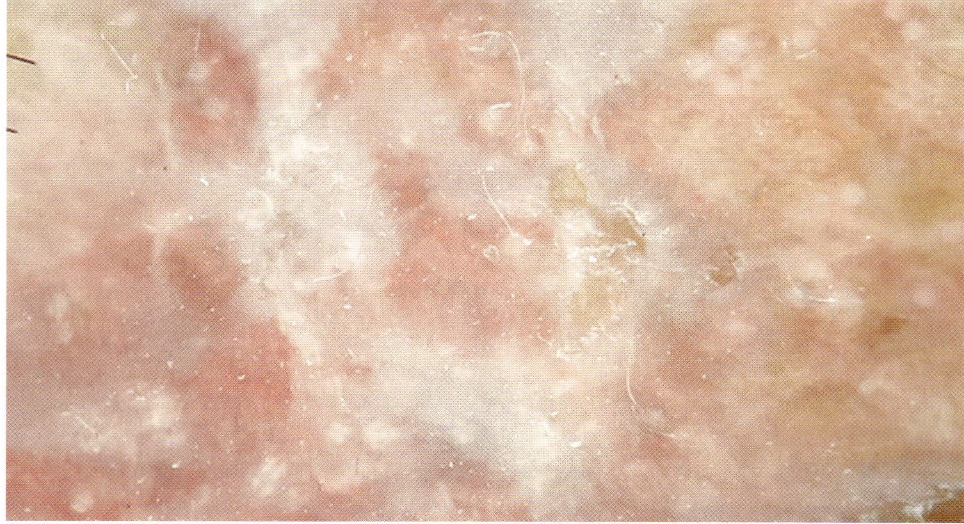

Fig. 23: Dermoscopy of Hailey–Hailey disease after treatment reveals whitish areas with few shiny white structures and rosettes.

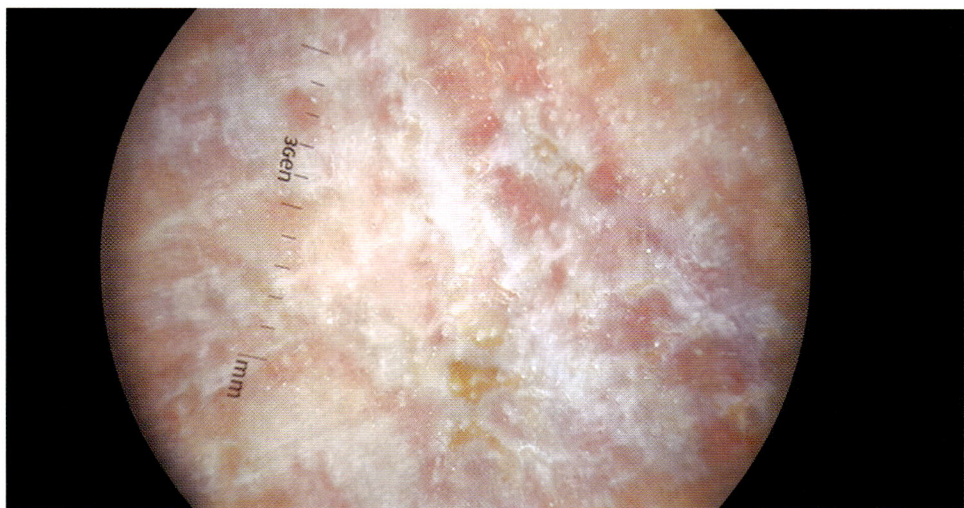

Fig. 24: Diffuse reticular yellow-white areas on dermoscopy of Hailey–Hailey suggest healing.

REFERENCES

1. Vasudevan B, Verma R, Badwal S, et al. Hailey-Hailey disease with skin lesions at unusual sites and a good response to acitretin. Indian J Dermatol Venereol Leprol. 2015;81(1):88-91.
2. Kelati A, Argenziano G, Mernissi FZ. Dermoscopic presentation of Hailey-Hailey disease. J Am Acad Dermatol. 2017;76:S31-3.

POROKERATOSIS

INTRODUCTION

Porokeratosis is a disorder of epidermal keratinization characterized by annular plaques surrounded by a keratotic border, which corresponds to a typical histopathologic feature, the cornoid lamella.[1]

KEY DERMOSCOPIC FEATURES (FIGS. 25 TO 34)[1-8]

- "White track" structure—annular peripheral whitish hyperkeratotic structure.
- The center of the lesion is atrophic which typically shows whitish or brownish color and may exhibit dotted or linear vessels according to the disease subtype and stage of progression.
- Dark-brown globules/dots.
- Hyperpigmented border.

DISCUSSION

The hallmark dermoscopic feature of all subtypes of porokeratosis is the "white track" structure, which appears as a well-defined, whitish, peripheral, and annular hyperkeratotic structure. The histopathologic hallmark of porokeratosis is the "cornoid lamella" which corresponds to the "white track" structure. The "white track" structure is similar to the outlines of a volcanic crater as observed from above; it may be hyperpigmented in disseminated superficial actinic porokeratosis.

The center of the lesion is typically whitish or brownish and may reveal circular or linear whitish and/or hyperpigmented tracks, blue-gray dots, and dotted or linear vessels.[4-10]

Yücel et al. reported a hyperpigmented border and dark-brown dots and globules on a brownish background in the center on dermoscopy of a case of linear porokeratosis.[2]

CASE 1 (FIGS. 25 TO 27)

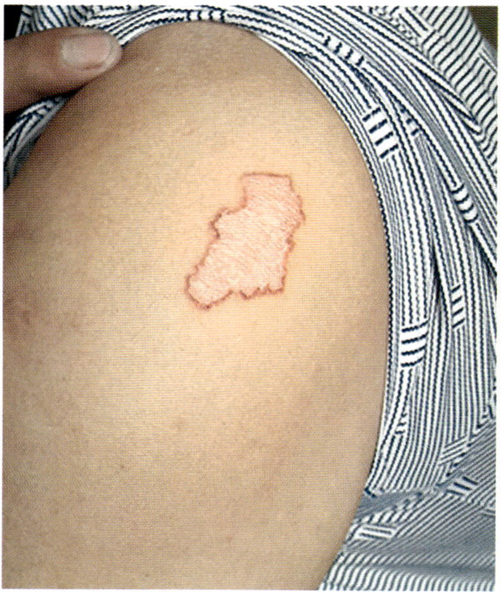

Fig. 25: A young male presented with a mildly pruritic lesion over the left arm since 9 months.

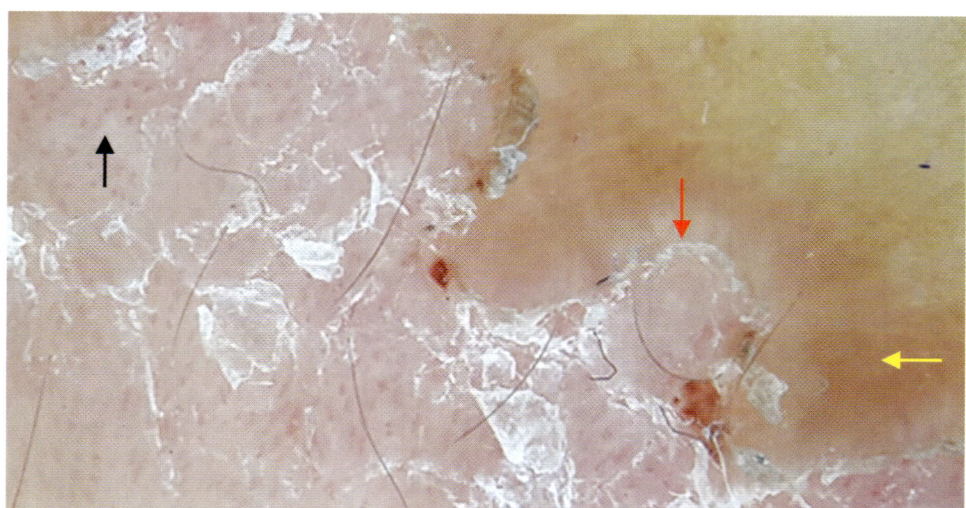

Fig. 26: Dermoscopy reveals a hyperpigmented border (yellow arrow) with white track appearance (red arrow). The center of the lesion is whitish with dotted vessels (black arrow).

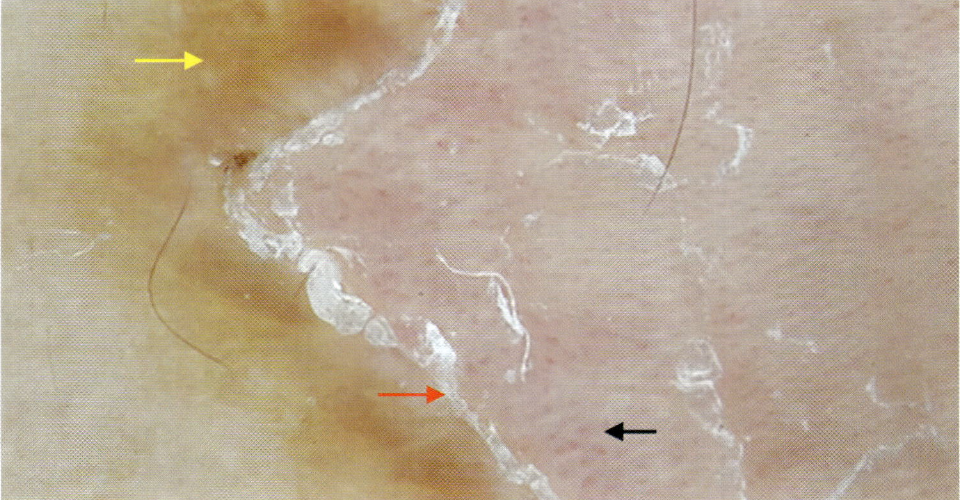

Fig. 27: Dermoscopy reveals a hyperpigmented border (yellow arrow) with white track appearance (red arrow). The center of the lesion is whitish with dotted and linear vessels (black arrow).

CASE 2 (FIGS. 28 AND 29)

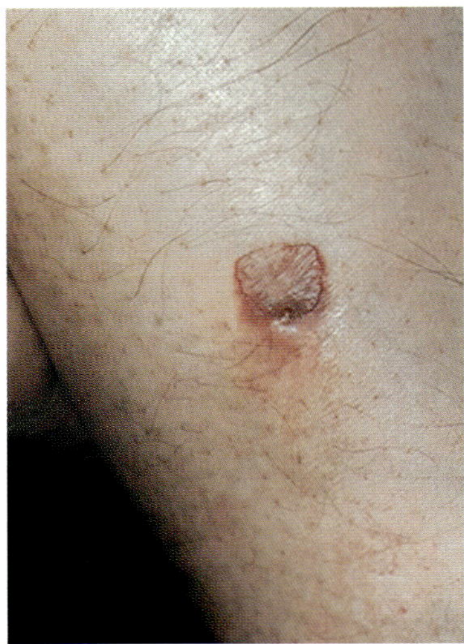

Fig. 28: A male patient presented with a hyperkeratotic annular plaque since 7 months, slowly increasing in size. Biopsy was done from the edge of the lesion following dermoscopy.

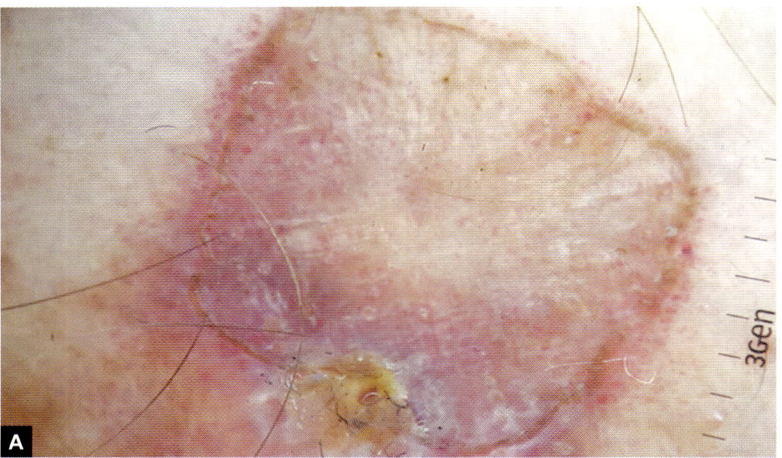

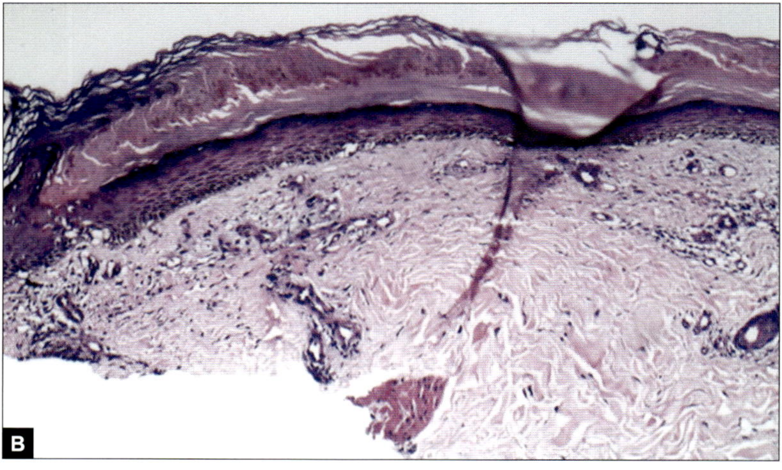

Figs. 29A and B: (A) Dermoscopy of the lesion clearly reveals (from outside to inside) hyperpigmented border, white track appearance, and brownish white center with dotted vessels; (B) In two to three small foci, the epidermis shows deep invaginations of the floor which lacks granular layer. Rising from the center of these invaginations is a tiny column of parakeratotic cells (cornoid lamella). At the bottom of this are seen scattered dyskeratotic cells.

CASE 3 (FIGS. 30 AND 31)

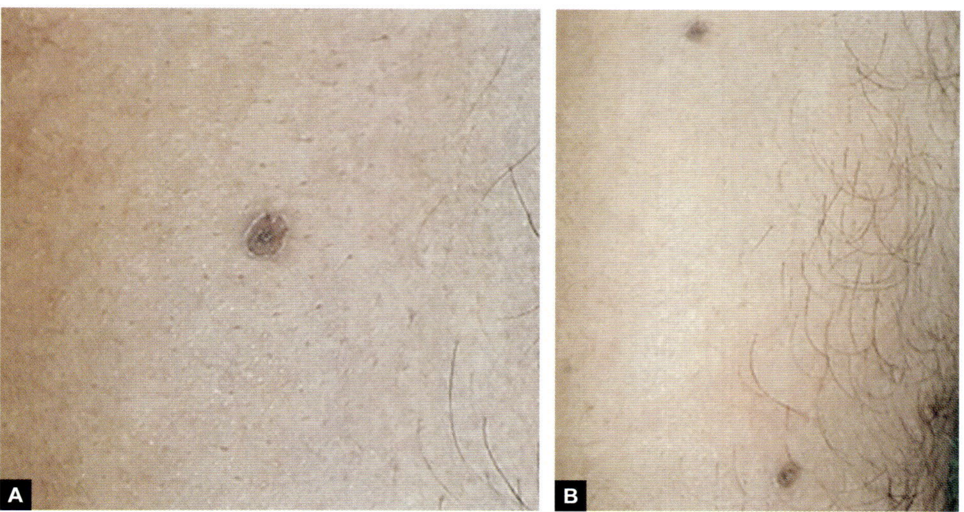

Figs. 30A and B: The patient presented with few blackish-brown rough rounded spots over the lower limbs since 4 months.

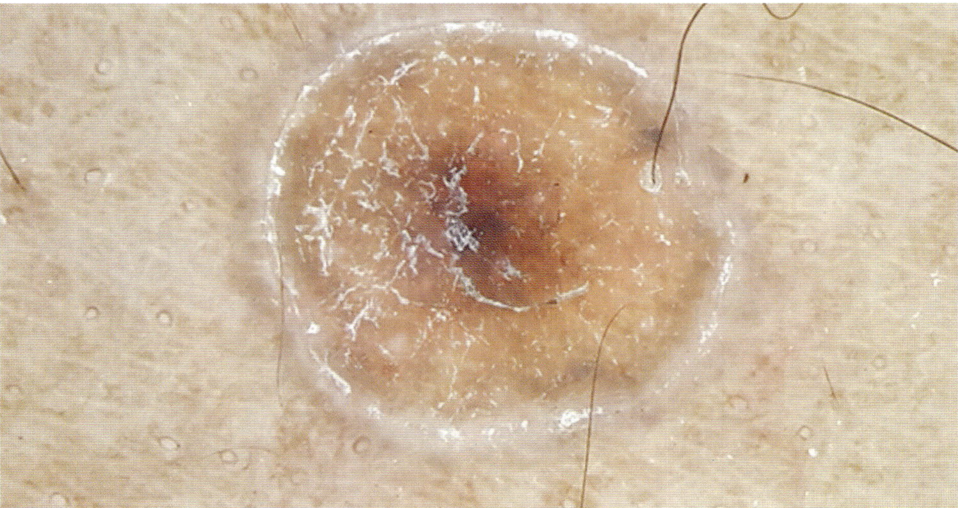

Fig. 31: Dermoscopy of the previous patient revealed hyperpigmented border, white track appearance which resembles diamond necklace sign with brownish center and dotted vessels.

CASE 4 (FIGS. 32 TO 34)

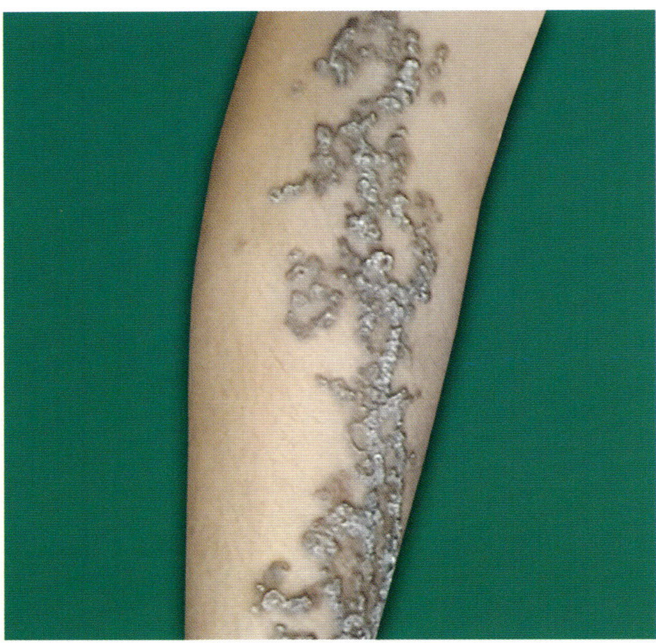

Fig. 32: A 9-year-old child presented with dirty looking warty papules over the lower limb in a linear fashion slowly increasing in extent since 3 years of age. The closest clinical differential is epidermal nevus.

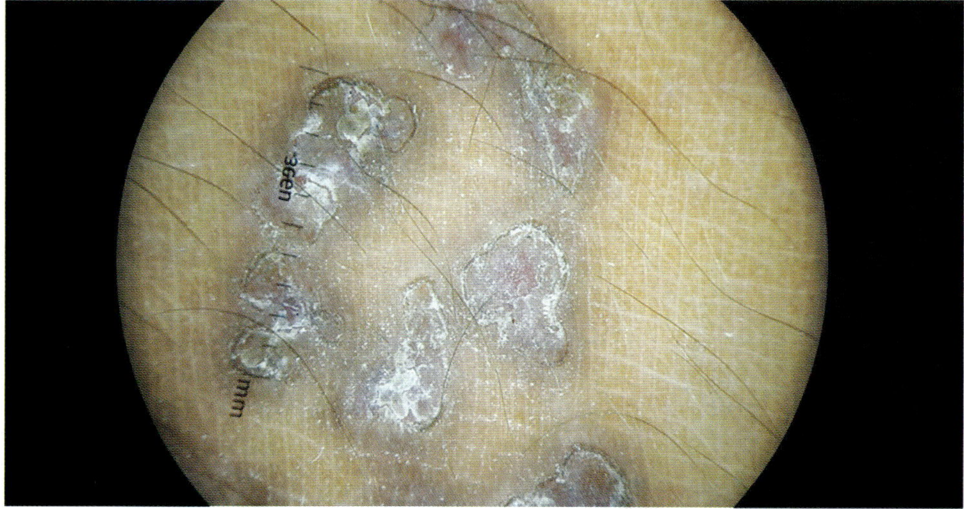

Fig. 33: Dermoscopy of the previous patient shows multiple annular lesions with hyperpigmented border, white track appearance, and atrophic center.

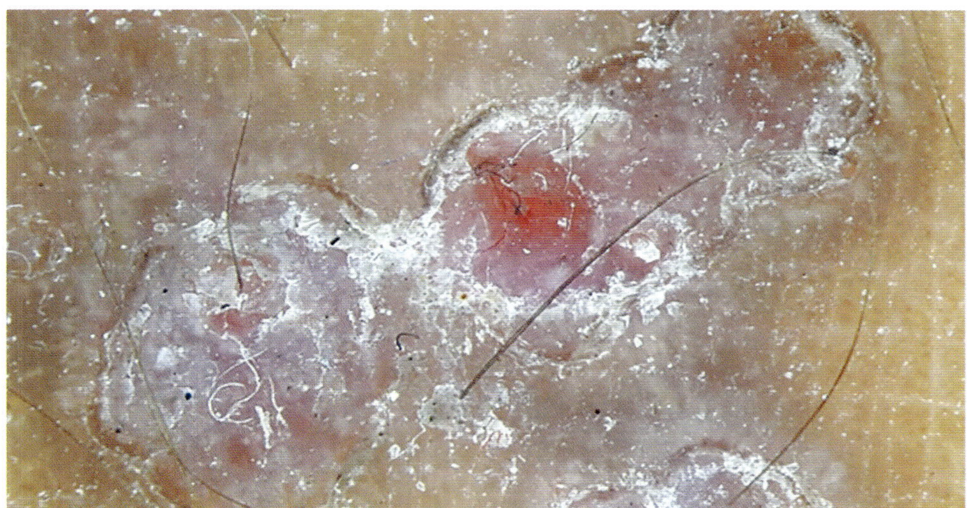

Fig. 34: On closer view in addition to the other features of porokeratosis, central erosion with sticky fiber sign is noted.

REFERENCES

1. Delfino M, Argenziano G, Nino M. Dermoscopy for the diagnosis of porokeratosis. J Eur Acad Dermatol Venereol. 2004;18:194-5.
2. Yüce A, Günaştı S, Maraklı SS, et al. A case of linear porokeratosis: dermoscopic and immunofluorescence findings. J Turk Acad Dermatol. 2008;2(2):82202c.
3. Pizzicheta MA, Canzonieri V, Massone C, et al. Clinical and dermoscopic features of porokeratosis of Mibelli. Arch Dermatol. 2009 145:91-2.
4. Zaballos P, Puig S, Malvehy J. Dermoscopy of disseminated superficial actinic porokeratosis. Arch Dermatol. 2004;140:1410.
5. Panasiti V, Rossi M, Curzio M, et al. Disseminated superficial actinic porokeratosis diagnosed by dermoscopy. Int J Dermatol. 2008 47:308-10.
6. Oiso N, Kawada A. Dermoscopic features in disseminated superficial actinic porokeratosis. Eur J Dermatol. 2011;21:439-40.
7. Uhara H, Kamijo F, Okuyama R, et al. Open pores with plugs in porokeratosis clearly visualized with the dermoscopic furrow ink test: report of 3 cases. Arch Dermatol. 2011;147:866-8.
8. Moscarella E, Longo C, Zalaudek I, et al. Dermoscopy and confocal microscopy clues in the diagnosis of psoriasis and porokeratosis. J Am Acad Dermatol. 2013;69:e231-3.
9. Hayashi Y, Ozeki M, Ishizaki S, et al. Inguinal porokeratosis in a Japanese man. Dermatol Pract Concept. 2013;3:29-31.
10. Vargas-Laguna E, Nagore E, Alfaro A, et al. Monitoring the evolution of a localized type of porokeratosis using dermatoscopy. Actas Dermosifiliogr. 2006;97:77-8.

CHAPTER 14

Vascular Lesions

Subrata Malakar

INTRODUCTION

Vascular lesions can be divided into two categories—(1) Tumors and (2) Malformations. Neoplasms of the vasculature cause vascular tumors, which include infantile hemangioma and pyogenic granuloma.[1]

Vascular malformations represent developmental anomalies without any endothelial proliferation that can further be categorized into capillary malformations (CMs) such as port-wine stain (PWS), venous, and lymphatic malformations. In contrast to infantile hemangiomas, vascular malformations are present since birth, persist for a lifetime, and do not regress.

REFERENCE

1. Paller A, Mancini A. Vascular disorders of infancy and childhood. In: Paller A, Mancini A (Eds). Hurwitz Clinical Pediatric Dermatology: A Textbook of Skin Disorders of Childhood and Adolescence. Philadelphia: Elsevier Saunders; 2005. pp. 307-44.

INFANTILE HEMANGIOMA PRECURSORS

INTRODUCTION

About 30–50% of hemangiomas are precursors and appear as either an area of pallor along with fine thread-like telangiectasias or a macular erythematous stain or a violaceous bruise-like area or a tiny scratch/ulcer (Figs. 1A, 2A and 3A).[1]

Most of the infantile hemangioma precursors (IHPs) develop into fully formed hemangiomas, but sometimes they do not proliferate or may proliferate focally in the peripheral region. They have initially been termed as abortive or minimal growth hemangiomas. These hemangiomas without a proliferative phase are glucose transporter-1 (GLUT-1) positive on immunohistochemistry.[2]

KEY DERMOSCOPIC FEATURES (FIGS. 1B, 1C, 2B AND 3B)[3]

- Red round globular vessels
- Red, comma-like vessels
- Red linear vessels.

DISCUSSION

Dermoscopic features of IHP are polymorphous showing red round globular vessels, comma vessels, and red linear vessels. Histopathology demonstrates: (i) Dilated vascular structures in the papillary dermis, (ii) Superficially dilated vasculature changing direction and transitioning to deep dilated horizontal subpapillary capillaries, and (iii) Dilated linear vascular structures in the subpapillary and upper reticular dermis. These histopathological features correspond to key dermoscopic features mentioned earlier; the red comma-like vessels on dermoscopy represent the transition between the other two types of vessels in the superficial papillary and subpapillary dermis (Fig. 3B).

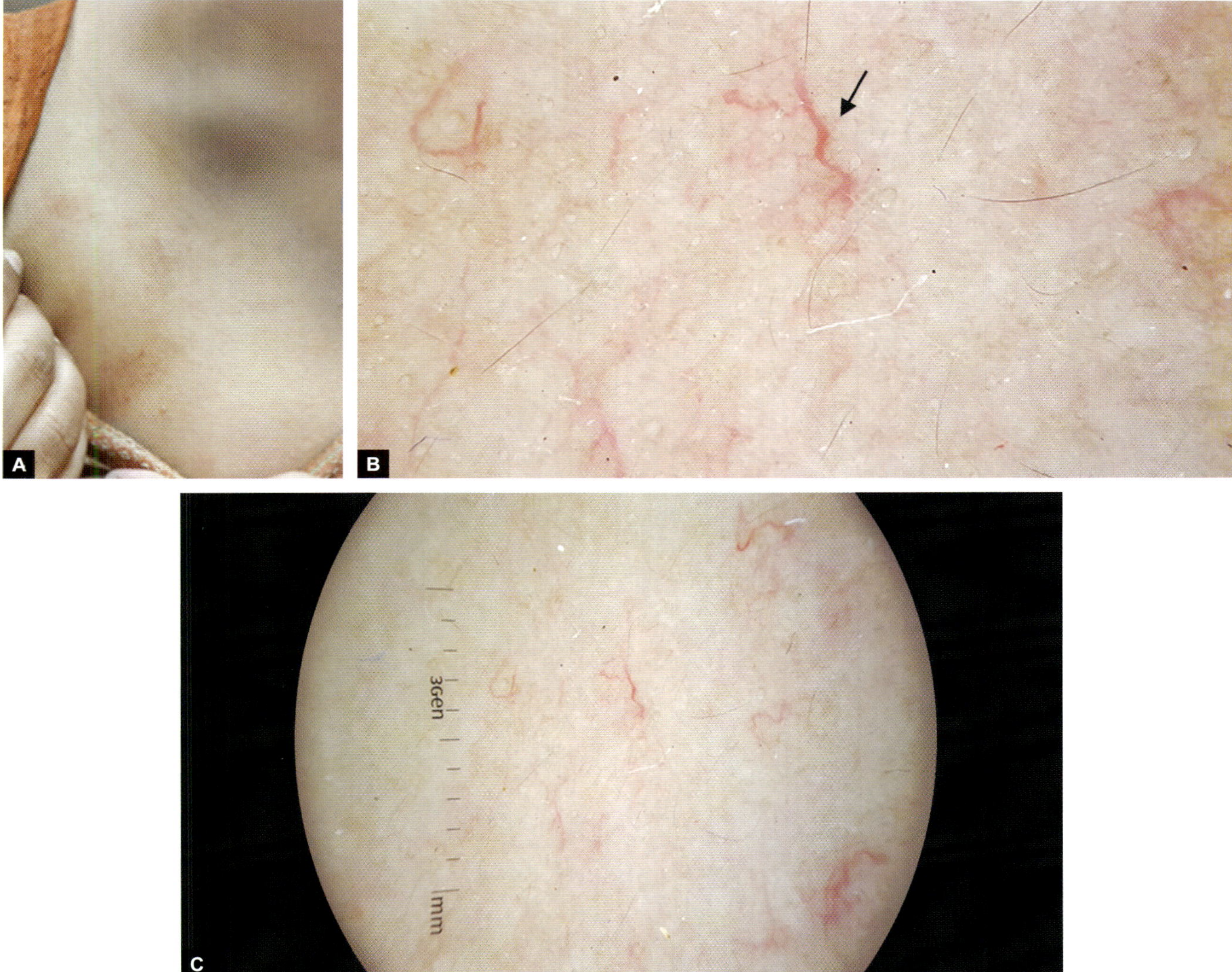

Figs. 1A to C: (A) Clinical picture of infantile hemangioma (IH) precursor showing macular erythematous stain on the upper chest present since infanthood; (B) Dermoscopy shows linear dilated vessels (arrow) which corresponds to vessels in the subpapillary plexus; and (C) Dermoscopic overview of IH precursor showing multiple dilated vessels, few of which are in focus while others being out of focus. In-focused vessels signify relatively superficially placed dermal vessels whereas the out of focus ones correlates with deep vessels of the subpapillary plexus.

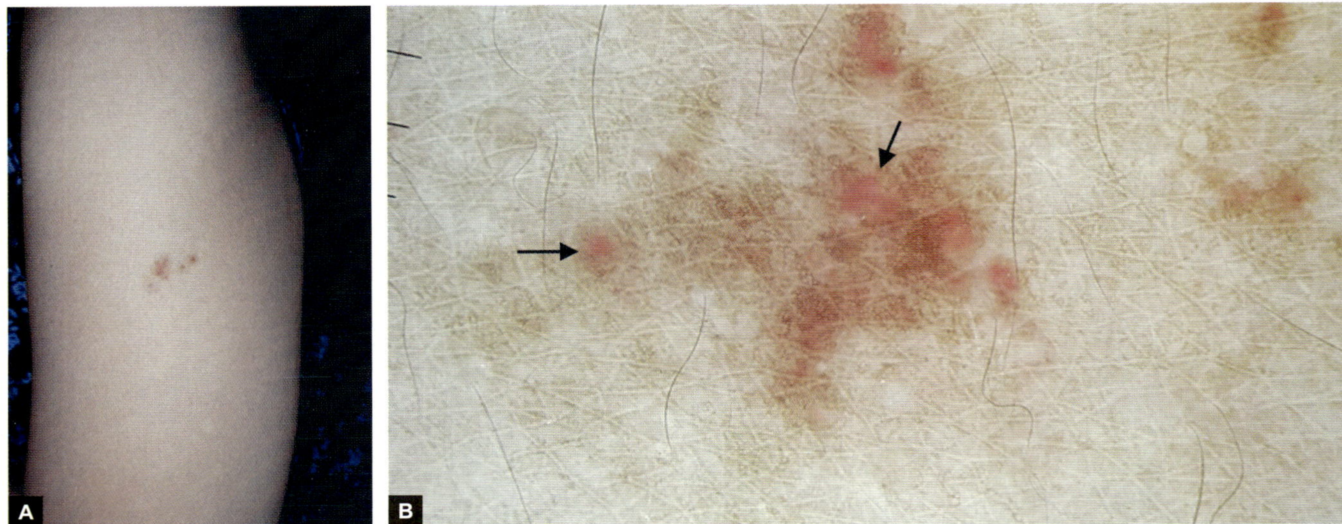

Figs. 2A and B: (A) An insignificant macular erythematous stain present since birth in a young girl; and (B) Dermoscopy of previous patient showing red round large globular vessels (arrows) signifying its location in the superficial dermis.

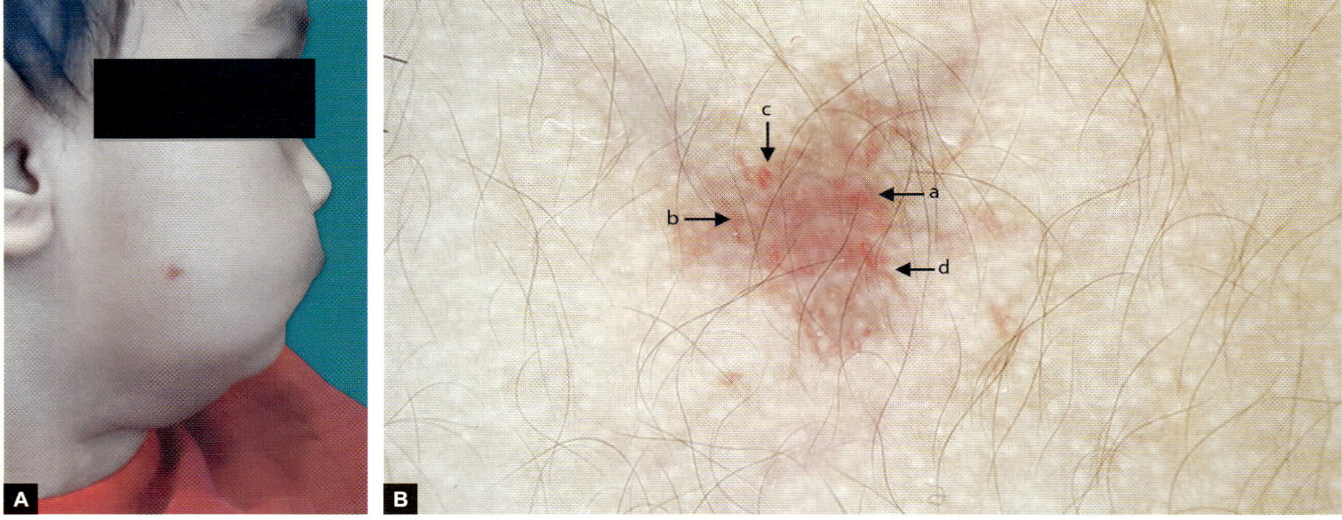

Figs. 3A and B: (A) A tiny erythematous papule on the right cheek of an infant; and (B) Dermoscopy reveals polymorphous appearance of vessels showing—(a) red round globular vessels, (b) red comma-shaped vessels, (c) twisted red capillaries, and (d) red linear vessels on an erythematous background.

REFERENCES

1. Hidano A, Nakajima S. Earliest features of the strawberry mark in the newborn. Br J Dermatol. 1972;87:138-44.
2. Corella F, Garcia-Navarro X, Ribe A, et al. Abortive or minimal-growth hemangiomas: immunohistochemical evidence that they represent true infantile hemangiomas. J Am Acad Dermatol. 2008;58:685-90.
3. Oiso N, Kimura M, Kawara S, et al. Clinical, dermoscopic, and histopathological features in a case of infantile hemangioma without proliferation. Pediatric Dermatol. 2011;28(1):66-8.

PYOGENIC GRANULOMA

INTRODUCTION

The term pyogenic granuloma (PG) is a misnomer; the lesions of PGs are neither pyogenic nor granulomatous. It consequently can be termed better as "lobular capillary hemangioma". The pathogenesis is not clear and it appears to be reactive in nature.

Pyogenic granuloma frequently presents as a solitary, rapidly growing papulonodule that has a tendency to bleed after trivial trauma (Figs. 4, 6, 8 and 10). Thus, diagnosis is fairly straightforward but occasionally common benign and malignant tumors may be confused with PG.[1,2]

KEY DERMOSCOPIC FEATURES (FIGS. 5, 7, 9, 11 AND 12) [3,4]

- Homogeneous reddish or reddish-white areas
- A whitish collarette which surrounds the reddish white area
- White rail lines
- Various vascular patterns such as hairpin, dotted, linear irregular, and polymorphous vessels
- Hemorrhagic crusts.

DISCUSSION

The most common dermoscopic pattern of PG is a homogeneous reddish or reddish-white area surrounded by a white collarette (in 85% of cases).[5] The reddish/reddish-white areas correspond histologically to proliferating capillaries and veins that are present in a myxoid stroma of PG. It is the most common dermoscopic sign associated with PG.[6]

The whitish collarette is located at the periphery of PG and is a ring-shaped squamous structure. The peripheral collarette represents hyperplastic epithelium that partially or totally embraces the proliferating blood vessels in pyogenic granuloma. It is the most specific structure for PG but has also been observed in clear cell acanthoma.[7]

Homogeneous reddish areas are often intersected by white rail lines, which appear dermoscopically as whitish streaks or bands. Histologically these rail lines correlate with the fibrous septae that surround the capillary tufts or lobules in advanced forms of pyogenic granuloma. These structures have a good specificity but low sensitivity. Similar feature has been observed in dermatofibroma (Figs. 5, 7 and 11).[8]

Additional criteria are various vascular patterns such as hairpin, dotted, linear irregular, polymorphous vessels, and hemorrhagic crusts (Fig. 12).

The four main dermoscopic features of PG in various combinations give rise to seven dermoscopic patterns, which have been described by Zaballos et al. (Table 1).[6]

Table 1: Seven dermoscopic patterns of pyogenic granuloma (PG).

Patterns	*Red homogeneous area*	*White collarette*	*White rail lines*	*Vascular structures*
P1	+	+		
P2	+		+	
P3	+			+
P4	+	+	+	
P5	+	+		+
P6	+		+	+
P7	+	+	+	+

After comparing all dermoscopic structures in PG, red homogeneous area is found to be present in all patterns. Zaballos et al. stated that P1, P4, and P5 are the most common patterns of PG.

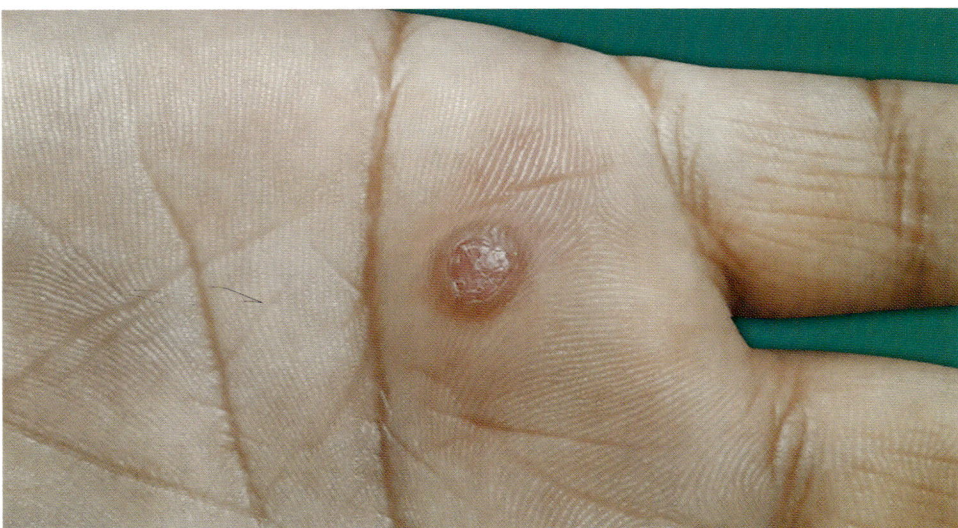

Fig. 4: Pyogenic granuloma over palm presenting as a solitary, red-brown, raised, and sessile nodule for 3 months. The base reveals a peripheral collarette of scale. Although it is solitary, multiple lesions of pyogenic granuloma are not uncommon.

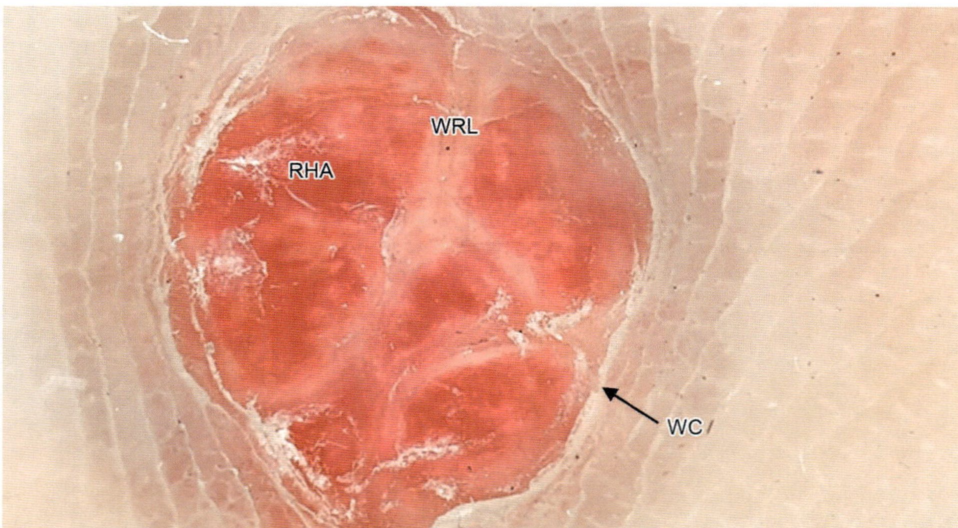

Fig. 5: P4—Dermoscopy shows white collarette (WC), red homogeneous area (RHA), and white rail lines (WRLs). The color of the red homogeneous area varies from completely red to reddish-white. Red homogeneous area is the most common dermoscopic feature of pyogenic granuloma. This pattern composed of WC, RHA, and WRL has been demonstrated to be 100% specific for pyogenic granuloma.

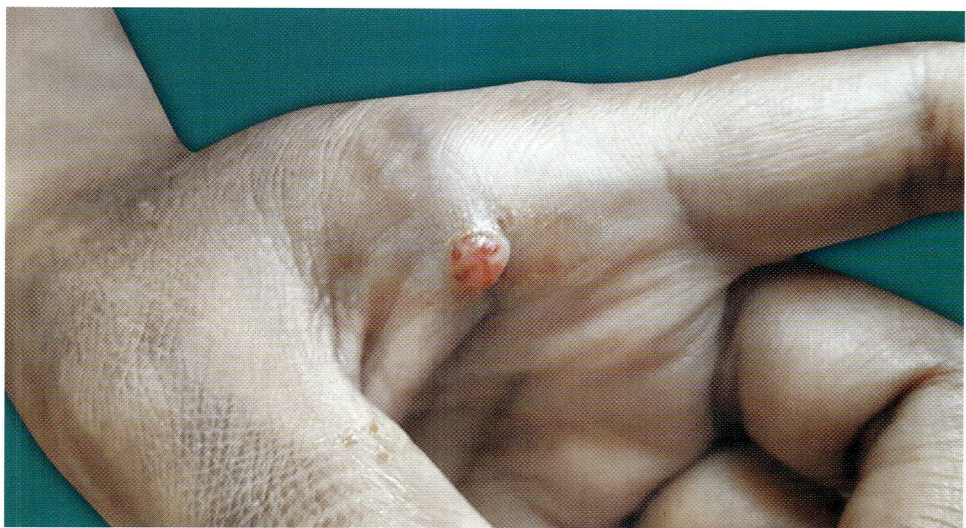

Fig. 6: Painless, glistening red nodule over palm that bleeds spontaneously or following trauma; duration being 2.5 months. Pyogenic granuloma (PG) usually evolves rapidly over a period of few weeks, most common sites being the head, neck, and extremities.

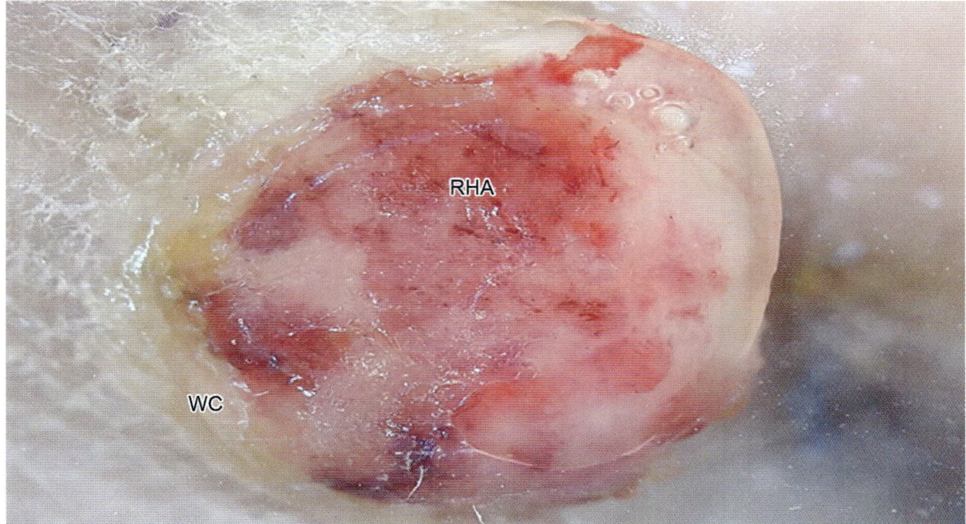

Fig. 7: P5—Dermoscopy reveals WC, RHA, and vascular structures. Vascular patterns seen in this picture are dotted, atypical, and hairpin vessels. (WC: White collarette; RHA: Red homogeneous area).

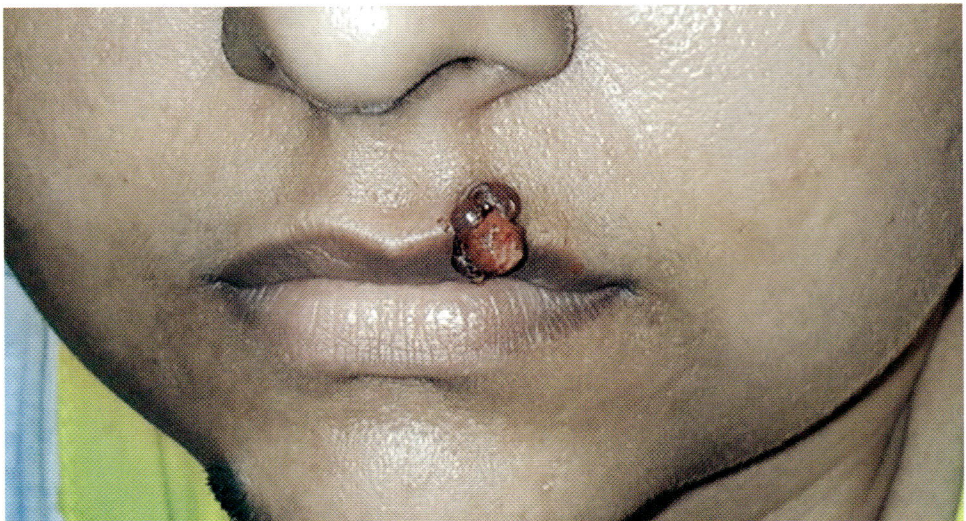

Fig. 8: Pyogenic granuloma (PG) is prone to ulceration and recurrent bleeding that usually makes the patient seek a medical consult. PGs most commonly appear in locations subject to trauma, especially fingers, face, and mucosal surfaces of the mouth.

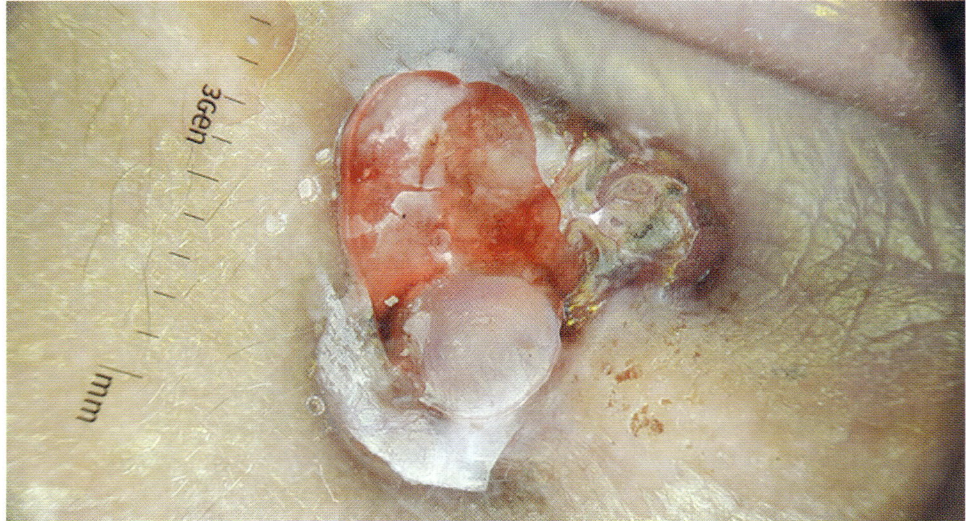

Fig. 9: P1—Pyogenic granulomas are frequently eroded and crusted. This feature may explain the dermoscopic finding of ulceration and crusts. Dermoscopic significance of this feature is very low as it is also a common feature in other tumors.

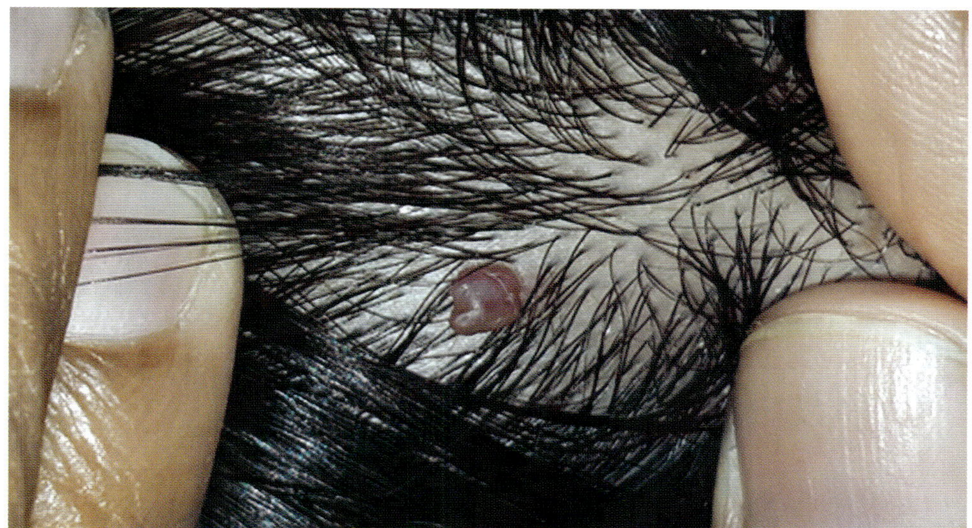

Fig. 10: A shiny red nodule of pyogenic granuloma (PG) on the scalp for 4 months. The possible factors which play a role in its development are trauma, infection, hormonal influences, and drugs such as systemic retinoids, etc.

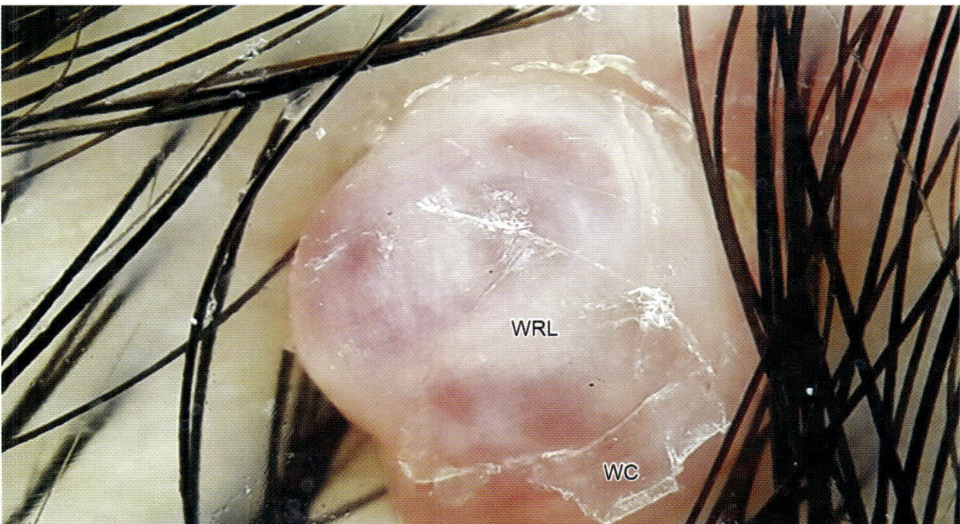

Fig. 11: P4—WC, RHA, and WRL. (RHA: Red homogeneous area; WC: White collarette; WRL: White rail line).

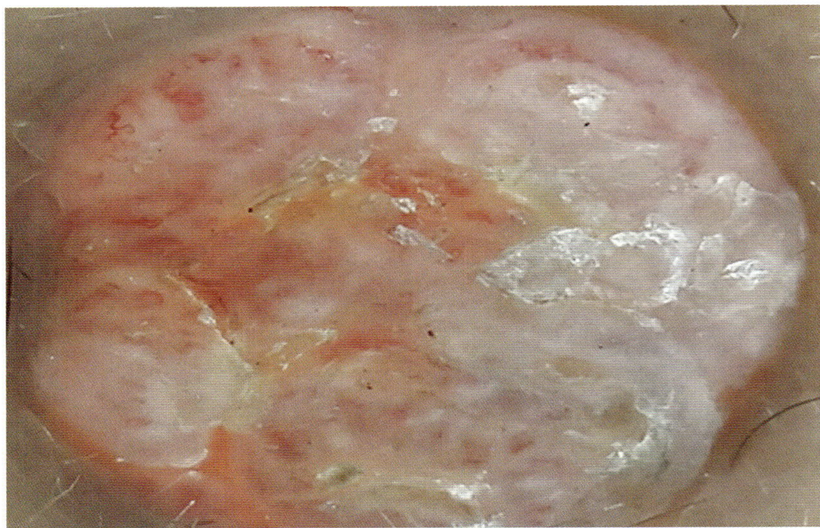

Fig. 12: Barring RHA, the most common vascular pattern in PG is linear irregular vessels. Hairpin vessels and atypical vessels are also observed. (PG: Pyogenic granuloma; RHA: Red homogeneous area).

KEYNOTE

None of the earlier features distinguish PG from amelanotic nodular melanoma. Hence, in the Western world, recommendation is excision of the all PGs followed by histopathological examination. But in the Indian subcontinent, biopsy can be avoided as melanoma is rare. Moreover, the classical history of bleeding post-trivial trauma in PGs as well as the characteristic dermoscopic findings is almost diagnostic of the condition. However, histopathological investigation remains to be the gold standard to exclude other possibilities.

REFERENCES

1. Pagliai KA, Cohen BA. Pyogenic granuloma in children. Paediatr Dermatol. 2004;21:10-3.
2. Requena L, Sangueza OP. Cutaneous vascular proliferation. Part II. Hyperplasias and benign neoplasms. J Am Acad Dermatol. 1997;37:887-919.
3. Zaballos P, Llambrich A, Cuellar F, et al. Dermoscopic findings in pyogenic granuloma. Br J Dermatol. 2006;154:1108-11.
4. Zaballos P, Salsench E, Puig S, et al. Dermoscopy of pyogenic granulomas. Arch Dermatol. 2007;143:824.
5. Martin JM, Bella-Navarro R, Jorda E. Vascular patterns in dermoscopy. Actas Dermosifiliogr. 2012;103(5):357-75.
6. Zaballos P, Carulla M, Ozdemir F, et al. Dermoscopy of pyogenic granuloma: a morphological study. Br J Dermatol. 2010;163:1229-37.
7. Bugatti L, Filosa G, Broganelli P, et al. Psoriasis-like dermoscopic pattern of clear cell acanthoma. J Eur Acad Dermatol Venereol. 2003;17:452-5.
8. Zaballos P, Llambrich A, Ara M, et al. Dermoscopic findings of haemosiderotic and aneurismal dermatofibroma: report of six patients. Br J Dermatol. 2006;154:244-50.

CAPILLARY MALFORMATIONS

INTRODUCTION

Capillary malformations include salmon patch and port-wine stain (PWS). PWS has widely been studied through a dermoscope. PWS presents as a macular stain, the color of which varies from pink to dark red (Figs. 13, 16 and 18). It is composed of dilated capillaries in the superficial and deep dermis. If the vessels are superficially placed the lesion looks bright red, whereas the stain appears pink in case of deeper but smaller vessels and purple in case of deeper but larger vessels.[1]

KEY DERMOSCOPIC FEATURES (FIGS. 14, 15, 17 AND 19)

- Red globules and dots
- Prominent red lines.

DISCUSSION

Red globules and dots correspond to perpendicular vessels in the papillary dermis whereas prominent red lines correlate with horizontal capillaries in the subpapillary plexus. Knowledge regarding the location of vessels in the dermis is essential with regard to the treatment outcome.

The lesions revealing a superficial pattern consisting of red globules and dots on dermoscopy respond well to pulsed dye laser.

KEYNOTE

Dermoscope is not only a useful tool for the selection of lesions for treatment; it also serves as a monitoring tool to record efficacy of the laser on PWS.

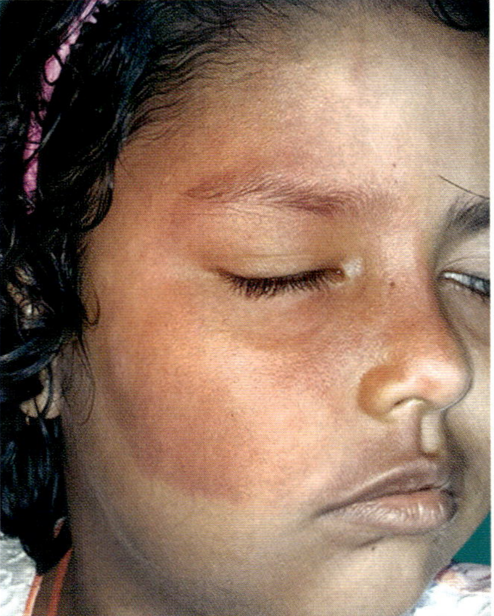

Fig. 13: Clinical picture of port-wine stain.

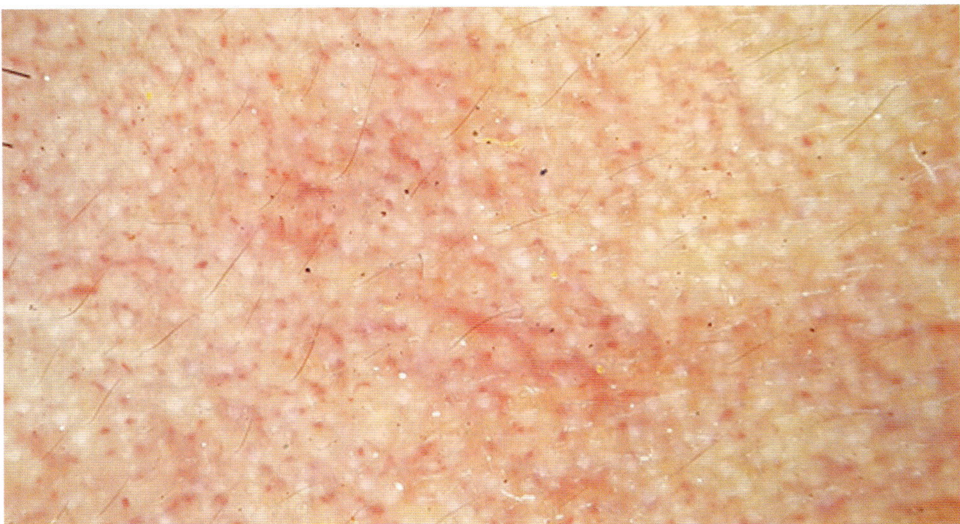

Fig. 14: Dermoscopy shows red globules and dots along with prominent red lines.

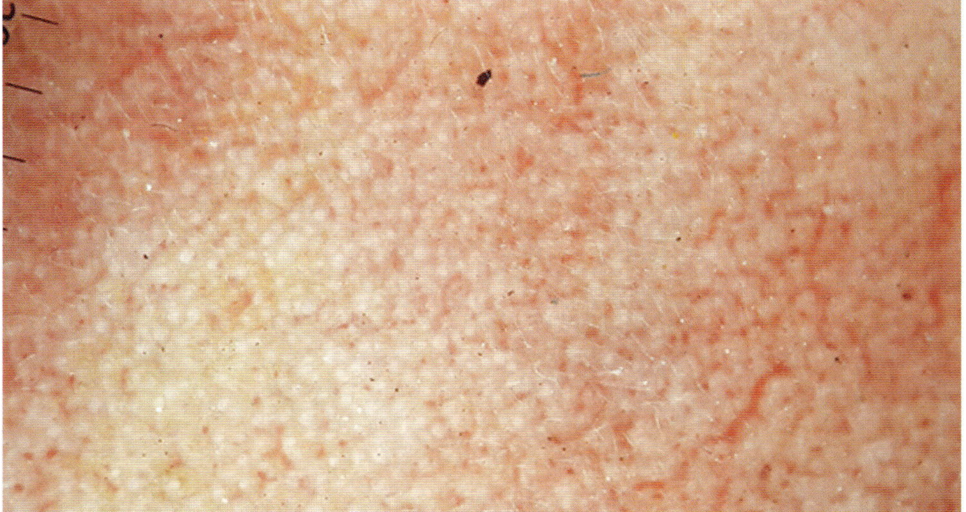

Fig. 15: Horizontal capillaries on dermoscopy signifies that the location of the vessels is in the subpapillary plexus.

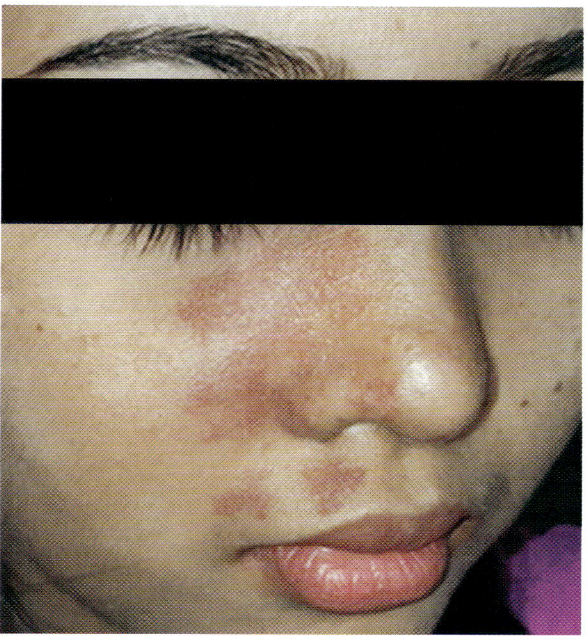

Fig. 16: Port-wine stain (PWS).

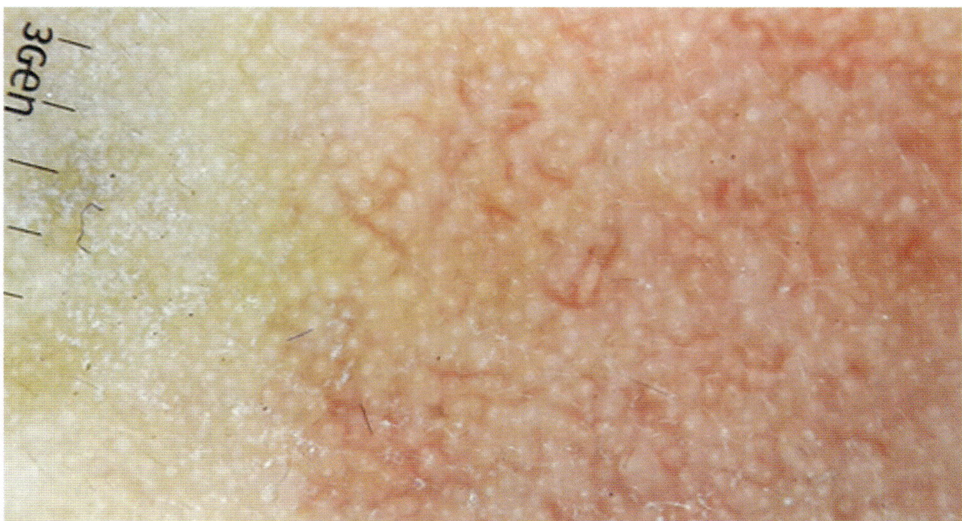

Fig. 17: Dermoscopy reveals mostly the prominent linear vessels. As the vessels are in a comparatively deeper plane, treatment with pulse dye laser here might lead to scarring.

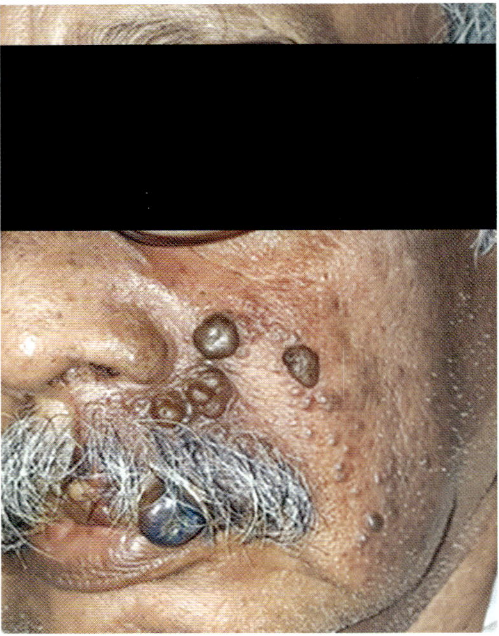

Fig. 18: An elderly patient with port-wine stain.

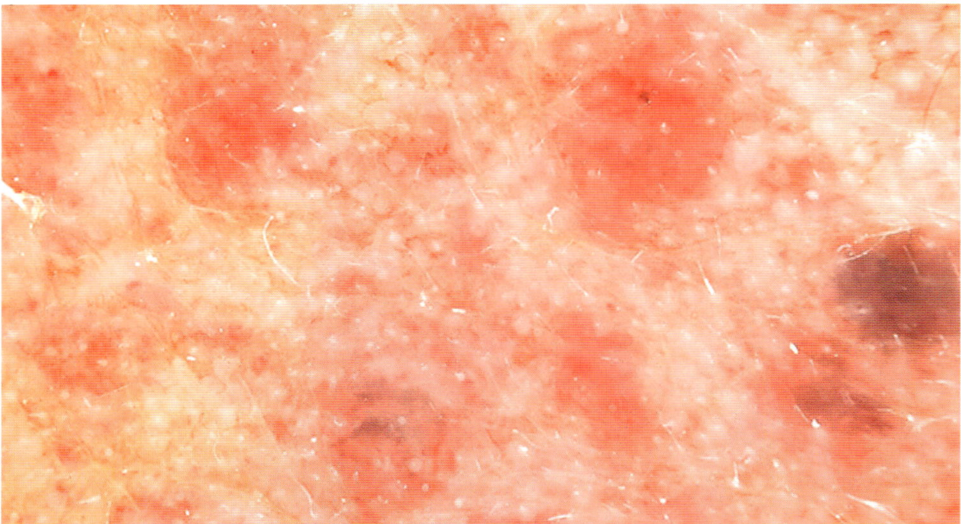

Fig. 19: Dermoscopy reveals larger globules of predominantly red color, with some purple.

REFERENCES

1. Sevila A, Nagore E, Botella-Estrada R, et al. Videomicroscopy of venular malformations (port-wine stain type): prediction of response to pulsed dye laser. Pediatr Dermatol. 2004;21:589-96.
2. Motley RJ, Lanigan SW, Katugampola GA. Videomicroscopy predicts outcome in treatment of port-wine stains. Arch Dermatol. 1997;133:921-2.

VENOUS LAKE

INTRODUCTION

A venous lake is usually a solitary, soft, compressible, and dark blue to violaceous small papule. It is commonly seen among elderly people and there is a predilection for sun-exposed areas such as lips, face including eyelids, and ears (Fig. 20).

It is an acquired form of vascular dilatation.

KEY DERMOSCOPIC FEATURES (FIG. 21)

- Homogeneous blue color
- Sometimes bluish-reddish appearance.

KEYNOTE

Dermoscope may be used to differentiate venous lake from melanocytic neoplasms.

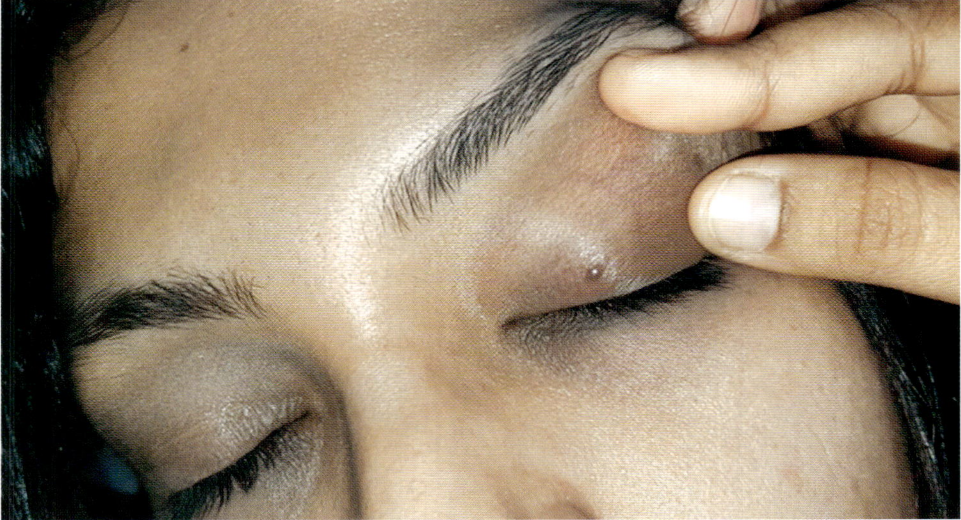

Fig. 20: A venous lake on left upper eyelid.

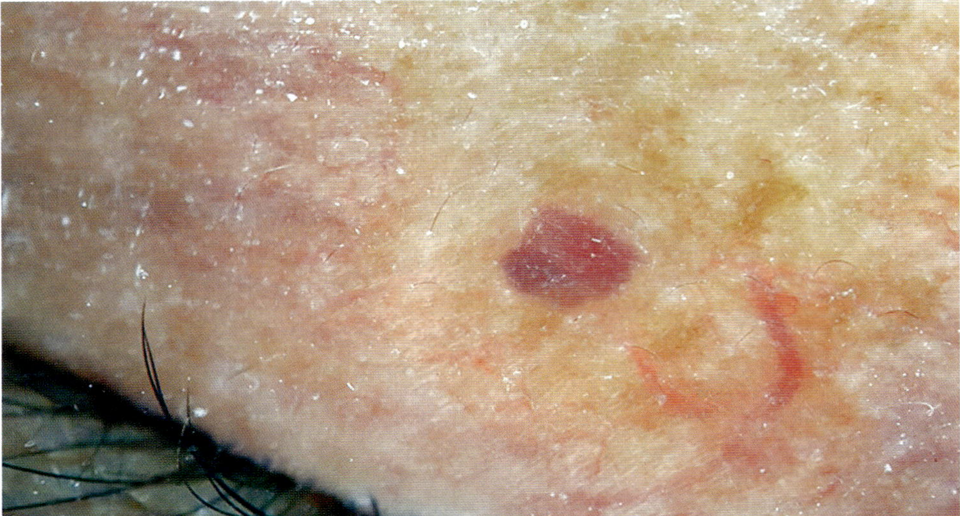

Fig. 21: Dermoscopy of the previous patient reveals homogeneous bluish-red area. Dermoscopy does not reveal any melanocytic criteria, thus ruling out melanocytic neoplasm.

LYMPHANGIOMA CIRCUMSCRIPTUM

INTRODUCTION

Lymphangiomas are congenital lymphatic malformations, accounting for 4% of all vascular tumors and have been classified into cutaneous lymphangioma circumscriptum (LC), cavernous lymphangiomas, and cystic hygromas. Cutaneous LC is the most common type and is described as superficial lymphatic malformation (SLM). It presents clinically as clusters of translucent vesicles; sometimes the vesicles contain varying amount of blood.[1] When cutaneous LC have a marked content of blood, it may be confused with hemangioma (Figs. 22, 25 and 27).[2] Histology of cutaneous LC shows thin-walled lymphatic vessels in the papillary and reticular dermis.

KEY DERMOSCOPIC FEATURES (FIGS. 23, 24, 26, 28 AND 29)[2,3]

- Yellow/brown lacunae surrounded by pale septa; thin linear vessels may or may not be visible
- Reddish to bluish lacunae
- Hypopyon-like lesions.

DISCUSSION

Lesions containing clear lymphatic fluid dermoscopically appear as yellow/brown lacunae surrounded by pale septa.

Varying amount of blood within the vesicle displays varied dermoscopic features, which range from focal reddish area to diffuse pink to violaceous-colored lacunae. The most plausible explanation to the presence of blood inside the lymphatic channel is microshunts between lymphatic channels and small blood vessels.[4]

The development of hypopyon-like structures in SLM is an interesting phenomenon. Over a period of time, the corpuscles, including erythrocytes, sediment at the bottom whereas serum lies at the upper part. This leads to a color transition from light to dark as you go from top to bottom in some lacunae, creating a similar effect that is seen in the eye, known as hypopyon.[2]

KEYNOTE

Cutaneous LC may sometimes contain marked amount of blood that mimics hemangioma. Consequently, it may be difficult to differentiate both conditions clinically and even dermoscopically. Hence, hypopyon-like feature can be a very useful dermoscopic pattern to differentiate between cutaneous LC from hemangioma.

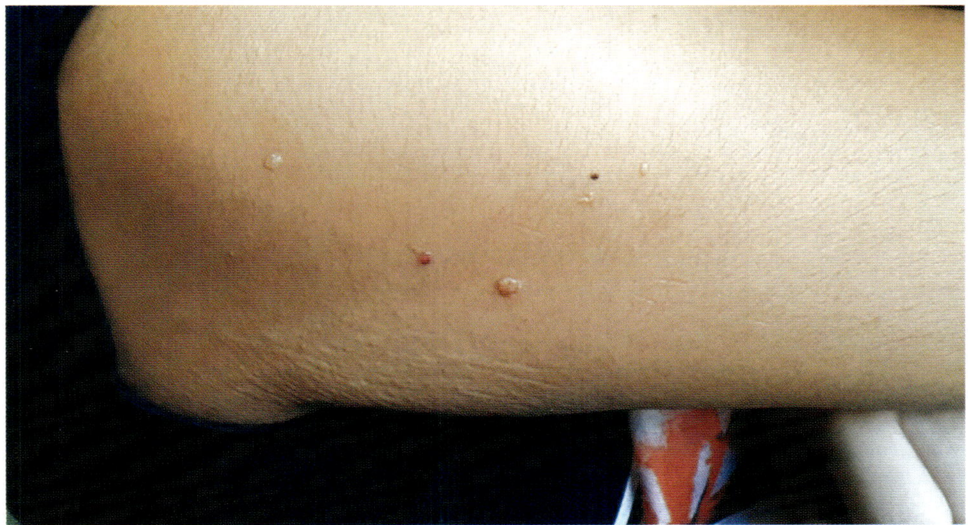

Fig. 22: Anomalies of the lymphatic system include lymphedema and lymphatic malformations (LMs). LMs are classified as microcystic, macrocystic, or combined.[5] Lymphangioma, lymphangioma circumscriptum, cavernous lymphangioma, and cystic hygroma are included in LMs. Macrocystic LMs are large interconnected lymphatic channels and cysts and include cystic hygromas and cavernous lymphangiomas, where a translucent mass lies under normal appearing skin. Microcystic LMs are common types of LMs composed of microscopic aggregations of small lymphatic channels. They present as plaques or nodules with superimposed cutaneous changes. Hemorrhages may occur within them. This clinical picture shows microcystic LM. Note: The multiple flesh colored, translucent papules with hemorrhagic changes in one of them.

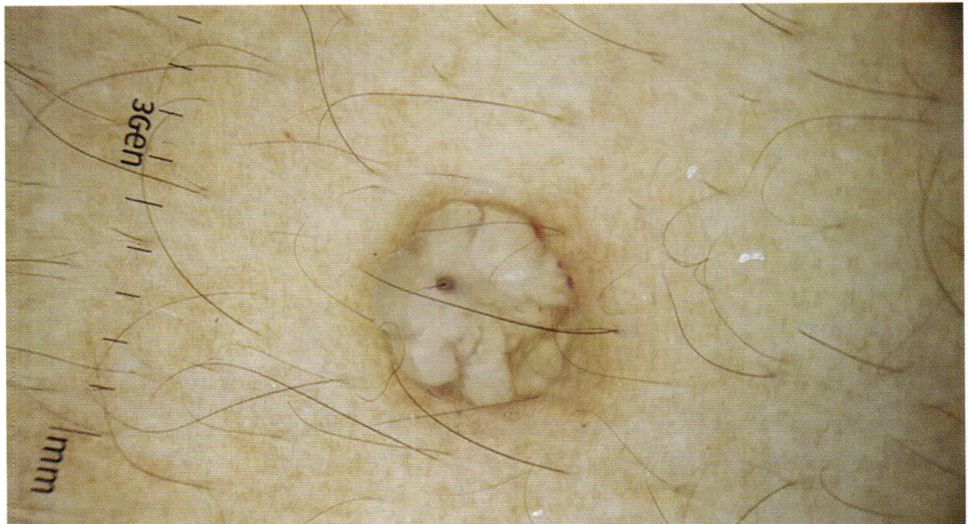

Fig. 23: Dermoscopy of microcystic lymphatic malformation (LM) shows yellow/brown lacunae surrounded by a pale septa.

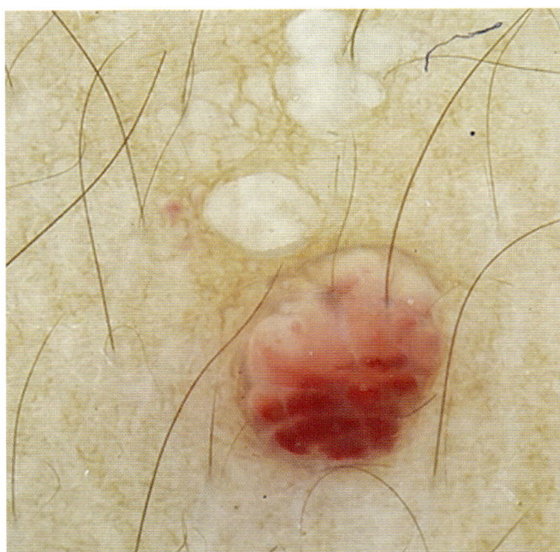

Fig. 24: Dermoscopy shows yellowish-white lacunae surrounded by a pale septa. One lacuna contains blood that has accumulated characteristically in its lowest part producing "hypopyon". It is termed as hypopyon because of its resemblance to the so-called "hypopyon sign" in ophthalmology.

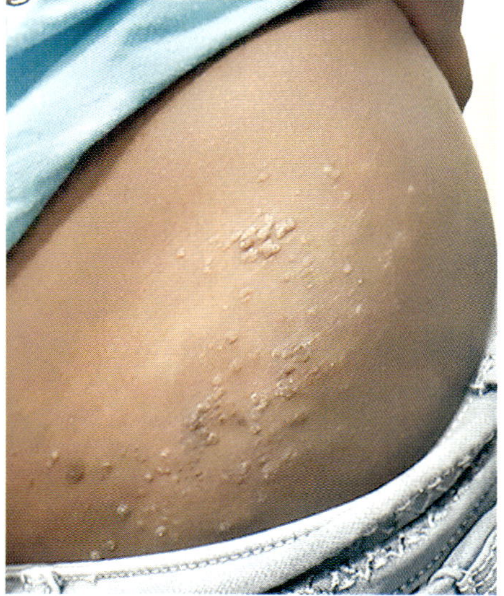

Fig. 25: Microcystic lymphatic malformation. Besides the flesh-colored translucent papules and hemorrhagic changes in some, the overlying skin has superimposed changes, accounting for the metaphoric analogy to frog spawn.

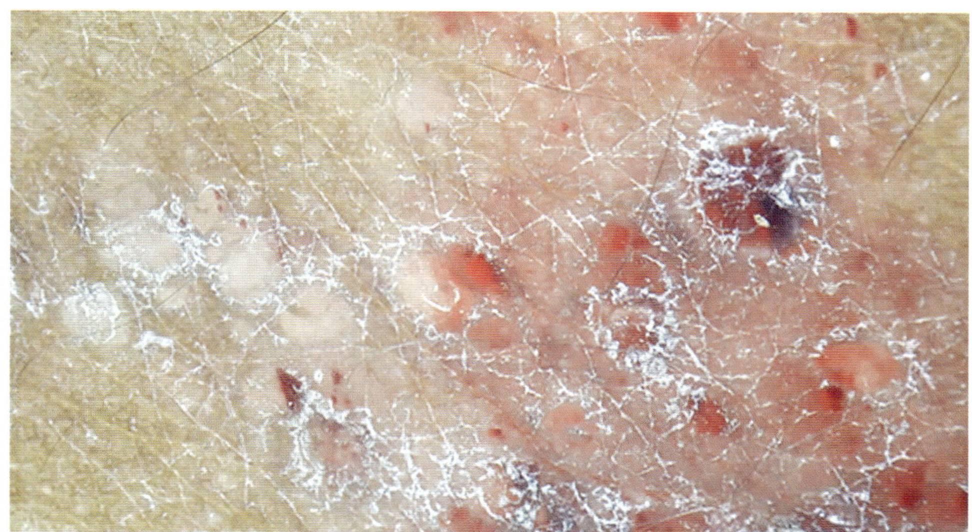

Fig. 26: Dermoscopy reveals yellow-white lacunae, red lacunae, and hypopyon-like structures.

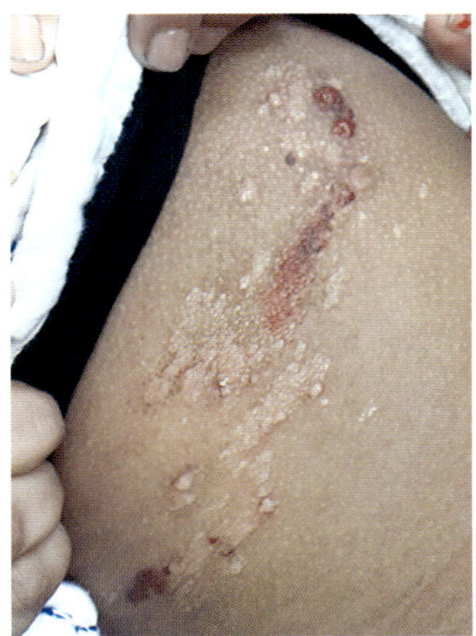

Fig. 27: Usually microcystic lymphatic malformations (LMs) are asymptomatic, but at times clear fluid might ooze from ruptured vesicles; also spontaneous episodes of bleeding may occur.

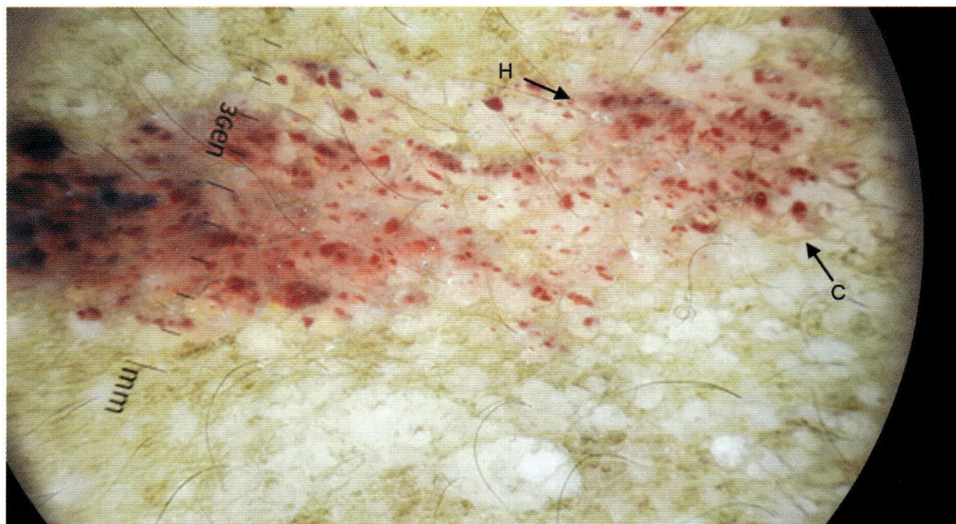

Fig. 28: Red lacunae are arranged in a linear fashion where multiple hypopyon-like structures are observed. Hypopyon-like structures may have different shapes like crescent (C), half and half (H), etc. In parallel with the red lacunae, white-yellow lacunae are also arranged linearly.

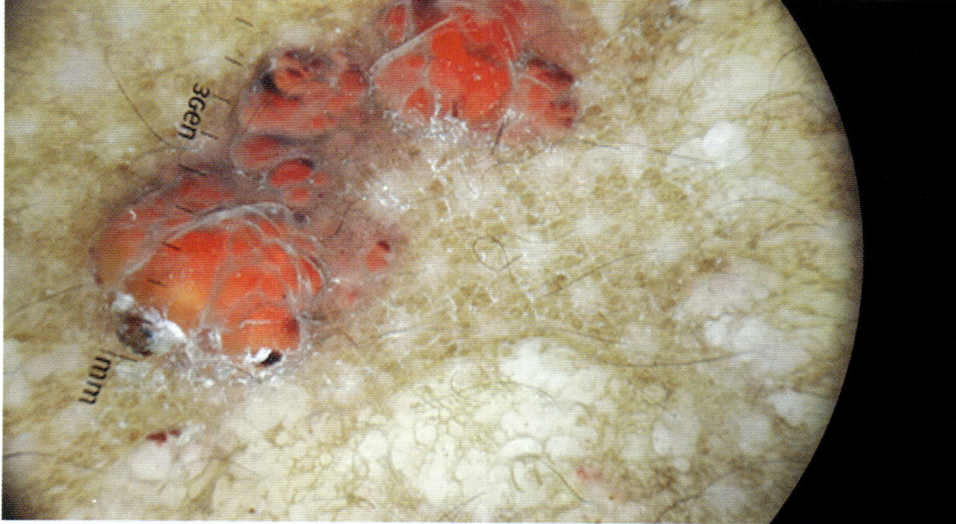

Fig. 29: On magnification, red lacunae are surrounded by multiple yellow-white lacunae with septa.

REFERENCES

1. Patel GA, Schwartz RA. Cutaneous lymphangioma circumscriptum: frog spawn on the skin. Int J Dermatol. 2009;48:1290-5.
2. Gencoglan G, Inanir I, Ermertcan AT. Hypopyon-like features: new dermoscopic criteria in the differential diagnosis of cutaneous lymphangioma circumscriptum and hemangiomas? J Eur Acad Dermatol Venereol. 2012;26:1023-5.
3. Massa AF, Moreira AI, Menezes N, et al. Cutaneous lymphangioma circumscriptum – dermoscopic features. An Bras Dermatol. 2015;90(2):262-4.
4. Franke FE, Steger K, Marks A, et al. Hobnail hemangiomas (targetoid hemosiderotic hemangiomas) are true lymphangiomas. J Cutan Pathol. 2004;31:362-7.
5. Paller A, Miancini A. Vascular disorders of infancy and childhood. In: Paller A, Miancini A (Eds). Hurwitz Clinical Paediatric Dermatology: A Textbook of Skin Disorders of Childhood and Adolescence. London: Elsevier; 2016. p. 304.

ANGIOKERATOMA

INTRODUCTION

Angiokeratomas (AKs) are vascular malformations of the upper dermis and present clinically as blue-black colored lesions (Fig. 30). Five clinical forms of AKs have been described such as: (1) Solitary and multiple AK, (2) AK circumscriptum, (3) AK of Mibelli, (4) AK of Fordyce, and (5) AK corporis diffusum (Fabry disease).[1]

KEY DERMOSCOPIC FEATURES (FIG. 31)[1,2]

- Dark lacunae and red lacunae
- Whitish veil
- Peripheral erythema
- Hemorrhagic crusts.

DISCUSSION

Dark lacunae are the hallmark dermoscopic feature of solitary AK and correspond histopathologically to partially or completely thrombosed dilated vessels.[2] Red lacunae refer to dilated vascular spaces without thrombosis in the upper dermis. The whitish veil represents hyperkeratosis and acanthosis. Additional dermoscopic features include erythema and hemorrhagic crusts.

Zaballos et al. described three patterns of dermoscopic AK.[2] Pattern 1 consists of red lacunae, dark lacunae, and whitish veil. Pattern 2 has peripheral erythema along with the features of pattern 1. Hemorrhagic crusts in addition to features of pattern 1 create pattern 3. The most common dermoscopic pattern is pattern 1.

KEYNOTE

Angiokeratomas are sometimes misdiagnosed as pigmented lesions such as malignant melanomas and Spitz nevi, nonpigmented lesions such as dermatofibromas, and vascular lesions such as angiomas and pyogenic granulomas. AKs being misdiagnosed as melanomas is not rare; however, melanomas dermoscopically do not show red and dark lacunae.[3]

Dermoscopic patterns such as red and blue lacunae and white veils of AKs easily differentiate it from other vascular and nonvascular lesions and thus a dermoscope is an essential tool for diagnosing AKs.

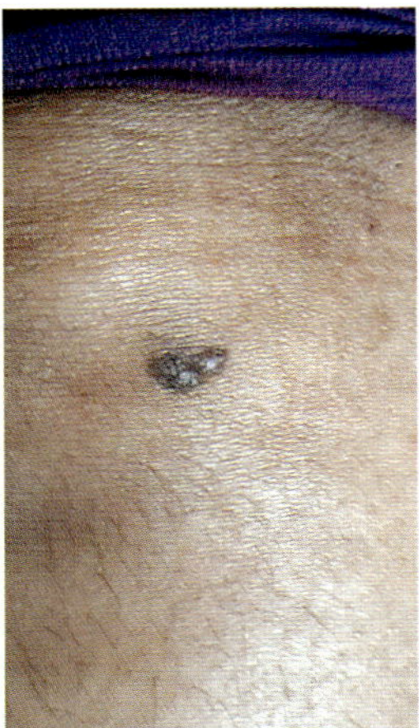

Fig. 30: Blue-red papulonodule over the knee with slight scaling on the surface. On histology, there are dilated thin-walled vessels in the upper dermis and the epidermis is hyperplastic.

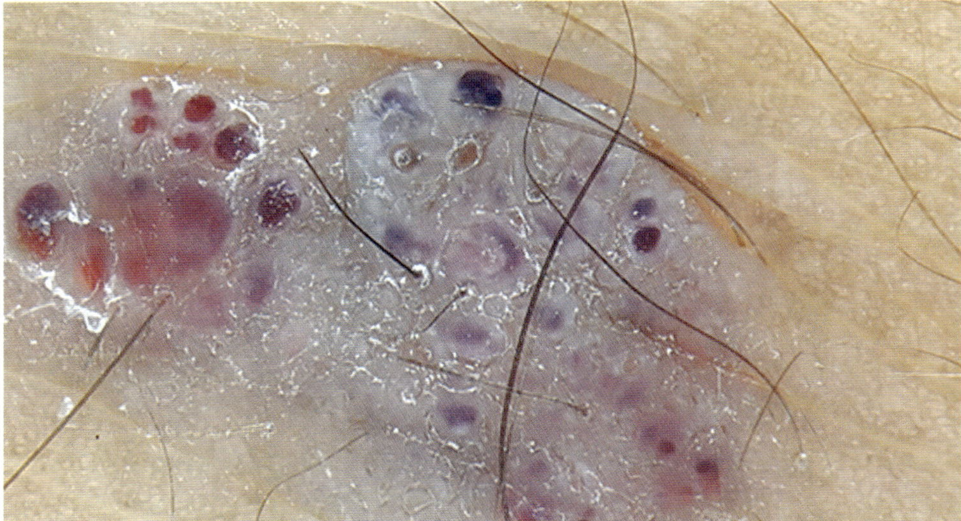

Fig. 31: Dermoscopically red and blue lacunae can easily be recognized. Red lacunae correspond to dilated vascular spaces without thrombosis whereas blue lacunae represent dilated blood vessels with thrombosis. The blue-white veil denotes hyperkeratosis and acanthosis.

REFERENCES

1. Wolf IH. Dermoscopic diagnosis of vascular lesions. Clin Dermatol. 2002;20:273-5.
2. Zaballos P, Daufi C, Puig S, et al. Dermoscopy of solitary angiokeratoma: a morphological study. Arch Dermatol. 2007;143:318-25.
3. Campos-do-Carmo G, Ramos-e-Silva M. Dermoscopy: basic concepts. Int J Dermatol. 2008;47:712-9.

ANGIOMA SERPIGINOSUM

INTRODUCTION

It is a rare acquired vascular malformation that involves the dermal capillaries. It usually appears on the lower extremities and buttocks and clinically present as tiny, partly compressible, and red to purple puncta. These tiny puncta develop in groups and spread by forming new satellite lesions at the periphery, thus resulting in a linear or serpiginous architect (Figs. 32 and 33).[1]

Histologically it shows thin-walled, dilated capillaries with neither erythrocyte extravasation nor hemosiderin deposition.[2]

KEY DERMOSCOPIC FEATURES (FIGS. 34 TO 37)[2]

- Minute, well-demarcated round to oval lacunae
- Lacunae are usually present in characteristic groups that form circles (personal observation).

DISCUSSION

Dermoscopy reveals lacunae distributed throughout the lesion. The lacunae are typically tiny, red, sharply demarcated, and round to oval in shape; although they could be linear.[2] Histologically, they correlate with the dilated thin-walled capillaries in the papillary and superficial dermis (Fig. 38).

Lacunae are usually present in characteristic groups. These groups are composed of tiny and larger lacunae that form a circular configuration. The largest lacuna, usually reddish or bluish color, lies in the center of the circle in most cases, may form a hemorrhagic crust (personal observation).

KEYNOTE

On diascopy, angioma serpiginosum shows incomplete blanching, thus may be confused with purpuric capillaritis such as Majocchi's disease.[2] Hence, the recognition of this dermoscopic pattern helps to distinguish angioma serpiginosum from purpuric dermatoses, thus avoiding unnecessary invasive procedures such as biopsy.[3]

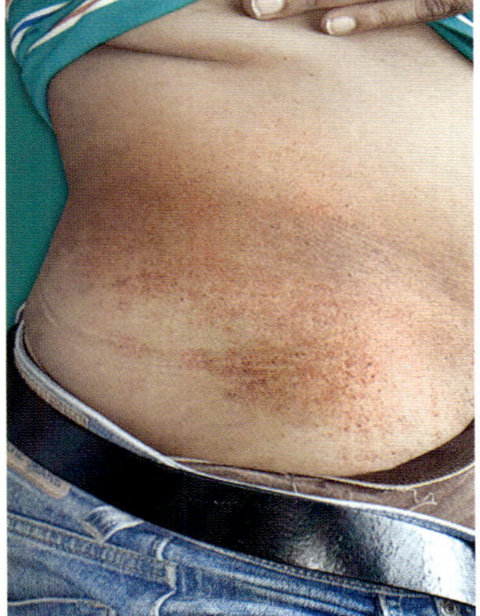

Fig. 32: A port-wine stain may be the first evidence of angioma serpiginosum. Years later, it enlarges in the form of tiny red satellites. Satellites spread and merge forming a serpiginous pattern. They are asymptomatic, progressive, and may be extensive in distribution.

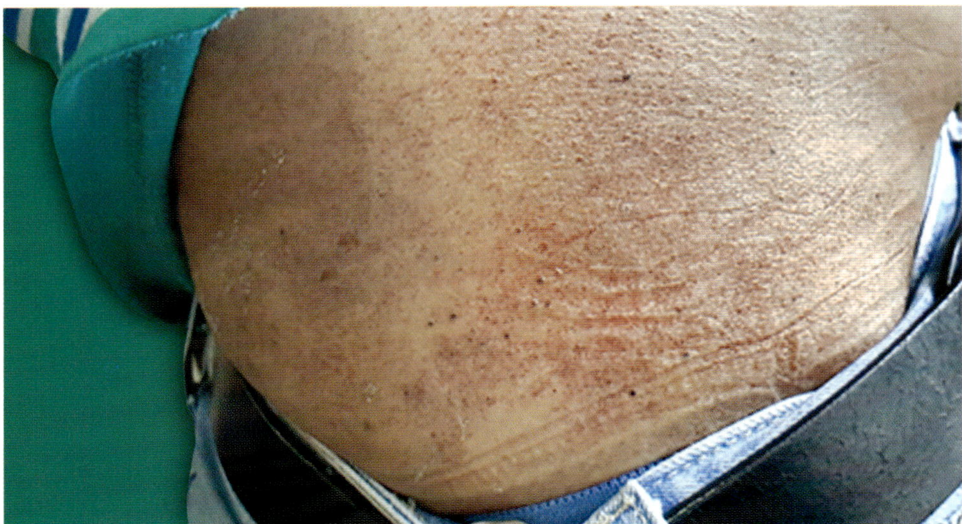

Fig. 33: Magnified view showing numerous red-purple puncta of 1 mm diameter. They are usually found grouped on the buttocks and lower extremities forming a serpiginous pattern.

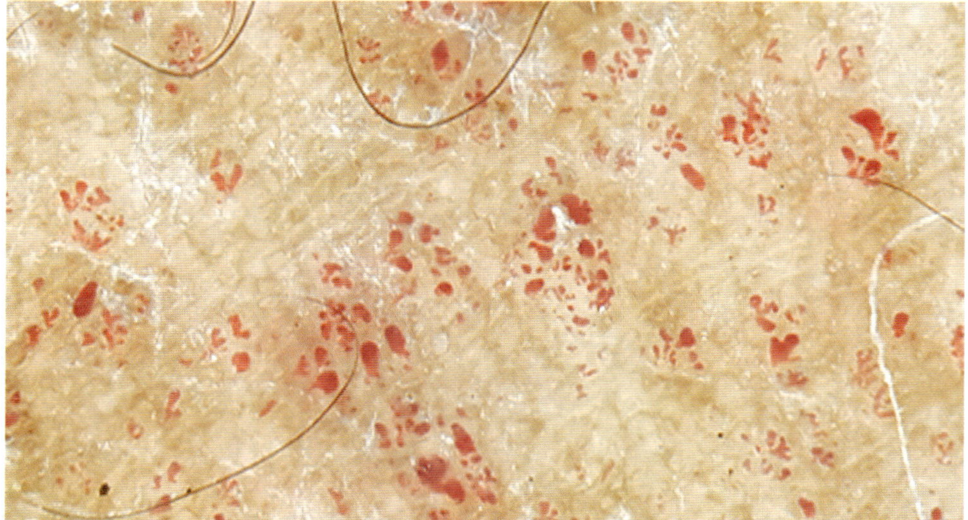

Fig. 34: Dermoscopy shows numerous sharply demarcated lacunae resembling a school of red fish in water. The lacunae are red and have many configurations such as oval, linear, comma, dots, etc.

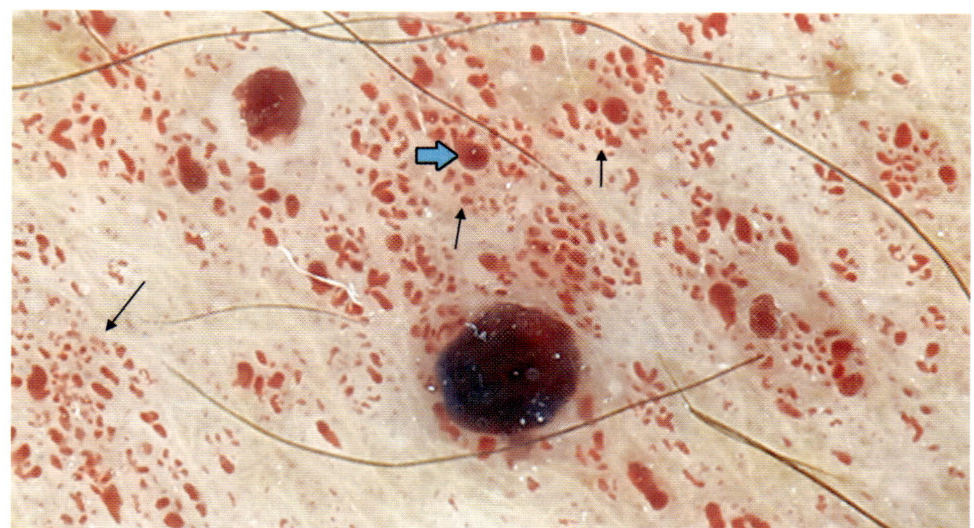

Fig. 35: Lacunae are usually present in characteristic groups. These groups comprise of tiny and larger lacunae that form a circular configuration (black arrows). The largest lacuna generally has a reddish or bluish color, lies in the center of the circle (thick arrow) in most cases.

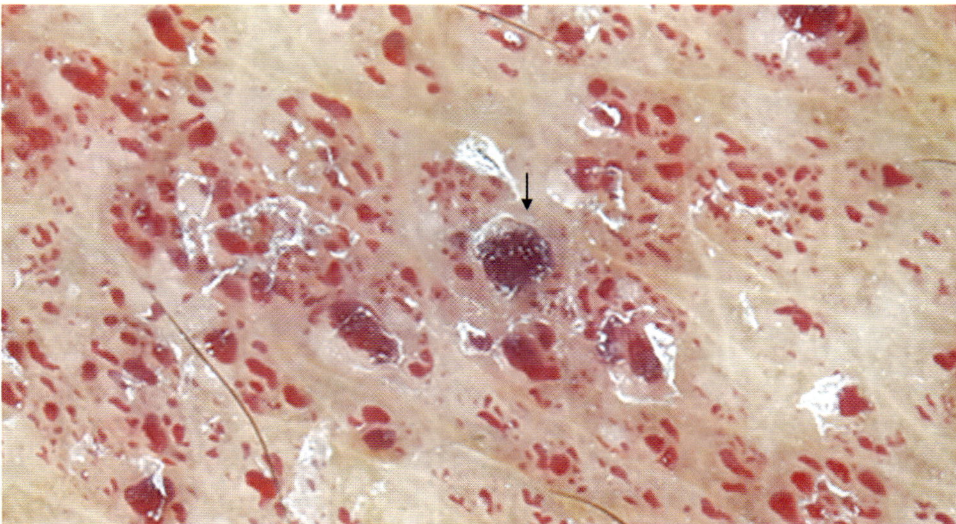

Fig. 36: Groups of lacunae may have a central hemorrhagic crust (arrow).

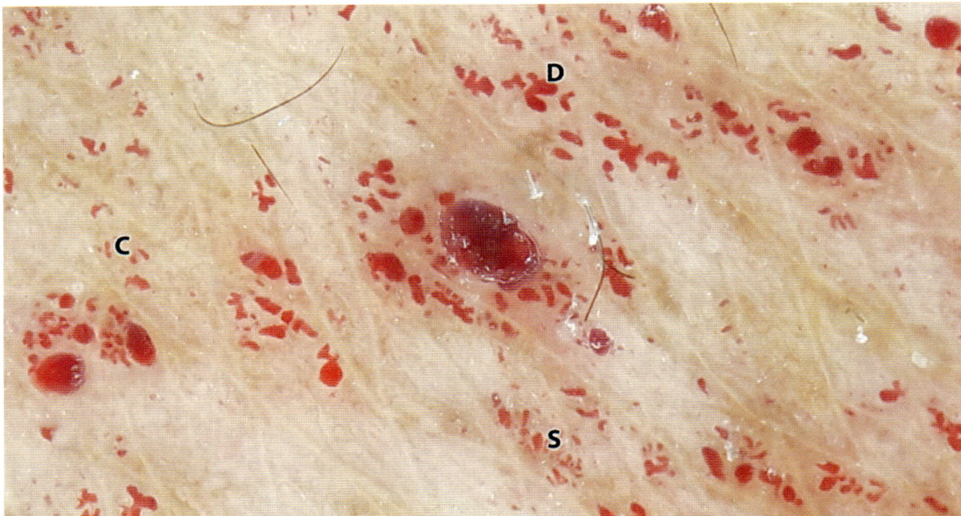

Fig. 37: Lacunae may be red or blue and apart from oval and linear, may have different shapes such as dumbbell (D), comma (C), spermatozoa (S), etc.

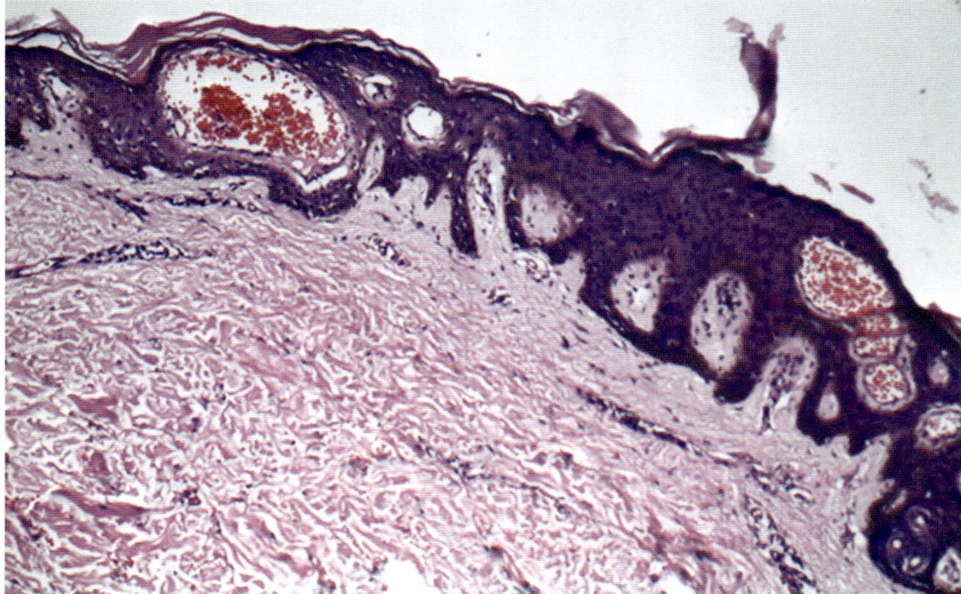

Fig. 38: Histopathology shows thin-walled capillaries in the papillary dermis engorged with erythrocytes.

REFERENCES

1. Paller A, Miancini A. Vascular disorders of infancy and childhood. In: Paller A, Miancini A (Eds). Hurwitz Clinical Paediatric Dermatology: A Textbook of Skin Disorders of Childhood and Adolescence. London: Elsevier; 2016. pp. 311-5.
2. Kuonen F, Gaide O. Clues in dermoscopy: dermoscopy of angioma serpiginosum. Eur J Dermatol. 2016;26(1):118.
3. Ohnishi T, Nagayama T, Morita T, et al. Angioma serpiginosum: a report of 2 cases identified using epiluminescence microscopy. Arch Dermatol. 1999;135:1366-8.

KAPOSI'S SARCOMA

INTRODUCTION

Kaposi's sarcoma presents as reddish to purplish macules, papules, and nodules over any cutaneous region or mucosae, lymph nodes, or other organs. Initially the lesions are small and painless, but later on they become painful and may ulcerate.

Histologically, Kaposi's sarcoma is a vascular tumor characterized by the proliferation of spindle cells and endothelial cells, which form closely arranged slit-like vascular spaces. They are divided into four clinical groups: (1) Classic or sporadic, (2) Immunocompromised, (3) Epidemic of acquired immunodeficiency syndrome (AIDS) related, and (4) Endemic (African).

KEY DERMOSCOPIC FEATURES[1]

- Bluish-reddish coloration
- Multicolored areas showing various colors of the rainbow spectrum
- Scaly surface
- Small brown globules.

DISCUSSION

Most commonly dermoscopy shows bluish-reddish coloration which represent the vascular nature of the tumor in less than 40% of cases, rainbow patterns, i.e. different colors juxtaposed next to each other are found. Hu et al. proposed that rainbow effect may be due to the optical phenomenon known as diffraction, which describes the bending of waves around small obstacles. Diffraction may cause white light to split into various wavelengths producing rainbow effect.

The scaly surface corresponds partly to eczematous changes, which develop in a small number of Kaposi's sarcoma.

Due to immature vascular structures significant amounts of erythrocytes may be extravasated, which overtime is engulfed by macrophages. Small brown globules on dermoscopy represent these hemosiderin-containing macrophages.

KEYNOTE

The rainbow pattern was once believed to be highly specific for Kaposi's sarcoma[1] but this peculiar phenomenon has been described in other conditions also, such as pyogenic granuloma, stasis dermatitis, melanoma, dermatofibromas, and lichen planus.[2]

REFERENCES

1. Hu SC, Ke CL, Lee CH, et al. Dermoscopy of Kaposi's sarcoma: areas exhibiting the multicolored rainbow pattern. J Eur Acad Dermatol Venereol. 2009;23(10):1128-32.
2. Martín JM. Vascularización en dermatoscopia. Actas Dermosifiliogr. 2012;103:357-75.

TARGETOID HEMOSIDEROTIC HEMANGIOMA

INTRODUCTION

It is a benign vascular tumor, which usually presents as a small, single lesion on the extremity, or trunk of a young and middle-aged person. The most common presentation is annular lesion with a central violaceous papule with a peripheral ecchymotic ring, thus exhibiting a targetoid appearance. It may have wide variation in clinical appearance.[1]

Histologically it is a biphasic vascular tumor exhibiting superficial telangiectasia lined by hobnail endothelial cells and deeper slit-like vascular spaces. Extravasated red blood cell (RBC) and variable amounts of hemosiderin are usually present between the dermal vasculature.[1]

KEY DERMOSCOPIC FEATURES[1]

- Central dark or red lacunae
- Peripheral homogeneous reddish, violaceous, or brownish area
- Sometimes a fine pigmented network.

DISCUSSION

Most targetoid hemosiderotic hemangioma (THH) do not clinically show a targetoid appearance. Dermoscopy is highly recommended as clinically and histologically it may be confused with melanoma, Kaposi's sarcoma, and angiosarcoma. Clinically, at times, it mimics dermatofibroma or melanocytic nevus.

KEYNOTE

Its name is derived from the extravasated hemosiderin that is found histopathologically. If targetoied appearance is missing clinically, the diagnosis is a dilemma and consequently THH is difficult to differentiate from melanocytic nevus, dermatofibroma, and melanoma. In a recent report dermoscopy was useful in correctly diagnosing THH in 77% cases.[2] However, attention must be paid to those cases that do not reveal targetoid appearance on dermoscopy.

REFERENCES

1. Bigham LG, Davis DM. Clinicopathologic challenge: targetoid hemosiderotic hemangioma. Int J Dermatol. 2008;47:991-2.
2. Zaballos P, Llambrich A, Del Pozo LJ, et al. Dermoscopy of targetoid hemosiderotic hemangioma: a morphological study of 35 cases. Dermatology. 2015;231(4):339-44.

LIVEDOID VASCULOPATHY

INTRODUCTION

Livedoid vasculopathy (LV) presents as purpuric papules that evolve into crusted ulcers which heal to form white atrophic scars known as atrophie blanche.[1-3] The lower legs, specially the dorsum of the feet and ankles are commonly affected (Fig. 39).[4] Not uncommonly venous stasis is also associated with LV. LV is a hypercoagulable state, leading to obstruction of small dermal blood vessels by intraluminal thrombi.

In the early stage of the disease hyaline thrombi form in the lumen of small vessels in the mid and papillary dermis associated with fibrinoid material in the vessel walls and perivascular stroma. In the advanced stage, dermal sclerosis and scarring with some dilated lymphatic vessels are seen.

KEY DERMOSCOPIC FEATURES (FIGS. 40 TO 45)[5]

- Ivory white areas
- Increased vascular structures (linear and glomerular vessels) in the periphery of the atrophic scars
- Rosettes
- Yellow-white lacunae surrounded by pale septa (personal observation).

DISCUSSION

- The central ivory white area corresponds to dermal fibrosis following healing of vasculitic ulcers.
- Vascular patterns observed in LV are telangiectatic linear and glomerular vessels surrounding the central ivory-white plaque. This might be because of dilatation and proliferation of vessels in response to thrombosis and ischemia of the central area.
- Glomerular vessels correspond histopathologically to the presence of grouped, convoluted, and dilated capillaries in the papillary dermis.
- The mechanisms responsible for the formation of glomerular vessels are chronic severe ischemia of the involved skin, which may promote angiogenesis and lead to an increased number of blood vessels in the surrounding skin.
- In advanced stage, yellow-white lacunae surrounded by pale septa are seen on dermoscopy which correspond to dermal sclerosis followed by dilated lymph spaces.

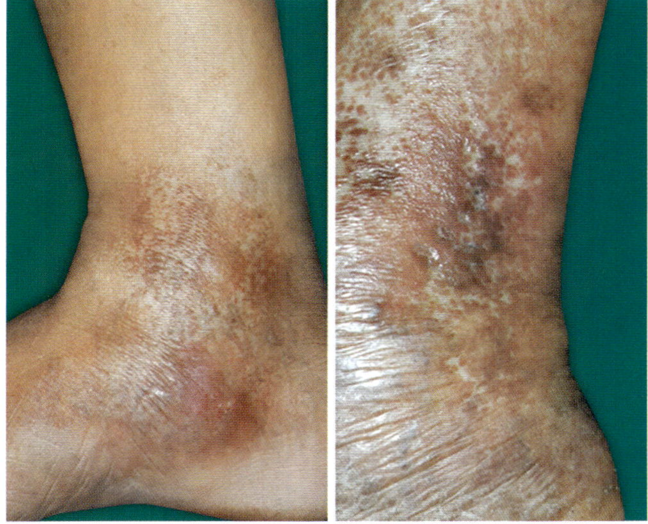

Fig. 39: Livedoid vasculopathy on the lower leg with white atrophic scar.

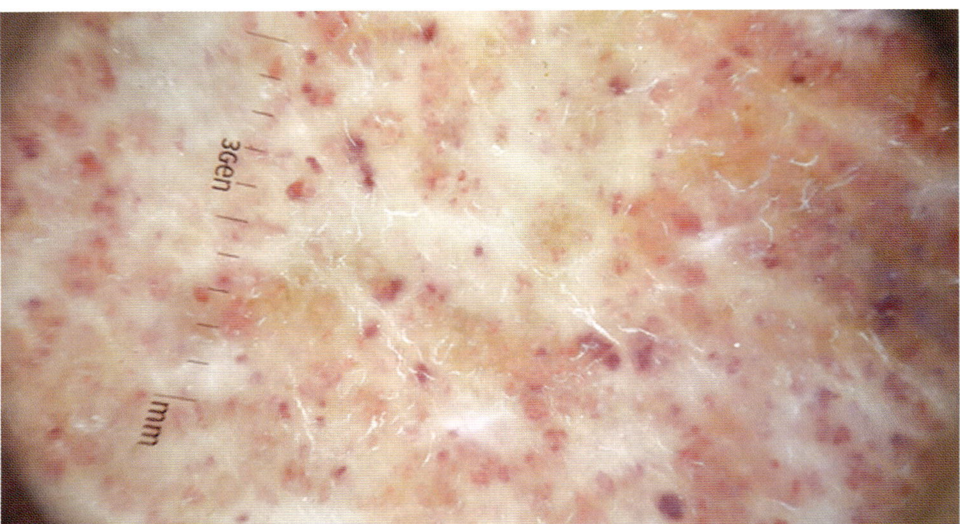

Fig. 40: Dermoscopy of livedoid vasculopathy is characterized by central whitish scar-like area or crusted ulceration and vascular structures. In this field, white shiny streaks are also visible which corresponds to dermal sclerosis in the late stage of the disease. Vascular structures consist mostly of glomerular vessels and some linear vessels.

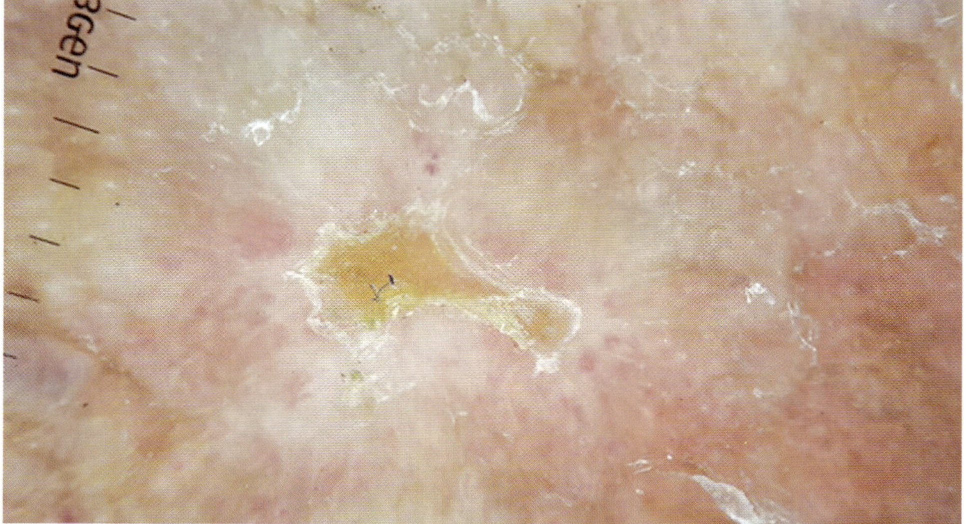

Fig. 41: Central crusted ulceration is the dominant feature of this dermoscopic field of livedoid vasculopathy (LV). Glomerular vessels and some faint linear vessels are also seen at the periphery of the central crust.

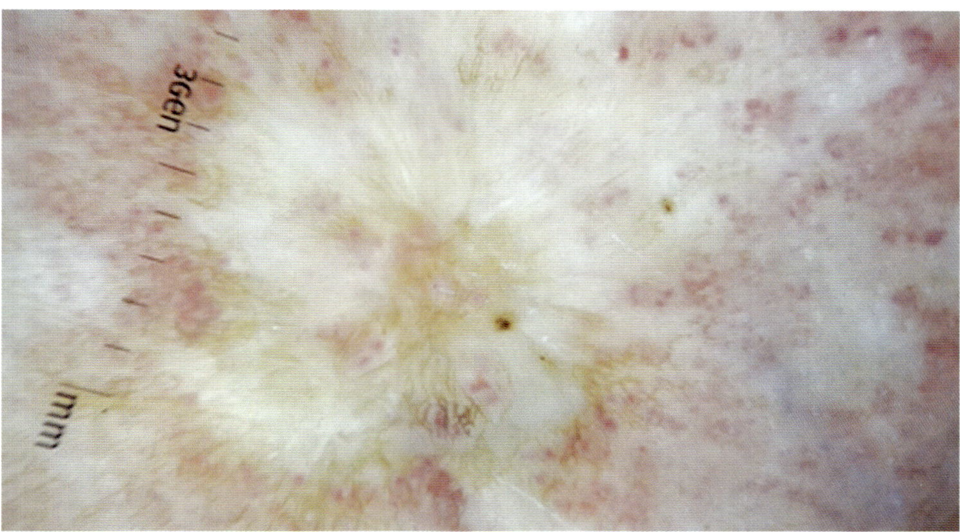

Fig. 42: Central whitish scar-like area along with peripheral vascular structures.

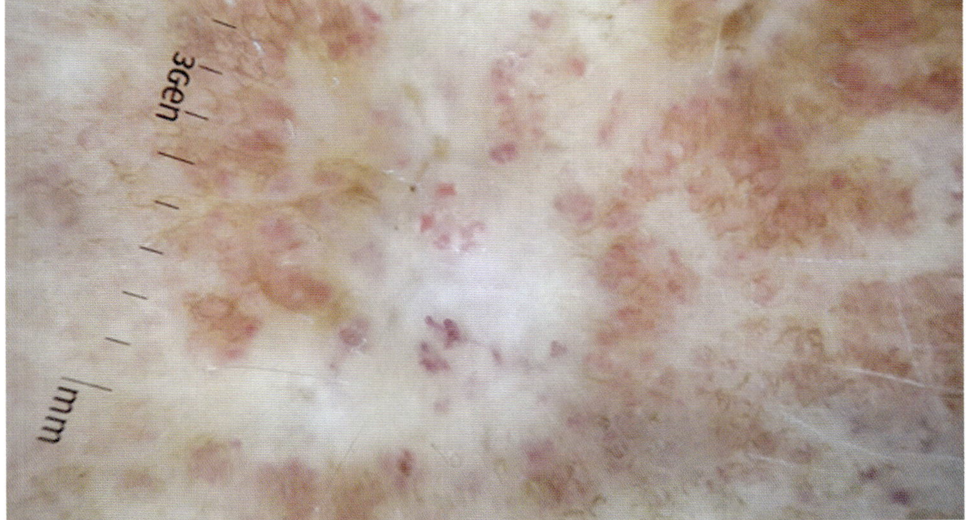

Fig. 43: White shiny streaks are present in the central whitish scar-like area; glomerular vessels are found in and around the central whitish scar-like area.

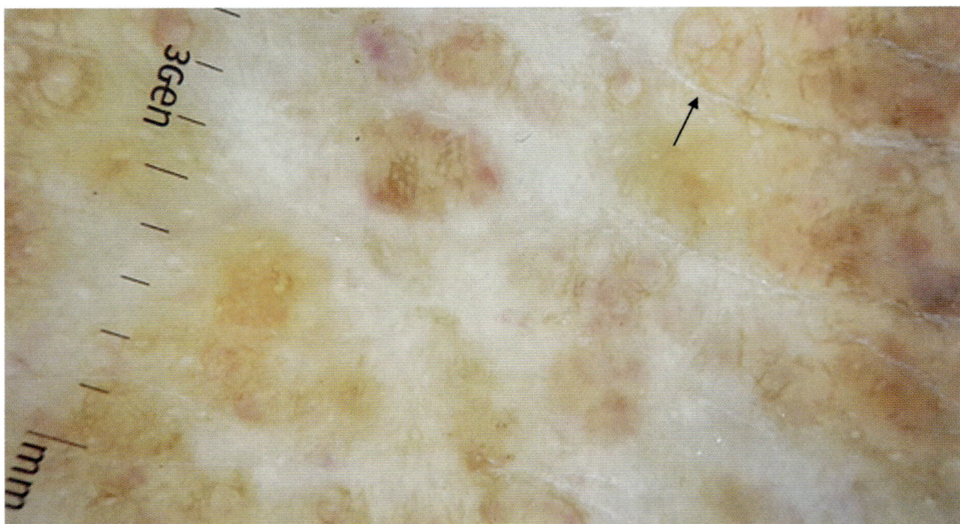

Fig. 44: Advanced stage of livedoid vasculopathy (LV) is characterized by dermal sclerosis with some dilated lymph vessels. Dermoscopy of the late stage LV may reveal yellow-white lacunae with peripheral septa (arrow) which correspond to dermal sclerosis with some dilated lymph vessels on histopathology.[4]

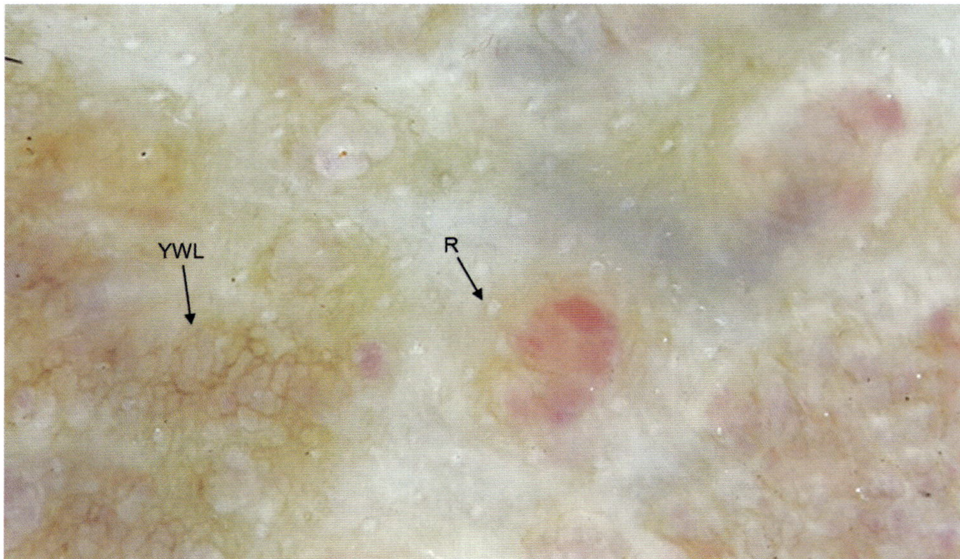

Fig. 45: Magnified dermoscopic image showing yellow-white lacunae (YWL) and rosettes (R).

REFERENCES

1. Alavi A, Hafner J, Dutz JP, et al. Livedoid vasculopathy: an in-depth analysis using a modified Delphi approach. J Am Acad Dermatol. 2013;69:1033-42.
2. Haunson GT, Judy DW, Prall NC, et al. Livedoid vasculopathy: review of pathogenesis, clinical presentation, diagnostic workup, and treatment. Cutis. 2012;90:302-6.
3. Criado PR, Rivitti EA, Sotto MN, et al. Livedoid vasculopathy: an intriguing cutaneous disease. An Bras Dermatol. 2011;86: 961-77.
4. Freedberg IM, Eisen AZ, Wolff K, et al. Fitzpatrick's Dermatology in General Medicine, 6th edition. New York: McGraw-Hill; 2003.
5. Chu-Sung S, Chen GS, Lin CL, et al. Dermoscopic features of livedoid vasculopathy. Medicine. 2017;96(11):e6284.

CHAPTER 15

Dermoscopic Surprises

Subrata Malakar, Purva Mehta

INTRODUCTION

Dermoscopy has revolutionized noninvasive methodology of clinical diagnosis in the field of dermatology. It not only exhibits the subsurface features invisible to the naked eye but also guides us to an accurate diagnosis. The discrepancy between clinical suspicion and the actual diagnosis can be highlighted by the simple yet effective use of a dermoscope.

CASE 1

Case 1A

A 40-year-old male presented with a lesion on the upper lip since a few years. The lesion was asymptomatic and static in nature. On cutaneous examination, there was a single, firm, sessile, skin-colored papular lesion measuring 0.5 × 0.5 cm in size, with two to three hair protruding from it (Fig. 1). On the basis of clinical examination, a differential diagnosis of compound nevus, verruca vulgaris, molluscum contagiosum, and seborrheic keratosis was made.

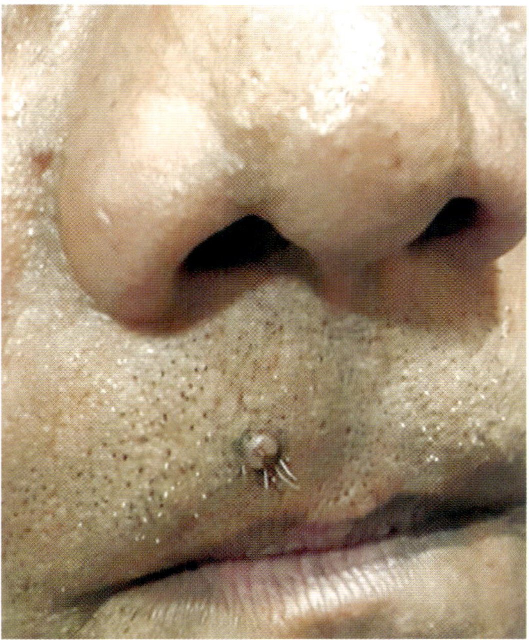

Fig. 1: Singular, firm, sessile, skin-colored papular lesion on the upper lip.

On dermoscopy, there was a white mass with central yellow keratin crusts surrounded by a paler dull white structureless zone. Blood spots were also noticeable in the center of the white keratin mass. At the periphery of the mass there was a radial distribution of hairpin blood vessels (Fig. 2).

Thus, dermoscopic examination clinched the diagnosis of keratoacanthoma.

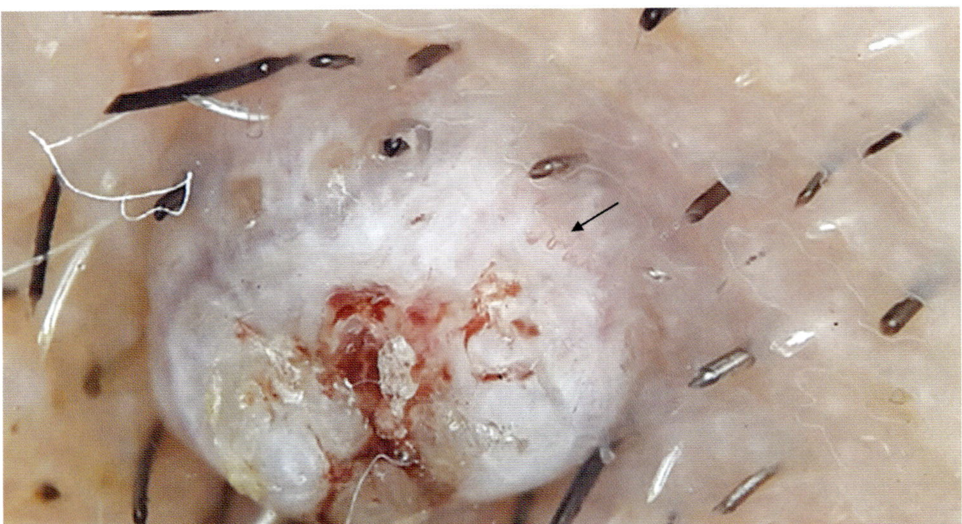

Fig. 2: White-colored structure with central yellow keratin crusts and blood spots with hairpin blood vessels (arrow) arranged along the periphery of the structure.

Case 1B

A 35-year-old female patient presented with a lesion on the nose since a couple of years. The lesion was asymptomatic in nature and static in size. Cutaneous examination revealed a single, firm, brown to black-colored sessile papule on the nose (Fig. 3). Considering the clinical appearance of the lesion, seborrheic keratosis, compound nevus, verruca vulgaris, and solitary fibrous papule of the nose were considered as differential diagnosis.

On dermoscopic examination, there was a dome-shaped white mass. At the center of this dome-shaped mass, there was a keratin plug which was surrounded by a white structureless zone. At the periphery of the mass, there were hairpin blood vessels (Fig. 4).

These dermoscopic features established the diagnosis of keratoacanthoma.

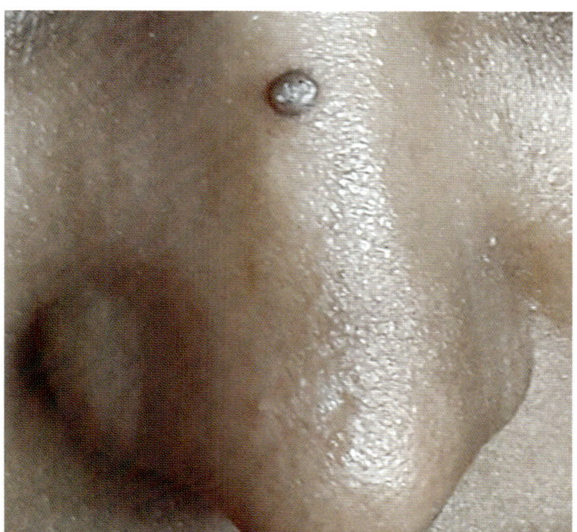

Fig. 3: Single, firm, brown to black-colored sessile papule on the nose.

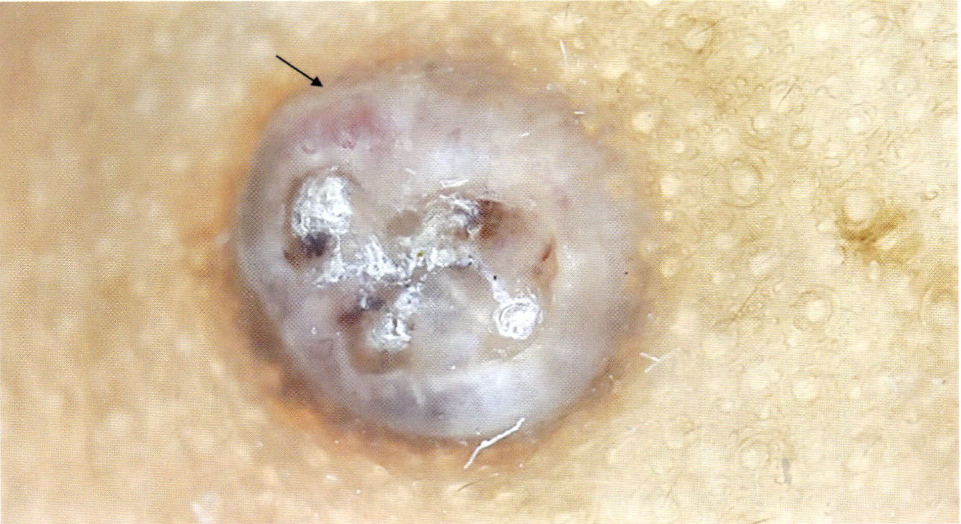

Fig. 4: Dome-shaped mass with central keratin and peripheral hairpin vessels (arrow).

Case 1C

A 43-year-old male presented with a lesion on his left forearm since few months. The lesion was essentially asymptomatic in nature with no change in size. Cutaneous examination revealed a solitary, skin-colored dome-shaped nodule with central scaling (Fig. 5). Clinical appearance led to differentials such as molluscum contagiosum, verruca vulgaris.

Dermoscopy revealed a white mass with central yellow keratin surrounded by a white structureless zone confirming the lesion to be keratoacanthoma and ruling out other clinical suspicions (Fig. 6).

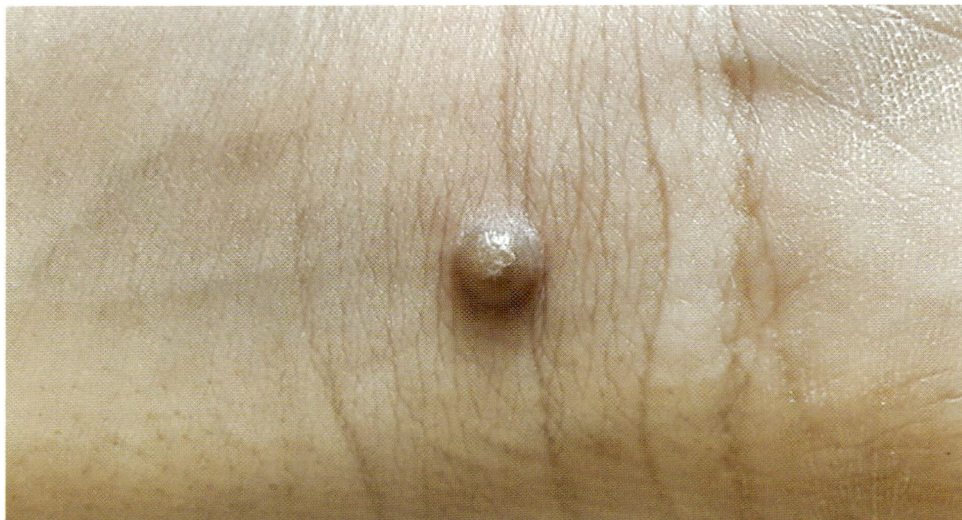

Fig. 5: Solitary, skin-colored dome-shaped nodule with central scaling.

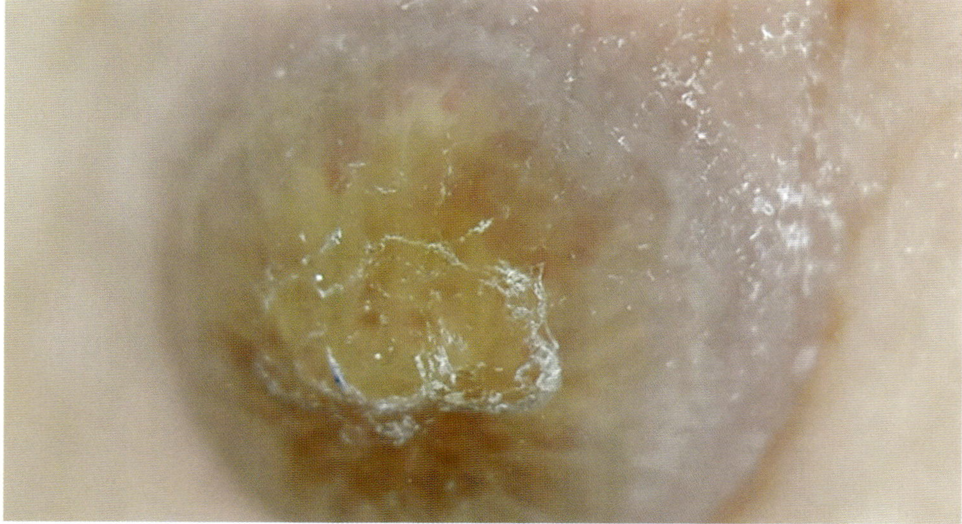

Fig. 6: White-colored mass with central yellow keratin surrounded by a white structureless zone and peripheral "out of focus" hairpin vessels.

DISCUSSION

The white mass with central blood spots and keratin crusts along with the characteristic peripheral arrangement of hairpin blood vessels is diagnostic of keratoacanthoma.[1] The peripheral arrangement of hairpin blood vessels favors a diagnosis of keratoacanthoma over seborrheic keratosis in which the hairpin vessels are evenly distributed throughout the lesion.[2] Dermoscopy ruled out compound nevus; as comma vessels which are a key dermoscopic feature of intradermal melanocytic nevi were missing.[3] The dermoscopic pattern of homogeneous dots and globules along with keratotic haloes was absent ruling out verruca vulgaris.[4] The absence of crown vessels at the periphery in a radial distribution ruled out molluscum contagiosum.[5]

CASE 2

A 45-year-old male presented with a lesion on the nose since a few months. The lesion was asymptomatic in nature but had gradually increased in size over the last 1 month. On cutaneous examination, there was a solitary, skin colored, and ovoid nodule measuring 1.5 × 1.5 cm on the nose (Fig. 7). The differential diagnosis was intradermal nevus or solitary fibrous papule of the nose.

Dermoscopy of the nasal lesion revealed arborizing telangiectatic vessels coursing throughout the lesion. These vessels were branching at irregular intervals into thin capillaries and were bright red in color. On closer examination, dermoscopy also highlighted that these arborizing vessels were sharp in focus and their borders were abruptly cutoff (Fig. 8)

The dermoscopic picture was diagnostic of basal cell carcinoma. Arborizing vessels are not a dermoscopic feature of either nevus or solitary fibrous papule of nose. The patient was then subjected to an excision biopsy and the excised specimen was sent for histopathological examination. Histological analysis showed nests of basaloid epithelial cells in the dermis with hyperchromatic nuclei and a peripheral palisading pattern all embedded in fibrous septae. Keratin pearls were also present in the dermis. Thus, histopathology confirmed dermoscopic findings and labeled the lesion to be keratotic basal cell carcinoma (Fig. 9).

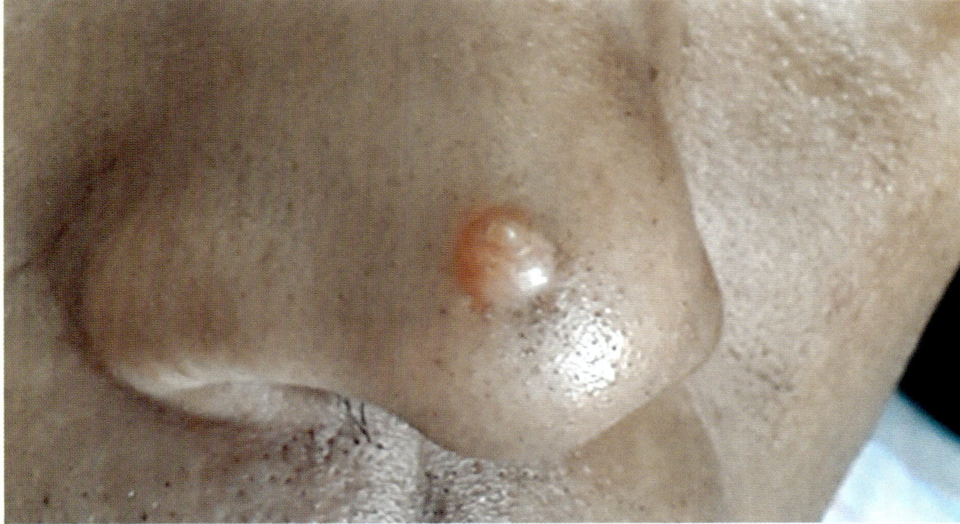

Fig. 7 Solitary, skin colored, and ovoid papulonodule on the nose.

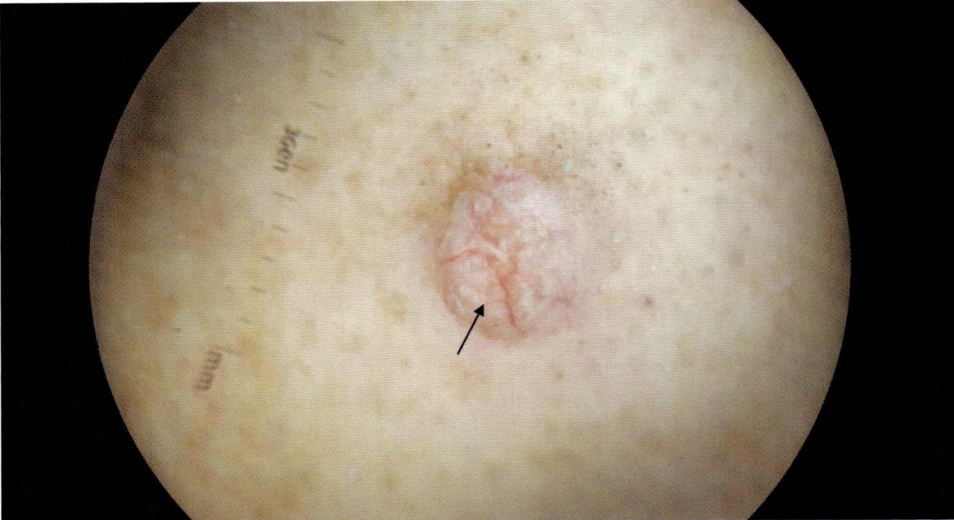

Fig. 8: Arborizing telangiectatic vessels (arrow) coursing throughout the lesion.

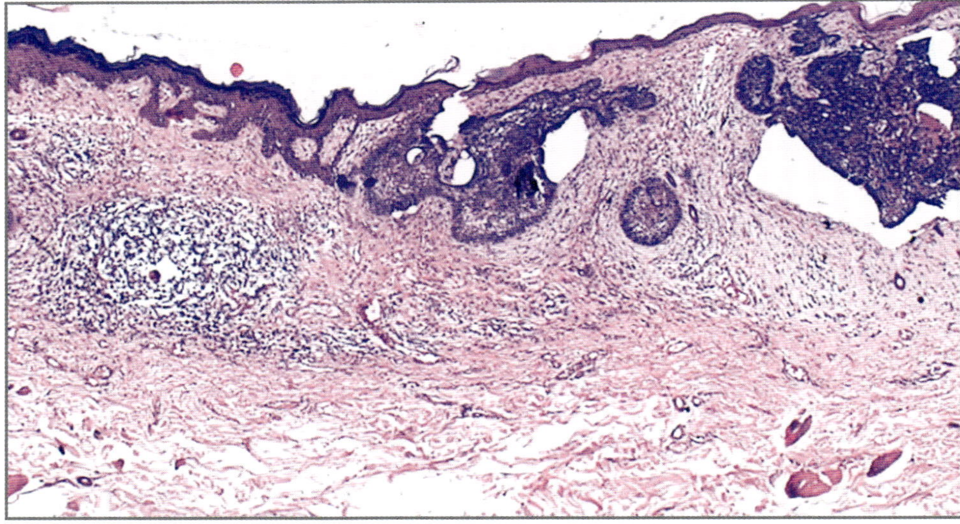

Fig. 9: Nests of basaloid cells in the dermis with hyperchromatic nuclei and a peripheral palisading pattern suggestive of basal cell carcinoma.

DISCUSSION

Identification of the vascular pattern is often imperative for the diagnosis of basal cell carcinoma as most of them are nonpigmented. Arborizing branching vessels which are hallmark for basal cell carcinoma are defined as large caliber vessels which are in focus and branch into finer secondary vessels. Arborizing branching vessels are a dermoscopic feature of both basal cell carcinoma and adnexal tumors. However, the clinical picture went against the diagnosis of an adnexal tumor as the lesion was solitary and larger in size whereas adnexal tumors tend to be multiple and smaller in size. The dermoscope also helps to pinpoint the location of the blood vessels by highlighting the color of the vessels and their characteristic morphology and architectural arrangement. The linear pattern of the blood vessels corresponds to the upper dermal plexus. The linearity of the blood vessels also suggested that they ran parallel to the skin surface whereas blood vessels that ran perpendicular to the skin surface would have been viewed as dots or loops. Also the vessels were bright red in color, prominent to the eye, and "in focus" reaffirming their location in the upper dermis. On the other hand, connective tissue in the dermis causes dispersion of light and this would make deeper dermal vessels appear as pink dots, less prominent, and out of focus.[2]

CASE 3

A 22-year-old female presented with a lesion on the right knee since several years. The lesion was asymptomatic and stable in size. Cutaneous examination revealed a single, gray to brown colored, lobulated mass measuring 1 × 0.5 cm in size on the right knee (Fig. 10). Clinical appearance led to a differential diagnosis of seborrheic keratosis and dermatofibroma.

On dermoscopy, there were several, round to oval well-demarcated red to blue lacunae with a whitish veil (Fig. 11). The dermoscopic features were diagnostic of angiokeratoma ruling out other clinical suspicions.

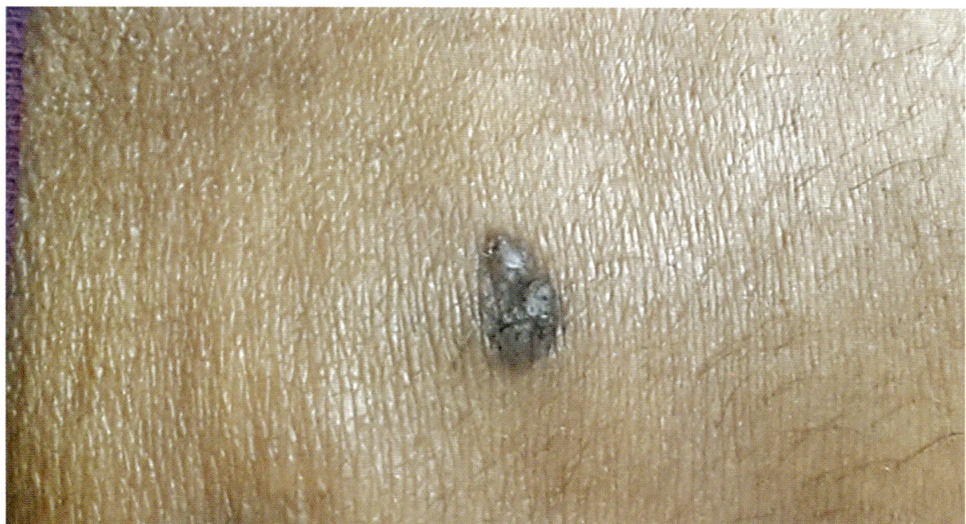

Fig. 10: Single, soft to firm, gray-brown lobulated mass on the right knee.

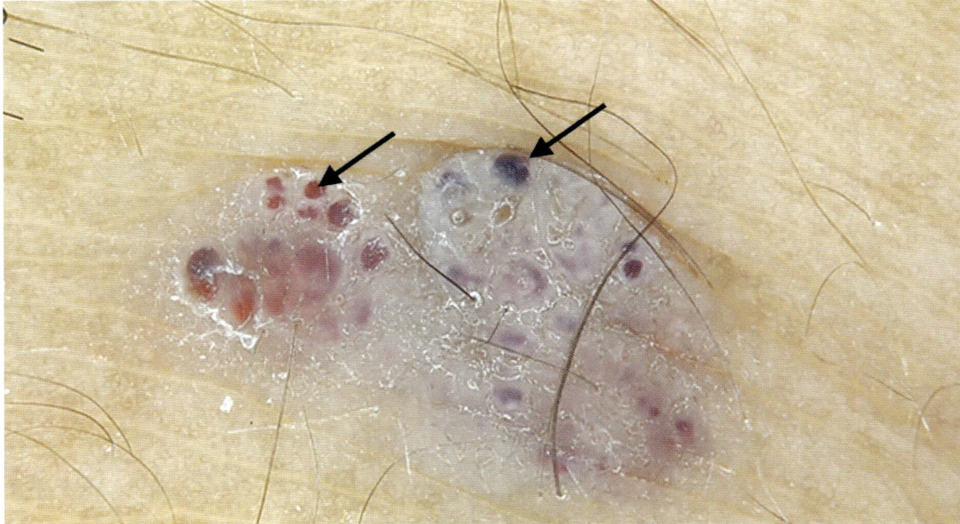

Fig. 11: Well demarcated, round to oval, red to blue lacunae (arrows) with a whitish veil.

DISCUSSION

The presence of red to blue lacunae with a whitish veil is diagnostic of angiokeratomas on dermoscopy. In this case, there was absence of diagnostic dermoscopic features of seborrheic keratosis such as cerebriform appearance, comedo-like openings, and milia-like cysts, etc.[6] Also the diagnostic dermoscopic features of dermatofibroma like pigment network and central white patch were missing.[7] The lacunae in angiokeratomas histologically correspond to dilated vessels which are either partially or completed thrombosed in the dermis. Hyperkeratosis and acanthosis are the histological markers for the whitish veil found on dermoscopy.[8]

In each case, dermoscopy revealed surprising findings underlining the fact that dermatological lesions have heterogeneous and atypical appearances and clinical acumen alone may not be sufficient. In such cases, the simple use of a noninvasive technique like dermoscopy can do wonders to lead to an accurate and informed diagnosis.

REFERENCES

1. Rosendahl C, Cameron A, Argenziano G, et al. Dermoscopy of squamous cell carcinoma and keratoacanthoma. Arch Dermatol. 2012;148(12):1-7.
2. Zalaudek I, Kreusch J, Giacomel J, et al. How to diagnose nonpigmented skin tumors: a review of vascular structures seen with dermoscopy: part I. Melanocytic skin tumors. J Am Acad Dermatol. 2010;63(3):361-74.
3. Argenziano G, Zalaudek I, Corona R, et al. Vascular structures in skin tumors: a dermoscopy study. Arch Dermatol. 2004;140(12):1485-9.
4. Bae JM, Kang H, Kim HO, et al. Differential diagnosis of plantar wart from corn, callus and healed wart with the aid of dermoscopy. Br J Dermatol. 2009;160(1):220-2.
5. Zalaudek I, Kreusch J, Giacomel J, et al. How to diagnose nonpigmented skin tumors: a review of vascular structures seen with dermoscopy: part II. Nonmelanocytic skin tumors. J Am Acad Dermatol. 2010;63(3):377-86.
6. Martin JM, Bella-Navarro R, Jordá E. Vascular patterns in dermoscopy. Actas Dermosifiliogr. 2012;103(5):357-75.
7. Arpaia N, Cassano N, Vena GA. Dermoscopic patterns of dermatofibroma. Dermatol Surg. 2005;31(10):1336-9.
8. Zaballos P, Daufi C, Puig S, et al. Dermoscopy of solitary angiokeratomas: a morphological study. Arch Dermatol. 2007;143(3): 318-25.

CHAPTER 16

Miscellaneous Dermatoses

Subrata Malakar, Samipa S Mukherjee, Priya Diwaker, Surit Malakar

ANETODERMA

INTRODUCTION

Anetoderma is a rarely encountered benign dermatological condition in which the elastic tissue in the dermis is lost, resulting in localized areas of flaccid or herniated saclike skin.[1] Currently, anetoderma is classified as either primary (idiopathic), or secondary anetoderma (which is associated with a variety of skin conditions, penicillamine use, or neonatal prematurity). Lesions appear on the upper arms, trunk, and thighs. This rare disorder occurs mainly in women aged 20–40 years, but is occasionally reported in younger and older patients of both sexes. In the most usual form, crops of round or oval, pink macules 0.5–1 centimeter in diameter develop on trunk, thighs and upper arms, less commonly on the neck and face and rarely elsewhere.[2]

KEY DERMOSCOPIC FEATURES (FIGS. 1A TO D)

- Erythematous background with partially obliterated pigment network
- Affected area has a translucent appearance as compared to the surrounding skin
- Multiple linear vessels.

DISCUSSION

The translucent nature of the skin noted on dermoscopy results from the loss of elastin tissue that is seen on histology in these lesions. The vasculature becomes visible due to thinning of the skin resulting from degradation of elastin. The background erythema results from the underlying inflammation. It may be postulated that the mild inflammation may interfere with the melanocytes in the basal layer leading to partial obliteration of the pigment network.

KEYNOTE

Dermoscopy may provide an important clinical clue toward the diagnosis of this rare entity by highlighting the translucent nature of the skin pointing toward the diagnosis.

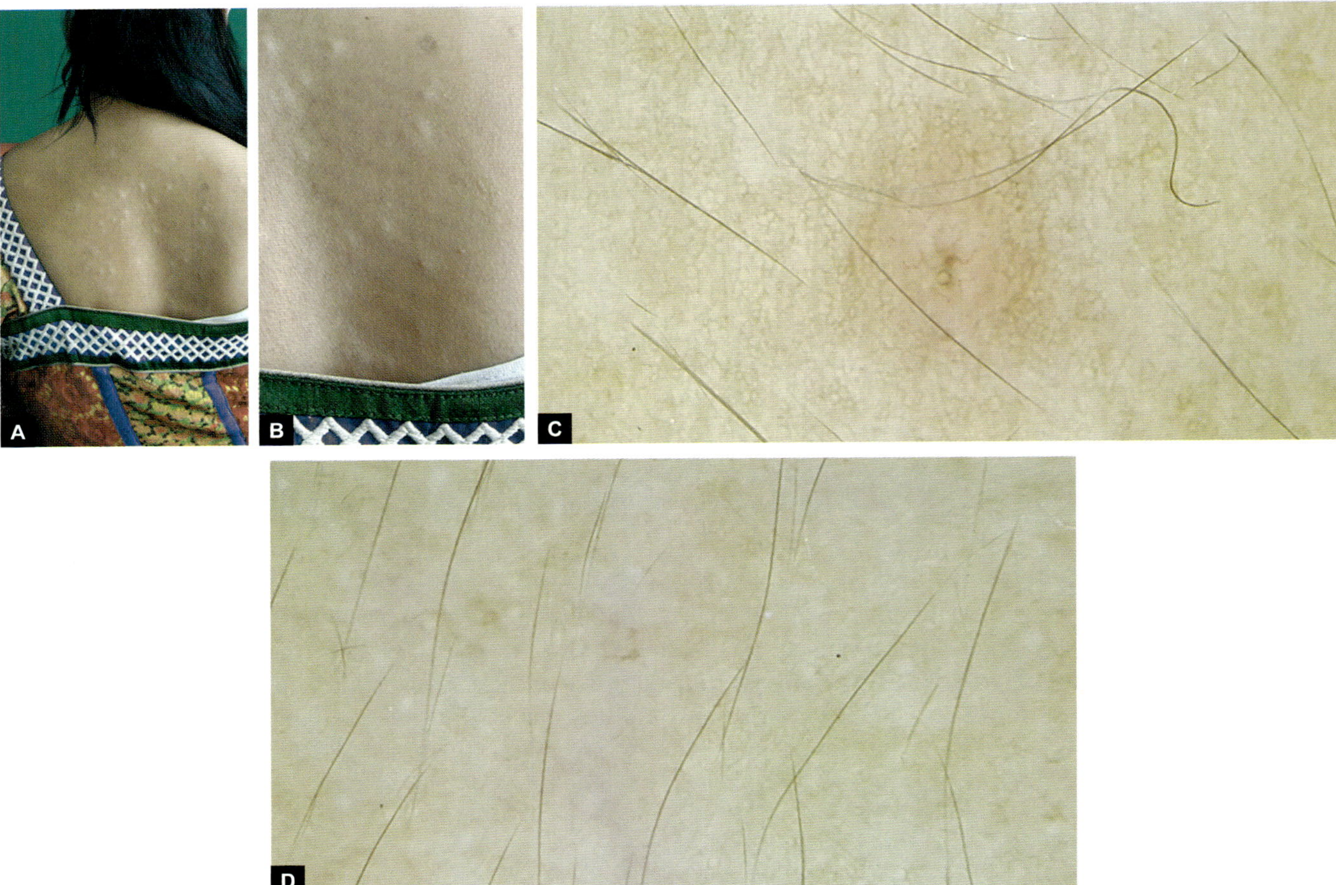

Figs. 1A to D: (A and B) A 32-year-old lady presented with slowly progressing asymptomatic lesions over the back since 1 year; (C) Dermoscopy shows a background of erythematous hue with partially obliterated pigment network. The skin of the affected area has a translucent appearance as compared to the surrounding skin; and (D) Multiple lesions are noted showing erythematous background with multiple linear vessels and translucent appearance of the skin. The vasculature becomes visible due to thinning of the skin resulting from degradation of elastin.

REFERENCES

1. Venencie PY, Winkelmann RK. Histopathologic findings in anetoderma. Arch Dermatol. 1984;120:1040-4.
2. Venencie PY, Winkelmann RK, Moore BA. Anetoderma: clinical findings, associations, and long term follow-up evaluations. Arch Dermatol. 1984;120:1032-9.

PROGRESSIVE CRIBRIFORM AND ZOSTERIFORM HYPERPIGMENTATION

INTRODUCTION

Progressive cribriform and zosteriform hyperpigmentation (PCZH) is a distinctive clinicopathological pigmentary disorder of the skin.[1] PCZH refers to an asymptomatic dermatosis consisting of a single area of uniformly tan, cribriform, macular pigmentation in a zosteriform distribution; histological pattern consisting of mild increase in melanin pigment in basal cell layer and complete absence of nevus cells.

KEY DERMOSCOPIC FEATURES (FIGS. 2 TO 6)

- Overview of the dermoscopic image reveals small islands of accentuated pigment.
- Dermoscopy of the hyperpigmented areas revealed accentuation of melanin network, areas with grayish homogeneous hyperpigmentation and brown dots and globules.
- Hyperpigmented lesions may show finger print-like structures.
- Rosettes were noted occasionally.

DISCUSSION

The accentuation of the melanin network on dermoscopy correlates histopathologically to hypermelanization of rete ridges.[2] Grayish homogeneous pigmented areas correlate with areas of pigment incontinence. Pigment incontinence has also been reported. The occurrence of rosettes could be attributed to the actinic area of distribution of lesions. This can be differentiated from lichen planus pigmentosus where the melanin network remains uncharacterized and pigmentary pattern is characterized by the presence of brown dots and globules with either diffuse or mixed pattern of pigmentation.

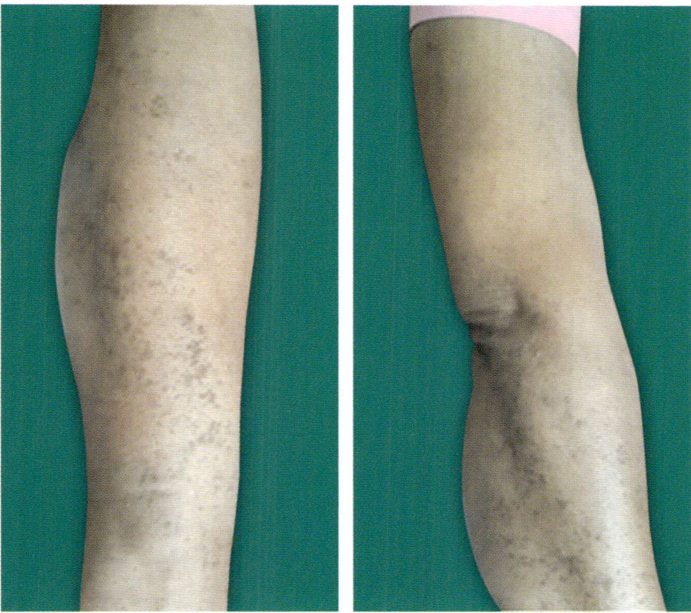

Fig. 2: An otherwise healthy 30-year-old lady presented to the dermatology outpatient department with a 4-year history of asymptomatic dark patches confined to the right side of her arm. Brownish macules with a cribriform configuration extended linearly from the lower part of right upper arm to the forearm area on the dorsal and ventral side.

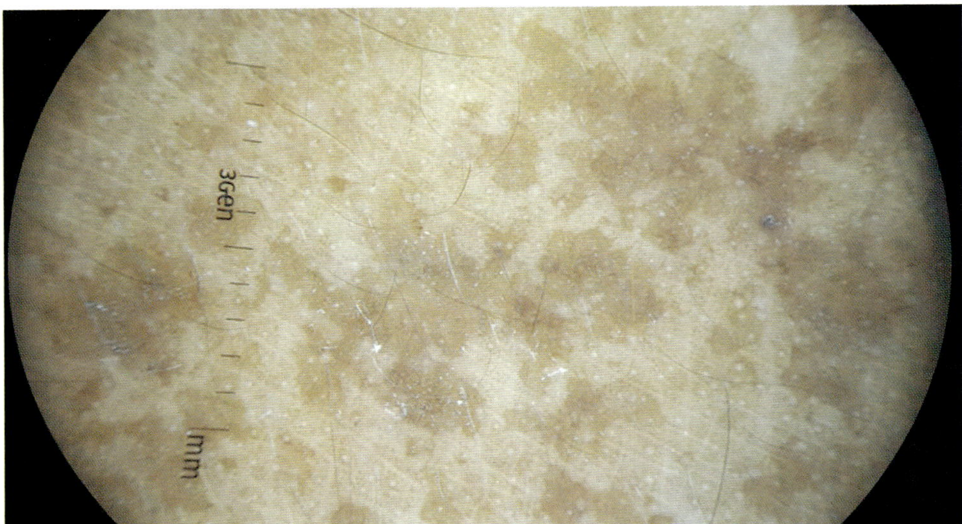

Fig. 3: Overview of the dermoscopic image reveals small islands of accentuated pigment.

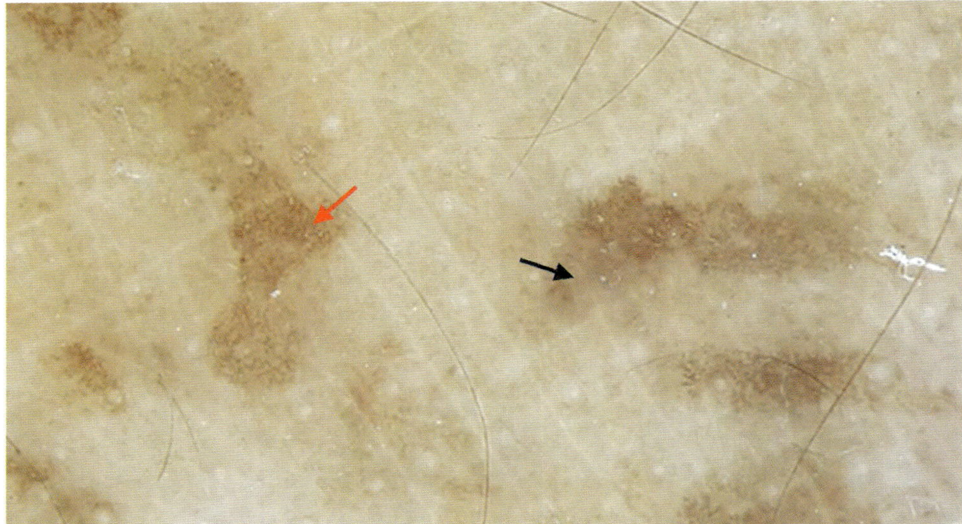

Fig. 4: Dermoscopy of the hyperpigmented areas revealed accentuation of melanin network (red arrow) and areas with greyish homogeneous hyperpigmentation (black arrow).

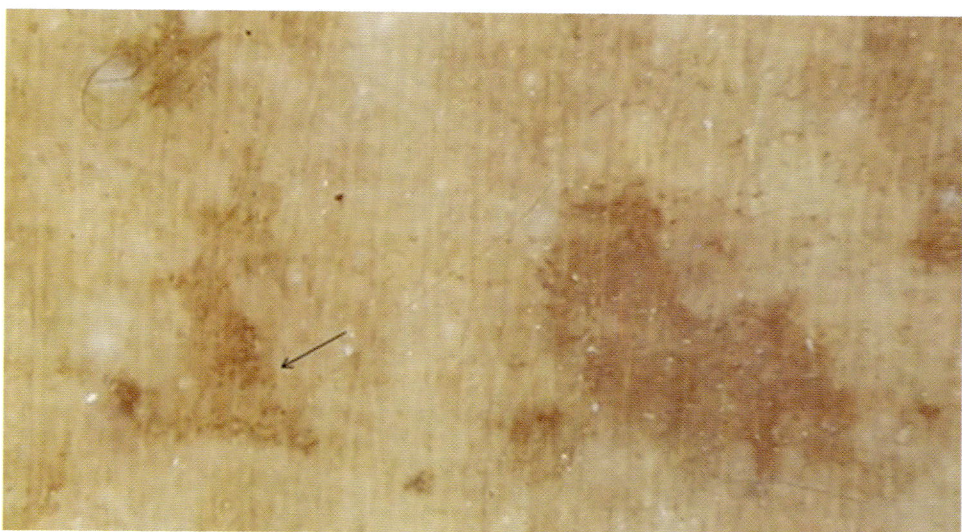

Fig. 5: Hyperpigmented areas showing brown dots and globules (arrow).

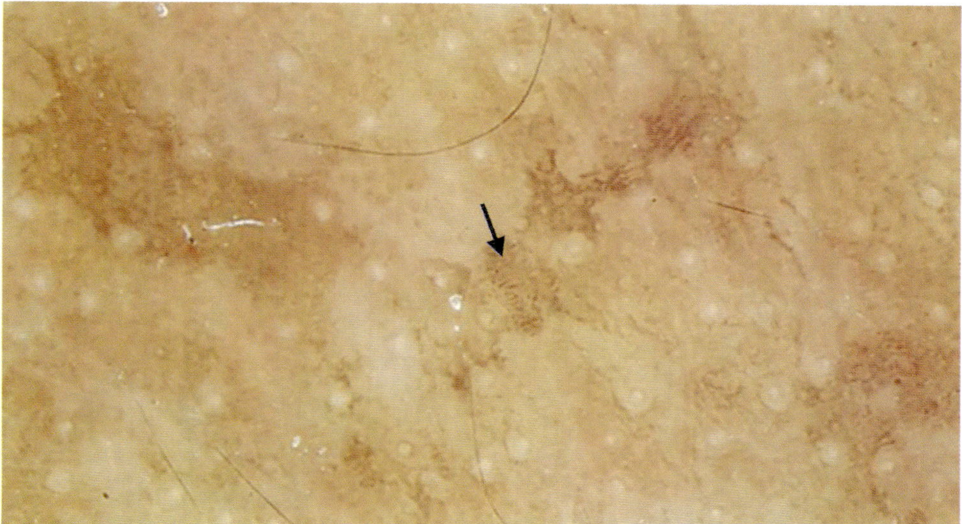

Fig. 6: Hyperpigmented lesions may show fingerprint-like structures (arrow).

KEYNOTE

A constellation of accentuation of melanin network, areas with grayish homogeneous hyperpigmentation, fingerprint-like structures along with clustered brown dots and globules could provide a clue toward this entity.

REFERENCES

1. Rower JM, Carr RD, Lowney ED. Progressive cribriform and zosteriform hyperpigmentation. Arch Dermatol. 1978;114:98-9.
2. Das A, Bandyopadhyay D, Mishra V, et al. Progressive cribriform and zosteriform hyperpigmentation. Indian J Dermatol Venereol Leprol. 2015;81:321-3.

ERYTHEMA MULTIFORME

INTRODUCTION

Erythema multiforme (EM) is an acute, self-limiting, inflammatory skin eruption that is usually triggered by drugs or infection. It presents with erythematous rashes on the skin having a typical target lesion. There may be involvement of the mucous membrane. This entity has now been separated from Stevens Johnson syndrome. The early stages of the target lesion may not be visible to the naked eye and dermoscopy helps as a rapid screening tool in this scenario.

KEY DERMOSCOPIC FEATURES (FIGS. 7 AND 8)[1]

- Central dusky zone shows clods of different colors such as red, blue, black, and purple.
- A plain featureless area correlating with the pale edematous zone.
- Homogeneous erythema represents the outer red ring.
- Few linear short vessels may be present.

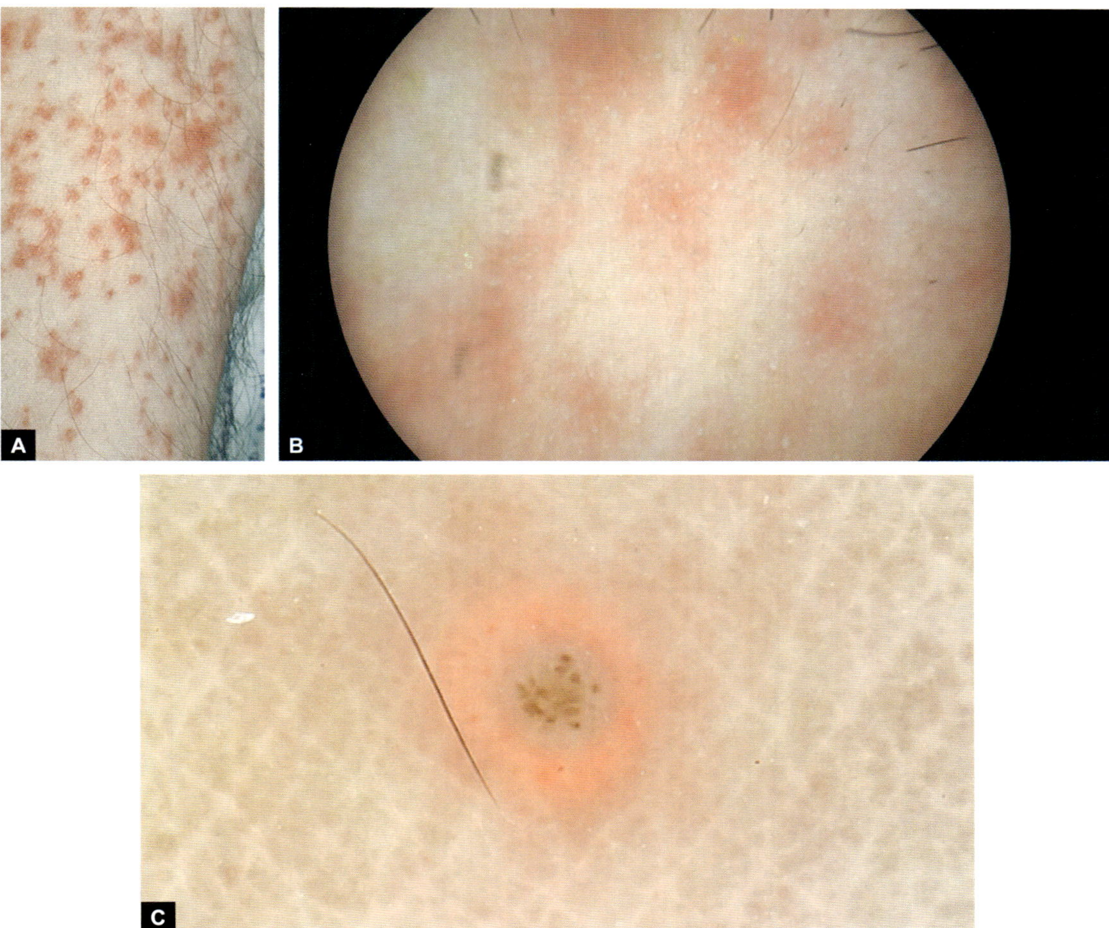

Figs. 7A to C: (A) The patient presented with classical erythema multiforme lesion showing target lesions and a few of them had central vesicles; (B) Dermoscopic overview shows patchy erythematous areas; and (C) Close-up view of the erythema reveals a central zone of variable color surrounded by a pale structureless zone followed by a zone of homogeneous erythema. On close inspection few vascular structures like linear and dotted vessels are seen.

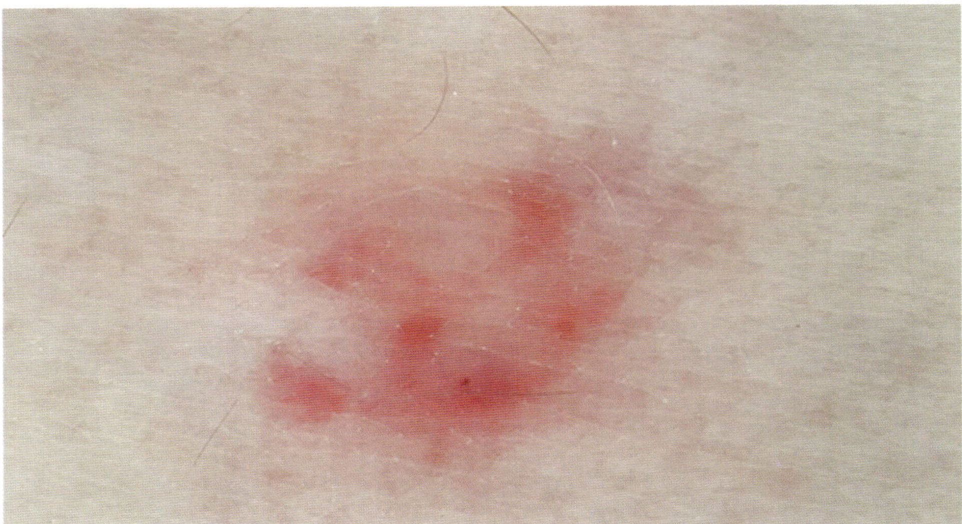

Fig. 8: Dermoscopy of another lesion with central vesiculation reveals a central colorless zone surrounded by patchy erythema.

KEYNOTE

It helps to differentiate EM from other purpuric conditions like leukocytoclastic vasculitis, etc.

REFERENCE

1. Kaliyadan F. Dermoscopy of erythema multiforme. Indian Dermatol Online J. 2017;8:75.

FORDYCE'S SPOTS

INTRODUCTION

They are small slightly elevated yellowish-white papules that can appear on the vermillion border of the lips or the inside of the cheeks. They can also be seen on the glans, shaft of penis or on the vulva in females. Fordyce's spots are visible sebaceous glands without hair follicle. Sometimes it can cause anxiety, where some people relate it to vitiligo.

Dermoscopy can be very convincing to assure the patient (Figs. 9 and 10).

KEY DERMOSCOPIC FEATURE

Closely set white granular structures resembling ice granules or sugar granules in a pot.

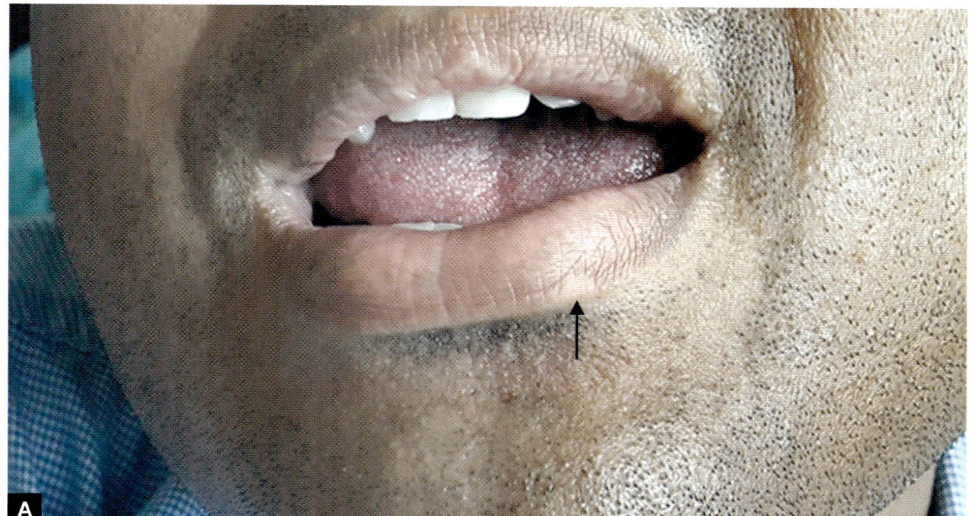

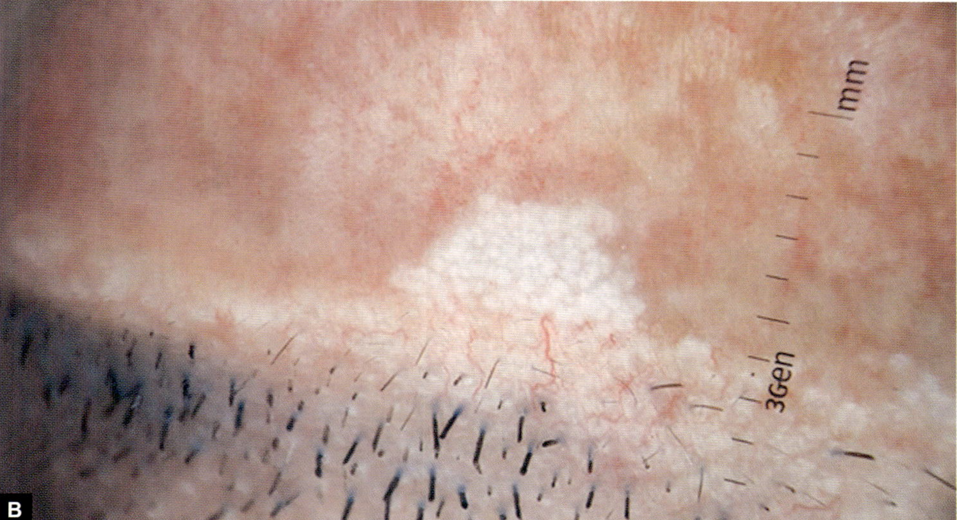

Figs. 9A and B: (A) A young male was apprehensive due to this (arrow) tiny hypopigmented patch on lower lip, which was being treated previously as vitiligo; and (B) On dermoscopy, closely set white granular structures were seen.

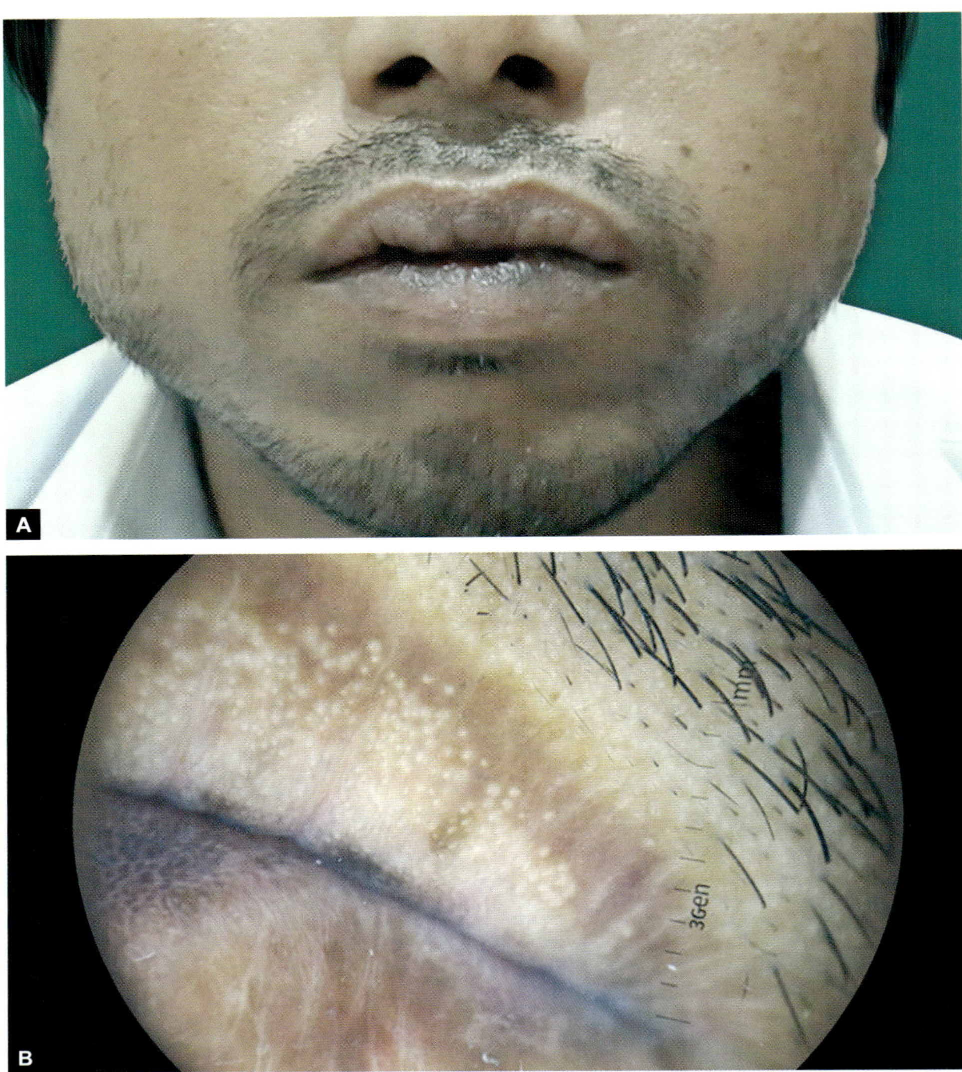

Figs. 10A and B: (A) Another patient presented with asymptomatic hypopigmented minute granular lesion over the upper lip; and (B) Dermoscopy reveals closely set white granular structures resembling ice granules or sugar granules in a pot.

FOREIGN BODY

INTRODUCTION

Reports state that up to 38% of soft tissue foreign bodies (STFBs) are neglected in initial clinical examinations in emergency departments, and 25% of all STFBs are presented weeks, months, and even years after a penetrating injury.[1,2] Only magnification can reassure that a disturbing skin lesion is free of a foreign substance, which can lead to a delay in the healing process.

KEY DERMOSCOPIC FEATURE

Suture knot often missed during naked eye examination is readily highlighted during routine dermoscopic screening (Figs. 11A and B).

KEY NOTE

Dermoscopy helps in unveiling the mystery of a hidden foreign body which maybe deceptive to the naked eye. Authors suggest routine dermoscopic examination of all the nodules where other investigations are negative before doing a biopsy.

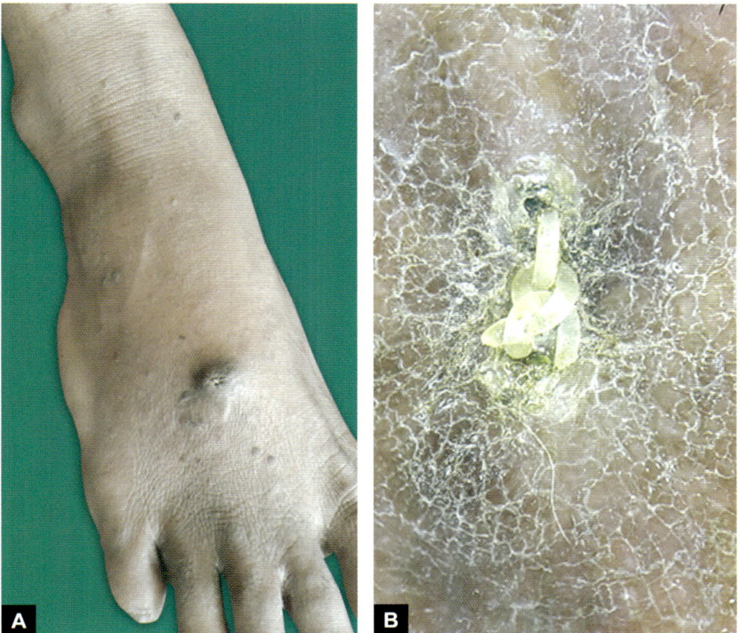

Figs. 11A and B: (A) Asymptomatic solitary hyperpigmented nodule over dorsum of foot since one and half years. Relevant investigations were negative. Not responding to conventional medications; and (B) Dermatoscopy showing suture knot in situ in the center of the nodule. Further history revealed an episode of incision and drainage followed by suturing which was forgotten by the patient.

REFERENCES

1. Anderson MA, Newmeyer WL 3rd, Kilgore ES Jr. Diagnosis and treatment of retained foreign bodies in the hand. Am J Surg. 1982;144:63-7.
2. Steele MT, Tran LV, Watson WA, et al. Retained glass foreign bodies in wounds: predictive value of wound characteristics, patient perception, and wound exploration. Am J Emerg Med. 1998;16:627-30.

TATTOO INK-INDUCED LICHENOID REACTION

INTRODUCTION

Cutaneous reactions to tattoos have been increasing in conjunction with the rise in popularity of tattoos. Complications of tattoos can have an impact on the quality of life. Cutaneous complications may be immediate or delayed. Examples of delayed reactions include allergic contact dermatitis, granulomatous dermatitis, lichenoid dermatitis, and pseudolymphomatous reactions.[1,2]

KEY DERMOSCOPIC FEATURES (FIGS. 12A TO D)

- Dermoscopy highlights the color of the tattoo
- Rosettes
- Plentiful white shiny structures.

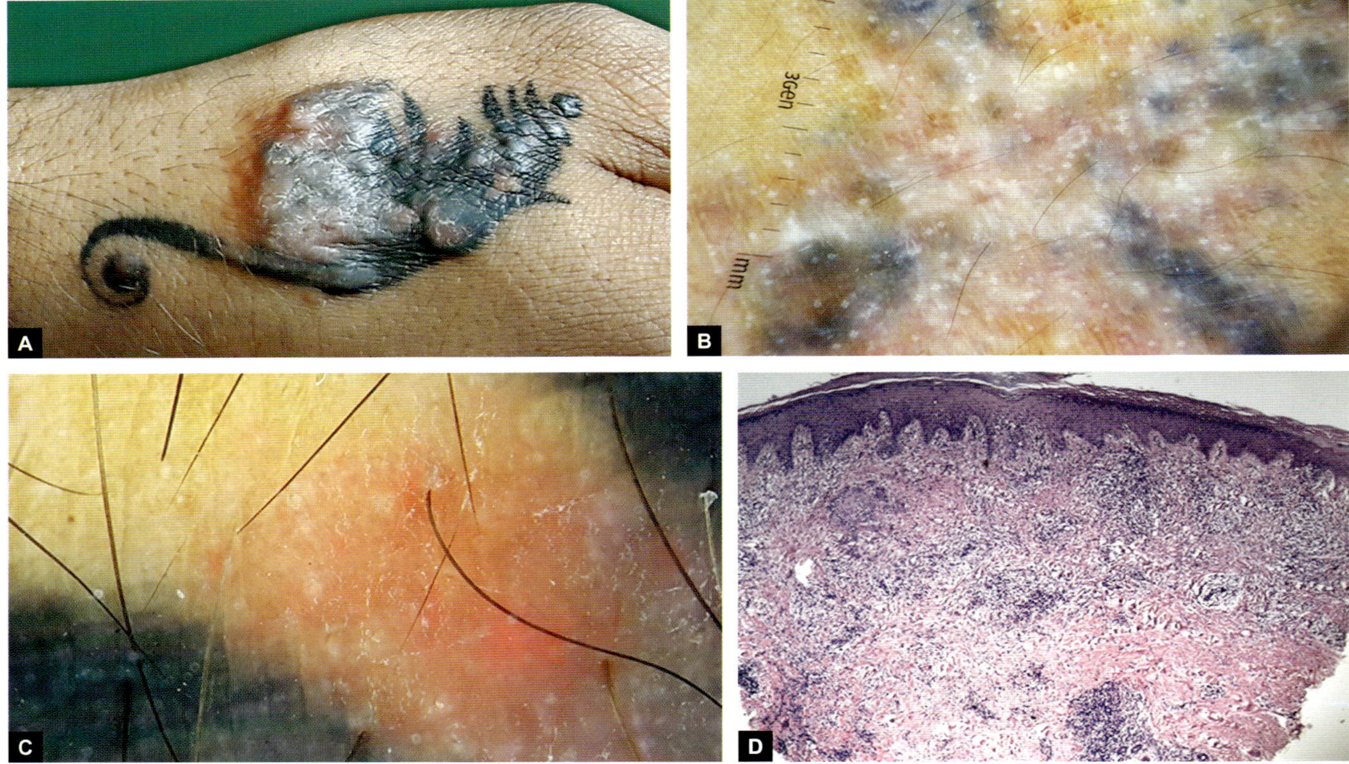

Figs. 12A to D: (A) A tattoo on the wrist of a male patient showing two colors- blue-black and red. The picture highlights the granulomatous reaction to red pigment (mercury). Granulomatous reaction can be seen after green and blue pigment as well but most common offending agent is red pigment; (B) Dermoscopy highlights the color of the tattoo and the field is studded with rosettes and plentiful white shiny structures; (C) This field reveals yellow orange background representing the granulomatous reaction with eccentric location of the tattoo pigment; and (D) Biopsy shows moderately dense superficial and perivascular lymphocytic infiltrate in lichenoid pattern. Note abundant granular pigment in upper and mid dermis in association with the lichenoid infiltrate.

REFERENCES

1. Mataix J, Silvestre JF. Cutaneous adverse reactions to tattoos and piercings. Actas Dermosifiliogr. 2009;100:643-56.
2. Jacob CI. Tattoo-associated dermatoses: a case report and review of the literature. Dermatol Surg. 2002;28:962-5.

JUVENILE XANTHOGRANULOMA

INTRODUCTION

Juvenile xanthogranuloma (JXG) is one of the common pediatric tumors and usually present as erythematous papules or nodules which undergo morphologic evolution to bright yellow-orange nodules; upon resolution it further evolves to form atrophic brown macules or patches.[1,2] Typically they present with one to multiple lesions on flexural areas or the scalp, but can be found anywhere on the body.

Classically there is dense dermal infiltration of vacuolated cells, along with Touton cells, and lymphocytes and eosinophils in varying proportion.[3] The quality of infiltrate varies with the clinical evolution of the lesion.

The term juvenile xanthogranuloma is a misnomer, simply xanthogranuloma is preferable.[3]

KEY DERMOSCOPIC FEATURES (FIGS. 13A TO C)[4,5]

- "Setting sun" appearance
- Clouds of pale yellow globules
- In darker skin, "setting sun" appearance is rarely visible, rather clouds of pale yellow globules is the main dermoscopic feature (personal observation)
- Whitish streak
- Linear and/or branched vessels.

DISCUSSION

Song et al. suggested a schematic overview of changing clinical presentation of JXG, along with corresponding dermoscopic patterns and histopathological maturation.

In the early evolutionary and fully developed stages of JXG, the setting sun appearance is the dermoscopic hallmark. The surrounding erythema decreases in the late regressive phase, thus setting sun become less apparent or absent. As the vacuolated cells of the early stage evolute to xanthomatized cells, yellow globular clouds manifest more. These yellow globular clouds are the consistent features of fully developed and late stages.

Whitish streaks become visible in the late regressive phase, which shows infiltration of spindle-shaped cells in variable amounts on histology.

In all the stages of JXG, linear, and branched vessels are observed in high percentage of cases. However the vessels and setting sun appearance is rarely visible in the darker skin probably due to the masking of the vessels and erythema by prominent melanocytic network and more melanin.

KEYNOTES

A thorough clinical examination along with a careful dermoscopy of the lesion avoids skin biopsy in JXG of the pediatric age group. Furthermore, follow-up dermoscopy allows a lot for the dermatologists who want to learn practical clues for the natural course of JXG.

Dermoscopy in darker skin rarely show the setting sun appearance, rather clouds of pale yellow color are the most common dermoscopic feature in them.

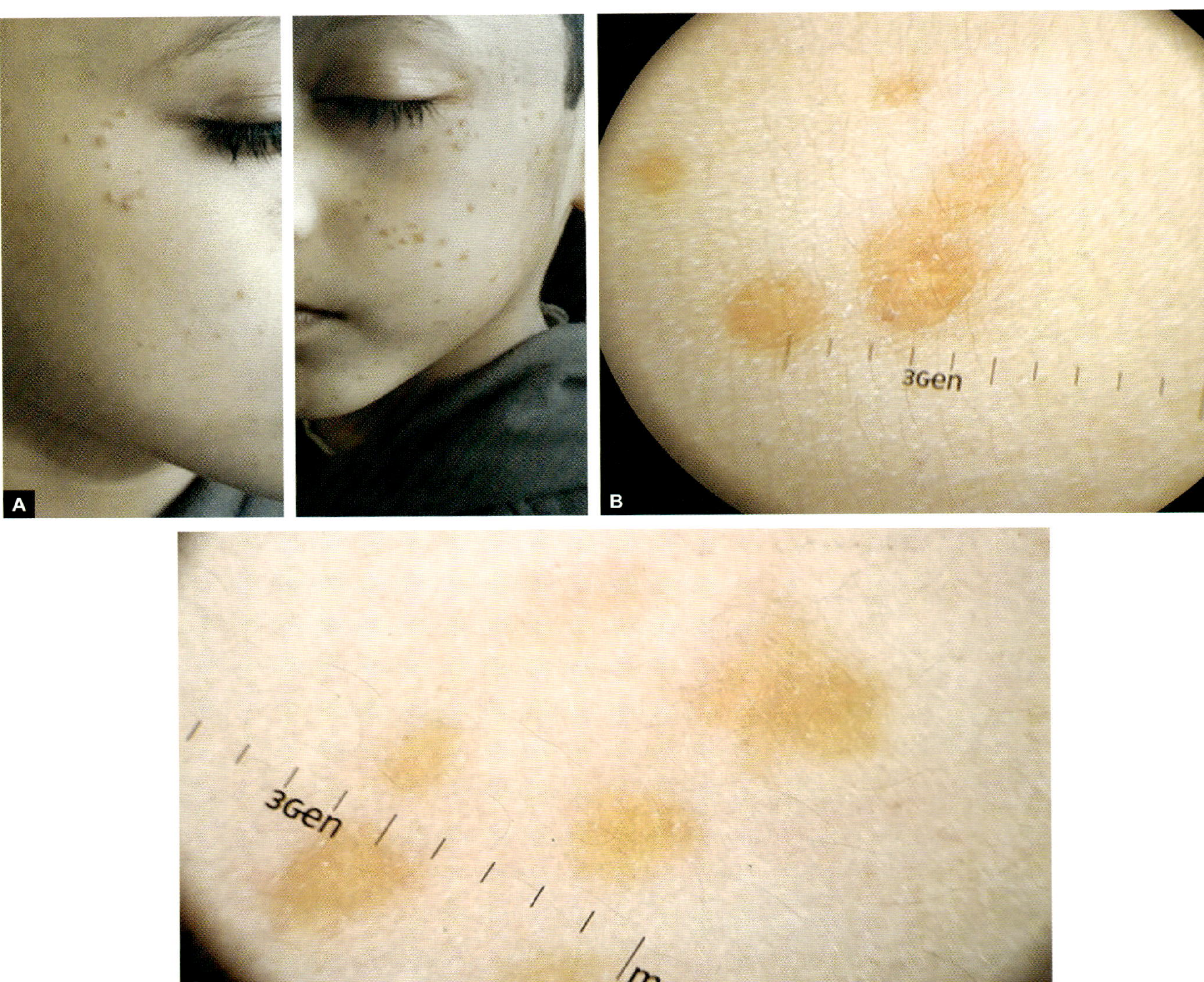

Figs. 13A to C: (A) A 6-year-old boy presented with asymptomatic yellow brown papules over the face of 8 months duration; (B) Clouds of pale yellow globules. In darker skin, "setting sun" appearance is rarely visible, rather clouds of pale yellow globules is the main dermoscopic feature (personal observation); and (C) Close-up view of the previous lesion shows yellow orange clouds.

REFERENCES

1. Hernandez-Martin A, Baselga E, Drolet BA, et al. Juvenile xanthogranuloma. J Am Acad Dermatol. 1997;36:355-67.
2. Janssen D, Harms D. Juvenile xanthogranuloma in childhood and adolescence: a clinicopathologic study of 129 patients from the kiel pediatric tumor registry. Am J Surg Pathol. 2005;29:21-8.
3. Burgdorf WHC, Gerami P, Yan A C. Benign and malignant tumors. In: Schachner L, Hansen RC (Eds). Pediatric Dermatology. Philadelphia: Elsevier; 2011. p. 1215.
4. Palmer A, Bowling J. Dermoscopic appearance of juvenile xanthogranuloma. Dermatology. 2007;215:256-9.
5. Rubegni P, Mandato F, Fimiani M. Juvenile xanthogranuloma: dermoscopic pattern. Dermatology. 2009;218:380.

LUPUS MILIARIS DISSEMINATUS FACIEI

INTRODUCTION

Lupus miliaris disseminatus faciei (LMDF) is a rare inflammatory and granulomatous disease of unknown etiology.[1] The patient presents with yellow to yellow brown papules on the face, classically on the eyelids. Considerable controversies exist with regards to the etiopathogenesis of this entity. Recently, it has been hypothesized to be a reaction to destroyed hair follicles.[2]

KEY DERMOSCOPIC FEATURES (FIGS. 14A TO C)

- Orange yellow background/erythematous background
- Follicular plugs
- Linear telangiectatic vessels/hairpin vessels

DISCUSSION

Keratotic plugs develop as a result of lateral pressure on the hair follicles.[3] Vascular pattern shows either hairpin or linear telangiectatic vessels or both. Vessels usually surround the follicular plugs. The granulomatous nature of the disease is suggested by the yellow orange background on dermoscopy.

KEYNOTE

Though dermoscopy gives a clue toward the diagnosis of granulomatous disease, it does not help to differentiate between the various granulomatous disorders, thereby mandating the need for biopsy in establishing the diagnosis of this entity.

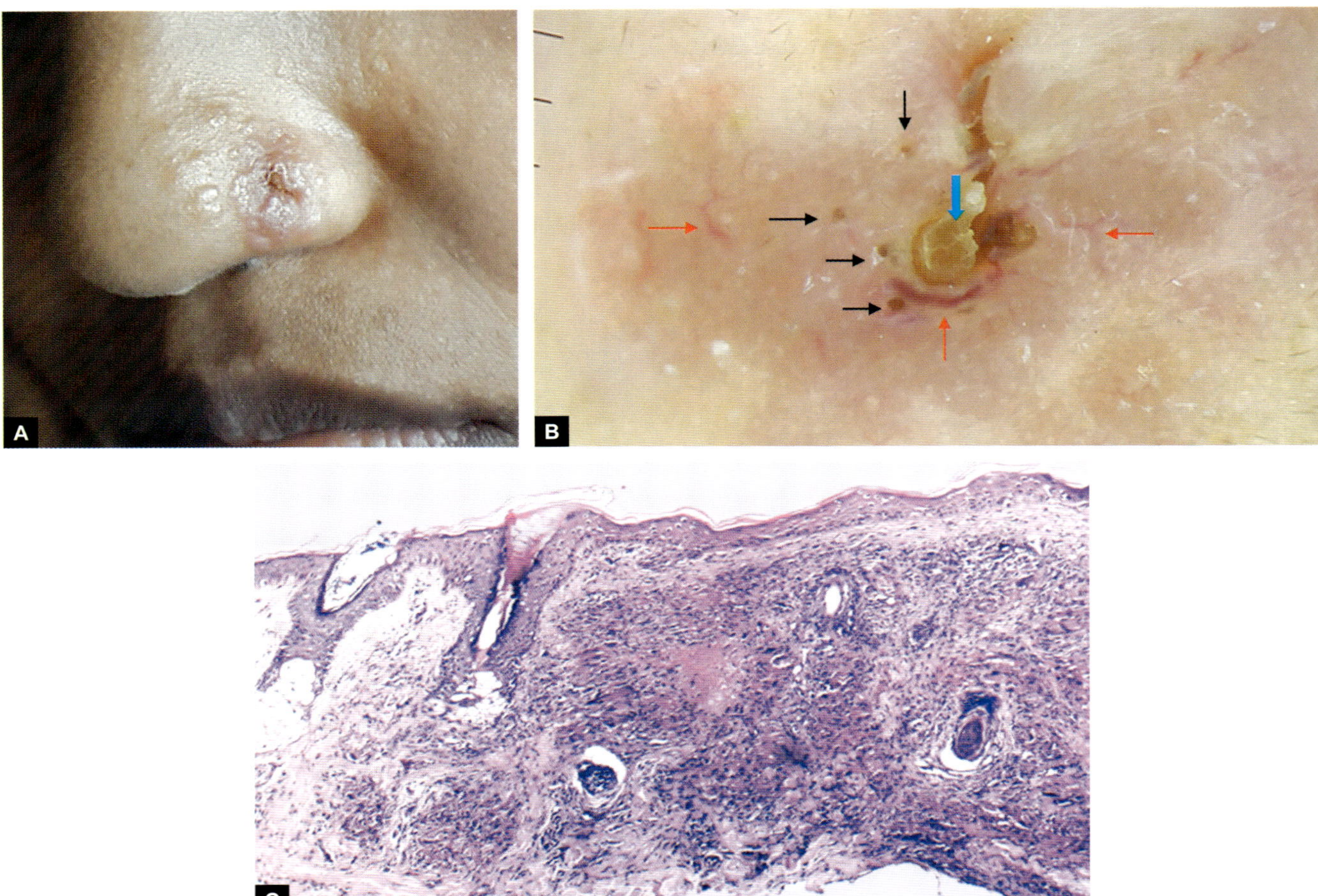

Figs. 14A to C: (A) An 18-year-old female patient presented with asymptomatic yellow brown-brown papules over the left nasal ala around the orifice for nose pin, of 1 year duration. The clinical differential diagnosis includes sarcoidosis, lupus vulgaris, sebaceous hyperplasia, cutaneous leishmaniasis, etc.; (B) Dermoscopy of the lesions show yellowish orange background denoting a granulomatous disorder. Other features in the field include vascular and nonvascular components like linear vessels, telangiectatic vessels (red arrows) and keratotic plugs (black arrows). Not a central large keratotic plug (blue arrow) surrounded by a prominent linear vessel; and (C) Biopsy shows single large focus of tuberculoid granuloma involving mid and deep reticular dermis. The granuloma consists of lymphocytes, epithelioid cells, Langhan's and foreign body giant cells and plasma cells. The center of the granuloma shows a large focus of fibrinoid necrosis. The periphery shows abundant fibroplasia. The rest of the dermis shows moderately dense perivascular and periappendiceal inflammatory infiltrate. Diagnosis: Lupus miliaris disseminatus faciei.

REFERENCES

1. Fox T. Disseminated follicular lupus (similating acne). Lancet. 1878;112:75-6.
2. Ayhan E, Alabalik U, Avci Y. Dermoscopic evaluation of two patients with lupus miliaris disseminatus faciei. Clin Exp Dermatol. 2014;39:500-2.
3. Llambrich A, Zaballos P, Terasa F, et al. Dermoscopy of cutaneous leishmaniasis. Br J Dermatol. 2009;60:756-61.

MILIA[1]

INTRODUCTION

Vascular structures in dermoscopy have an important role to play in the categorization of lesions as benign or malignant. Some of the more characteristic findings like crown vessel, comma vessels can help in narrowing down the diagnosis further. Although there has been significant work in dermoscopy for pigmentary disorders, there is a paucity in literature with regards to vascular patterns in common dermatological conditions. Milia[1] although easy to diagnose most of the times, can mimic sebaceous hyperplasia, molluscum contagiosum and at times basal cell carcinoma. Dermoscopy forms an easy aid to rule out the other differentials in case of diagnostic dilemma.

KEY DERMOSCOPIC FEATURES (FIGS. 15 TO 17)

- Yellow white structureless areas
- Arborizing vessels originating at the periphery and crossing the entire length of the lesion.

DISCUSSION

Superficial vessels are not seen in dermatoscopy of a normal facial skin, however, when present, one must think of inflammatory conditions, basal cell carcinoma or topical steroid induced skin atrophy. The vessels in the papillary dermis are visible as dots due to their orientation in a vertical direction and proliferation may be seen in conditions like psoriasis. The subpapillary plexus vessels are oriented horizontally and become visible in inflammatory conditions or when the skin is stretched. In milia there is stretching of the overlying skin leading to apparent upliftment of the subcapillary plexus thereby making these vessels visible of which the pattern has been described.

A milia can be differentiated from a molluscum contagiosum by the absence of crown vessels, mixed flower pattern of vessels and absence of the central orifice. The dermoscopy of sebaceous hyperplasia has been described as a combination of yellowish nodules with crown vessels that are not arborizing.

KEYNOTE

In-focus arborizing vessels are not the monopoly of basal cell carcinoma. It may also be seen in milia and adnexal tumors. Careful search for yellowish-white structureless areas, negative features of basal cell carcinoma and clinical correlation clinches the diagnosis of milia.

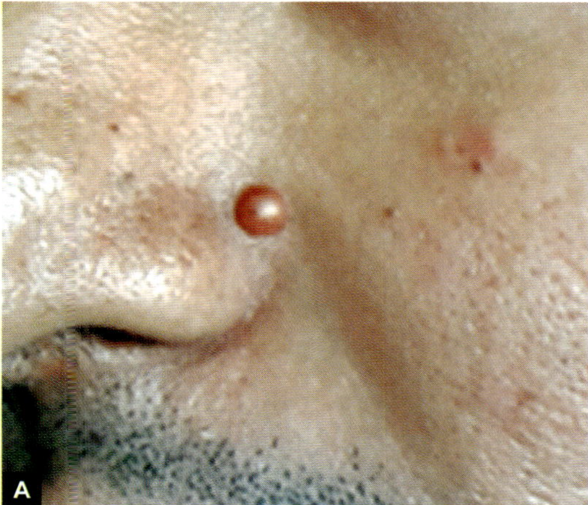

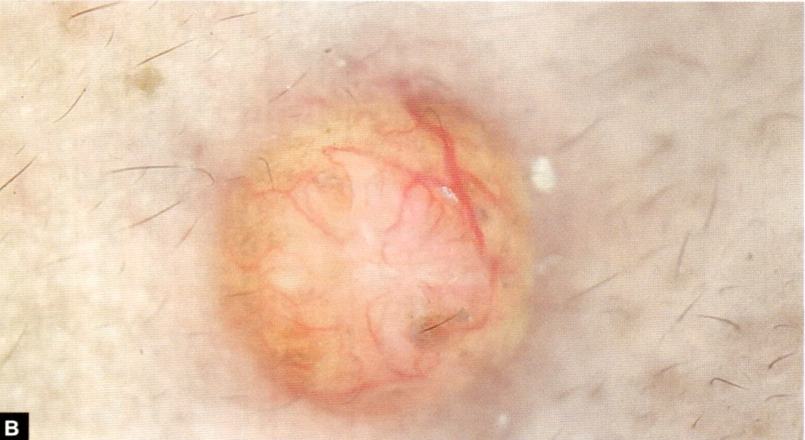

Figs. 15A and B: (A) This papulonodule may have several differential diagnosis ranging from sebaceous hyperplasia, milia to the more sinister basal cell carcinoma. To rule out the possibilities histopathology serves as a gold standard; and (B) Dermoscopy of the previous patient shows in focus arborizing vessels at the background of yellow orange areas. Basal cell carcinoma (BCC) was ruled out due to the absence of additional dermoscopic features such as maple leaf pattern, blue ovoid nests, white shiny structures, etc.

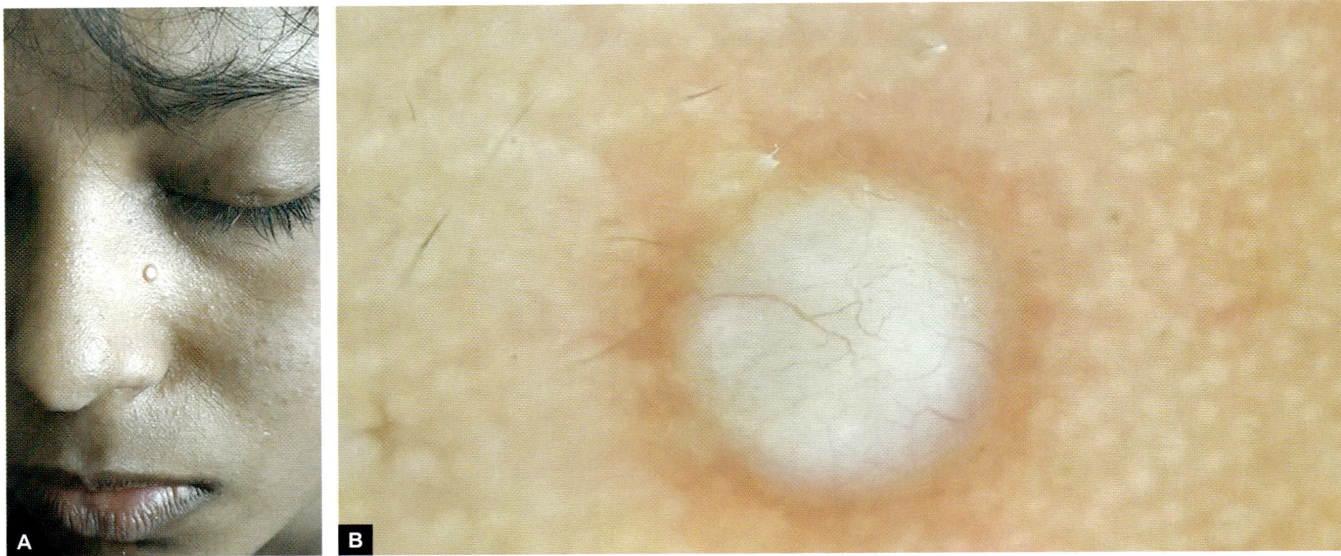

Figs. 16A and B: (A) This patient presented with an asymptomatic lesion over the left side of the nose; and (B) Dermoscopy of the lesion shows yellow white structureless areas with arborizing vessels crossing the midline of the lesion. Kindly note that the usual report of arborizing vessels is mostly associated with basal cell carcinoma.

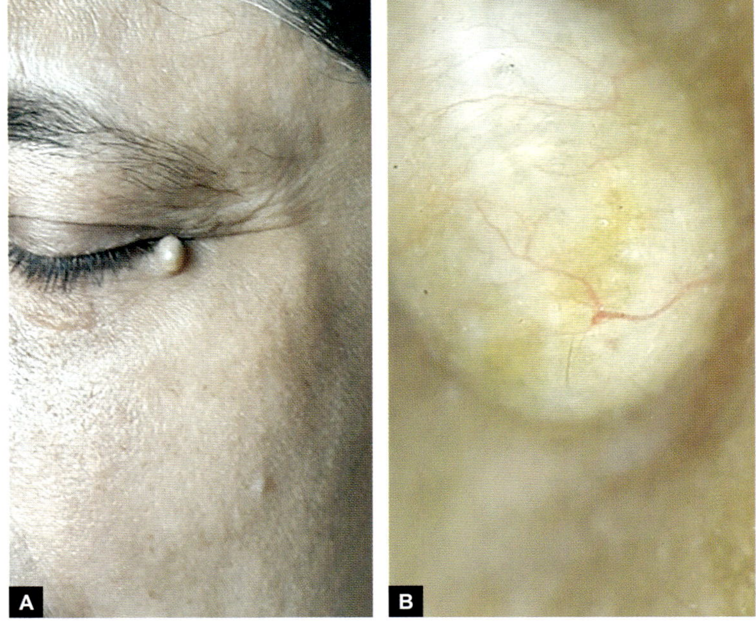

Figs. 17A and B: (A) Yellowish hued to skin colored papulonodule over the outer corner of the left eye in a middle-aged man; and (B) Dermoscopy shows yellow white structureless areas and arborizing vessels arising from the periphery of the lesion and traversing the length.

REFERENCE

1. Malakar S, Mukherjee SS. Vascular pattern of milia on dermatoscopy. Our Dermatol Online. 2017;8:497-8.

NOTALGIA PARESTHETICA

INTRODUCTION

Notalgia paresthetica (NP) is defined as an isolated mononeuropathy usually associated with paresthesia or nagging localized itch or "itch-like" sensation that involves the skin over the scapula or subscapular paravertebral region.

There is sensory nerve entrapment involving the posterior rami of the T2 to T6 nerve root which may be associated with vertebrae degeneration. Due to paresthesia it leads to chronic pruritus and friction of the affected area resulting in a circumscribed hyperpigmented patch that resembles macular amyloidosis clinically.[1] NP is unilateral in most of the cases, only rarely it is found to be bilateral which helps in differentiating it from macular amyloidosis.

On histology, basal hyperpigmentation and pigmentary incontinence are found. In some cases, dermal amyloidosis is described. This may be the result of prolonged irritation and friction followed by degeneration of keratinocytes which ultimately lead to production of amyloid from degraded keratin.

KEY DERMOSCOPIC FEATURES (FIGS. 18 AND 19)

- Alternate hypo- and hyperpigmented patches are present throughout the entire lesion.
- Hyperpigmented patches show different patterns of pigmentation of brown or slate gray color. The pigment pattern may take the formation of irregular nets, may have central hypo- or hyperpigmented hub surrounded by pigment configurations of different shapes and patterns.
- Hypopigmented patches may be devoid of any characteristics, but have shiny white streaks in few of them.

DISCUSSION

Shiny white streaks correspond to the amyloid fibrils which may be deposited in NP.[2] The amyloid fibrils are deposited extracellularly and are characterized by abnormally polymerized, cytokeratin-derived material. Arnold and Bowling recently reported that the amyloid materials are birefringent and when visualized by polarized dermoscopy appear as shiny white streaks.[3] Pigmentation of various patterns can be correlated with the basal pigmentation and scattered melanophages/pigmentary incontinence.

KEYNOTE

Notalgia paresthetica resembles macular amyloidosis clinically and also dermoscopically, however its unilateral distribution more commonly on the back provides an important clue to diagnosis. Shiny streaks have not been described in macular amyloidosis. In lichen amyloidosis shiny white structures are abundant.

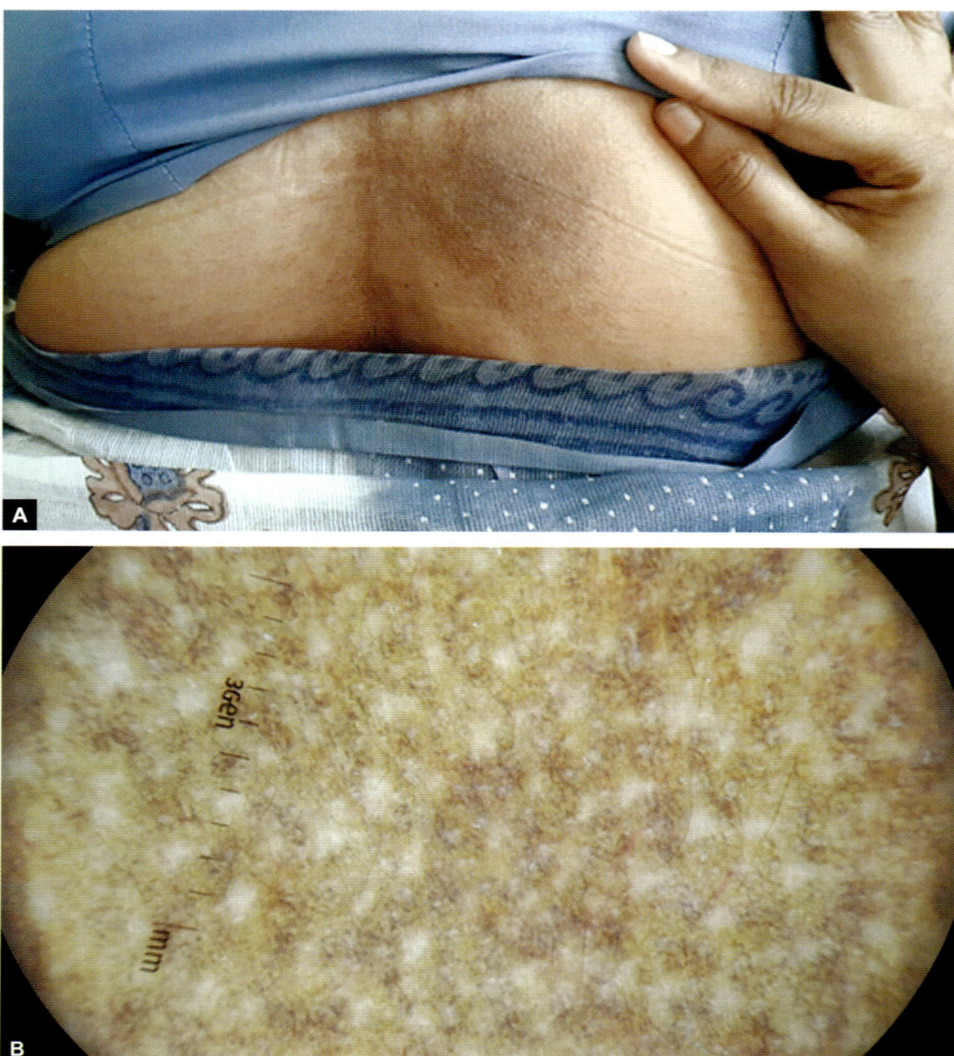

Figs. 18A and B: (A) A case of notalgia paresthetica (NP) in an elderly lady. NP usually presents unilaterally, which clinically mimics macular amyloidosis (MA). The main difference from MA is its unilateral presentation and some unusual associated symptoms like itching, burning and unusual sensations. The most accepted hypothesis is compression of the nerves at the vertebral spinous openings; (B) Dermoscopic overview of the lesion shows alternate hypo- and hyperpigmented patches throughout the lesion.

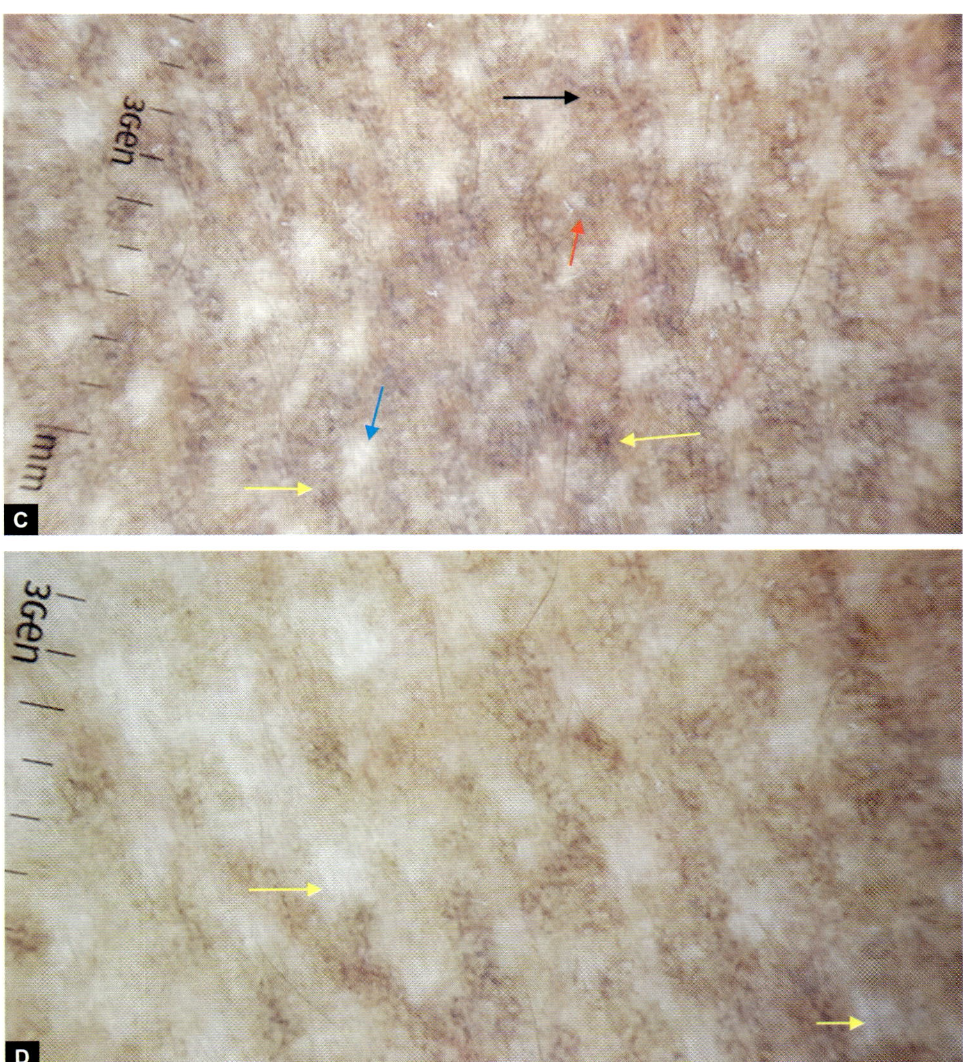

Figs. 8C and D: (C) Hyperpigmented patches show different patterns of pigmentation of brown or slate gray color. The pigment pattern may take the formation of irregular nets (black arrow), may have central hypo- (red arrow) or hyperpigmented hub (yellow arrows) surrounded by pigment configurations of different shapes and patterns. Shiny white streaks (blue arrow) are also seen; and (D) Another field showing shiny white streaks (yellow arrows). Pigmentation of various patterns revealed by dermoscopy corresponds to the basal pigmentation and scattered melanophages or pigmentary incontinence.

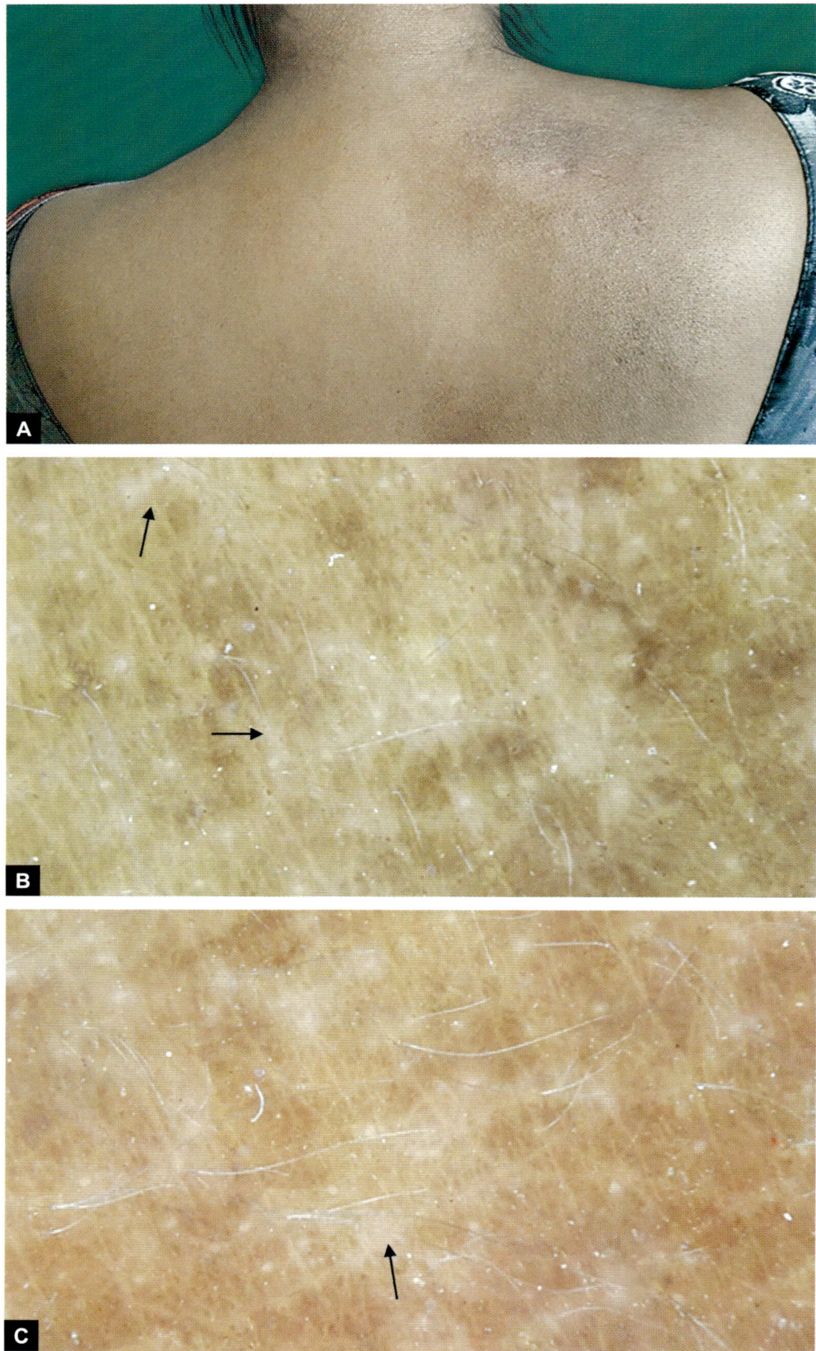

Figs. 19A to C: (A) A middle-aged lady presented with a hyperpigmented patch on the right upper back with an unusual sensation of 1 year duration; (B) Dermoscopic field shows alternate hypo- and hyperpigmented patches. On close examination shiny white streaks (arrows) are visible in some of the hypopigmented patches; and (C) Note the shiny white streaks (arrow) in some hypopigmented patches.

REFERENCES

1. Raison-Peyron N, Meunier L, Acevedo M, et al. Notalgia paresthetica: clinical, physiopathological and therapeutic aspects. A study of 12 cases. J Eur Acad Dermatol Venereol. 1999;12:215-21.
2. Shin J, Kim YC. Neuropathic itch of the back: a case of notalgia paresthetica. Ann Dermatol. 2014;26:392-94.
3. Arnold SJ, Bowling J. Shiny white streaks' in lichen amyloidosis: a clue to diagnosis. Australas J Dermatol.. 2012;53:272-3.

PIGMENTED PURPURIC DERMATOSES

INTRODUCTION

Pigmented purpuric dermatosis (PPD) is a chronic skin disorder characterized by symmetrical petechial and pigmented macules, often confined to the lower limbs. It results from the extravasation of erythrocytes in the skin due to increased venous pressure and marked hemosiderin deposition. The differential diagnosis of PPD includes stasis pigmentation, scurvy, leukocytoclastic vasculitis, drug hypersensitivity reactions, hyperglobulinemic purpura, early mycosis fungoides, and purpuric clothing dermatitis.

KEY DERMOSCOPIC FEATURES (FIGS. 20 AND 21)

- Purpuric dots and globules
- Yellow orange or yellow brown or coppery-red background
- Linear telangiectatic vessels
- Brown dots and globules.

KEYNOTE

Dermoscopy can serve as an important noninvasive diagnostic tool to rule out other purpuric dermatoses.

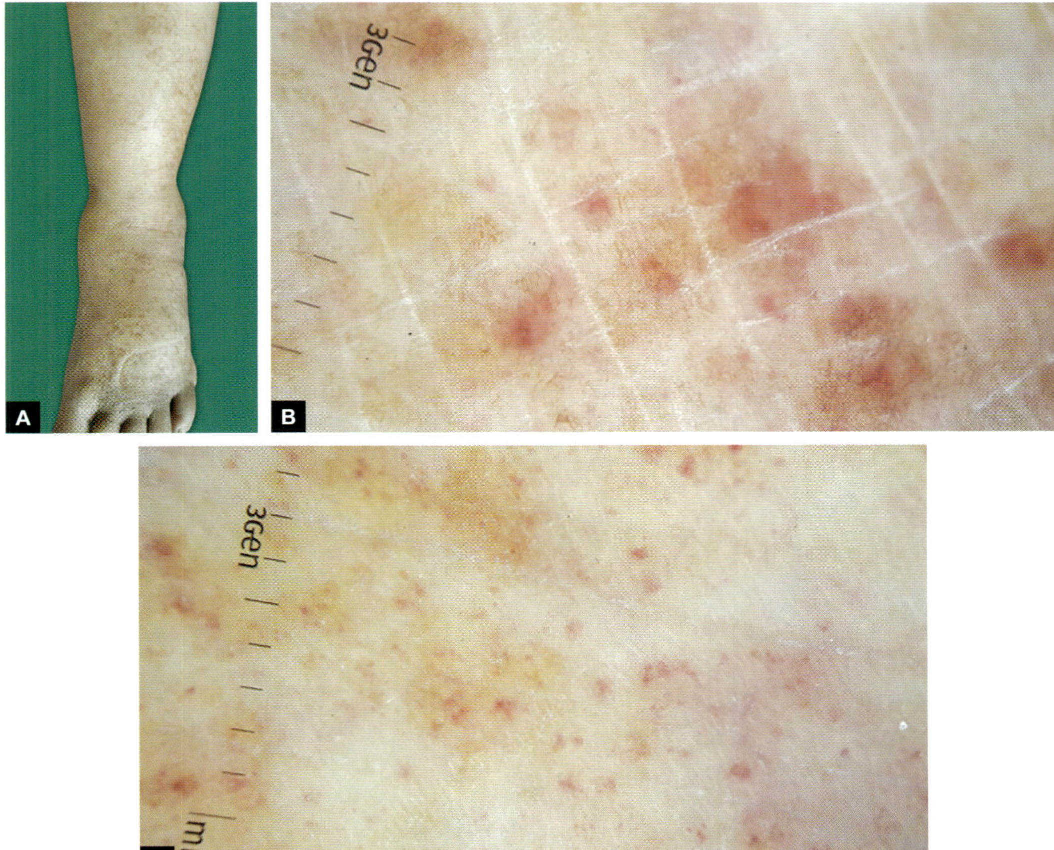

Figs. 20A to C: (A) A middle-aged-obese lady presented with pigmented patches over bilateral lower limbs with minimal itching of 2 years duration; (B) Dermoscopy of the lesions revealed a yellow-brown background, purpuric red dots and patches; and (C) Dermoscopy shows coppery red-background on the left half of the field and erythematous hue on the right half of the field with scattered purpuric dots and globules.

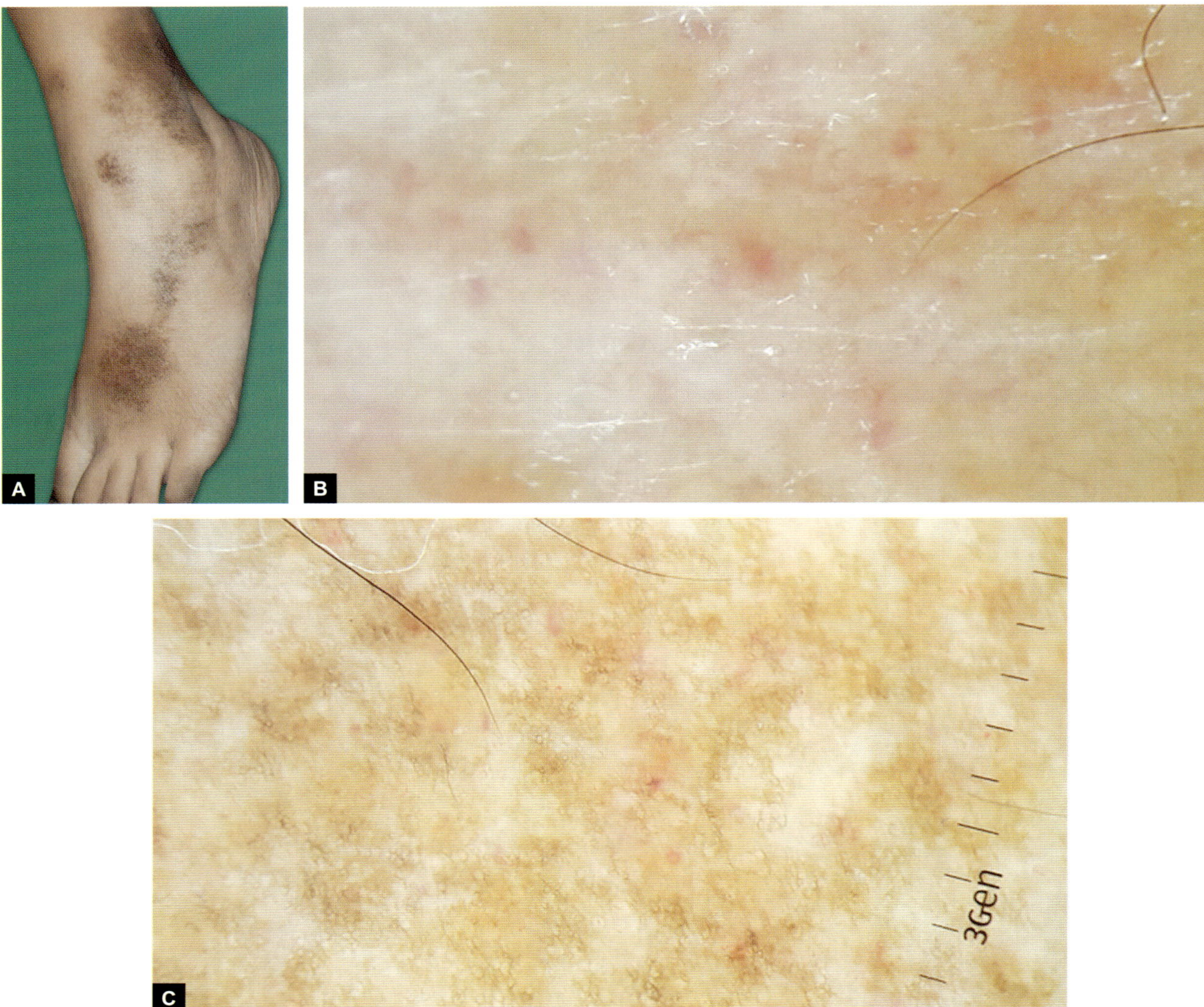

Figs. 21A to C: (A) A middle-aged man with history of long duration of standing hours presented with pigmented patches on the left leg extending from just above the ankle to the dorsum of the foot; (B) Dermoscopy shows yellow-brown background with purpuric dots and globules; and (C) Dermoscopy shows coppery-red background with purpuric patches.

SENILE COMEDONES

INTRODUCTION

Senile comedones are a feature of the older age group predominantly affecting the periocular area. They may be present alone or as a part of Favre–Racouchot syndrome in the elderly.

KEY DERMOSCOPIC FEATURES (FIGS. 22A AND B)

- Comedo-like openings with brown black follicular plugging
- Yellowish hue in the background may be suggestive of photodamage.

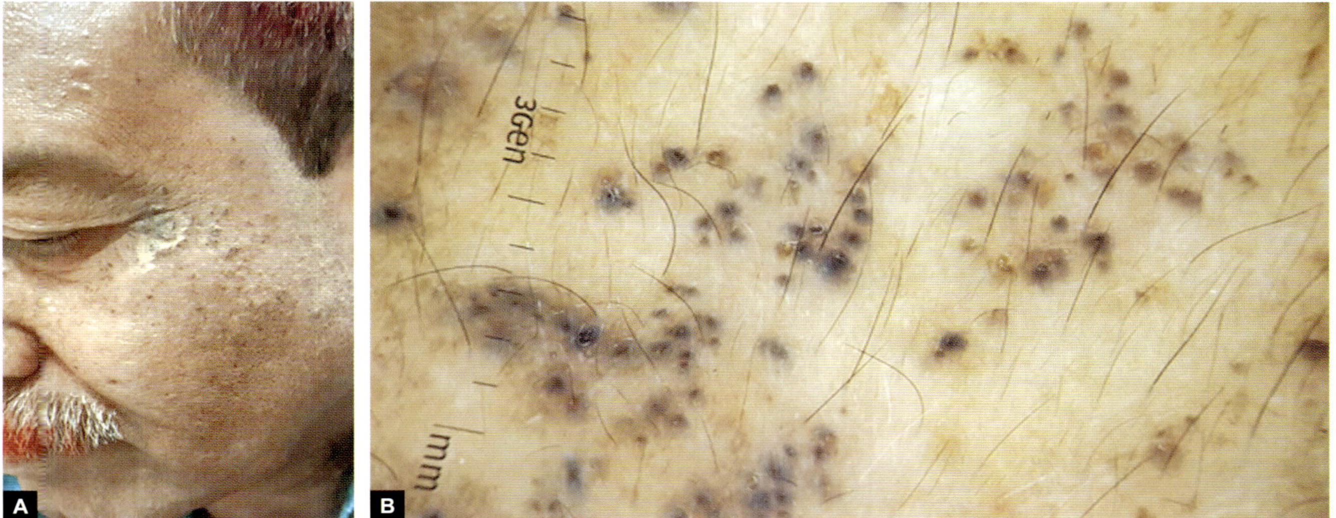

Figs. 22A and B: (A) A 65-year-old male presented with asymptomatic black dots around the left periocular area; and (B) Comedo-like openings with brown black follicular plugging against a yellowish hued background (suggestive of photoaging). Please note that other features of seborrheic keratosis are absent.

TERRA FIRMA-FORME DERMATOSIS

INTRODUCTION

Terra firma-forme dermatosis (TFFD) belongs to the group of "dirty dermatoses" that is not uncommon in clinical practice. By excluding other dirty appearing disorders such as acanthosis nigricans, a strong clinical suspicion and using dermoscopy, the diagnosis is usually instant.

KEY DERMOSCOPIC FEATURES (FIGS. 23A TO C)[1]

- Large polygonal plate-like brown scales arranged in a mosaic or tile-like pattern.
- The brown scales are interrupted by furrows.

DISCUSSION[2]

Clinically it can closely mimic pityriasis versicolor (PV), confluent and reticulated papillomatosis (CRP), frictional melanosis (FM) and macular amyloidosis. Dermoscopy is highly helpful to differentiate it from these conditions. PV on dermoscopy shows fine whitish scaling mainly distributed in net-like fashion. CRP typically displays whitish scaling associated with brownish polygonal flat globules separated by pale striae creating a cobblestone appearance or sulci and gyri pattern. In FM brownish structureless area are seen in a reticular fashion, whereas MA is characterized by hub and spoke pattern.

KEYNOTE

It is not uncommonly a misdiagnosed and underestimated condition. Clinical suspicion, dermoscopy, and alcohol swab test is the key to successful diagnosis and treatment.

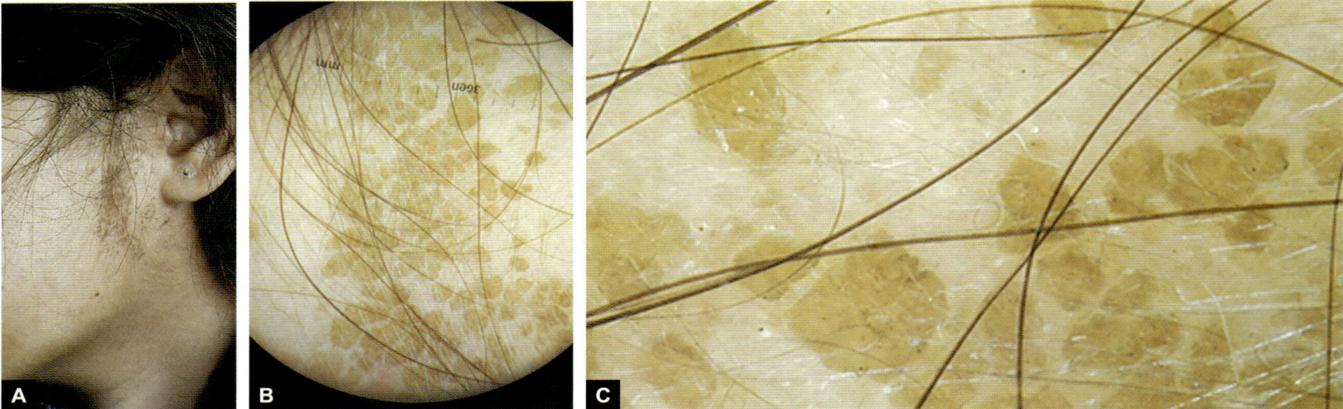

Figs. 23A to C: (A) A 20-year-old female presented with a hyperpigmented patch on the left preauricular area of 3 months duration; (B) Dermoscopy reveals large polygonal plate-like brown scales arranged in a mosaic or tile-like pattern. The brown scales are interrupted by furrows; and (C) Magnified view of the previous image shows distinct polygonal large plate-like scales separated by furrows.

REFERENCES

1. Errichetti E, Stinco G. Dermoscopy in terra firma-forme dermatosis and dermatosis neglecta. Int J Dermatol. 2017;1481-3.
2. Errichetti E, Stinco G. Dermoscopy in general dermatology: a practical overview. Dermatol Ther (Heidelb). 2016;6:471-507.

TELANGIECTASIA ERUPTIVA MACULARIS PERSTANS

INTRODUCTION

Telangiectasia macularis eruptiva perstans (TMEP) is a rare form of cutaneous mastocytosis that affects predominantly adults and usually presents as erythematous-brown macules with telangiectasias, located on the trunk and upper limbs. Darier sign is usually absent.[1,2]

Dermoscopy reveals a characteristic reticular vascular pattern that helps to differentiate TMEP from other forms of mastocytosis.

Histopathological examination shows dilated vessels with moderate inflammatory reaction, mainly composed of mast cells.

KEY DERMOSCOPIC FEATURES (FIGS. 24A TO C)

- Reticular vascular pattern
- Delicate pigment network
- Yellow-brown background.

DISCUSSION

Dermoscopy shows a characteristic vascular pattern, the reticular pattern that corresponds to dilatation and vascular proliferation associated with the presence of mast cells in the dermis. Vano-Galvan et al. evaluated the dermoscopic findings of 127 patients with cutaneous mastocytosis and described four distinct patterns: (1) pigmented network, (2) yellow-orange amorphous area, (3) brown amorphous area, and (4) telangiectasia with reticular pattern.[3]

KEYNOTE

Dermoscopy reveals a characteristic reticular vascular pattern that helps to differentiate TMEP from other forms of mastocytosis.

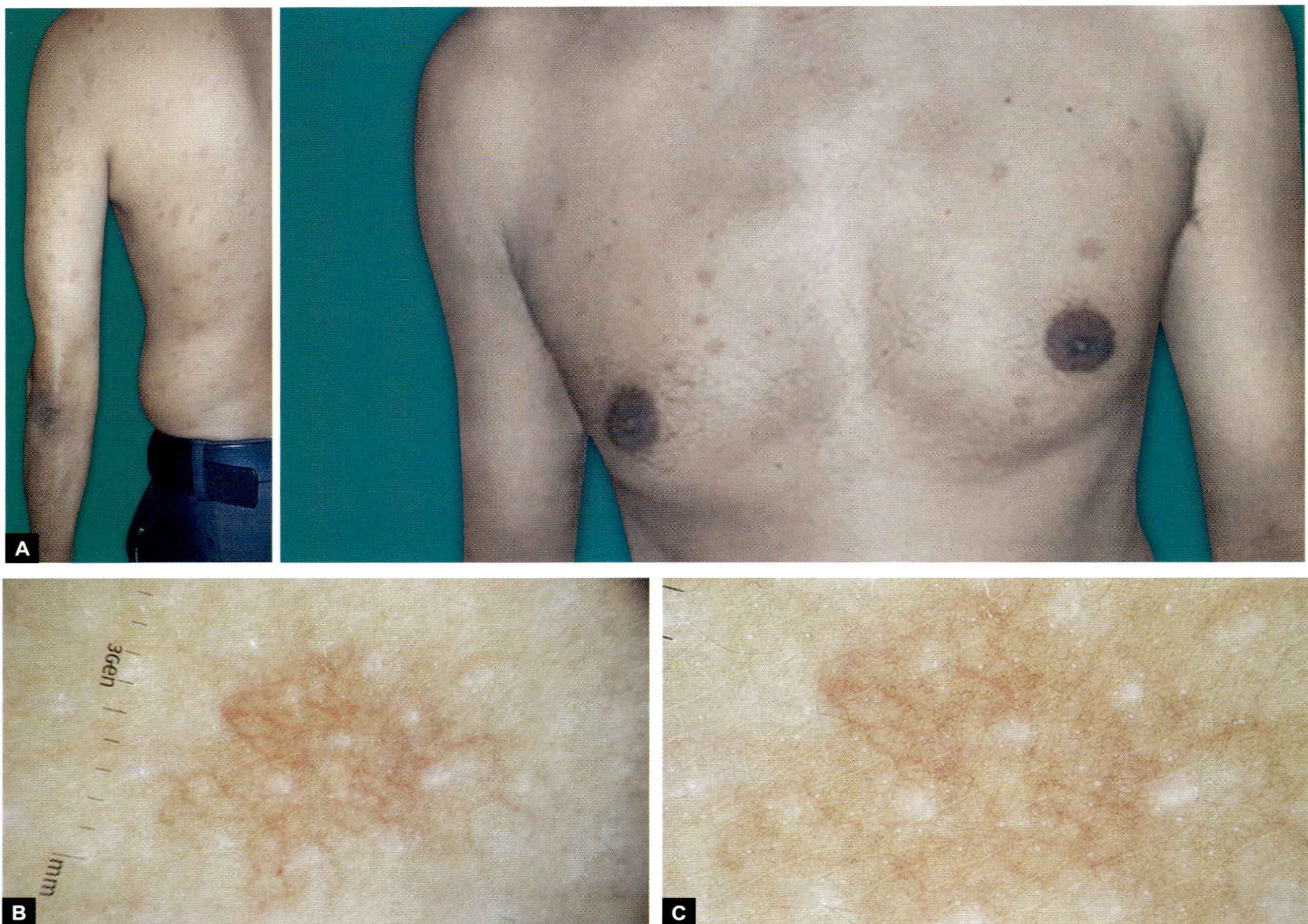

Figs. 24A to C: (A) Erythematous-brownish macules over trunk; (B) Mild erythema, thin and tortuous linear vessels, delicate pigment network, yellow-brown background; and (C) Close-up view of the previous dermoscopic picture.

REFERENCES

1. Maluf LC, Barros JA, Machado Filho CD. Mastocytosis. An Bras Dermatol. 2009;84:213-25.
2. Carvalho IM, Friedman H, Medeiros BM. Telangiectasia macularis etuptiva perstans: a case report. An Bras Dermatol. 2013;76:611-4.
3. Vano-Galvan S, Alvarez-Twose I, De las Heras E, et al. Dermoscopic features of skin lesions in patients with mastocytosis. Arch Dermatol. 2011;147:932-40.

CHAPTER 17

Dysplastic Nevi

Sushrut Save

INTRODUCTION

Dysplastic (atypical, clark) nevi are benign acquired melanocytic proliferations, which, not only morphologically resemble a melanoma, but also have an increased propensity of developing de novo melanoma.[1,2]

Despite the fact that clinically, dysplastic nevi share some or even all of the ABCDE (A, asymmetry; B, border irregularity; C, color variability; D, Diameter more than 6 mm; and E, evolving) characteristics of melanoma, majority of dysplastic nevi may be diagnosed as benign melanocytic neoplasms using a dermoscope and need not be biopsied.[1,2]

Dermoscopically, pattern analysis, which involves determining the global dermoscopic pattern depending upon presence or absence of pigment network, globules, homogeneous areas, and pin-pointing the presence of characteristic local features, helps to discriminate atypical nevi from melanomas.

DERMOSCOPIC FEATURES[1-7]

The clue to histological atypia appears to be related to various dermoscopic patterns, which involve different structural features and pigment distribution. Usually a patient with multiple atypical nevi will have a predominance of only one dermoscopic pattern.

Possible dermoscopic patterns in atypical nevi include:[2,7,8]

- *Reticular:* This pattern is observed in congenital nevi, usually those distributed on the lower extremity, acquired nevi, junctional nevus, and lentiginous nevus (zaladeuk, dermoscopic criteria). Histologically it corresponds to the junctional nests of melanocytes.
- *Reticular diffuse:* Diffuse honeycomb-like pigment network, with uniform thickness and color of the lines, which fades out at the periphery, and is a sign of benign nature. Holes of the network are uniform in size, and are a reflection of the paucity of pigment in the suprapapillary epidermis.
- *Reticular patchy:* The network lacks continuity as it is interrupted by presence of homogeneous structureless areas.
- *Peripheral reticular with central hypopigmentation (annular type):* Uniform peripheral pigment network with central homogeneous hypopigmented (not bony-milky white, structureless) area. This pattern is commonly seen in fair skin.
- *Peripheral reticular with central hyperpigmentation (black lamella):* Relatively uniform peripheral pigment network with a central homogeneous and dark blotch corresponding to pigmented parakeratosis. This dark blotch can be removed by tape stripping which allows visualization of the underlying reticular pattern. Usually seen in dark skin.
- *Globular:* Characterized by globules, uniform in appearance and distributed symmetrically throughout the lesion, and correlates histologically with junctional and dermal large nests of melanocytes. Commonly observed in congenital nevus, compound nevus, and dermal nevus.
- *Peripheral reticular with central globules:* It suggestive of congenital origin
- *Peripheral globules with central reticular or homogeneous area:* It suggestive of acquired growing nevus that has not yet become senescent.

- *Starburst:* This pattern is manifested by the presence of globules, tiered one on top of other, in the periphery of the lesion, or it may present as radial streaks or pseudopods at the perimeter of the lesion resembling an exploding star. On histopathology it corresponds to the confluent junctional melanocytes and is commonly observed in Spitz nevus and Reed nevus (Fig. 1).
- *Homogeneous tan, brown, or blue pigmentation:* It is characterized by prominent diffuse structureless (homogeneous) pigmentation, with or without the presence of reticular pigment network or globular pattern. In the fair skin the pattern usually appears as tan in color and represents acquired nevus, while it represents a congenital nevus when it is dark brown in color. The blue color represents blue nevus and is histologically characterized by the presence of dermal dendritic melanocytes.

TWO COMPONENTS

Characterized by the presence of two different patterns (reticuloglobular, reticulohomogeneous, or globular homogeneous). One half of the lesion displays one pattern while the other half is represented by a different pattern.[1]

Multicomponent dysplastic nevi are represented by three or more patterns, namely reticular, globular, and homogeneous. These nevi may also exhibit other structures such as network, streaks, negative pigment network, chrysalis, etc. As long as these structures are arranged symmetrically and in an organized manner, the lesion usually tends to correspond to dysplastic nevus on histopathology.[1]

As long as the lesions manifests one of the abovementioned benign patterns in the presence or absence of any atypical structure in a uniform distribution and symmetrical manner, the lesion can be considered benign. However, if the lesion manifests an overall benign pattern along with the presence of a melanoma-specific structure (Box 1), then the lesion needs to be subjected to biopsy. The decision to biopsy the lesion further depends upon the fact whether the dermoscopic pattern of the lesion is outlier or not, i.e. whether it is manifested by a pattern similar to the other neighboring nevi or not.[1,2]

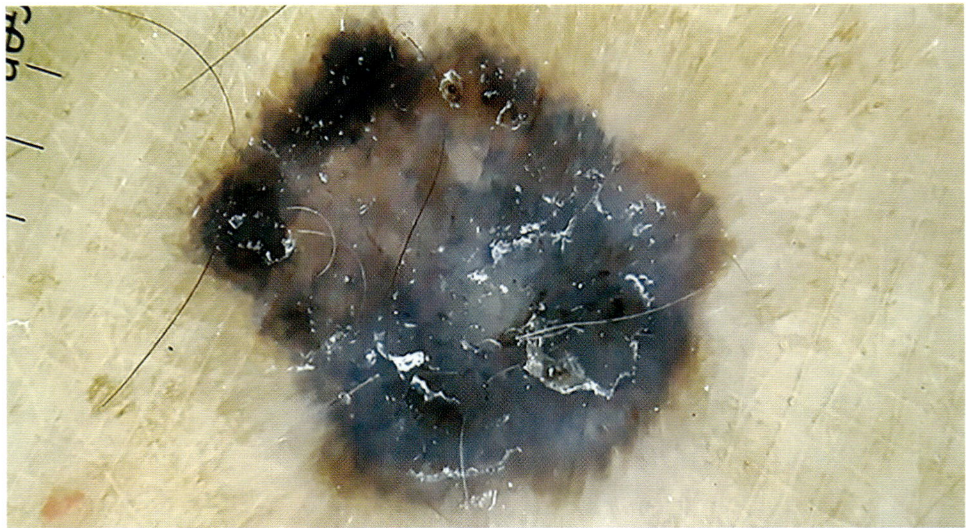

Fig. 1: Radial streaming present around the lesion resembling an exploding star. It may be found in dysplastic nevi, Spitz nevi, etc.

Box 1: Melanoma-specific structures.

- Atypical pigment network
- Radial streaming/pseudopods
- Negative pigment network
- Crystalline
- Atypical dots and globules
- Irregular blotches
- Blue-white veil
- Regression structures, peppering
- Atypical vascular structure
- Peripheral brown structureless areas.

REFERENCES

1. Marghoob AA, Kopf AW. Dysplastic (atypical) nevi. In: Marghoob AA, Malvehy J, Braun RP (Eds). Atlas of Dermoscopy, 2nd edition. London: Informa Healthcare; 2012. pp. 159-70.
2. Hofmann-Wellenhof R, Blum A, Wolf IH, et al. Dermoscopic classification of Clark's nevi (atypical melanocytic nevi). Clin Dermatol. 2002;20(3):255-8.
3. Wang SQ, Kopf AW, Koenig K, et al. Detection of melanomas in patients followed up with total cutaneous examinations, total cutaneous photography, and dermoscopy. J Am Acad Dermatol. 2005;50(1):15-20.
4. Menzies SW, Gutenev A, Avramidis M, et al. Short-term digital surface microscopic monitoring of atypical or changing melanocytic lesions. Arch Dermatol. 2001;137(12):1583-9.
5. Seidenari S, Pellacani G, Martella A, et al. Instrument-, age- and site-dependent variations of dermoscopic patterns of congenital melanocytic nevi: a multicentre study. Br J Dermatol. 2006;155(1):56-61.
6. Changchien L, Dusza SW, Agero AL, et al. Age- and site-specific variation in the dermoscopic patterns of congenital melanocytic nevi: an aid to accurate classification and assessment of melanocytic nevi. Arch Dermatol. 2007;143(8):1007-14.
7. Zalaudek I, Docimo G, Argenziano G. Using dermoscopic criteria and patient-related factors for the management of pigmented melanocytic nevi. Arch Dermatol. 2009;145(7):816-26.
8. Ashfaq A, Marghoob AA, Kopf AW. Dysplastic nevi. In: Marghoob AA, Malvehy J, Braun RP (Eds). Atlas of Dermoscopy. London: Informa Healthcare; 2012. p. 159.

CHAPTER 18

Dermoscopy in Diagnostic Dilemmas

Subrata Malakar, Samipa S Mukherjee

INTRODUCTION

Throughout the journey in dermatology so far histopathology has been considered as a gold standard in diagnostic dilemmas. However, the downtime for histopathology results serves as a disadvantage which can be solved by using dermoscope in many cases. With the advent of the science of dermoscopy definition of more and more disease-specific diagnostic dermoscopic criteria's serves to alleviate the need for biopsy. In addition in conditions where patient refuses a biopsy or in instances where performing a biopsy may not be feasible dermoscopy provides important clues in the diagnosis, for example, the visualization of a yellow-orange color points to a granulomatous etiology thus mandating and stressing the need for a biopsy. Similarly observing the Wickham's striae determines the diagnosis obviating the need for biopsy. It serves as a bridge between the clinical and histopathological tale in a dermatological disorder. In instances where there is a clinical dilemma this instrument serves as an important deciding factor in correlating the clinical and histopathologic picture. The histopathological changes manifest as clinical features of different dermatological conditions, which is further visualized with more definition under the dermoscope as various patterns, like fibrosis in histopathology is seen as white structureless areas under the dermoscope or alteration of collagen is manifested as white shiny streaks under the dermoscope. Dermoscopy helps in solving the puzzle of a clinical case by providing important clues and evidences pointing toward or against a particular diagnosis.

CASE 1

A 57-year-old male presented to the outpatient department with white patches on the neck and upper chest area of 3 years duration. Examination revealed depigmented macular lesions over the neck and chest (Fig. 1).

Clinical Differentials

- Vitiligo
- Postinflammatory depigmentation
- Idiopathic guttate hypomelanosis (IGH)
  Dermoscopic examination reveals depigmentation with petaloid appearance (Fig. 2).

Final Diagnosis

Idiopathic guttate hypomelanosis.

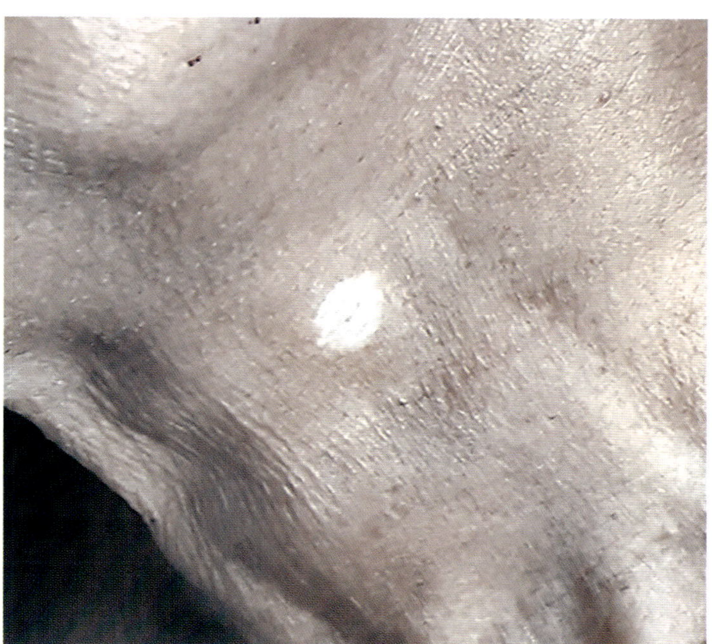

Fig. 1: Depigmented macular lesions and white patches over the neck.

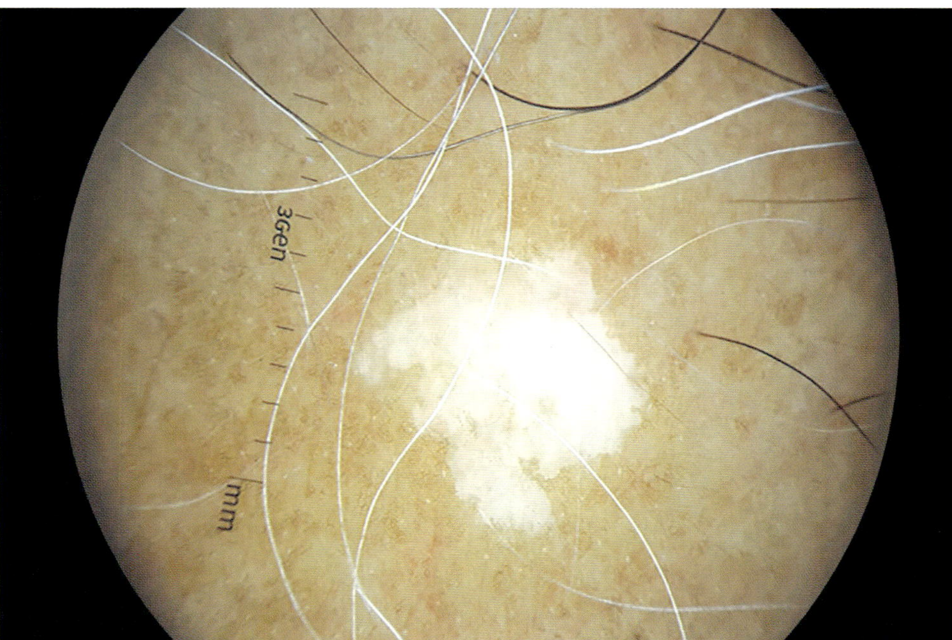

Fig 2: Depigmentation with petaloid appearance.

CASE 2

A middle-aged man presented to the outpatient department with itchy lesions over the leg of 1.5 years duration. He was treated with multiple topical medications elsewhere for varying period of time with temporary relief. Examination revealed hyperpigmented keratotic papules and plaques with few depigmented scar-like areas (Fig. 3).

Clinical Differentials

- Lichen simplex chronicus
- Hypertrophic lichen planus
- Treatment modified psoriasis.

Dermoscopic examination reveals areas of hemorrhage, white corn pearls in clusters against a violaceous background, and rippling scales (Fig. 4).

Final Diagnosis

Hypertrophic lichen planus.

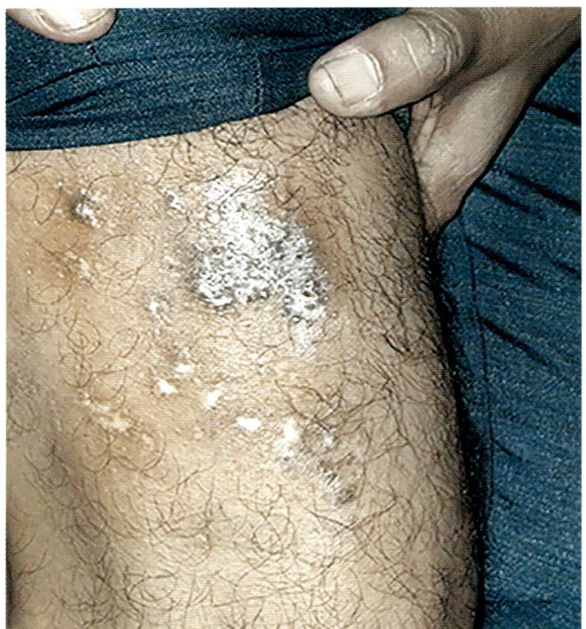

Fig. 3: Hyperpigmented keratotic papules and plaques with few depigmented scar-like areas.

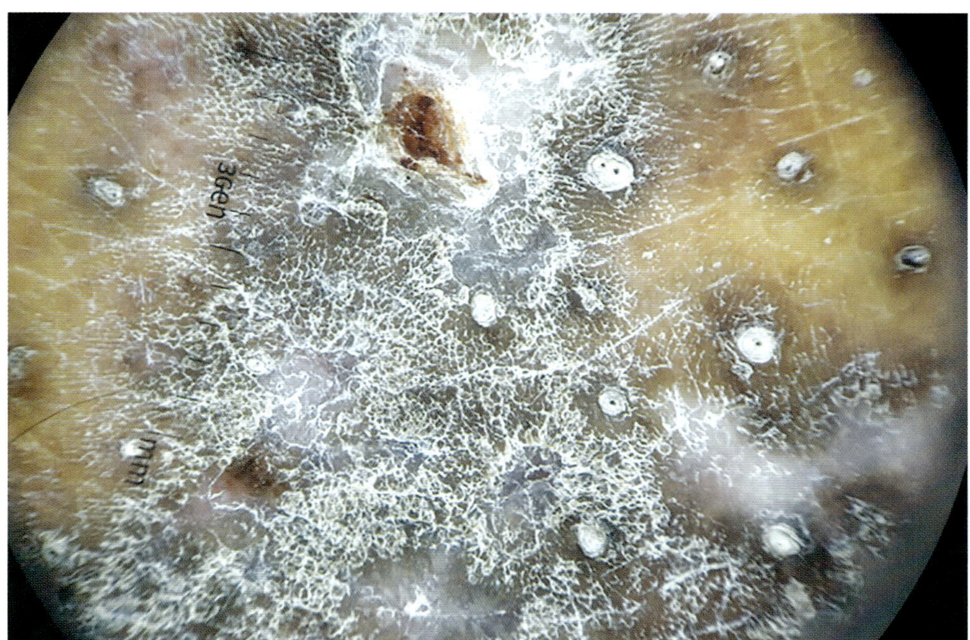

Fig. 4: White corn pearls in clusters against a violaceous background, and rippling scales.

CASE 3

An 13-year-old female presented to the skin outpatient department with a raised lesion located over the outer aspect of the upper arm area of about 2 years duration. She denied any history of preceding lesion prior to the onset of the current lesion. The lesion remained relatively static in size and extent over the entire duration and the patient was not concerned regarding this. Examination revealed erythematous to brownish firm raised, nontender lesion over the outer aspect of the upper arm. Dimple sign was negative (Fig. 5).

Clinical Differentials

- Dermatofibroma
- Keloid
- Granulomatous disorders.

Dermoscopy reveals diffuse erythema over the entire lesion with absence of white scar-like areas in the center and faint pigmentary network in the surrounding which are features of dermatofibroma (Fig. 6).

Final Diagnosis

The erythematous hue present throughout the lesion can be attributed to the increased vascularity in a *keloid*.

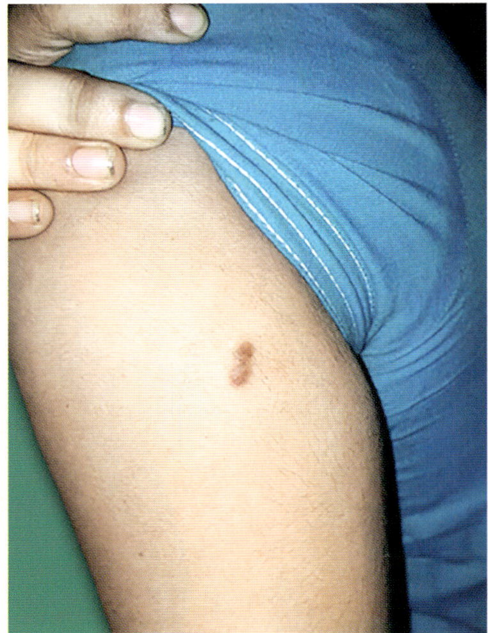

Fig. 5: Erythematous to brownish firm raised, nontender lesion over the outer aspect of the upper arm.

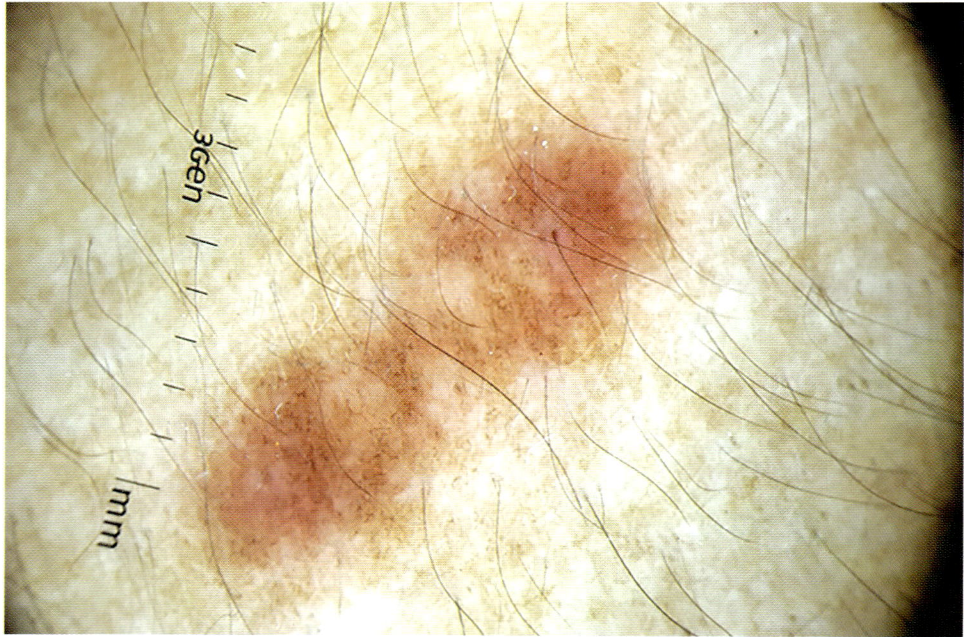

Fig. 6: Diffuse erythema over the entire lesion with absence of white scar-like areas in the center and faint pigmentary network.

CASE 4

A 27-year-old male patient presented with itchy lesions over the lateral aspect of the left lower limb since 9 months. The lesions disappeared on usage of topical medications but recurred on stopping. Examination revealed well-defined plaque with a dull erythematous to violaceous hue with moderate scaling. Auspitz sign was negative, Wickham's striae were not appreciable to the naked eye (Fig. 7).

Clinical Differentials

- Dry discoid eczema
- Lichen planus
- Psoriasis.

Dermoscopic examination revealed a dull erythematous background with red dots and globules distributed in a uniform pattern with diffuse scaling (Fig. 8).

Final Diagnosis

Psoriasis.

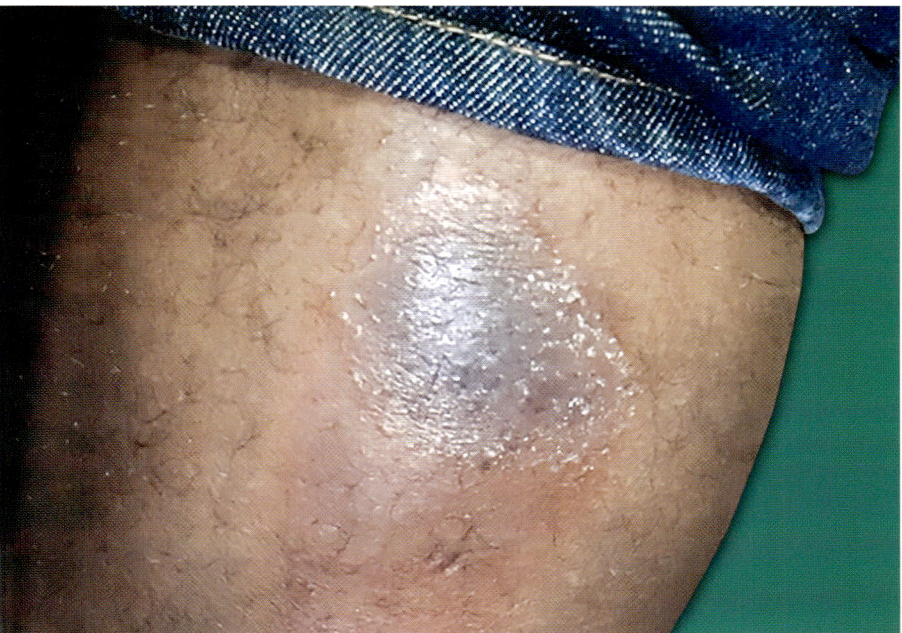

Fig. 7: Itchy lesions over the lateral aspect of the left lower limb.

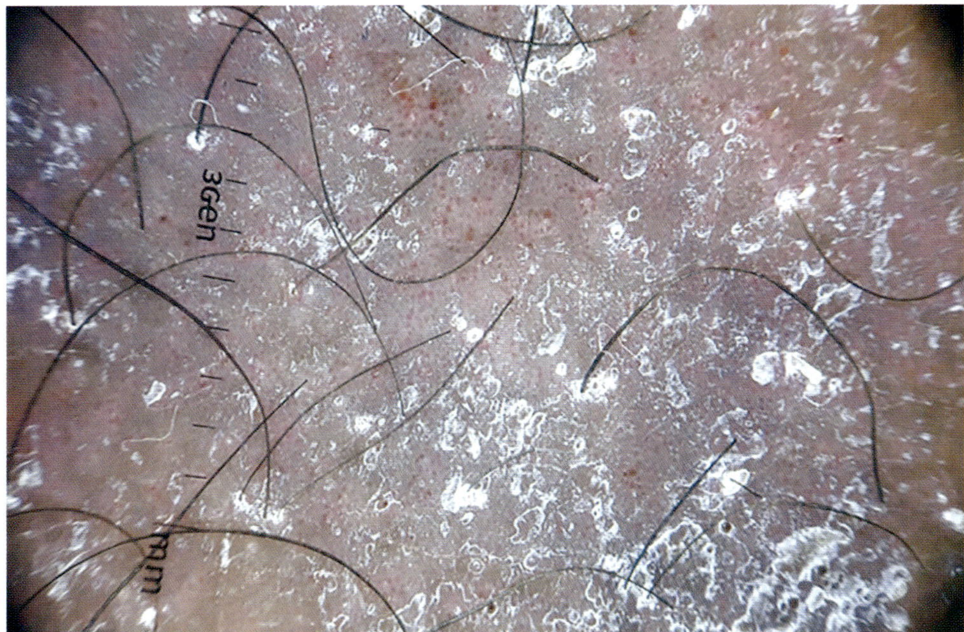

Fig. 8: Dull erythematous background with red dots and globules distributed in a uniform pattern.

CASE 5

A patient presented with mildly itchy lesion over the anterior aspect of the lower limb of 6 months duration. Examination revealed dull erythematous annular plaque (Fig. 9). Note the biopsy site.

Clinical Differentials

- Discoid eczema
- Psoriasis
- Differentials for other annular lesions.

Dermoscopy of the lesion clearly reveals (from outside to inside) hyperpigmented border, white track appearance, and brownish-white center with dotted vessels (Fig. 10).

Final Diagnosis

Porokeratosis.

Histopathology confirmed the diagnosis of porokeratosis (Fig. 11).

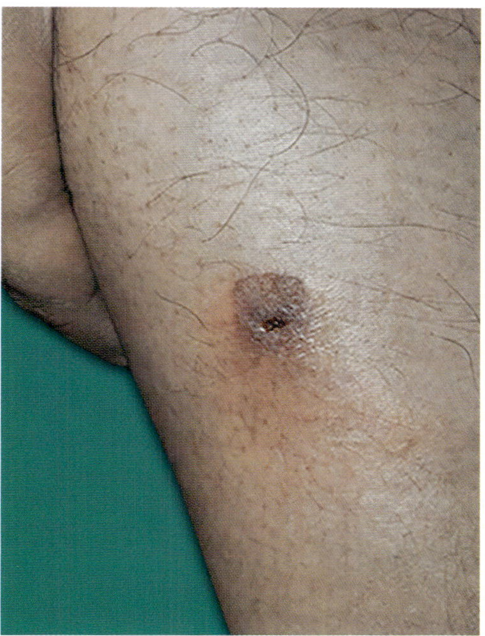

Fig. 9: Dull erythematous annular plaque over the anterior aspect of the lower limb.

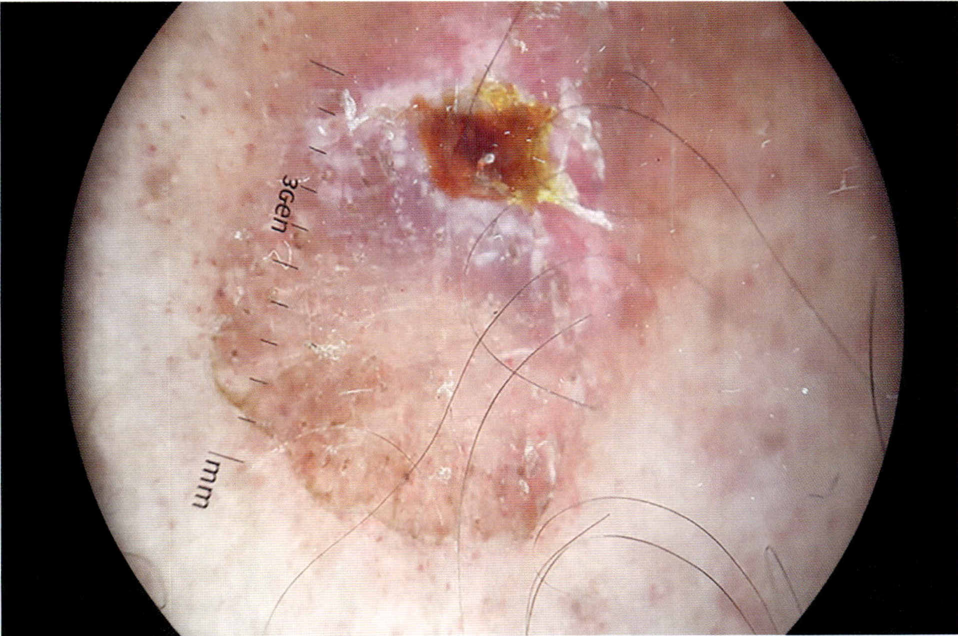

Fig. 10: Lesion reveals hyperpigmented border, white track appearance, and brownish-white center with dotted vessels.

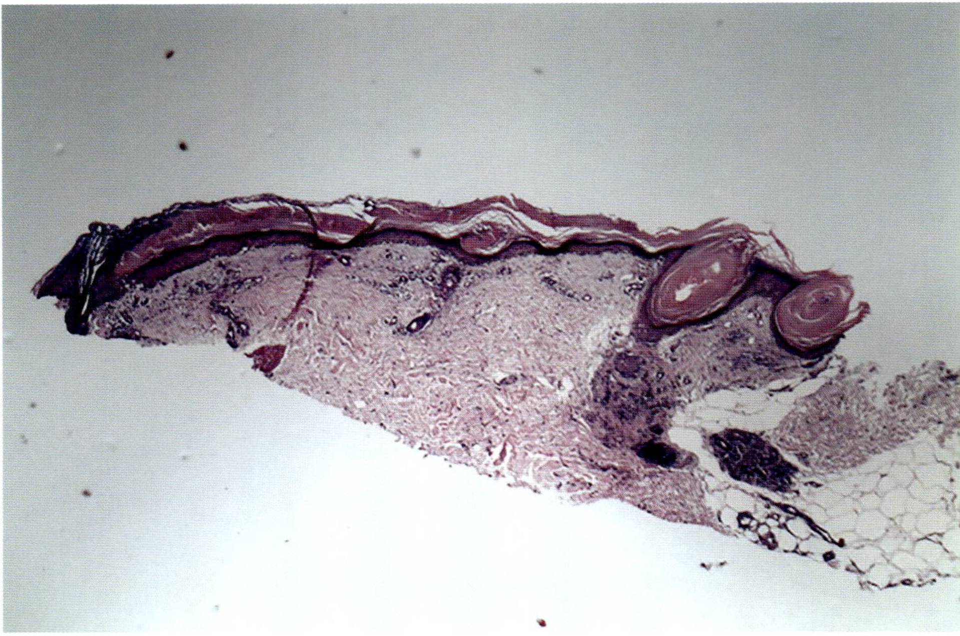

Fig. 11: Histopathology confirmed the diagnosis of porokeratosis.

CASE 6

A 44-year well-defined old male patient presented with a hyperpigmented patch over the forehead of about 6 years duration which was slowly increasing in size. He wanted a removal of the same due to cosmetic concerns. Examination revealed a bluish-black smooth surfaced plaque over the forehead (Fig. 12).

Clinical Differentials

- Melanocytic nevus
- Seborrheic keratosis.

Dermoscopic examination revealed a melanocytic pattern showing central homogeneous pigmentation and peripheral reticular melanocytic network (Fig. 13). Note the absence of features of seborrheic keratosis, such as milia-like cysts, cerebriform pattern, and comedo-like openings.

Final Diagnosis

Note the dermoscopically enhanced hypertrichosis which is suggestive of hairy melanocytic nevus.

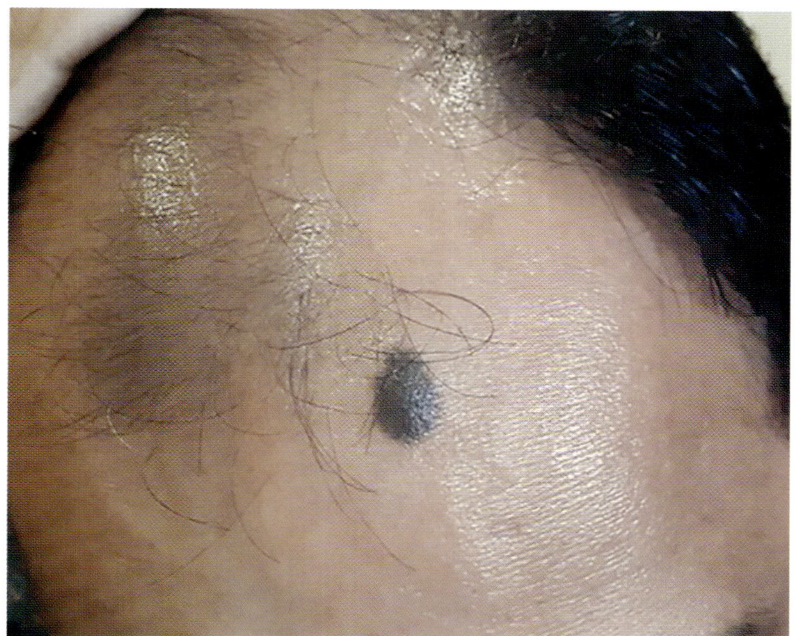

Fig. 12: Bluish-black smooth surfaced plaque over the forehead.

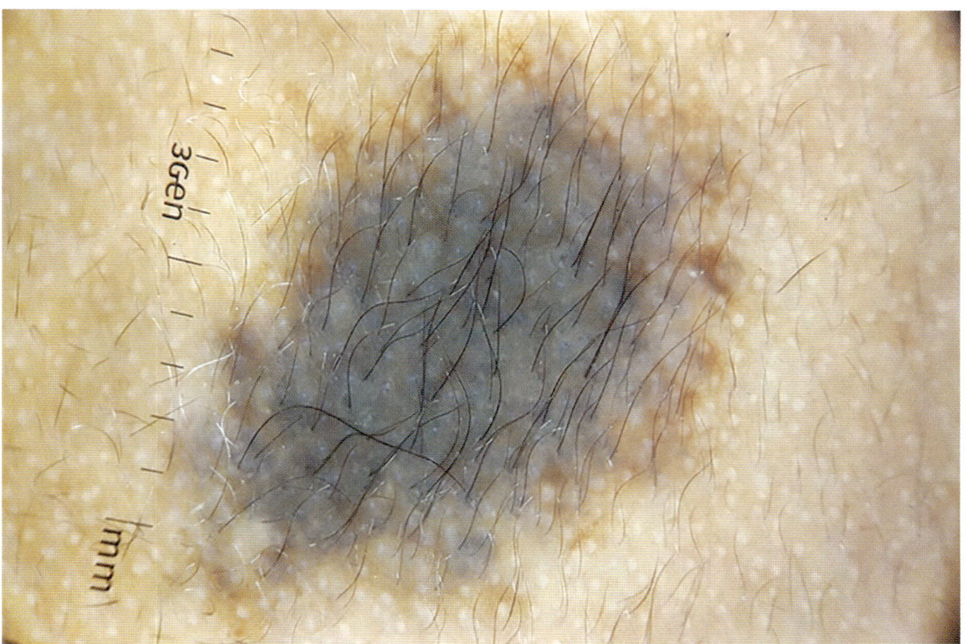

Fig. 13: Melanocytic pattern showing central homogeneous pigmentation and peripheral reticular melanocytic network.

CASE 7

A 60-year-old male patient presented with a slow growing hyperpigmented lesion just below the left tear trough area. Clinical examination revealed a bluish hued lobulated, firm, and nontender nodule with minimal surface changes on one end of the lesion (Fig. 14).

Clinical Differentials

- Senile comedones
- Basal cell carcinoma
- Compound nevus.

  Dermoscopy revealed cerebriform appearance with milia-like cysts and comedo-like openings (Fig. 15).

Final Diagnosis

Seborrheic keratosis.

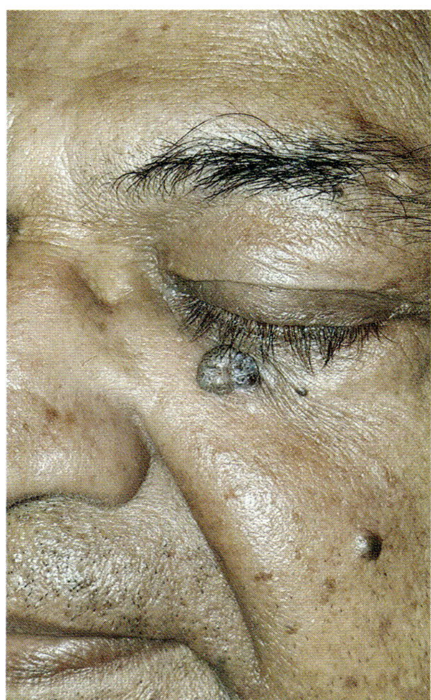

Fig. 14: Bluish hued lobulated, firm, and nontender nodule just below the left tear trough area.

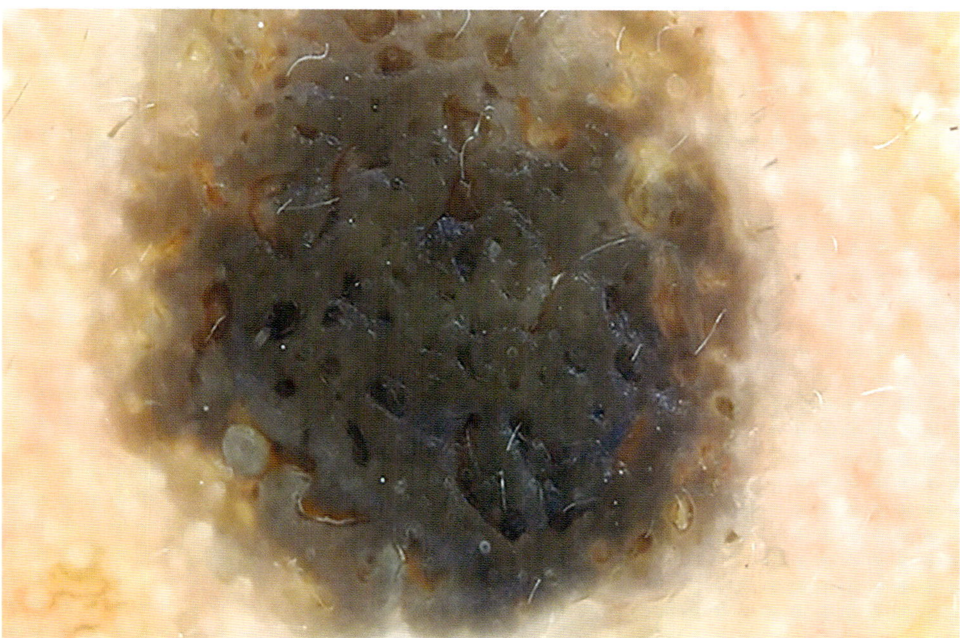

Fig. 15: Cerebriform appearance with milia-like cysts and comedo-like openings.

CASE 8

A 22-year-old male patient presented with a mildly pruritic lesion over the posterior aspect of the lower limb. Examination revealed erythematous annular plaque with minimal scaling over the lesion (Fig. 16).

Clinical Differentials

Discoid eczema.

Dermoscopy revealed uniform red dots, with white scaling, and dermoscopic Auspitz sign (Fig. 17).

Final Diagnosis

Psoriasis.

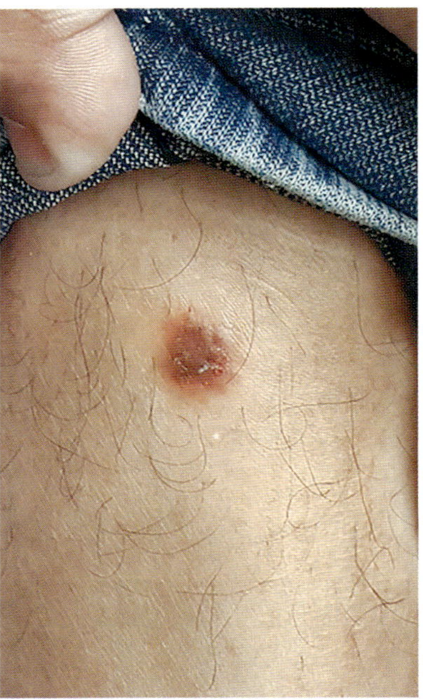

Fig. 16: Erythematous annular plaque with mildly pruritic lesion over the posterior aspect of the lower limb.

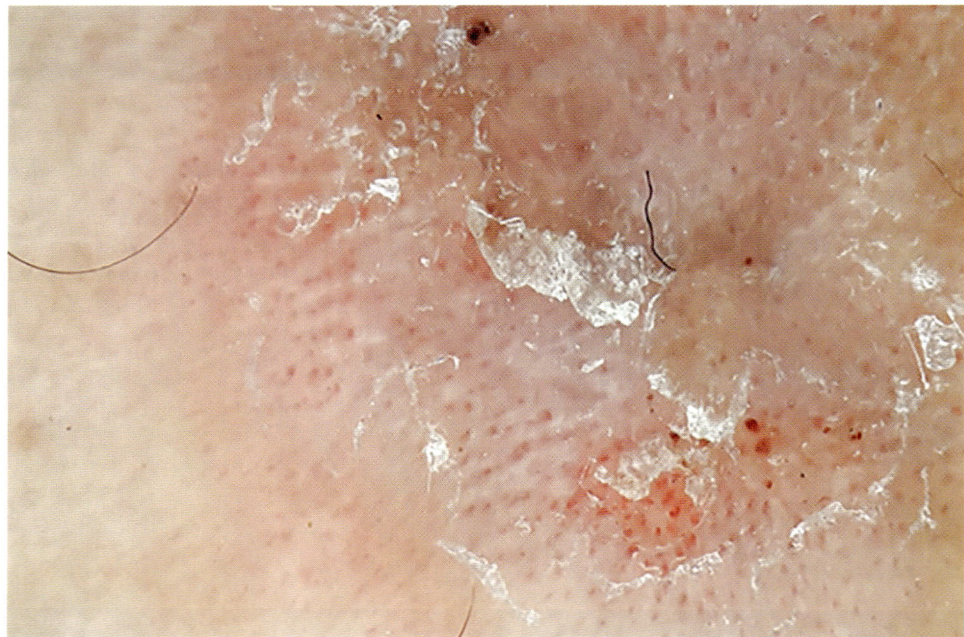

Fig. 17: Uniform red dots, with white scaling, and dermoscopic Auspitz sign.

CASE 9

A middle-aged lady presented with a lesion over the scalp of 10 months duration slowly increasing in size (Fig. 18). She denied any history of trauma preceding the lesion and bleeding from the lesion.

Clinical Differentials

- Pyogenic granuloma
- Wart
- Adnexal tumors.

Dermoscopy reveals large white keratotic halos with areas of hemorrhage (Fig. 19).

Final Diagnosis

Verruca vulgaris.

Biopsy shows an epidermal proliferation with marked papillomatosis, hypergranulosis, and hyperkeratosis (Fig. 20). The epidermis shows incurving of peripheral rete ridges and in foci has vacuolation of cytoplasm of upper spinous cells. The granular layer shows coarse keratohyalin granules and the stratum corneum shows marked and compact orthohyperkeratosis with vertical columns of parakeratosis topping hyperplastic dermal papillae. The thickened and elongated dermal papillae show tortuous and dilated capillaries. Sparse perivascular lymphocytic infiltrate is also present in the dermis and encroaches on the epidermis at places. Impression: Verruca vulgaris.

KEYNOTE

In case of clinical dilemmas dermoscopy serves as the first filter in routine practice. Histopathology should be resorted to in cases of persisting dilemma even after doing dermoscopy thus saving time and increasing the feasibility of a confirmed diagnosis. Dermoscopy many a times opens the possibility of an out of the box diagnosis and may take a nonsuspecting clinician by surprise (vide Chapter on Dermoscopic Surprises).

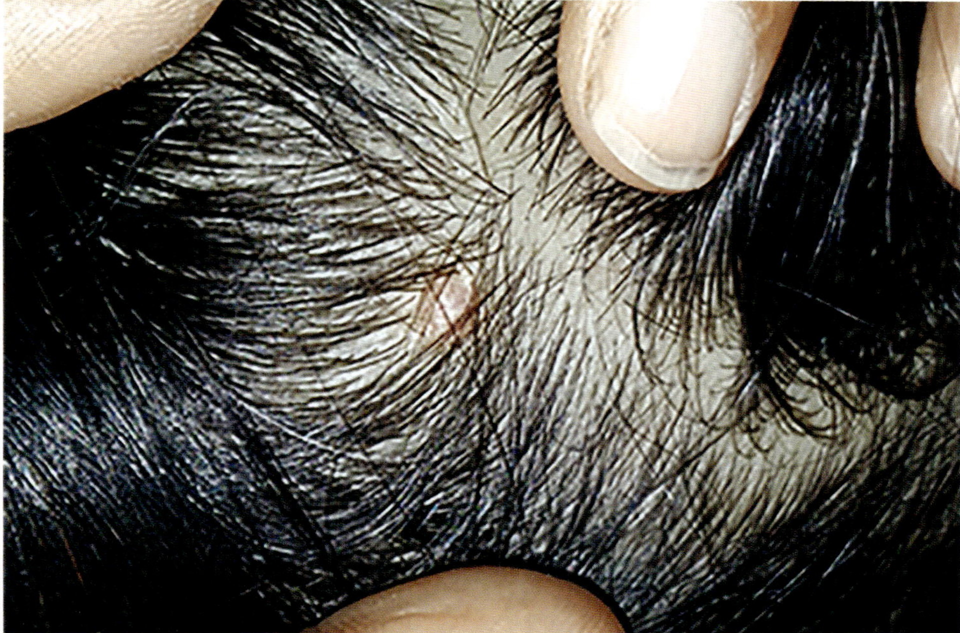

Fig. 18: Lesion over the scalp in a middle-aged lady.

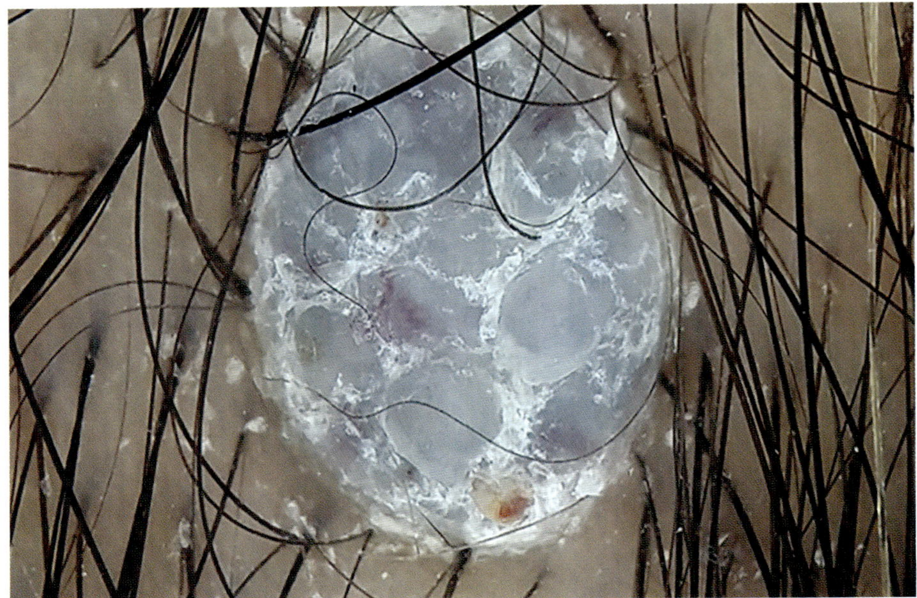

Fig. 19: Large white keratotic halos with areas of hemorrhage.

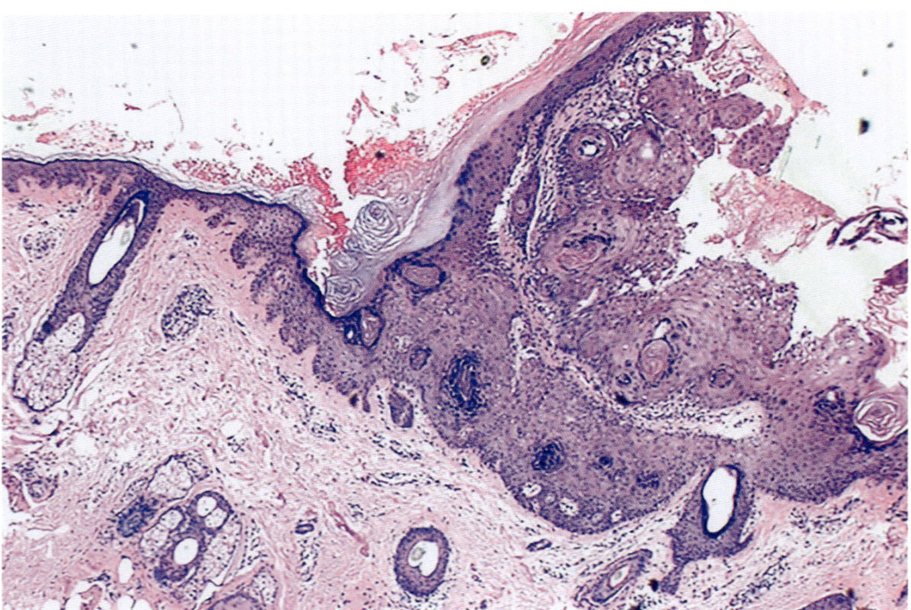

Fig. 20: Epidermal proliferation with marked papillomatosis, hypergranulosis, and hyperkeratosis.

CHAPTER 19

Dermoscopy in Therapeutic Monitoring and Follow-up

Subrata Malakar, Samipa S Mukherjee

INTRODUCTION

Dermoscopy provides an important clue not only to the diagnosis but also towards the monitoring of the condition once treatment is initiated. The subtle changes associated with clearance of lesion or response to treatment may not be visible to the naked eye, and this is better appreciated on dermoscopy (Figs. 1 to 13).

It not only reveals the stages of regression of the skin condition, but even cutaneous side effects like development of hypopigmentation post topical corticosteroid application may be picked up on dermoscopy very easily.

Dermoscopic evaluation of the disease during its course of treatment not only helps to decide maintenance therapy, but also helps in modification of drug dosages.

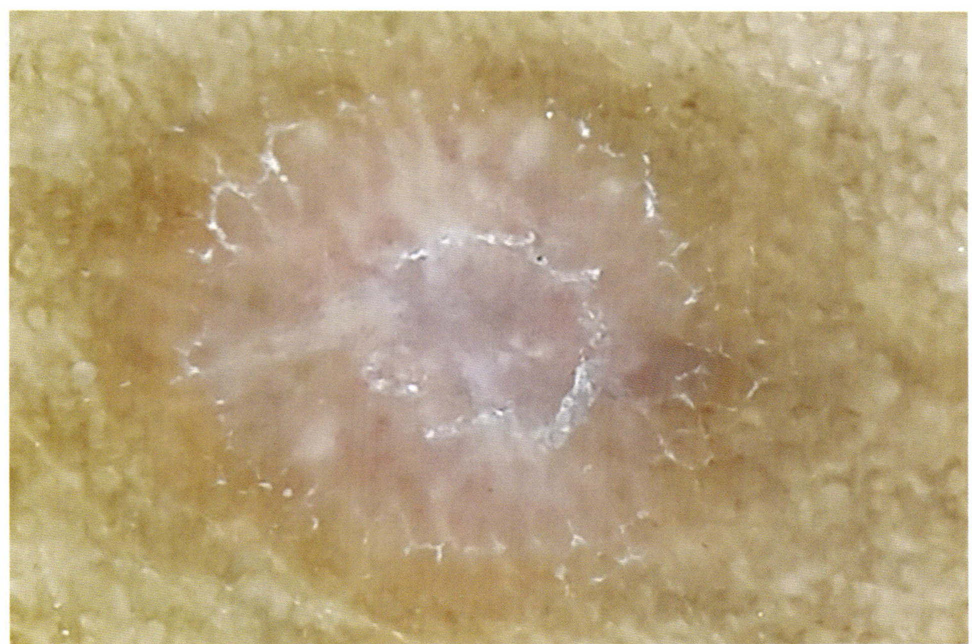

Fig. 1: Dermoscopy of lichen planus, showing radial streaming and few globular Wickham's striae (WS), violaceous background, and starburst pattern.

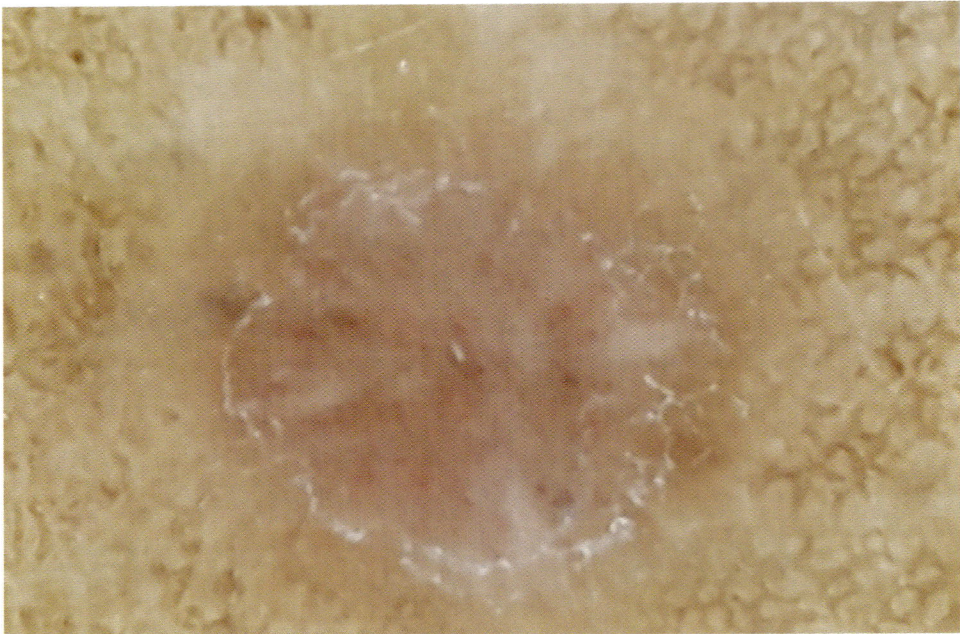

Fig. 2: The same lesion three weeks after treatment. Wickham's striae (WS) has reduced significantly. Note, the violaceous background has completely disappeared.

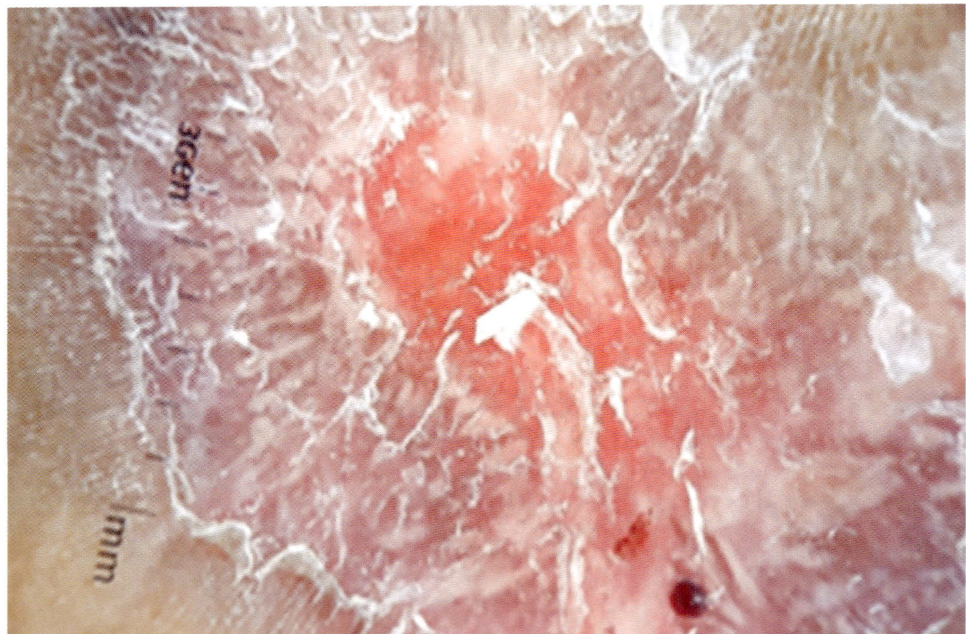

Fig. 3: In annular lichen planus, the pattern of Wickham's striae (WS) is predominantly radial streaming. In the extreme right of this dermoscopic field, globular pattern mixed with few linear pattern of WS can be observed. The background is red while the special feature starburst pattern is obvious.

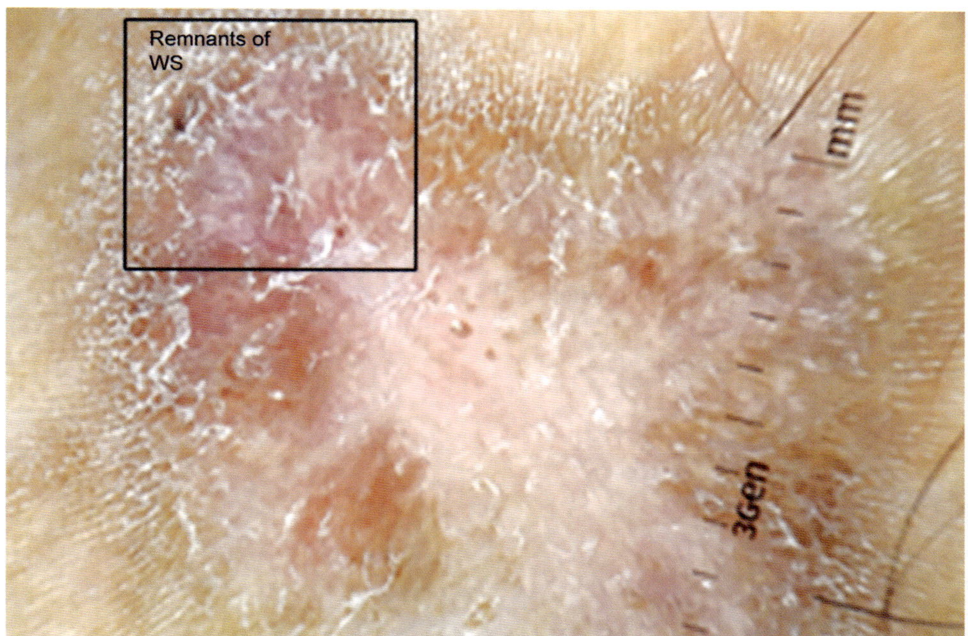

Fig. 4: Same lesion after 4 weeks of treatment. Remnant of Wickham's striae (WS) can be seen in the upper left part of this field while background erythema has cleared completely. Remember WS is an activation marker in lichen planus (LP) lesion.

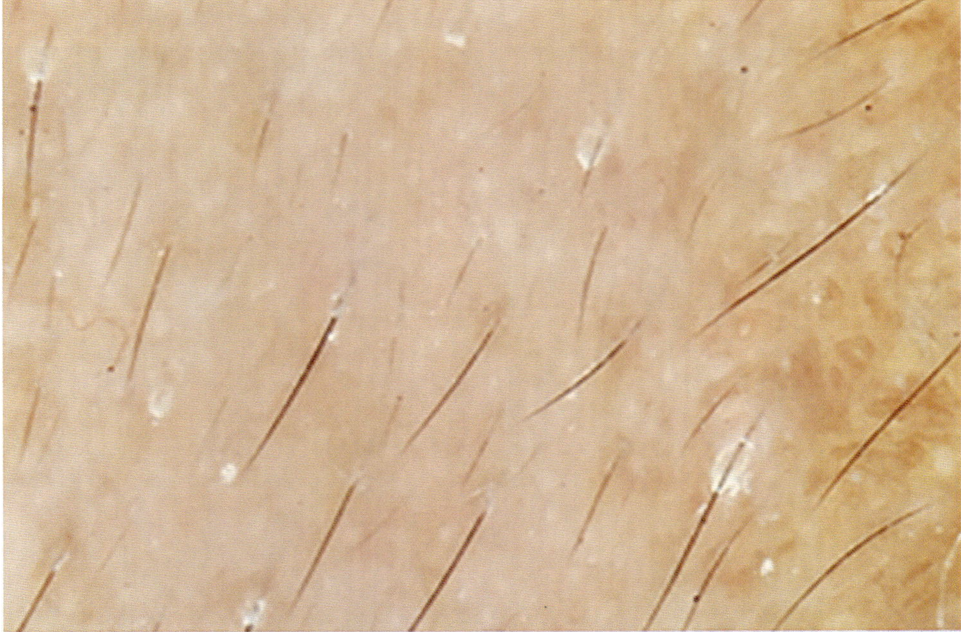

Fig. 5: White spicules of Demodex in the infundibulum of the facial hairs. The protruding part of spicules are the tails of Demodex.

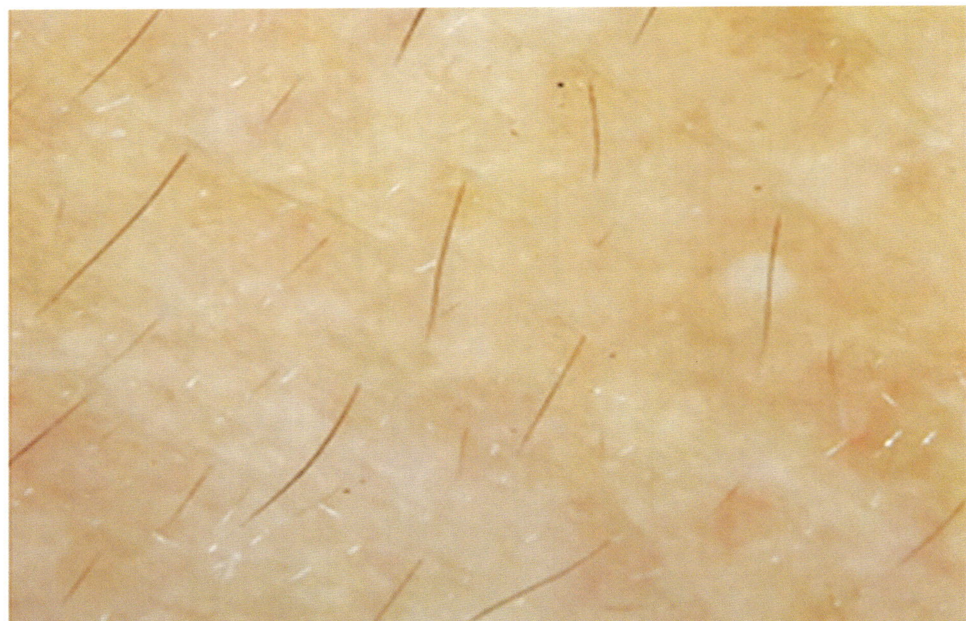

Fig. 6: Trichoscopic follow-up after 2 weeks of treatment with oral and topical ivermectin. Improvement is highly significant with no trace of demodex.

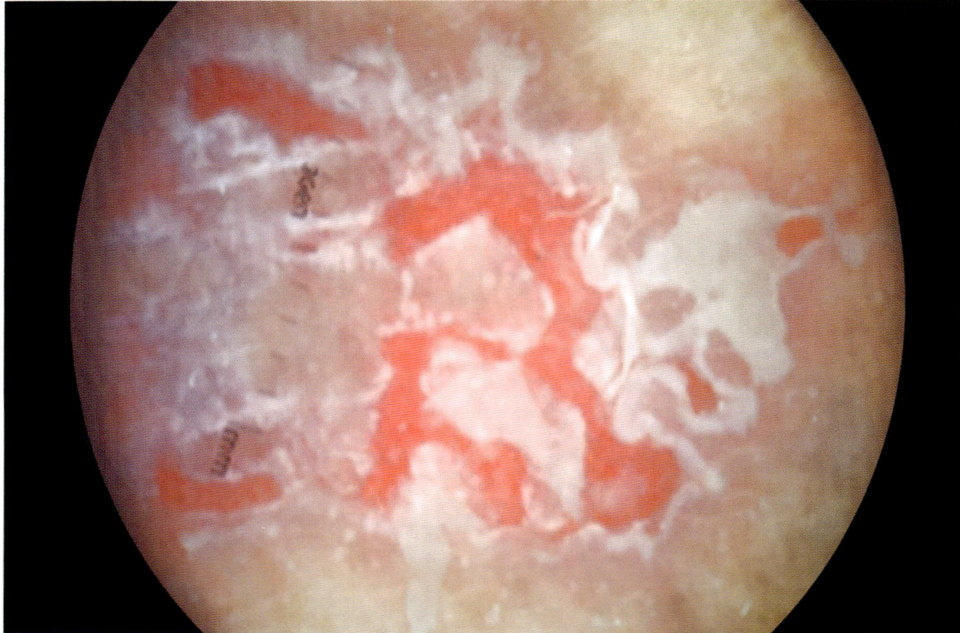

Fig. 7: A case of Hailey-Hailey disease. Dermoscopy shows pink and white areas which resemble clouds.

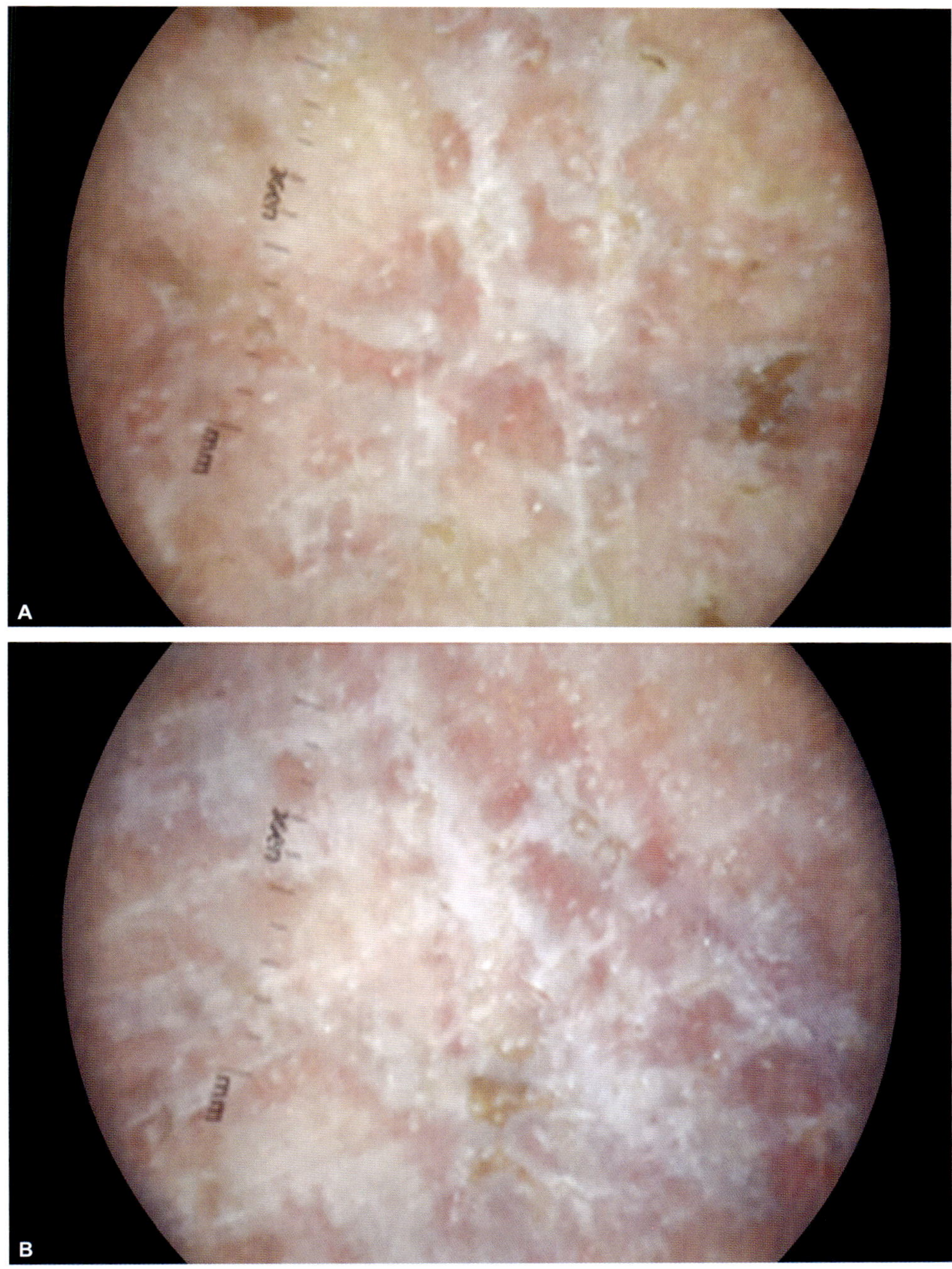

Figs. 8A and B: The same lesion, after treatment. (A) The earlier pink and white areas resolved posttreatment (oral retinoids) and (B) thereafter shows reticular yellow-white pattern on dermoscopy.

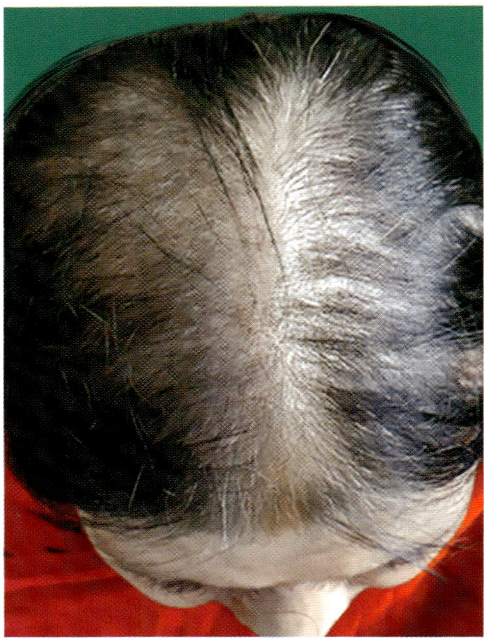

Fig. 9: SLE 1. A case of systemic lupus erythematosus (SLE) with diffuse hair loss.

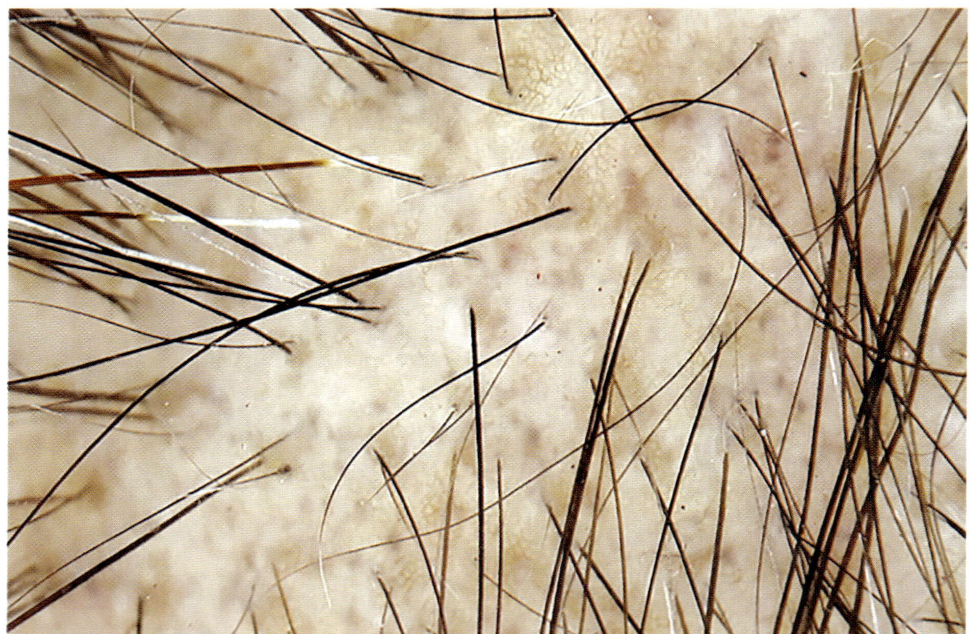

Fig. 10: SLE 2. Trichoscopy shows blue-gray dots in a speckled pattern. As there is interface dermatitis in systemic lupus erythematosus (SLE), melanin incontinence occurs all throughout the dermis including perifollicular area. Lichen plano pilaris (LPP) differs from SLE in that, there is only perifollicular incontinence of melanin in the former, resulting in blue-gray target pattern.

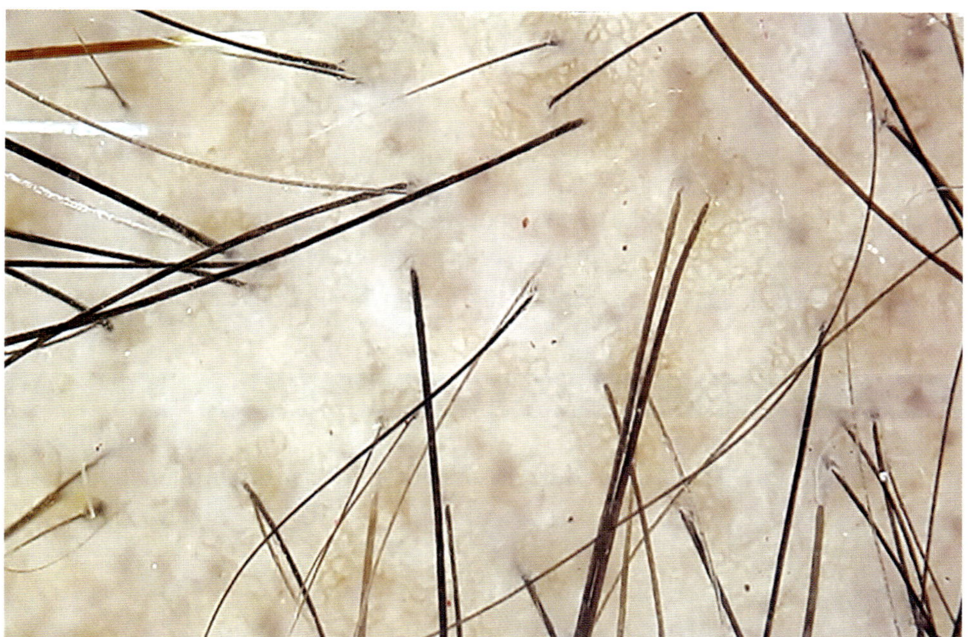

Fig. 11: S_E 3. Another field from same patient showing blue-gray dots in speckled pattern. Note, there is loss of hair density.

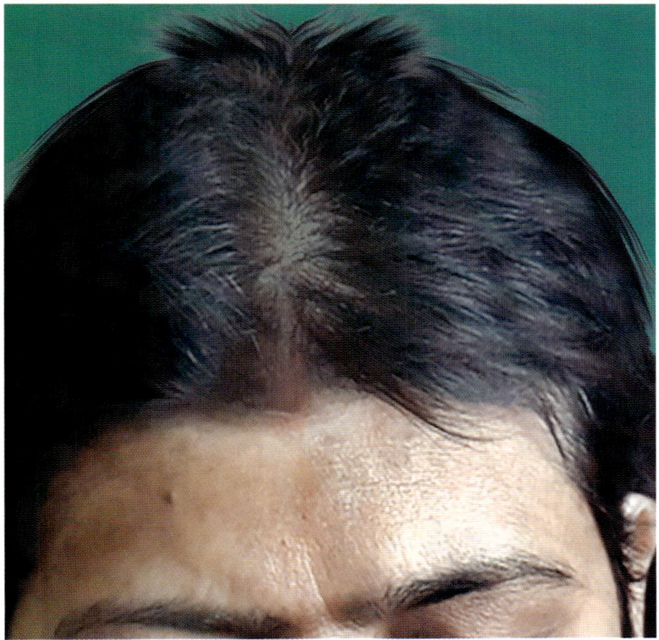

Fig. 12: SLE 4. Same patient after treatment for 3 months showing remarkable improvement in hair density along with improvement of other parameters of systemic lupus erythematosus (SLE).

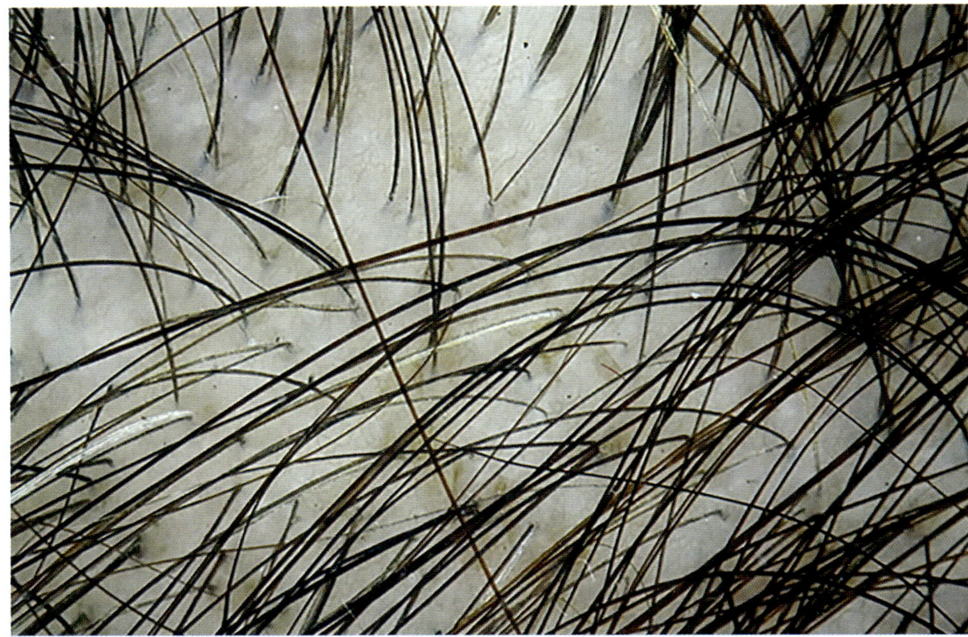

Fig. 13: SLE 5. This is the image of trichoscopic follow-up of the previous patient. Blue-gray dots in a speckled pattern are not observed after 3 months of treatment. Hairs have become dense.

KEYNOTES

- Along with invasive investigative parameters, recent developments in the noninvasive investigative tools help in monitoring the therapeutic outcome in various dermatological disorders with zero downtime.
- The various parameters to be monitored include pigmentary patterns, vascular pattern, and hair diameter and density.

CHAPTER 20

Algorithms

Samipa S Mukherjee

Flowchart 1: Dermoscopic diagnosis of a skin lesion.

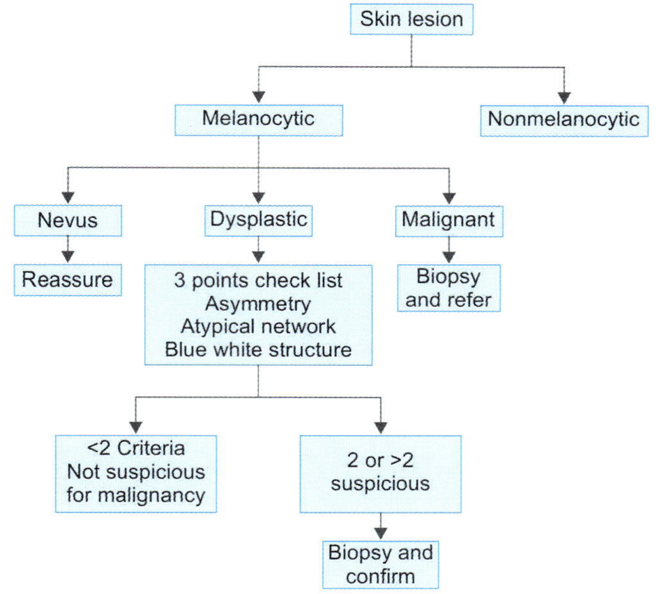

Flowchart 2: Approach to papulosquamous disorders.

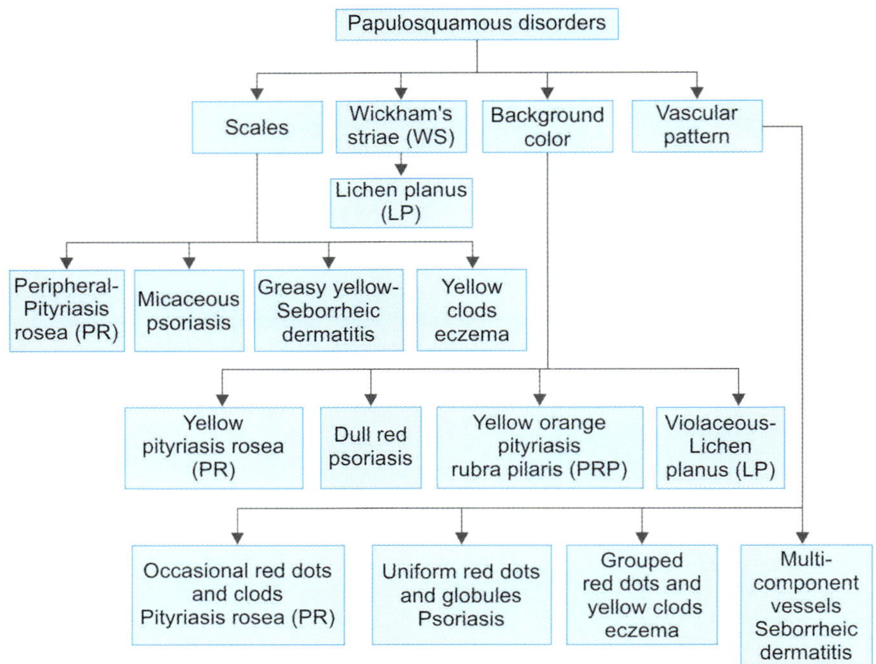

Flowchart 3: Approach to yellow orange colored areas.

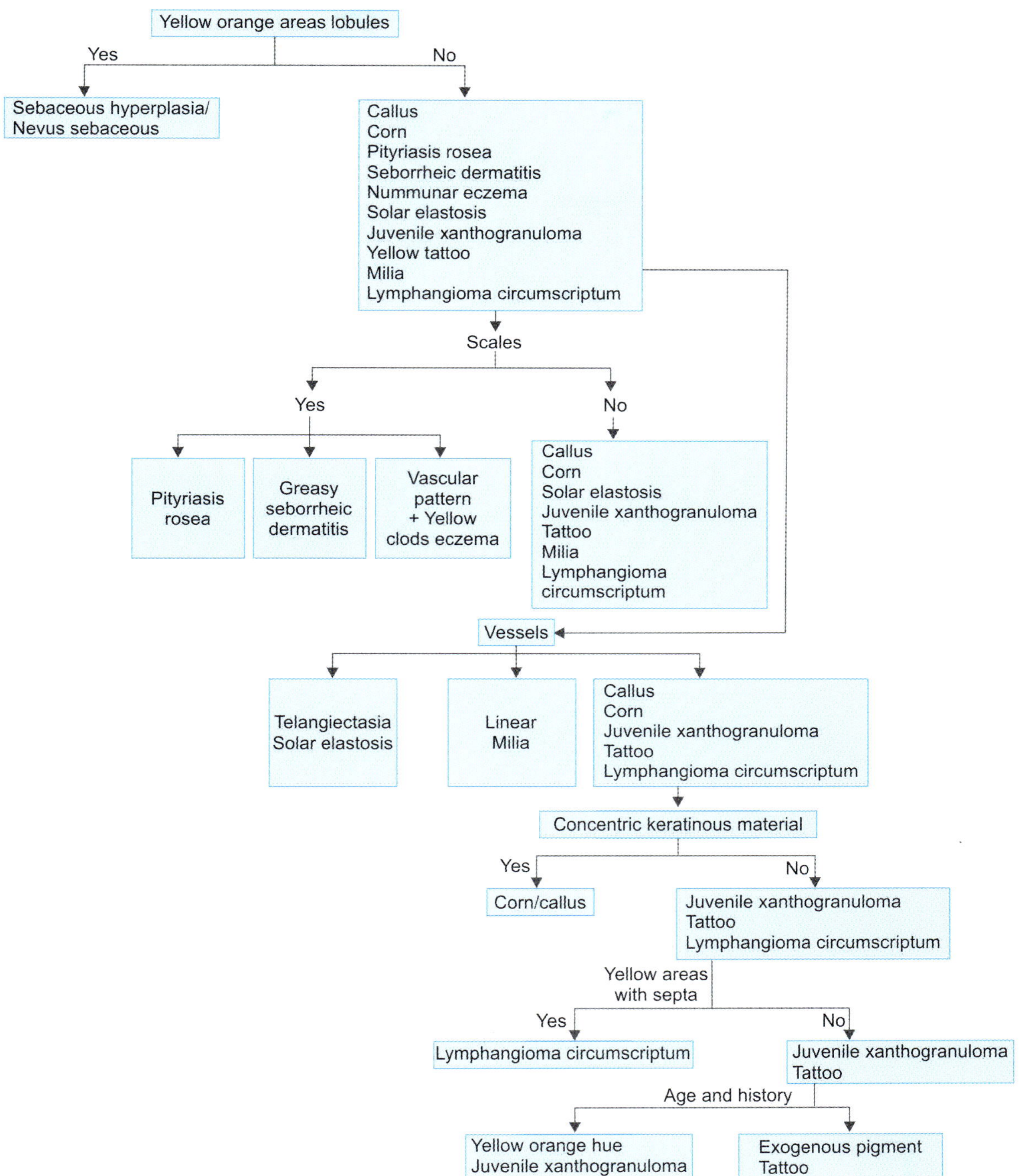

Flowchart 4: Approach to orange colored areas.

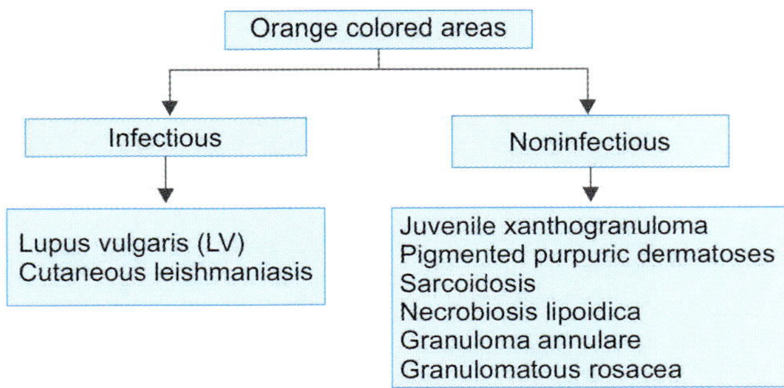

Index

Page numbers followed by *b* refer to box, *f* refer to figure and *t* refer to table

A

B

C

M

N

O

P

R

S

T

U

V

W

Y

Z